Pharmaceutics: Insights into Pharmaceutical Product Development

Pharmaceutics: Insights into Pharmaceutical Product Development

Edited by Brendon Krauss

hayle
medical

New York

Hayle Medical,
750 Third Avenue, 9th Floor,
New York, NY 10017, USA

Visit us on the World Wide Web at:
www.haylemedical.com

ISBN: 978-1-63241-439-7

Cataloging-in-Publication Data

Pharmaceutics : insights into pharmaceutical product development / edited by Brendon Krauss.
   p. cm.
Includes bibliographical references and index.
ISBN 978-1-63241-439-7
1. Drugs. 2. Pharmacy. 3. Pharmaceutical technology. 4. Therapeutics. 5. Pharmaceutical industry.
I. Krauss, Brendon.
RS79 .P43 2017
615.1--dc23

Table of Contents

Preface

Pharmaceutics is defined as the design and manufacture of safe and consumable drugs from new chemical entities. This book on pharmaceutics discusses effective drug delivery systems and pharmaceutical formulation for drug manufacture. Relation of drugs to the body as well as the conversion of pure chemical substances into dosage-based prescription drugs is also related to pharmaceutics. Sub-branches of pharmaceutics include pharmaceutical technology, pharmacy sciences and pharmaceutical manufacturing. This book is a valuable compilation of topics, ranging from the basic to the most complex advancements in this field. It will prove useful for students and teachers in the field of pharmacology, medicinal chemistry and drug delivery systems. This book is meant for students who are looking for an elaborated written script on pharmaceutics.

After months of intensive research and writing, this book is the end result of all who devoted their time and efforts in the initiation and progress of this book. It will surely be a source of reference in enhancing the required knowledge of the new developments in the area. During the course of developing this book, certain measures such as accuracy, authenticity and research focused analytical studies were given preference in order to produce a comprehensive book in the area of study.

This book would not have been possible without the efforts of the authors and the publisher. I extend my sincere thanks to them. Secondly, I express my gratitude to my family and well-wishers. And most importantly, I thank my students for constantly expressing their willingness and curiosity in enhancing their knowledge in the field, which encourages me to take up further research projects for the advancement of the area.

Editor

Lifting the Mask: Identification of New Small Molecule Inhibitors of Uropathogenic *Escherichia coli* Group 2 Capsule Biogenesis

Carlos C. Goller[1,9], Mehreen Arshad[1,9], James W. Noah[2], Subramaniam Ananthan[2], Carrie W. Evans[2], N. Miranda Nebane[2], Lynn Rasmussen[2], Melinda Sosa[2], Nichole A. Tower[2], E. Lucile White[2], Benjamin Neuenswander[3], Patrick Porubsky[3], Brooks E. Maki[3], Steven A. Rogers[3], Frank Schoenen[3], Patrick C. Seed[1,4,5]*

1 Department. of Pediatrics, Duke University School of Medicine, Durham, North Carolina, United States of America, 2 Southern Research Specialized Biocontainment Screening Center, Southern Research Institute, Birmingham, Alabama, United States of America, 3 Specialized Chemistry Center, University of Kansas, Lawrence, Kansas, United States of America, 4 Department of Molecular Genetics and Microbiology, Duke University School of Medicine, Durham, North Carolina, United States of America, 5 Center for Microbial Pathogenesis, Duke University School of Medicine, Durham, North Carolina, United States of America

Abstract

Uropathogenic *Escherichia coli* (UPEC) is the leading cause of community-acquired urinary tract infections (UTIs), with over 100 million UTIs occurring annually throughout the world. Increasing antimicrobial resistance among UPEC limits ambulatory care options, delays effective treatment, and may increase overall morbidity and mortality from complications such as urosepsis. The polysaccharide capsules of UPEC are an attractive target a therapeutic, based on their importance in defense against the host immune responses; however, the large number of antigenic types has limited their incorporation into vaccine development. The objective of this study was to identify small-molecule inhibitors of UPEC capsule biogenesis. A large-scale screening effort entailing 338,740 compounds was conducted in a cell-based, phenotypic screen for inhibition of capsule biogenesis in UPEC. The primary and concentration-response assays yielded 29 putative inhibitors of capsule biogenesis, of which 6 were selected for further studies. Secondary confirmatory assays identified two highly active agents, named DU003 and DU011, with 50% inhibitory concentrations of 1.0 µM and 0.69 µM, respectively. Confirmatory assays for capsular antigen and biochemical measurement of capsular sugars verified the inhibitory action of both compounds and demonstrated minimal toxicity and off-target effects. Serum sensitivity assays demonstrated that both compounds produced significant bacterial death upon exposure to active human serum. DU011 administration in mice provided near complete protection against a lethal systemic infection with the prototypic UPEC K1 isolate UTI89. This work has provided a conceptually new class of molecules to combat UPEC infection, and future studies will establish the molecular basis for their action along with efficacy in UTI and other UPEC infections.

Editor: Mikael Skurnik, University of Helsinki, Finland

Funding: This work was supported by NIH grant R03MH090791 (PI, Seed) and the NIH Molecular Libraries Probe Production Centers Network grant 5U54HG005031 (PI, Jeffrey Aubé). The funders had no role in study design, data collection and analysis, decision to publish, or preparation of the manuscript.

Competing Interests: The authors have declared that no competing interests exist.

* Email: patrick.seed@duke.edu

9 These authors contributed equally to this work.

Introduction

Urinary tract infection (UTI) is the second leading infection in humans [1] and the most common bacterial infection in the ambulatory care setting in the United States, accounting for up to 8.6 million health care visits in 2007 [2]. Of the major causes of UTIs, *Escherichia coli* (*E. coli*) is by far the primary etiology, producing over 74.2% and 65.5% of UTIs in ambulatory and hospitalized patients, respectively [3–5]. Twenty-five to forty percent of first-time community-acquired UTIs are followed by recurrences caused by the same clone of UPEC [3,6,7]. In addition, *E. coli* also accounts for a significant proportion of sepsis and meningitis of the young and old, with the infections originating from the urinary tract or direct translocation from the gut into the bloodstream [8]. With over 100 million UTIs

occurring annually throughout the world, including more than 10 million cases in U.S. adolescents and adults (per NIDDK data, [9]), UPEC accounts for substantial medical costs and morbidity worldwide.

Among all UTI cases, approximately 40-times more are treated in the outpatient setting relative to inpatient care [7]. Rising antibiotic resistance is a serious problem affecting the clinical utility of the drugs commonly available for outpatient treatment of UTIs (e.g., [10]). In the last decade, widespread use of antibiotics has resulted in an increase in resistance of *E. coli* to commonly used oral antibiotics. Whereas ampicillin and amoxicillin were once the standard of treatment in uncomplicated UTI, the rates of resistance are approaching 50% in certain parts of North America [4]. Resistance rates have also dramatically increased among

UPEC against trimethoprim-sulfamethaxozole (TMP-SMX), currently the first line therapy for outpatient treatment of UTI [11,12]. Resistance to TMP-SMX has been emerging among urinary tract isolates with rates in excess of 20% in some areas. The Infectious Diseases Society of America (IDSA) now recommends that in regions where resistance to TMP-SMX exceeds 20%, TMP-SMX should no longer be used for empirical therapy [13]. Ciprofloxacin and other fluoroquinolones are used routinely, but resistance to these agents is also on the rise (e.g., [14,15]), and fluoroquinolone-resistant isolates of *E. coli* are often multidrug resistant [16].

Almost all UTI treated in the community occur in individuals with normal, robust immune responses to infection. Thus, a new approach to therapy may be development and institution of UTI-specific therapeutics that render microbes vulnerable to host clearance mechanisms such as the innate immunity. Multiple innate defense mechanisms are thought to participate in clearance of bacteria from the urinary tract. A robust pro-inflammatory cytokine response of IL-6 and IL-8 results from TLR4-LPS stimulation [17–21]. Subsequently, neutrophils are recruited into the urinary tract, producing pyuria. Complement levels increase during inflammatory conditions in the urinary tract [22] and may be an important mechanism of defense. Antimicrobial peptides (AP), including the cationic 3–5 kDa peptides called defensins, are abundant in the urine [23]. AP form pores in phospholipid bilayers but require access to the bacterial outer membrane for function [24]. Similar immune responses are activated and effective in limiting the spread of UPEC from the urinary tract to produce more disseminated disease.

The effectiveness of the innate immune response against bacteria such as *E. coli* may, however, be severely hindered by bacterial factors such as polysaccharide capsule. Capsules are well-established virulence factors for a variety of pathogens and serve to protect the cell from opsonophagocytosis and complement-mediated killing [25,26]. In murine models, prior research has demonstrated that the K capsule of *E. coli* is a preeminent virulence determinant during UTI and bacteremia [27–29], as well as critical for formation of intracellular bacterial communities within the murine model of UTI. K capsules, also called K antigens, are enveloping structures composed of acidic, high-molecular-weight polysaccharides. Llobet *et al.* demonstrated that highly acidic polysaccharide capsules of *K. pneumoniae*, *P. aeruginosa*, and *S. pneumoniae* interact strongly with AP, acting as "sponges" to sequester and neutralize the AP [30]. Furthermore in murine models of UTI, we have found that K capsule contributes to multiple aspects of UTI pathogenesis, including intracellular replication [28], making inhibition of capsule biosynthesis a novel target for attenuation of UPEC virulence.

Inhibiting K capsule production may sensitize the organism to various components of the immune system. Proof-of-concept evidence comes from the demonstration that injection of purified K1 endosialiase, which enzymatically degrades the *E. coli* K1 capsule, prevented sepsis and meningitis after intraperitoneal infection of neonatal rats with *E. coli* K1 [29]. However, endosialidases may have limited therapeutic applications due to their antigenicity, poor bioavailability, and potential action on sialidated host proteins and lipids with shared linkages as the capsular sialic acids (such as those present in neural tissues, [31]). Furthermore, endosialidase has a very narrow biochemical target range, limiting its application to specific K antigen types. Chemical inhibition of K capsule production may achieve similar therapeutic results without most of these limitations.

The genomic organization of Group 2 K capsules is highly conserved with operons for assembly, export, and synthesis genes.

The synthesis genes vary encoding a variety of saccharide-modifying enzymes that together change the polysaccharide composition. The assembly and export genes are conserved and encode for a multi-subunit export channel that spans the inner membrane and periplasm to direct the polysaccharide capsule through an outer membrane pore where the capsule is linked to the outer membrane through end lipidation [32]. Similarly genetic regulation of the Group 2 capsule operons is highly conserved with two promoters solely driving transcription of all of the genes needed for capsule expression [33–35]. Thus, small molecules inhibiting the conserved aspects of the export channel or regulation of its expression would be expected to block encapsulation of a range of serotypically diverse Group 2 encapsulated UPEC.

Here we extend our discovery process for new capsule small molecule inhibitors. We previously described a facile assay for the identification of such inhibitors that, when employed against a modest number of bioactive small molecules, revealed an inhibitor of K1 and K5 Group 2 capsule biogenesis designated as C7 [36]. We now describe the application of the assay to a large magnitude, high-throughput screen for additional broad-spectrum capsule inhibitors from which we found multiple new, chemically distinct, and highly active molecules with promising therapeutic characteristics.

Methods

Bacterial strains, phage, and growth conditions

All *E. coli* strains and phage used in the present study are listed in Table 1. Unless otherwise indicated, bacteria were routinely grown at 37°C in Luria-Bertani medium (LB) with shaking at 250 rpm. LB was supplemented with 1% dimethyl sulfoxide (DMSO; Acros) with or without compound. Phage lysates were prepared from 50 mL cultures of *E. coli* strains UTI89 (for K1F phage), MG1655 (for T7 phage) or DS17 (for K5 phage) and stored at 4°C over several drops of chloroform as described [37].

Screen for inhibitors of bacterial capsule biogenesis

Primary assay.   The primary assay consisted of detection of the presence and absence of the K1 capsule on the *E. coli* urinary tract isolate UTI89 under growth conditions with compounds from a large chemical library. The assay was conducted as previously described [36] with the following modifications. The primary assay was conducted in 1,536-well plate format. UTI89 Δ*kpsM*, an isogenic K1 capsule export mutant, was included as an unencapsulated control. Tetracycline, 50 μM, was used as a negative growth control. A 1:75 dilution of overnight cultures were made in LB broth containing 0.5% DMSO, and 3 μL of this culture was added to each plate well, and plates were incubated, inverted, at 37°C for 2 hr. K1F phage stock was diluted 1:8 in LB Broth containing 0.5% DMSO, and 1.5 μL of diluted phage (or media only) was added to the pre-plated test compound wells and appropriate control wells. The plates were centrifuged briefly, and then were incubated, inverted, at 37°C for an additional 2 hr. To increase sensitivity of detection of viable bacteria, 1 μL of a 1:2 dilution of AlamarBlue reagent (Invitrogen, #DAL1100) in LB broth was added to each plate well. Alamar Blue, resazurin, is converted in living cells to the fluorescent molecule, resorufin. The plates were again centrifuged briefly, and then were further incubated, inverted, at 37°C for 30 min. Resorufin fluorescence was measured using excitation of 560 nm and emission of 590 nm, as per the manufacturer's recommendations.

Compounds from the NIH Molecular Libraries Small Molecule Repository (MLSMR) were utilized in the primary assay. The

Table 1. Bacterial strains and phage used in this study.

Strain/phage	Description or relevant genotype	Reference
Bacterial strains		
UTI89	K1 *Escherichia coli* cystitis isolate	[49]
UTI89 ΔRegion I	Region I (*kps*) K1 capsule mutant	[28]
UTI89 ΔRegion II	Region II (*neu*) K1 capsule synthesis mutant	[28]
UTI89 Δ*kpsM*	K1 capsule export mutant	[28]
DS17	*Escherichia coli* K5 pyelonephritis isolate; K5 encapsulated, susceptible to K5 specific phage	[50]
EV36	K-12/K1 hybrid produced by conjugation with an Hfr *kps*⁺ strain; K1 encapsulated, susceptible to K1-specific phage.	[51]
CFT073	K2 *Escherichia coli* urosepsis isolate	[52]
536	K15 *Escherichia coli* urinary tract isolate	[53]
Phage		
T7 phage (T7φ)	Inhibited by K1 capsule	[54]
K1F phage (K1Fφ)	K1 capsule specific	[55]
K5 phage (K5φ)	K5 capsule specific	[56]

MLSMR collection of over 300,000 compounds generically grouped into one of the following five categories: (a) specialty sets, comprising bioactive compounds such as known drugs and toxins, (b) non-commercial compounds, mainly from academic labs, (c) targeted libraries, (d) natural products, and (e) diversity compounds [38]. The MLSMR library covers a diverse sample of the chemical space occupied by drugs and natural products, but only narrowly represents combinatorial chemical space [39]. Compounds or vehicle control (DMSO) were diluted to a final well concentration of 1:200 in assay media. Compounds (22.5 nL in 100% DMSO) were dispensed to assay plates using an Echo non-contact dispenser (Labcyte). Compounds from the libraries were added to the plates at a final concentration of 50 µM, before the addition of bacteria or phage. Each compound was tested as a single point, and ~1,200 compounds were tested per plate. A positive hit was defined by the compound producing greater than a 50% inhibition of K1F phage-induced lysis. Compound hits were further confirmed using an optical density-based detection method in a 96-well format as previously described [36].

Concentration-response to chemical inhibition. Concentration-response testing (concentration range = 0.58–300 µM) was used to confirm and characterize the primary screen hits, which was necessary to determine the number of compounds advanced to secondary screens. Compounds were plated in 1536-well microplates, and the concentration-response efficacy assay was performed as described for the primary screen, with the exception that each compound was tested in duplicate at 10 concentration points starting from 300 µM and continuing to lower concentrations by 2-fold serial dilutions. The strain UTI89 Δ*kpsM*, a K1 capsule export mutant, was evaluated with the wild-type strain as a phage-insensitive control (mimicking 100% capsule inhibition).

T7 phage counter assay. This secondary assay was performed as previously described [36] and was used to distinguish compounds with phage inhibitory effects from true polysaccharide capsule inhibitors. T7 phage has a nearly identical genome to K1F phage and thus a similar life cycle [40]; however, T7 phage does not encode for an endosialidase, and its entry into *E. coli* is inhibited by K capsules. Thus, the presence of a capsule inhibits T7-mediated lysis [41]. In this assay, an increase in phage-induced

lysis correlates to a decrease in capsule formation. True inhibitors of capsule yielded bacteria that were susceptible to T7 phage and lysed within 2 hr of the addition of phage. However, compounds inhibiting phage replication did not promote bacterial lysis. The positive control molecule C7 (100 µM final well concentration) was used in this screen.

Pan Assay Interference Compound (PAINS) analysis. Groups of compound substructural features are associated with compound biological promiscuity, and compounds containing these features arise as frequent hits in biochemical high throughput screens. These molecules have been described as PAINS [42]. To determine if molecules of interest were within chemical groups with known non-specific interference with the bioassays, the structures for compounds DU001, DU003, DU005, DU007, DU008, and DU011 were retrieved from PubChem and saved in the Structure Data Format (SDF). The structures were then compared to the SYBYL PAINS compounds library, to see which, if any, of the compounds contain PAINS functional groups [43].

Cytotoxicity. Testing was performed essentially as previously described [36,44]. Concentration-response testing was performed over a range 0.58–300 µM in a 386 well plate format. Bladder carcinoma 5637 cells (ATCC HTB-9) were added to the compounds, and 72 hrs later cell viability was measured using CellTiter Glo (Promega). The 50% toxic concentration (TC$_{50}$) was determined and compared to the IC$_{50}$ to calculate the therapeutic index. Hyamine was used as a positive cytotoxic control. All wells contained 0.5% DMSO.

Evaluation of off-target effects. Off target effects of lead molecules of interest were evaluated using the LeadProfilingScreen commercial assay at Eurofins Panlabs (Bothell, Washington). Reference standards were run as an integral part of each assay to ensure the validity of the results obtained. Assay results are presented as the percent inhibition of specific binding or activity (for n = 2 replicates) for the probe compound tested at a concentration of 10 µM. Details regarding the individual assays and methods are provided in File S1.

Orcinol assay for released capsule material. Orcinol reactivity was used as a biochemical confirmation of altered extracellular capsule after compound treatment. UTI89 or an isogenic capsule mutant was grown in 100 µM of test compound or 1% DMSO. The assay was performed as previously described [36]. The molecule C7 (100 µM final concentration) was used as a positive control. The assay was performed 3 times with replicate samples.

K1 antigen dot blot. K1 antigen was detected by dot blot assays of culture extracts probed with anti-K1 H46 serum. The assay was performed as previously described [36]. The experiment was repeated twice with similar results, and a representative dot blot is shown.

Visualization of capsule using Alcian blue staining. Overnight cultures of clinical *E. coli* strains were diluted 1:100 in the presence of 1% DMSO or 100 µM DU011. Cultures were grown for ~6 hrs (OD$_{600}$ = 1.2) at 37°C. Samples were centrifuged at 13,200 RPM for 5 min. The medium was removed and the cells were resuspended in 500 µL of Tris-Acetate (pH 5) and shaken for 1 hr at 37°C. Samples were re-centrifuged, and the supernatant was concentrated ~100 fold in Amicon 3K microconcentrators. The preparations were separated on a 7.5% SDS-PAGE gel and stained with 0.125% Alcian blue as previously described [45].

K5 phage assay. This assay determined if compounds found to be active in the K1F, T7, orcinol, and K1 antigen dot blot secondary assays were able to also inhibit K5 capsule biogenesis. The assay was performed in a method identical to the T7 assay test [36]. *E. coli* strain DS17, a pyelonephritis clinical isolate expressing a K5 capsule and susceptible to K5 phage (K5), was used as a K5 prototypic test strain. The degree of inhibition of phage-mediated lysis was determined based on the absorbance (OD$_{600}$).

Human serum sensitization by capsule inhibitor treatment. Overnight cultures of UTI89 were diluted 1:100 and grown with or without 50 µM compound for approximately 1.5 hrs on a shaker at 37°C. Then 25 µL of anonymous, non-identified, sterile filtered pooled human serum (purchased from Equitech Bio) was added per 100 µL of growth media. This was returned to the shaker for another 3 hrs, after which 20 µL of 5 mg/mL MTT (3-(4,5-Dimethylthiazol-2-yl)-2,5- diphenyltetra-zolium bromide) was added. MTT is reduced to purple formazan by bacterial reductase enzymes, thus measuring viable bacteria. This was shaken for another 15 min at 37°C. The sample was spun to remove the growth media, followed by two washes with PBS. The formazan crystals were dissolved in 100 µL of DMSO and measured at OD$_{570}$.

Murine UPEC sepsis model and treatment with DU011. Groups of five 6–7 week old C57BL/6NCr female mice (purchased from Frederick National Laboratory for Cancer Research) were injected subcutaneously twice daily with 100 µL of 1% DMSO (vehicle control) or DU011 (1 mg/ml) starting 12 hrs prior to the intra peritoneal infection. Weights were recorded twice daily to monitor health of the animals and tolerance to the compound. Mice were challenged by intraperitoneal injection with 10^8 CFU of the indicated *E. coli* UTI89 in 100 µL of PBS. Briefly, cultures were prepared by diluting overnight cultures (18 hrs) 1:100 into 3 mL of LB supplemented with 1% DMSO final or 100 µM DU011 (1% DMSO final). Shaken cultures were grown at 37°C for 6 hours to an OD$_{600}$ of 1.2, and then cells were pelleted and resuspended in 1 mL of PBS. Absorbance was adjusted to OD$_{600}$ of 0.8 in PBS, and the cultures were then diluted 1:10 in sterile PBS. Animals were also given an intraperitoneal dose of 1% DMSO or DU011, in a site different than the administration of bacteria, to ensure sufficient systemic delivery of drug. Animal survival was assessed after 12 hours. Surviving mice were re-dosed according to the treatment groups and continued to be monitored. The experiment was concluded 48 hours post infection. The entire experiment was repeated with similar results.

Throughout each experiment, animals were monitored each 6 hours from the time of infection until conclusion for serious morbidity, including ruffled fur, decreased activity, slowed respirations, and ill appearance. Animals were provided gel packs for easily accessible additional hydration throughout the experiments. When a moribund state was suspected or anticipated by these criteria, animals were immediately euthanized to minimize potential pain and/or suffering. Of the total animals with an outcome categorized as death, the following numbers were euthanized for terminal morbidity prior to septic death (euthanized/total deaths): 3/10, no prior treatment; 3/5 prior chemical treatment of bacteria alone; 0/2 prior chemical treatment of mice alone. Euthanasia for all animals was through complete respiratory cessation using the inhaled anesthetic isoflurane followed by secondary assurance of death using bilateral thoracotomy. All animal experiments were conducted with prior approval from the Institutional Animal Care and Use Committee of Duke University.

Statistical analyses

Results were calculated as averages and standard deviations of the means using the Graph Pad Prism 5 software package (San Diego, CA). Nonparametric t-tests were used for statistical analysis of data and calculation of *p*-values using Graph Pad Prism 5 or Graph Pad online calculators. Significant differences are highlighted with a single asterisk when the p value is less than 0.05, with two asterisks when the p value is less than 0.01, and three asterisks when the p value is less than 0.001.

Results

Primary screen for novel capsule inhibitors

Our initial screen of 2,195 compounds from the Developmental Therapeutics Program at the National Cancer Institute successfully identified a small-molecule inhibitor of uropathogenic *E. coli* Group 2 capsule biogenesis. We described this compound, termed C7, in a previous report as proof-of-principle that small-molecule inhibition of capsule biogenesis is possible and that these novel anti-infectives can block encapsulation and attenuate a pathogen through exposure to host innate immune factors [36]. Based on this proof-of-concept, the primary assay was adapted to a 1,536-well format with the modifications for high-throughput screening necessary to search for additional active molecules in significantly larger chemical repositories. The K1 encapsulated strain of uropathogenic *E. coli* UTI89 was grown in a 1,536-well plate format in the presence of 50 µM compounds. After an initial growth step, K1F phage specific for K1 capsule was added. Compounds with no effect on capsule biogenesis allowed the growth of organisms with an intact capsule that were subsequently lysed by the addition of the K1F phage. However, those compounds that presumably inhibited capsule biogenesis and allowed growth of the unencapsulated organism did not lyse with the addition of the K1F phage. These compounds were then selected for a secondary assay.

In total, 338,740 compounds were screened in the primary assay (using K1F phage), and 1,767 compounds associated with resistance to phage lysis (0.52% of total) were tested in concentration-response format. Of these, 29 compounds passed concentration-response validation (1.6% of compounds passing the primary screen), and 6 were selected after demonstrating high activity in the T7 phage secondary assay, the reciprocal phage assay in which chemical unencapsulation sensitizes a K1:K12 hybrid strain, EV36, to lysis by the T7 phage. Concentration response curves for 2 of these compounds are shown in Figure 1. Compounds with promising chemical structures and low cytotoxicity to cultured bladder epithelial cells were selected for further characterization. As seen in Table 2, the activity of these compound hits in primary and secondary assays is consistent with molecules with capsule inhibitory action. Cytotoxicity data further indicate that these molecules are non-toxic to cultured bladder epithelial cells. Furthermore, these new compounds, designated DU001, DU003, DU005, DU007, DU008, and DU011, are more active in the phage assays than the original proof-of-concept agent C7, with IC_{50} values in the micromolar range.

Identification of potential Pan Assay Interference Compounds (PAINS) among capsule inhibitor hits

A number of compound substructural features have been identified that are associated with compound biological promiscuity, and, in particular, compounds with certain structural features appear as frequent hits in biochemical high throughput screens. These molecules have been described as PAINS {Merging Citations}. Although PAINS may remain useful hits, we sought to prioritize the compound hits DU001, DU003, DU005, DU007, DU008, and DU011 by identifying and removing PAINS-like molecules from our prioritization. Three of the six most active and selective compound hits, DU005, DU007, and DU008, are considered PAINS [40], and thus were not submitted for additional biological characterization.

Confirmation of primary hits and spectrum of activity

Compounds were further characterized by determining biochemically the level of surface capsule upon compound treatment of a wild-type K1 encapsulated UPEC strain. We used mild-acid to release capsule from cultures of UTI89 grown in the presence of 100 µM compound. We then used the orcinol reagent to quantify the amount of released material. As shown in Figure 2A, orcinol

reactivity as % of wild-type for compound treatment indicates that cultures treated with capsule inhibitors had decreased surface reactive material, similar to levels observed for capsule synthesis and assembly mutants.

As another independent measure of capsule inhibition by the DU compounds, K1 antigen was evaluated using whole-cell dot blots with anti-K1 serum. In all cases, treatment with these molecules reduced reactivity to levels resembling those of genetic capsule mutants (Figure 2B). The combined results from the phage, orcinol, and immune-dot blots demonstrate that these molecules inhibit normal capsule production and assembly, significantly reducing the amount of surface assembled capsule.

A major consideration was whether the inhibitors of K1 encapsulation were also able to inhibit the production of other important *E. coli* Group 2 capsule types. To confirm the range of activity, we first demonstrated that treatment with each of confirmed inhibitory molecules also inhibited K5 phage infection of a K5 capsule-expressing strain, DS17 (Figure 3A). We next determined if leading capsule inhibitors would also inhibit the production of capsule in non-K1 serotypes. Capsular material was isolated from strains 536 (K15 serotype), CFT073 (K2 serotype) and DS17 (K5 serotype), and UTI89 (K1 serotype) in the presence and absence of capsule inhibitors. Capsule was isolated from the same amount of bacteria after growth in vehicle or with inhibitor DU011 (200 µM). Isolated material was separated on a polyacrylamide gel and stained with the cationic dye alcian blue. As shown in Figure 3B, capsule was reduced in each strain following growth with DU011, regardless of serotype. Although visibly reduced in capsule after growth in DU011, the reduction in capsular material from treated CFT073 appeared slightly less than the other serotypes tested. A similar reduction in extracted capsule was also seen with DU003 (data not shown).

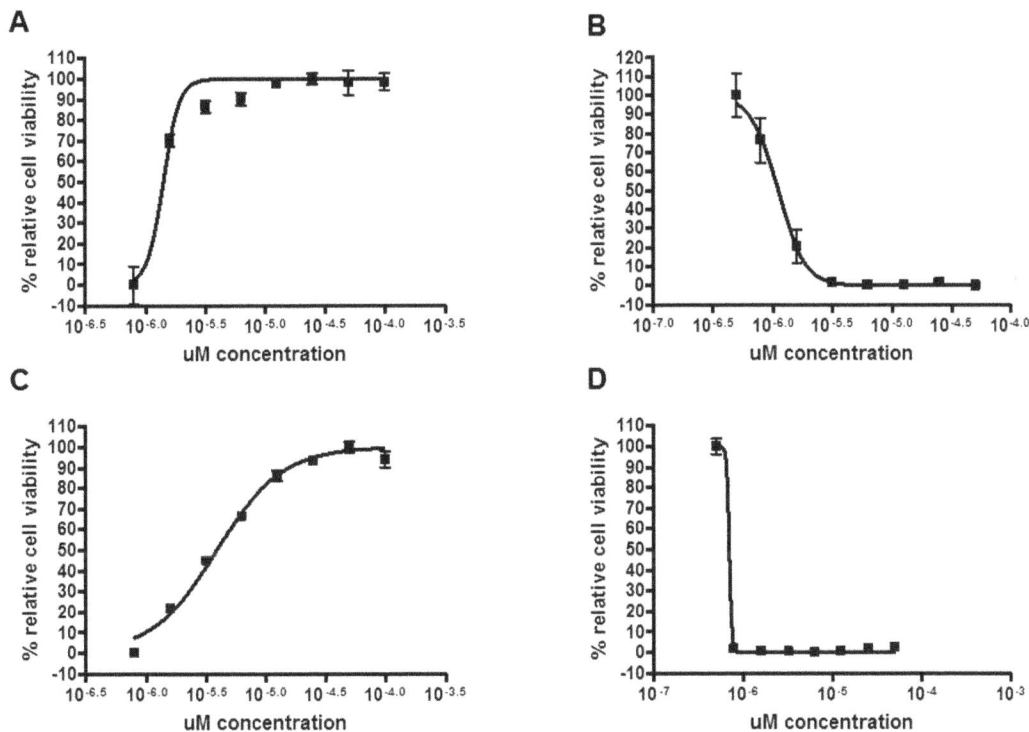

Figure 1. Concentration-response inhibition of K1 and T7 phage-mediated cell lysis. K1 (**A, C**) and T7 (**B, D**) phage activity in *E. coli* strain UTI89 or EV36 (K1:K-12 hybrid strain), respectively, following treatment with various concentrations of DU003 (**A, B**) or DU011 (**C, D**).

Table 2. Structure, K1 and T7 phage activity, cytotoxicity, and selectivity of capsule inhibitor compounds.

Compound	CID	IC50 K1 phage (in μM)	IC50 T7 phage (in μM)	Cytotoxicity (CC50 in μM)	Selectivity (CC50/IC50)
DU001	1247114	10.6±2.0	0.26±0.18	>100	>9.4
DU003	18109210	1.38±0.02	1.0±0.03	239±89	183
DU005	24235566	26.1±1.57	1.57±0.01	>100	>3.8
DU007	46254879	22.6±5.4	2.5±0.02	>100	4.4
DU008	4483668	3.3±0.76	0.54±0.7	45.08	13.7
DU011	23602075	4.5±2.5	0.69±0.78	51.6±13.6	13.3

Values shown correspond to the average of at least 3 replicates ± SEM. CID indicates the PubChem Compound Identification.

Chemical inhibition sensitized UPEC to serum-mediated killing

Capsule offers protection against serum-mediated killing. In order to test whether compound treatment of UPEC increased serum-mediated killing, an *in vitro* serum resistance assay was used. As shown in Figure 4, pooled human serum decreased the amount of viable UPEC as measured by an MTT metabolic activity assay. Treatment of UPEC with either 50 μM DU003 or DU011 further increased serum-mediated killing, thus significantly reducing the measurable bacteria as compared to DMSO treated cells (p = 0.0067). This decrease was similar to the serum sensitivity observed for a genetic capsule mutant (Δneu).

DU003 & DU011 are biologically selective

DU003 and DU011 were submitted to the Eurofins Panlabs LeadProfilingScreen to assess off-target pharmacology [42]. Both compounds were tested in duplicate at 10 μM concentration and showed no significant activity across the panel of 68 targets (i.e., < 32% inhibition for DU011 and <30% inhibition for DU003, except for one target, the norepinephrine transporter, for which 58% inhibition was observed; full data and assays are provided in File S1). In review of PubChem data, DU011 (CID23602075) is reported to have shown activity in only 21 of 467 (4.5%, as of September 5, 2013) bioassays in which it was tested (assays unrelated to the current project). Per PubChem, DU003 (CID18109210) is reported to have shown activity in only 5 of 427 (1.2%, as of September 5, 2013) bioassays in which it was tested (assays unrelated to the current project). Together, these

results suggest that DU011 and DU003 are not biologically promiscuous compounds.

Attenuation of *E. coli* disseminated infection by DU011

In order to test the ability of these compounds to prevent lethal systemic *E. coli* infection in mice, we selected DU011 for animal testing based on its favorable solubility, permeability, and plasma and microsome stability profiles (Table 3). As shown in Figure 5A, C57BL/6 mice were administered DU011 or 1% DMSO 12 hours prior to lethal challenge with 10^8 CFU of UPEC UTI89 by intraperitoneal injection. All previously untreated mice receiving non-pretreated bacteria were moribund or died within 24 hr post-infection. In contrast, pretreatment of the bacteria and mice with DU011 conferred complete protection with 100% survival for the duration of the experiments (48 hrs) and recovery of pre-infection weights (Figure 5B), similar to the 100% survival of animals administered UTI89 ΔRII, an unencapsulated isogenic mutant (data not shown). Administration of subcutaneous DU011 and untreated UTI89 provided 80% survival with stabilization of weights at the end of the experiment. Pre-treatment of bacteria without pretreatment of the mice produced 50% survival with ongoing weight loss among surviving animals. Mice tolerated DU011 without evident side effects. These data indicate that pretreatment of mice with DU011 was able to significantly reduce mortality due to disseminated *E. coli* infection, demonstrating the potency of polysaccharide inhibition *in vivo*.

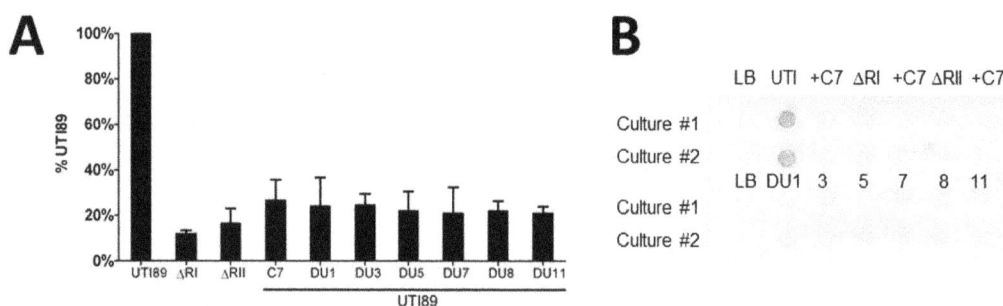

Figure 2. Biochemical and immunologic verification of *E. coli* Group 2 capsule inhibition through small molecules. A) Orcinol reactivity of capsular material released by mild acid treatment of cultures grown with 1% DMSO vehicle (UTI89 and genetic capsule mutants) or 100 μM C7, DU001, DU003, DU005, DU007, DU008, or DU011. Data represent independent experiments performed in duplicate. Treatment of K1 strain UTI89 with compounds reduces amount of orcinol-reactive polysaccharides on surface of bacteria by ~80%. **B)** Whole-cell anti-K1 dot blots of cultures of UTI89 or indicated genetic capsule mutants treated with 1% DMSO or 100 μM DU001, DU003, DU005, DU007, DU008, or DU011 indicate that treatment of cultures with compounds reduces K1 reactive material to levels comparable to those of genetic capsule mutants. ΔRI and ΔRII indicate a complete deletion of Region I of the capsule *kps* and Region II capsule *neu* loci, respectively.

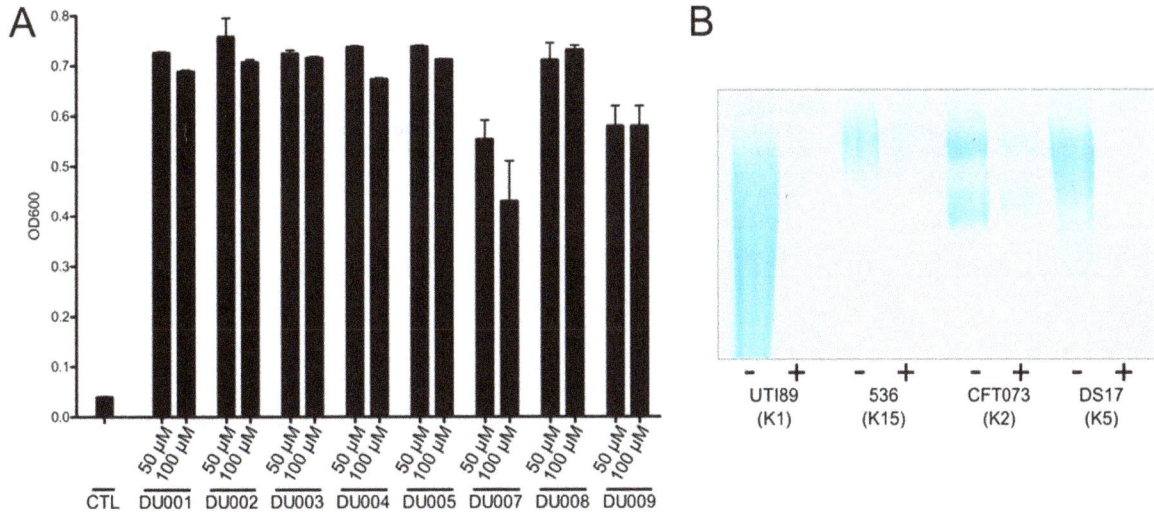

Figure 3. Inhibitor treatment decreases capsule production in different pathogenic *E. coli* serotypes. A) K5 *E. coli* was grown in vehicle or with different inhibitors (50 and 100 μM) and then challenged with K5 lytic phage, which results in cell death in the presence of capsule. Growth was measured by absorbance at OD_{600}. **B**) Capsular material was isolated from multiple strains grown with and without inhibitor DU011 (200 μM). Capsule preparations were performed in at least 3 independent trials. A single representative image is shown.

Discussion

E. coli infections play a significant role in community-acquired UTI with substantial morbidity and associated costs. With a diminishing arsenal of antibiotics available for the treatment of UTI, new therapeutics are in great demand. Anti-virulence agents

capable of specifically attenuating a pathogenic organism during its infectious cycle hold great potential as they may spare the microbiota in commensal niches.

Previous work in our lab and in others has highlighted the importance of capsular polysaccharides in the pathogenesis of uropathogenic *E. coli* [27–29]. Group 2 and 3 capsules are highly

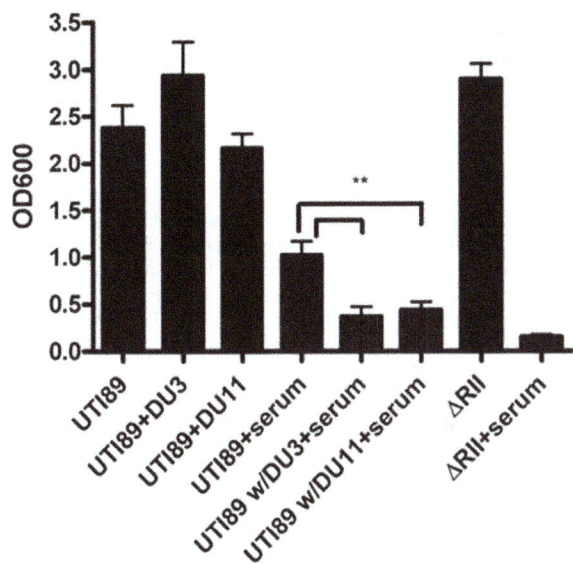

Figure 4. Capsule inhibitors sensitize UPEC K1 strain to serum-mediated killing. *E. coli* UTI89 and genetic capsule mutants were grown in the presence and absence of DU003 or DU011 at 50 μM and exposed to human serum. Bacterial metabolism and viability was measured using MTT (3-(4,5-Dimethylthiazol-2-yl)-2,5- diphenyltetrazolium bromide). UTI89 grown in the presence of 50 μM DU003 or DU011 were significantly more sensitive to pooled human serum compared to control UTI89 (** p = 0.0067). This was similar to the serum sensitivity of the capsule mutant UTI89 ΔRII. ΔRI and ΔRII indicate a complete deletion of Region I of the capsule *kps* and Region II capsule *neu* loci, respectively.

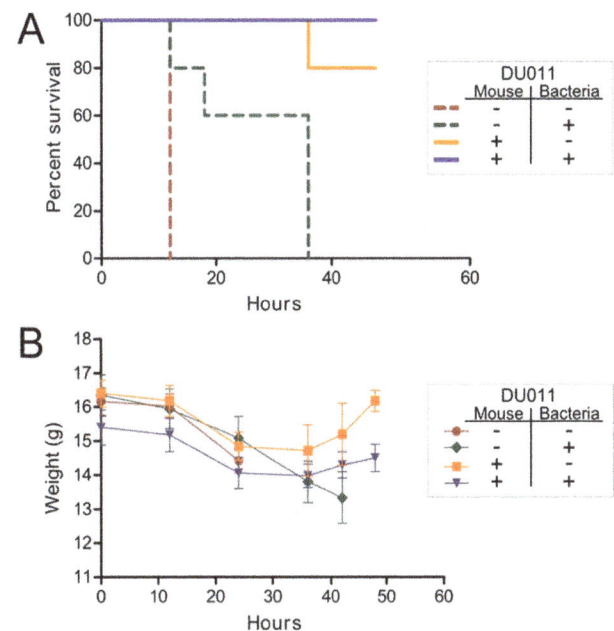

Figure 5. DU011 protects mice against a lethal dose of K1 *E. coli*. A) C57BL/6 mice were administered subcutaneous 1% DMSO (control) or DU011 (100 μL of 1 mg/ml in 1% DMSO) 12 hours prior to lethal intraperitoneal injection with 10^8 CFU of UTI89 prepared in media containing 1% DMSO or DU011 (200 μM in 1% DMSO). Surviving animals continued to receive DMSO or DU011 each 12 hours through the course of the experiment, according to their groups (**B**) Weight was monitored during DMSO and DU011 administration and after infection.

Table 3. Solubility, permeability and plasma and microsome stability.

Compound	PubChem CID	Aqueous Solubility[1] (μg/mL)	Hepatic Microsome Stability[2] (Human/Mouse)	Aqueous Solubility[3] (μg/mL)	PAMPA Permeability Pe[4] ($\times10-6$ cm/s) (Donor pH: 5.0/6.2/7.4)	Plasma Stability[5] (Human/Mouse)
DU001	1247114	<0.01	38.73/0.56	<0.01	749/1303/566	90.09/92.69
DU003	18109210	104.1	57.86/14.57	>126	35/183/230	100/86.86
DU011	23602075	92.6	89.64/74.32	68	14/209/52	95.31/78.39

[1]Measured in 1× PBS.
[2]Percent remaining at 1 hr.
[3]Measured in LB medium.
[4]Acceptor pH: 7.4.
[5]Percent remaining at 3 hrs.

conserved and represent the predominant circulating capsule types [46]. We have previously described the identification and characterization of a novel agent designated C7 that is active (IC_{50} between 12.5–25 μM), blocks the production of K1 and K5 capsule biogenesis, and lacks obvious toxicity to cultured bladder epithelial cells [36]. We have since conducted a high-throughput screen for additional broad-spectrum capsule inhibitors, finding several structurally distinct and highly active new molecules with promising therapeutic characteristics.

Herein, we described the initial identification and characterization of these new small molecules. This group of capsule inhibitors features lower IC_{50} values and improved solubility, permeability, and plasma and microsome stability profiles (Table 3; File S2). We have demonstrated their activity in assays with human serum (Figure 4). Most importantly, dosing of mice with DU011 had no detectable adverse effects on the animals and protected against a lethal *E. coli* systemic challenge (Figure 5). This new approach may provide the basis for the next pre-clinical steps to test these inhibitors as UTI-specific therapeutics that render microbes vulnerable to host clearance mechanisms such as innate immunity, enhancing the adaptive immune responses in the process by allowing greater engagement of the immune system. While dosing and delivery will need to be evaluated in future pre-clinical pharmacokinetic and pharmacodynamics studies, we believe these data highlight the potential use of capsule inhibitors as specific anti-virulence therapeutics. The compounds listed in Tables 2 and 3 are synthetically amenable lead compounds and work is currently underway to improve upon their properties. Synthesis of large lots of DU011 and other compound hits has made animal testing possible as well as facilitated work on the mechanism of action of these compounds. This will aid in the identification of their biological target and will advance our understanding of capsule biogenesis and regulation in *E. coli* and other organisms with similarly conserved capsule loci. This could lead to the attenuation of diverse encapsulated organisms sharing similar capsule assembly and regulatory mechanisms. The generation of novel highly active small-molecule inhibitors of

capsule biogenesis will also aid in our understanding of the role of the innate and adaptive immune systems in control of encapsulated bacterial pathogens during systemic infections. A better understanding of how DU003, DU011 and others affect the interaction of the bacterium with host immune responses will significantly aid in the development better anti-infectives that not only attenuate the organism, but also actively engage the host immune system to promote clearance.

Supporting Information

File S1 Ricera LeadProfiling Screen Data Tables. Data for screens of off target effects by DU003 and DU011 are provided.

File S2 Experimental procedures for aqueous and LB medium solubility, hepatic microsome stability, PAMPA permeability, and plasma stability. Additional methodological details are provided for these assays.

Acknowledgments

The authors thank Richard Silver for kindly provided the horse Group B meningococcal antiserum (H46), K1F bacteriophage, and useful *E. coli* strains. The authors thank Dr. Ian Roberts for kindly providing the K5 bacteriophage used in these studies. Portions of this work regarding DU03 and DU011 were previously described in official Probe Reports submitted to the NIH upon project completion. The official Probe Reports have been made available online by the NIH, free of charge [47,48].

Author Contributions

Conceived and designed the experiments: CCG MA PCS FS JWN. Performed the experiments: CCG MA FS JWN PP SAR PCS. Analyzed the data: CCG MA PCS FS JWN ELW NAT. Contributed reagents/materials/analysis tools: SA CWE NMN LR MS BN BEM PCS. Wrote the paper: CCG MA PCS FS JWN.

References

1. NKUDIC (2005) Urinary Tract Infections in Adults.

2. Schappert S, Rechtsteiner E (2011) Ambulatory medical care utilization estimates for 2007. Vital and health statistics. Series 13.

3. Foxman B (2010) The epidemiology of urinary tract infection. Nat Rev Urol 7: 653–660. doi:10.1038/nrurol.2010.190.

4. Gupta K, Scholes D, Stamm WE (1999) Increasing prevalence of antimicrobial resistance among uropathogens causing acute uncomplicated cystitis in women. Jama 281: 736–738. doi:jbr80382 [pii].

5. Ma JF, Shortliffe LMD (2004) Urinary tract infection in children: etiology and epidemiology. Urol Clin North Am 31: 517–26, ix–x. doi:10.1016/j.ucl.2004.04.016.

6. Hooton TM, Scholes D, Stapleton AE, Roberts PL, Winter C, et al. (2000) A prospective study of asymptomatic bacteriuria in sexually active young women. N Engl J Med 343: 992–997. doi:10.1056/NEJM200010053431402.

7. Foxman B, Brown P (2003) Epidemiology of urinary tract infections: transmission and risk factors, incidence, and costs. Infect Dis Clin North Am 17: 227–241.

8. Gaschignard J, Levy C, Romain O, Cohen R, Bingen E, et al. (2011) Neonatal Bacterial Meningitis: 444 Cases in 7 Years. Pediatr Infect Dis J 30: 212–217.

9. Litwin M, Saigal C (2007) Introduction. In: Litwin M, Saigal C, editors. Urologic Diseases in America. Washington, D.C: NIH. pp. 3–7.

10. King T, Abedin A, Belal M (2012) Rise of multi-resistant urinary tract infections. BJU Int 110: 300–301. doi:10.1111/j.1464-410X.2012.11142.x.

11. Olson RP, Harrell LJ, Kaye KS (2009) Antibiotic resistance in urinary isolates of Escherichia coli from college women with urinary tract infections. Antimicrob Agents Chemother 53: 1285–1286.

12. Edlin RS, Shapiro DJ, Hersh AL, Copp HL (2013) Antibiotic resistance patterns of outpatient pediatric urinary tract infections. J Urol 190: 222–227. doi:10.1016/j.juro.2013.01.069.

13. Gupta K, Hooton TM, Naber KG, Wullt B, Colgan R, et al. (2011) International clinical practice guidelines for the treatment of acute uncomplicated cystitis and pyelonephritis in women: A 2010 update by the Infectious Diseases Society of America and the European Society for Microbiology and Infectious Diseases. Clin Infect Dis 52: e103–20. doi:ciq257 [pii] 10.1093/cid/ciq257.

14. Yang Q, Zhang H, Wang Y, Xu Y, Chen M, et al. (2013) A 10 year surveillance for antimicrobial susceptibility of Escherichia coli and Klebsiella pneumoniae in community- and hospital-associated intra-abdominal infections in China. J Med Microbiol 62: 1343–1349. doi:10.1099/jmm.0.059816-0.

15. Gupta K, Hooton TM, Stamm WE (2005) Isolation of fluoroquinolone-resistant rectal Escherichia coli after treatment of acute uncomplicated cystitis. J Antimicrob Chemother 56: 243–246.

16. Karlowsky JA, Hoban DJ, Decorby MR, Laing NM, Zhanel GG (2006) Fluoroquinolone-resistant urinary isolates of Escherichia coli from outpatients are frequently multidrug resistant: results from the North American Urinary Tract Infection Collaborative Alliance-Quinolone Resistance study. Antimicrob Agents Chemother 50: 2251–2254.

17. Hang L, Wullt B, Shen Z, Karpman D, Svanborg C (1998) Cytokine repertoire of epithelial cells lining the human urinary tract. J Urol 159: 2185–2192.

18. Schilling JD, Mulvey MA, Vincent CD, Lorenz RG, Hultgren SJ (2001) Bacterial invasion augments epithelial cytokine responses to Escherichia coli through a lipopolysaccharide-dependent mechanism. J Immunol 166: 1148–1155.

19. Hedges S, Anderson P, Lidin-Janson G, de Man P, Svanborg C (1991) Interleukin-6 response to deliberate colonization of the human urinary tract with gram-negative bacteria. Infect Immun 59: 421–427.

20. Svanborg C, Agace W, Hedges S, Linder H, Svensson M (1993) Bacterial adherence and epithelial cell cytokine production. Zentralbl Bakteriol 278: 359–364.

21. Schilling JD, Martin SM, Hung CS, Lorenz RG, Hultgren SJ (2003) Toll-like receptor 4 on stromal and hematopoietic cells mediates innate resistance to uropathogenic Escherichia coli. Proc Natl Acad Sci U S A 100: 4203–4208.

22. Li K, Sacks SH, Sheerin NS (2008) The classical complement pathway plays a critical role in the opsonisation of uropathogenic Escherichia coli. Mol Immunol 45: 954–962.

23. Valore E V, Park CH, Quayle AJ, Wiles KR, McCray Jr PB, et al. (1998) Human beta-defensin-1: an antimicrobial peptide of urogenital tissues. J Clin Invest 101: 1633–1642.

24. Ali ASM, Townes CL, Hall J, Pickard RS (2009) Maintaining a sterile urinary tract: the role of antimicrobial peptides. J Urol 182: 21–28. doi:10.1016/j.juro.2009.02.124.

25. Roberts IS (1995) Bacterial polysaccharides in sickness and in health. The 1995 Fleming Lecture. Microbiology 141 (Pt 9: 2023–2031.

26. Roberts IS (1996) The biochemistry and genetics of capsular polysaccharide production in bacteria. Annu Rev Microbiol 50: 285–315.

27. Buckles EL, Wang X, Lane MC, Lockatell C V, Johnson DE, et al. (2009) Role of the K2 capsule in Escherichia coli urinary tract infection and serum resistance. J Infect Dis 199: 1689–1697. doi:10.1086/598524.

28. Anderson GG, Goller CC, Justice S, Hultgren SJ, Seed PC (2010) Polysaccharide Capsule and Sialic Acid-Mediated Regulation Promote Biofilm-like Intracellular Bacterial Communities During Cystitis. Infect Immun 78: 963–975. doi:IAI.00925-09 [pii] 10.1128/IAI.00925-09.

29. Mushtaq N, Redpath MB, Luzio JP, Taylor PW (2005) Treatment of experimental Escherichia coli infection with recombinant bacteriophage-derived capsule depolymerase. J Antimicrob Chemother 56: 160–165.

30. Llobet E, Tomas JM, Bengoechea JA (2008) Capsule polysaccharide is a bacterial decoy for antimicrobial peptides. Microbiology 154: 3877–3886. doi:154/12/3877 [pii] 10.1099/mic.0.2008/022301-0.

31. Varki A (2008) Sialic acids in human health and disease. Trends Mol Med 14: 351–360. doi:10.1016/j.molmed.2008.06.002.

32. Vimr ER, Steenbergen SM (2009) Early molecular-recognition events in the synthesis and export of group 2 capsular polysaccharides. Microbiology 155: 9–15. doi:10.1099/mic.0.023564-0.

33. Rowe S, Hodson N, Griffiths G, Roberts IS (2000) Regulation of the Escherichia coli K5 capsule gene cluster: evidence for the roles of H-NS, BipA, and integration host factor in regulation of group 2 capsule gene clusters in pathogenic E. coli. J Bacteriol 182: 2741–2745.

34. Whitfield C, Roberts IS (1999) Structure, assembly and regulation of expression of capsules in Escherichia coli. Mol Microbiol 31: 1307–1319.

35. Stevens MP, Clarke BR, Roberts IS (1997) Regulation of the Escherichia coli K5 capsule gene cluster by transcription antitermination. Mol Microbiol 24: 1001–1012.

36. Goller CC, Seed PC (2010) High-Throughput Identification of Chemical Inhibitors of E. coli Group 2 Capsule Biogenesis as Anti-virulence Agents. PLoS One 5(7): e11642. doi:10.1371/journal.pone.0011642.

37. Sambrook Fritsch EF, Maniatis TJ (1989) Molecular Cloning: A Laboratory Manual. 2nd ed. Cold Spring Harbor, NY: Cold Spring Harbor. p.

38. Molecular Libraries Program: Pathways to Discovery (2014). Available:http://mli.nih.gov/mli/compound-repository/mlsmr-compounds/.

39. Singh N, Guha R, Giulianotti MA, Pinilla C, Houghten RA, et al. (2009) Chemoinformatic analysis of combinatorial libraries, drugs, natural products, and molecular libraries small molecule repository. J Chem Inf Model 49: 1010–1024. doi:10.1021/ci800426u.

40. Scholl D, Merril C (2005) The genome of bacteriophage K1F, a T7-like phage that has acquired the ability to replicate on K1 strains of Escherichia coli. J Bacteriol 187: 8499–8503.

41. Scholl D, Adhya S, Merril C (2005) Escherichia coli K1's capsule is a barrier to bacteriophage T7. Appl Env Microbiol 71: 4872–4874.

42. Baell JB (2010) Observations on screening-based research and some concerning trends in the literature. Future Med Chem 2: 1529–1546. doi:10.4155/fmc.10.237.

43. Baell JB, Holloway GA (2010) New substructure filters for removal of pan assay interference compounds (PAINS) from screening libraries and for their exclusion in bioassays. J Med Chem 53: 2719–2740. doi:10.1021/jm901137j.

44. Noah JW, Severson W, Noah DL, Rasmussen L, White EL, et al. (2007) A cell-based luminescence assay is effective for high-throughput screening of potential influenza antivirals. Antiviral Res 73: 50–59. doi:10.1016/j.antiviral.2006.07.006.

45. YAMADA K (1963) Staining of sulphated polysaccharides by means of alcian blue. Nature 198: 799–800.

46. Johnson JR (1991) Virulence factors in Escherichia coli urinary tract infection. Clin Microbiol Rev 4: 80–128.

47. Noah JW, Anathan S, Evans C, Nebane M, Rasmussen L, et al. (2013) 3-(2,6-difluorobenzamido)-5-(4-ethoxyphenyl) thiophene-2-carboxylic acid inhibits E.coli UT189 bacterial capsule biogenesis.

48. Noah JW, Anathan S, Evans C, Nebane M, Rasmussen L, et al. (2013) N-(pyridin-4-yl)benzo[d]thiazole-6-carboxamide inhibits E. coli UT189 bacterial capsule biogenesis.

49. Mulvey MA, Lopez-Boado YS, Wilson CL, Roth R, Parks WC, et al. (1998) Induction and evasion of host defenses by type 1-piliated uropathogenic Escherichia coli. Science (80-) 282: 1494–1497.

50. Roberts JA, Kaack MB, Baskin G, Marklund BI, Normark S (1997) Epitopes of the P-fimbrial adhesin of E. coli cause different urinary tract infections. J Urol 158: 1610–1613. doi:S0022-5347(01)64290-3 [pii].

51. Vimr ER, Troy FA (1985) Regulation of sialic acid metabolism in Escherichia coli: role of N-acylneuraminate pyruvate-lyase. J Bacteriol 164: 854–860.

52. Mobley HL, Jarvis KG, Elwood JP, Whittle DI, Lockatell C V, et al. (1993) Isogenic P-fimbrial deletion mutants of pyelonephritogenic Escherichia coli: the role of alpha Gal(1–4) beta Gal binding in virulence of a wild-type strain. Mol Microbiol 10: 143–155.

53. Hacker J, Bender L, Ott M, Wingender J, Lund B, et al. (1990) Deletions of chromosomal regions coding for fimbriae and hemolysins occur in vitro and in vivo in various extraintestinal Escherichia coli isolates. Microb Pathog 8: 213–225.

54. Serwer P (1974) Fast sedimenting bacteriophage T7 DNA from T7-infected Escherichia coli. Virology 59: 70–88.

55. Vimr ER, McCoy RD, Vollger HF, Wilkison NC, Troy FA (1984) Use of prokaryotic-derived probes to identify poly(sialic acid) in neonatal neuronal membranes. Proc Natl Acad Sci U S A 81: 1971–1975.

56. Gupta DS, Jann B, Schmidt G, Golecki JR, Ørskov I, et al. (1982) Coliphage K5, specific for E. coli exhibiting the capsular K5 antigen. FEMS Microbiol Lett 14: 75–78. doi:10.1111/j.1574-6968.1982.tb08638.x.

2

Preparation, Characterization, *In Vitro* Release and Degradation of Cathelicidin-BF-30-PLGA Microspheres

Lili Li[1⁹], Qifeng Wang[2⁹], Hongli Li[1], Mingwei Yuan[1], Minglong Yuan[1]*

1 Engineering Research Center of Biopolymer Functional Materials of Yunnan, Yunnan University of Nationalities, Kunming, Yunnan, China, **2** Department of Radiation Oncology, Sichuan Cancer Hospital, Chengdu, Sichuan, China

Abstract

Cathelicidin-BF-30 (BF-30), a water-soluble peptide isolated from the snake venom of Bungarus fasciatus containing 30 amino acid residues, was incorporated in poly(D,L-lactide-co-glycolide) (PLGA) 75:25 microspheres (MS) prepared by a water in oil in water W/O/W emulsification solvent extraction method. The aim of this work was to investigate the stability of BF-30 after encapsulation. D-trehalose was used as an excipient to stabilize the peptide. The MS obtained were mostly under 2 μm in size and the encapsulation efficiency was 88.50±1.29%. The secondary structure of the peptide released *in vitro* was determined to be nearly the same as the native peptide using Circular Dichroism (CD). The ability of BF-30 to inhibit the growth of Escherichia coli was also maintained. The cellular relative growth and hemolysis rates were 92.16±3.55% and 3.52±0.45% respectively.

Editor: Jie Zheng, University of Akron, United States of America

Funding: This work was supported by the National Natural Science Foundation of China (31160198, 31360417), the Applied Basic Research Key Project of Yunnan (2013FA039), the Applied Basic Research Project of Yunnan (2011FB084), the High-End Technology Professionals Introduction Plan in Yunnan province (2010CI119). The funders had role in study design, data collection and analysis, decision to publish, or preparation of the manuscript.

Competing Interests: The authors have declared that no competing interests exist.

* Email: yml@188.com

⁹ These authors contributed equally to this work.

Introduction

BF-30 is a 30-residue peptide isolated from the venom of the snake *Bungarus fasciatus*, which exhibits broad antimicrobial activity against bacteria and fungi. The peptide has strong antibacterial activity that has been identified *in vitro* against *Pseudomonas aeruginosain* in infected burns [1,2]. BF-30 has a short onset of action when acting against P. aeruginosa and the drug-resistant bacteria, S. aureus. However, the peptide has a short half-life in serum [3], which may be caused by proteases present in serum [4]. Attempts have been made to increase the stability of BF-30 by chemical modification of the peptide through pegylation to extend the half-life [5,6]. However, pegylation is a chemical modification method for increasing the stability of peptide by conjugating PEG to peptide or protein, the process may have an effect on the therapeutic effect of the peptide [3]. An alternative route to improve stability is to formulate the chemically intact peptide in a suitable carrier vehicle [3].

Microsphere (MS)-based peptide polymer conjugation has proved to be a good delivery system for the encapsulation of other similar animal-based peptides [7,8]. Hence this system was investigated as a potential method to encapsulate BF-30 for use in inhibiting the growth of bacteria. Figure 1 shows the preparation procedure of BF-30 loaded microspheres by W/O/W solvent extraction method, which containing twice emulsification and then solvent extraction by isopropanol solution.

Biomacromolecular therapeutics are a type of improved drugs that have been developed in recent years and biodegradable polymers such as polylactide have been used widely in protein and peptide delivery systems [7,8,9,10]. As most biomolecular materials are hydrophilic, the MS are made by the water/oil/water emulsification solvent extraction method. In recent years, several kinds of novel polymers have been made to be used in drug delivery systems [11]. Of these polymers, poly(D,L-lactide-co-glycolide) (PLGA) has been in use the longest and has been approved by the US FDA for medical use [12]. In addition, MS containing luteinizing hormone-releasing hormone (LH-RH) formed using PLGA have been commercialized [9].

The aim of this research is to encapsulate BF-30 in PLGA MS, allowing a steady release of the peptide, while maintaining its activity.

Materials and Methods

Materials

PLGA 75:25 with a weight average molecular mass (Mw) of 1.85×10^4 Da and a polydispersity index of 1.30 was prepared through condensation polymerization in our lab. Polyvinyl Acetate (PVA, Mw = 75,000 Da, 88% alcoholysis, biochemical reagent) was purchased from Shanghai Jingchun Reagent Company Limited (Shanghai, China). Dichloromethane and isopropanol (analytical grade) were purchased from Tianjin Damao Chemical Reagent Factory (Tianjin, China). Sodium azide, trifluoroacetic acid, disodium hydrogen phosphate, monopotassium phosphate, and sodium chloride (analytical grade) were purchased from

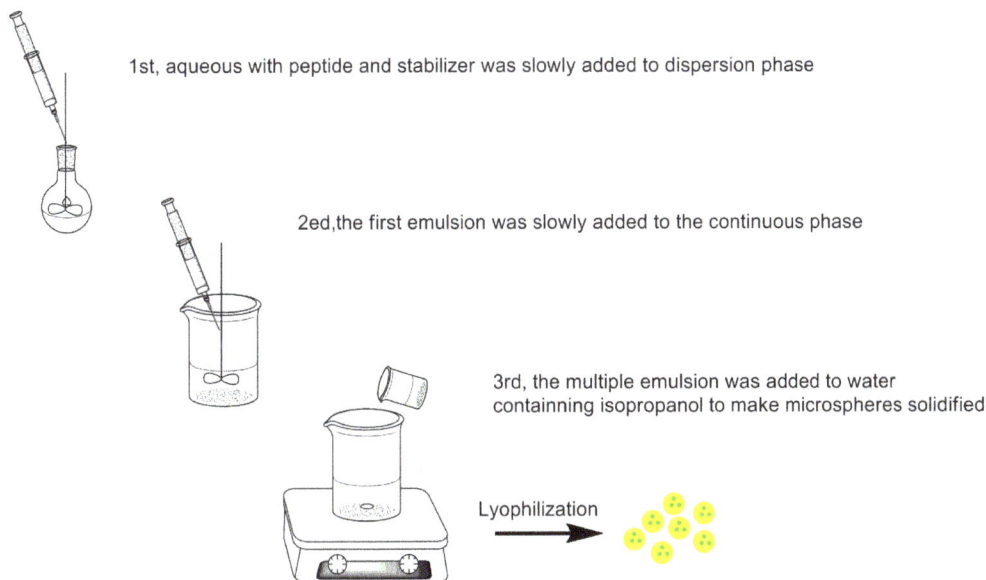

Figure 1. The process of preparing the microspheres.

Chengdu Kelon Reagent Company (Chengdu, China). Acetonitrile (HPLC grade) was from MREDA Technology Inc (US). BF-30 (KFFRKLKKSVKKRAKEFFKKPRVIGVSIPF) with a Mw of 3637.50 Da was synthesized using solid phase synthesis by GL Biochem (Shanghai, China). Male rabbit (2.0 kg) was obtained from the Laboratory Animal Unit of Kunming Medical University (Kunming, China). Animal was anesthetized with pentobarbitone sodium (200 mg/kg,i.p.). Then drew blood from rabbit pericardium to heparinized tubes. All experiments about animals performed in this study were approved by the Committee on the Use of Live Animals in Teaching and Research of Yunnan University of Nationalities.

Preparation of BF-30 loaded PLGA MS

BF-30 MS were prepared by dispersion followed by solvent extraction and evaporation according to the methods described in early articles by Ogawa and He [9,13]. Briefly, 0.50 mL BF-30 solution in water (20 mg/mL) with excipient trehalose was slowly added to a solution of 5 mL of 16% (w/v) PLGA in dichloromethane (DCM) in an ice-bath under high-speed homogenization with Tween80 as surfactant. Then, the obtained emulsion was injected into a 1% PVA solution (the continuous phase) under the conditions described above. After the second emulsion process, the double emulsion was added to a 5% isopropanol solution to solidify the MS, then the MS were obtained by centrifugation for 10 min at 5000 rpm and washed with 0.30% mannitol/water solution three times.

Surface morphology and size analysis

The surface morphology of the MS was analyzed using a JEM-100CX (HATACHI S-3000N, Japan) Scanning Electronic Microscope (SEM) and E-1010 Ion sputtering apparatus (HATACHI, Japan). Freeze-dried MS were placed on a metal stub, which was coated with conducting resin. The particle size and mean diameter distribution (polydispersity index) of the MS were measured by laser diffraction analysis using a Mastersizer 2000 (Malvern, UK). The preparation of the sample was as follows: the microparticles were dispersed in distilled water, then a dilute solution of uniformly dispersed microspheres were obtained by ultrasonic vibration. The samples were measured three times to calculate the mean diameter and polydispersity index (PDI).

Encapsulation efficiency (EE) and microspheres yield rate

High encapsulation efficiency of MS was a key index of an excellent MS delivery system, and was the ratio between the amount of peptide entrapment and peptide added in the process of preparing MS. The amount of peptide entrapment was measured by dissolving 50 mg MS in 2.00 mL DCM (n = 3), then extracting the peptide twice with 2.0 mL Phosphate Buffer Solution containing Tween (PBST) (pH 7.40, 10 mM, containing 0.02% NaN_3, 0.02% Tween80, and 150 mM NaCl) according to the method of OGAWA [9]. The concentration of peptide in the water phase was measured by HPLC, compared with a standard curve data of known concentrations of BF-30 solutions. In order to determine the amount of peptide loss during the inefficient extraction process, a certain amount (m_1) of peptide solution was added into PLGA/DCM solution with the same concentration of MS preparing process. The BF-30 concentration in extraction liquid was measured in triplicate for three different batches, and different calibration values for inefficient extraction were detected for each sample as the method of Li [14]. The yield rate is another index of a delivery system which relates to the amount of microspheres obtained. The peptide entrapment efficiency was calculated according to the equation below.

$$\text{Encapsulation Efficiency (\%)} = \frac{\text{Peptide in microspheres (mg)}}{\text{Peptide added (mg)}} \times 100\% \tag{1}$$

$$\text{Extraction Efficiency (\%)} = \frac{\text{Peptide in extraction solution(mg)}}{m_1 \text{(mg)}} \times 100\% \tag{2}$$

$$microspheres\ yield(\%)$$

$$= \frac{lypholizied\ microspheres(mg)}{peptide\ added(mg) + polymer\ added(mg)} \times 100\% \quad (3)$$

In vitro release study

The MS loaded with BF-30 were incubated in a capped centrifugal tube containing 10 mL PBST (n = 3), kept at 37 °C and shaken at 120 rpm. At predetermined intervals, the tubes were removed and the samples were centrifuged at 3000 rpm for 10 min. Supernatant (1 mL) was extracted and an equal amount of fresh PBST was added. The peptide concentration in the supernatant was determined by the method described above.

$$Q = C_n \times V_t + V_s \sum C_{n-1} \quad (4)$$

Q: cumulative release (μg)

C_n: concentration of the release medium (μg/mL) at time t

V_t:volume of the release medium, V_t = 10 mL

V_s: volume of solution obtained from the release medium for testing, V_s = 1 mL

The release profile was obtained by plotting the cumulative release rate ($Q/m_2 \times 100\%$) versus the release time.

Each experiment was repeated three times and the result is presented as the mean value of the three samples. The error bars in the plot show the standard deviation of the data.

In vitro degradation study

The in vitro degradation study was similar to the release study, except that at the predetermined intervals, the degradation medium in the tubes was removed and the degraded MS were washed with distilled water to rinse off the buffer salt.

HPLC and CD analysis

The concentration of the peptide extracted in the water phase was measured using reverse-phase HPLC (Agilent Technologies 1200 Series, Waters, xTerra, RP18, 5 μm, 4.6×250 mm column). The elution phase was A: water with 0.10% (v/v) trifluoroacetic acid and B: acetonitrile with 0.10% (v/v) trifluoroacetic acid; UV detection was at 220 nm [15]. The concentration of the acetonitrile phase was raised from 21.00% to 46.00% over 25 min using a linear gradient, and the sample size was 25 μL.

The peptide conformational change during the release period was measured on a far-UV (190–280 nm) Circular Dichroism Spectrometer Chirascan (Applied Photophysics Limited) at ambi-

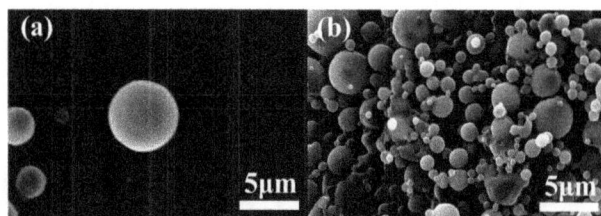

Figure 3. The size distribution histogram of the MS.

ent temperature in a quartz cell (path length 0.05 cm) [16,17] and compared with the native peptide.

In vitro cytotoxicity analysis

The in vitro cytotoxicity of the peptide-loaded PLGA MS was characterized by the MTT (3-(4,5-dimethylthiazol-2-yl)-2,5-diphe-nyltetrazolium bromide) method, inendothelial cells at a concentration of 120 μg/mL (n = 5) [18,19], under the conditions described by Shen [19]. The MTT method is based on the theory that succinate dehydrogenase in the mitochondria reduces dissolved MTT to a purple, water-insoluble formazan product in living cells, but not in dead cells. In detail, endothelial cells were grown at 37 °C under a 5% CO_2 atmosphere in RPMI-1640 medium in a 96-well plate, supplemented with 10% calf serum in a fully humidified incubator. After 24 h, the culture medium was removed, MTT was added, and the samples were incubated for another 4 h. DMSO was added to dissolve the formazan crystals, and the optical density at 570 nm was measured on Multiskan Go spectrophotometer (Thermo, USA) with PBST as negative control. Each sample was prepared in triplicate. The cellular relative growth rate (RGR) indicating the ratio of living cells during the test was calculated according to the following equation:

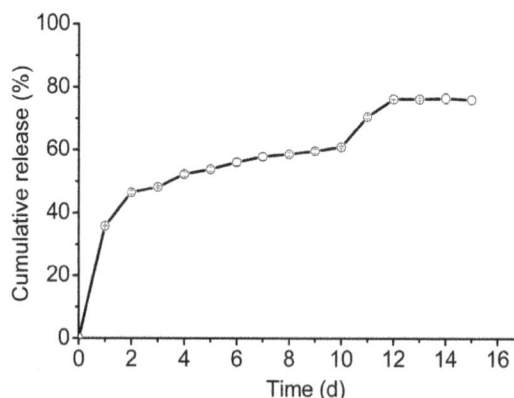

Figure 2. Morphology of peptide-loaded PLGA MS. (a) High magnification, (b) low magnification.

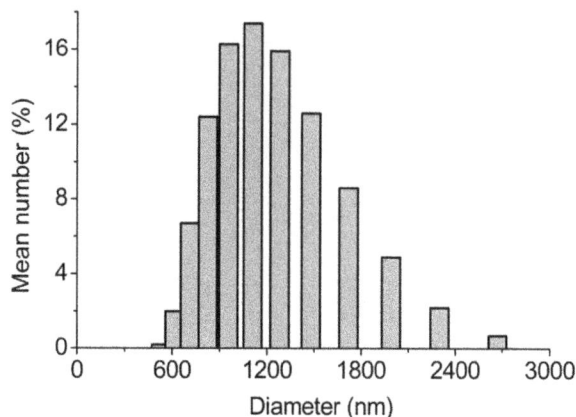

Figure 4. The release profile of the MS in PBST (pH = 7.40).

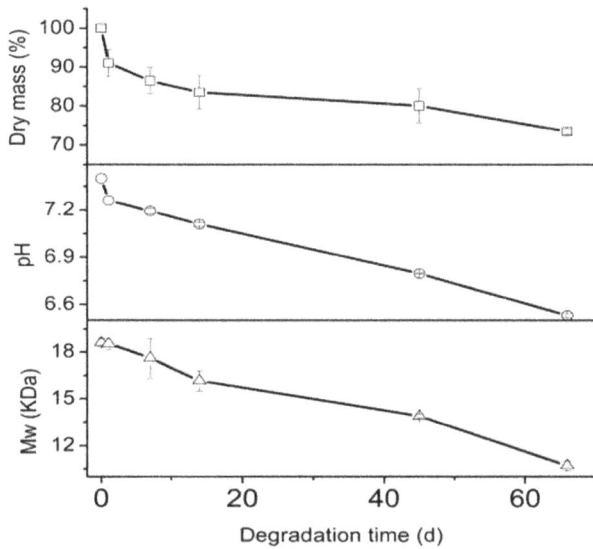

Figure 5. The degradation profiles of MS in PBST (pH = 7.40): pH, Mw, and dry mass – release time profiles.

$$RGR(\%) = \frac{Abs_{samples}}{Abs_{negative\ control}} \times 100\% \qquad (5)$$

In vitro hemolysis test

A hemolysis test was carried out to measure the ability of the biomaterial to destroy red blood cells when contacted with blood. The rate was quantified by measuring the suspension absorbance at 541 nm, which was consistent with the ferrohemoglobin released by destroyed red cells [20]. The hemolysis activity of BF-30-loaded PLGA MS was tested according to the method of Shen [19]. The hemolysis was quantified spectrophotometrically according to the method of Shen [19]and Fischer [16]. Blood obtained from rabbit pericardium was collected in heparinized tubes (n = 3), then centrifuged at 1500 rpm for 10 min on Eppendorf centrifuges (Germany, 5417R) to acquire rabbit red blood cells (RRBCs). Discarding the serum above by suction, the RRBCs were found deep in the centrifuge tube. Suspensions of the red blood cells were obtained by washing the RRBCs with a sterile physiological saline solution until the absorbance value of the positive control supernatant was located in the range 0.5–0.6 at 541 nm.

The hemolysis rate was calculated according to the following equation:

$$Hemolysis\ rate(\%) = \frac{Abs_{material} - Abs_{negative\ control}}{Abs_{positive\ control} - Abs_{negative\ control}} \times 100\% \quad (6)$$

The sterile physiological saline solution and distilled water were the negative and positive controls respectively, and the corresponding hemolysis rates were 0% and 100% respectively.

Biological activity

The ability of the released peptide to inhibit the growth of *Escherichia coli* was investigated according to the method of Kim

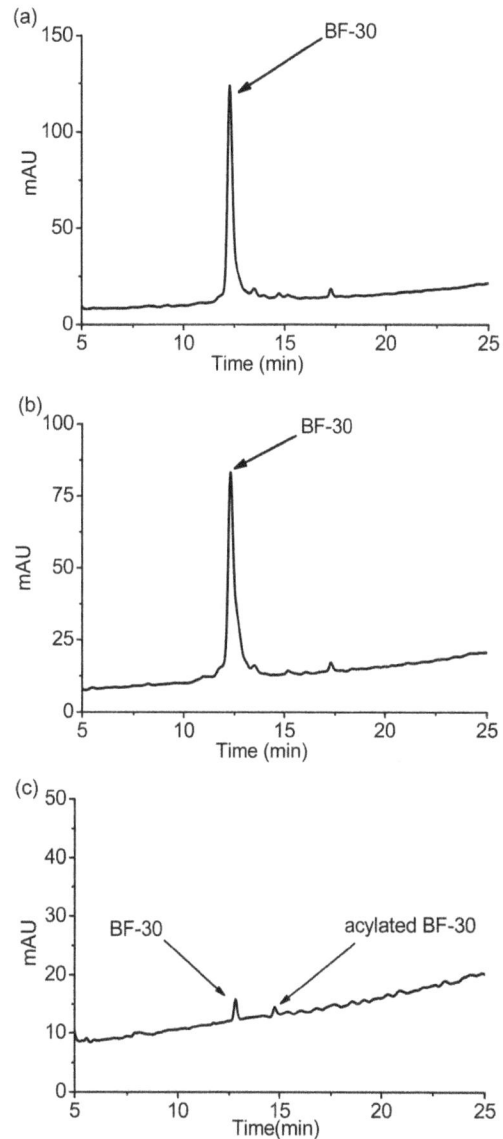

Figure 6. The elution curves of (a) the native BF-30 and (b) the peptide released on the 11th day, (c) the peptide released on the 10th day.

[21]. The freeze-dried *Escherichia coli*, purchased from Guangdong Huankai Microbial SCI & Tech. Co. Ltd. (Cat. No. FSCC 149005, Lot. No. A0144B), were reconstituted in a brain-heart infusion broth. The bacterial solution was diluted to between 0.10 and 0.20 at OD625, an absorbance of half the McFarland standard. The absorbance value at 625 nm of the bacteria solution is proportional to the concentration of the bacteria in the solution [21]. Diluted bacterial solution (0.10 mL) was added to 96-well plates with 0.10 mL of the released peptide solution (n = 3), then incubated on a shaker at a constant temperature of 37°C and a rotation speed of 80 rpm. The absorbances at 625 nm were measured after 5 and 24 h. The percentage of bacterial inhibition was calculated according to the absorbance difference between the bacteria solution with and without the peptide after 5 and 24 h incubation using the equation:

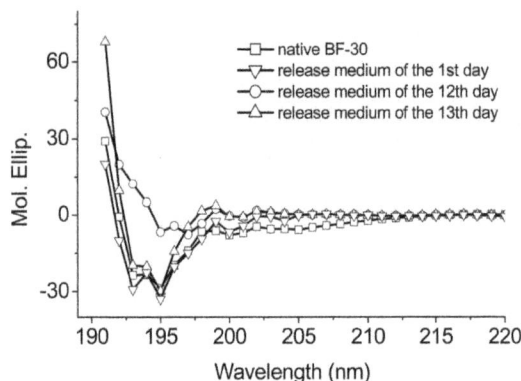

Figure 7. The CD spectra of the peptide released from the MS at different times compared with the native BF-30.

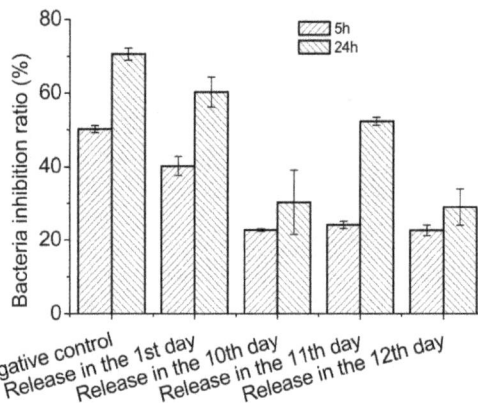

Figure 8. Antimicrobial activity against Escherichia coli of the native BF-30 and the peptide released from the microspheres on the 1st, 10th, 11th, and 12th days.

$$\text{Bacterial inhibition rate}(\%) = \frac{\text{Absc} - \text{Abss}}{\text{Absc}} \times 100\% \quad (7)$$

A_{bsc} and A_{bss} stand for the absorbance at 625 nm of the control group solution and the release medium with peptide, respectively.

Results and Discussion

Morphology characterization

Microspheres prepared by the W/O/W emulsion/solvent evaporation/extraction method with a high yield of $76.64 \pm 8.07\%$ according to the equation (3). SEM was used to investigate the morphology of the microspheres. Figure 2 shows the SEM images of lyophilized PLGA MS; most of the MS had spherical and smooth surfaces, but a few MS appeared pitted. As seen in Figure 2 (b), PLGA (75:25) had little nonmicrosphere-forming ratio.

The MS size and size distribution were studied in a microsphere–water solution using Mastersizer 2000. As shown in Figure 3, the size of all microspheres obtained ranged from 500 to 3000 nm, with a mean diameter of 1460 ± 14.02 nm. The majority of MS had a mean diameter between 800 and 1500 nm, in the submicro range [22], and a PDI of 0.24, which was<0.30. This means a narrow size distribution.MS with a diameter under 50 μm contribute to a steady release rate and decrease the burst release, thus the release kinetics would be close to a zero-order release mode [23,24].

Encapsulation and in vitro release of BF-30 loaded PLGA MS

In our study, the concentration of the peptide had a liner range of 55.50 to 333 μg/mL, as measured by HPLC according to the standard curve equation: $y = 4.88x - 74.80$, $R^2 = 0.9991$; where y is the peak area and x is the concentration of the peptide (μg/mL). The encapsulation efficiency indicates the ratio of the actual amount of peptide encapsulated in the MS. In this study, the encapsulation efficiency was $88.50 \pm 1.29\%$, which was the calibration value according to inefficient extraction ratio $62.66 \pm 0.86\%$. Figure 4 shows the release profile of the BF-30 loaded PLGA MS. The release profile indicated the burst release was nearly 40% over the first release day, which may relate to peptide adsorbed on the surface of the MS [25,26]. The peptide entrapped in the MS was released gradually with the degradation

of polymer. The release process of the peptide containing three phases: the first burst release, lag and the second burst release. The second burst release often due to the erosion of polymer matrix [27]. At the end, $76.60 \pm 1.70\%$ of the peptide encapsulated in the MS had been released.

In vitro degradation and erosion of PLGA MS

Figure 5 shows a continued degradation of PLGA MS over 60 days with a significant drop in the pH value of the release medium and the dry mass (%). MS dry mass and Mw decreased during the first few degradation days were apparent, dry mass loss from 100% to 91% in the first day, the Mw of the BF-30 loaded microspheres dropped visibly from 18.50 to 17.60 KDa, which indicated that MS had undergone apparent degradation. As a result of acidic degradation products of PLGA-(lactic acid and glycolic acid) monomers and oligomers [24], pH value of the degradation medium dropped from 7.40 to 7.26, followed by a slower degradation process over the remaining 60 days.

HPLC and CD analysis

As shown in Figure 6, the HPLC elution curve of the peptide released on the 11th day(b) is similar to the native peptide(a), with the same retention time of 12.30 min. Curve (c) represents the peptide released in the 10th day, which containing two peaks, peptide and acylated peptide. The HPLC results indicated that the peptide released on the 11th day has the same polarity as the native peptide, but produced some acylated peptide on the 10th day [28].

PLGA degraded to acidic compounds, including lactic and glycolic acids over time, which resulted in the observed decrease in the pH value of the degradation medium. Peptide would precipitate and assemble when the pH value of the medium is close to the isoelectric point. Fortunately, the isoelectric point of 11.79 for BF-30 is far above the observed pH value of the degradation medium. Thus the peptide in the MS would not precipitate and assemble and so most peptide encapsulated would be released [29]. Furthermore, Figure 7 shows that the far-UV CD spectrum of the peptide in the release medium of the 1st day and of the later period of the release process, the 12th and 13th days, matching that of the native peptide. This demonstrates that the released BF-30 retains its α-helical secondary structure [30], indicating that the structure of BF-30 has not changed during the release process.

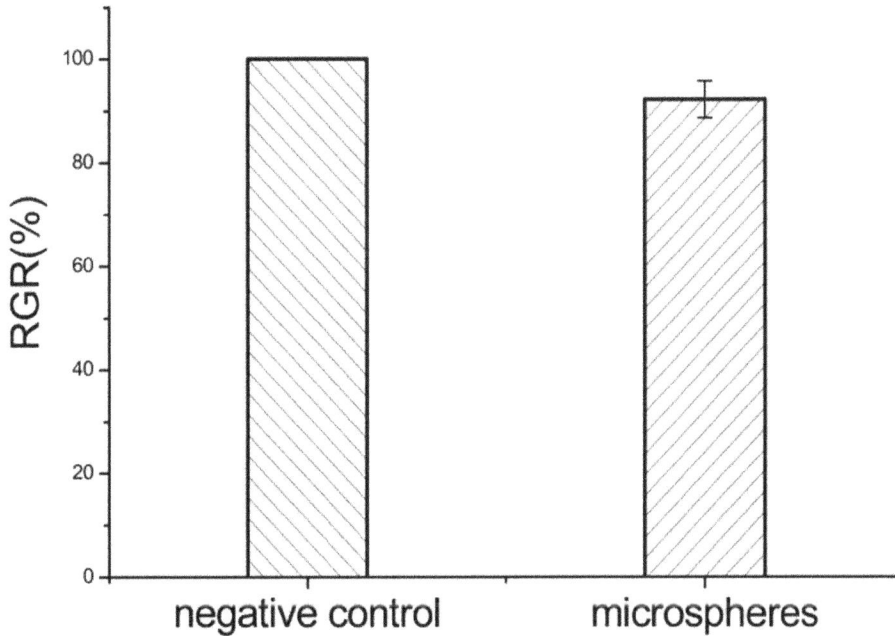

Figure 9. Cytotoxicity of the MS. PBST was used as the negative control.

Antimicrobial activity of the released peptide

To test the biological effect of the released peptide, we investigated the activity of release medium on the 1st, 10th, 11th, and 12th days against *Escherichia coli*, which is sensitive to BF-30 [1,2]. As shown in Figure 8, the released medium of the 1st, 10th, 11th and 12th days were efficient in inhibiting the growth of *Escherichia coli*. The inhibition ratios and the peptide concentrations were 35.84±0.15%, 63.93±0.32%, 70.60±0.57%, 76.32±0.03%, and 25.50±0.34, 17.91±0.20, 19.70±0.10, 19.47±0.10 μg/mL on days 1, 10, 11, and 12 respectively, while the concentration of native peptide for antimicrobial test was 35 μg/mL. The inhibition ratio of the native peptide was higher than the 1st, 10th, 11th, 12th days in all, and the 10th day was lower than the 11th and the 12th day; this may be caused by a lower peptide concentration in the 10th day, the acylated peptide, and the degradation of the MS, which makes the system unstable. We can see from Figure 6 that the 10th day containing acylated

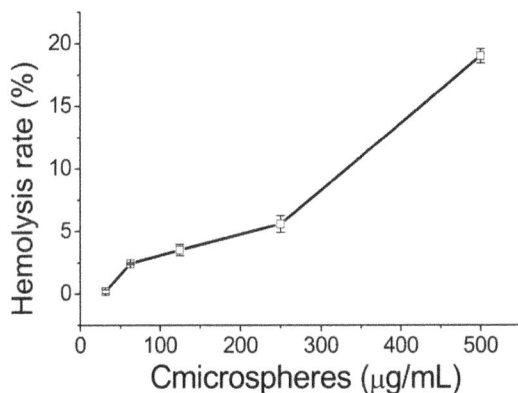

Figure 10. The hemolysis rate of BF-30-loaded PLGA MS at different concentrations.

peptide with lower concentration, and the 11th day containing unbroken peptide compared with native peptide HPLC curves, but a little change in the 12th day according to Figure 7. We can see from Figure 4 that the 11th and the 12th day were during the second burst release process. The peptide concentration in the release medium and the inhibition ratio on the 11th day were higher than on the 10th and 12th days. Also, peptide in release medium of the 1st day maintained its bioactivity according to Figure 8. The ability of the release medium to inhibit the growth of *Escherichia* was apparent after 24 h incubation with dilute bacteria solution. This means that the peptide has retained its bioactivity during the release period and the PLGA MS delivery system has the potential to protect the fragile peptide from adverse conditions.

In vitro cytotoxicity analysis

A concentration of 120 μg/mL was used for cytotoxicity testing based on the amount of peptide encapsulated in the microspheres and the minimal inhibitory concentration (MIC) of 0.15 μg/mL for *Escherichia coli* [1].

After 48 h, the water-insoluble formazan formed by MTT in living cells was dissolved in dimethyl sulfoxide and the absorbance value of the samples at 570 nm was measured by absorbance spectroscopy on a Multiskan Go spectrophotometer (Thermo, USA). Figure 9 shows the results of the MTT assay, using PBST as the negative control. The BF-30-loaded microspheres showed 92.16±3.55% RGR, which indicated that no toxicity occurred at the concentration tested (120 μg/mL).

In vitro hemolysis

Figure 10 shows the hemolysis level of microspheres at different concentrations. The OD value of the negative control, corresponding to 0% hemolysis, was 0.04±0.0003 and the value for the positive control, corresponding to 100% hemolysis, was 0.39±0.005. The hemolysis rate was 3.52±0.45%, which was lower than the ISO criterion of 5% [13], when the concentration of the microspheres was 125 μg/mL. These results indicate that the BF-30-loaded PLGA microspheres are safe when in contact with blood at the efficient concentration of 125 µg/mL.

Conclusions

The antimicrobial peptide BF-30 of animal origin, which has antimicrobial activity, has been encapsulated into PLGA microspheres by the W/O/W double emulsion method with high encapsulation efficiency. The surface morphology of the MS was found to be spherical with a narrow size distribution. The delivery system released peptide over more than 15 days. The peptide retained its α-helix secondary structure during the release period. The BF-30 peptide released from the microspheres was found to be effective in inhibiting the growth of *Escherichia coli*, which means

that the PLGA microsphere delivery system protected the peptide in terms of both structural stability and antimicrobial activity. In addition, the cytotoxicity and biocompatibility of the MS system was found to be within acceptable limits. In summary, the BF-30-PLGA microspheres hold great potential for use as an antimicrobial agent and the system may be useful for encapsulating other sensitive peptide-based drugs.

Author Contributions

Performed the experiments: LLL QFW. Contributed to the writing of the manuscript: LLL MLY. Revised the manuscript: HLL. Assisted to prepare the polymer material PLGA: MWY.

References

1. Wang Y, Hong J, Liu X, Yang H, Liu R, et al. (2008) Snake cathelicidin from Bungarus fasciatus is a potent peptide antibiotics. PLoS ONE 3: e3217.
2. Zhou H, Dou J, Wang J, Chen L, Wang H, et al. (2011) The antibacterial activity of BF-30 *in vitro* and in infected burned rats is through interference with cytoplasmic membrane integrity. Peptides 32: 1131–1138.
3. Zetterberg MM, Reijmar K, Pränting M, Engström Å, Andersson DI, et al. (2011) PEG-stabilized lipid disks as carriers for amphiphilic antimicrobial peptides. Journal of Controlled Release 156: 323–328.
4. Hamamoto K, Kida Y, Zhang Y, Shimizu T, Kuwano K (2002) Antimicrobial activity and stability to proteolysis of small linear cationic peptides with D-amino acid substitutions. Microbiology and immunology 46: 741–749.
5. Kim TH, Lee H, Park TG (2002) Pegylated recombinant human epidermal growth factor (rhEGF) for sustained release from biodegradable PLGA microspheres. Biomaterials 23: 2311–2317.
6. Monkarsh SP, Ma Y, Aglione A, Bailon P, Ciolek D, et al. (1997) Positional isomers of monopegylated interferon α-2a: Isolation, characterization, and biological activity. Analytical biochemistry 247: 434–440.
7. Fude C, Dongmei C, Anjin T, Mingshi Y, Kai S, et al. (2005) Preparation and characterization of melittin-loaded poly (dl-lactic acid) or poly (dl-lactic-co-glycolic acid) microspheres made by the double emulsion method. Journal of Controlled Release 107: 310–319.
8. Trindade RA, Kiyohara PK, de Araujo PS, Bueno da Costa MH (2012) PLGA microspheres containing bee venom proteins for preventive immunotherapy. International Journal of Pharmaceutics 423: 124–133.
9. Ogawa Y, Yamamoto M, Okada H, Yashiki T, Shimamoto T (1988) A new technique to efficiently entrap leuprolide acetate into microcapsules of polylactic acid or copoly (lactic/glycolic) acid. Chemical & pharmaceutical bulletin 36: 1095–1103.
10. Yeh M-K, Coombes A, Jenkins P, Davis S (1995) A novel emulsification-solvent extraction technique for production of protein loaded biodegradable microparticles for vaccine and drug delivery. Journal of Controlled Release 33: 437–445.
11. Sun H, Meng F, Dias AA, Hendriks M, Feijen J, et al. (2011) α-Amino acid containing degradable polymers as functional biomaterials: rational design, synthetic pathway, and biomedical applications. Biomacromolecules 12: 1937–1955.
12. Jain RA (2000) The manufacturing techniques of various drug loaded biodegradable poly(lactide-co-glycolide) (PLGA) devices. Biomaterials 21: 2475–2490.
13. He Z, Xiong L (2011) Drug Controlled Release and Biological Behavior of Poly(D,L-Lactide-Co-Glycolide) Microspheres. Journal of Macromolecular Science, Part B 50: 1154–1161.
14. Li X-h, Z Y-h (2000) Influence of process parameters on the protein stability encapsulated in poly-D,L-lactide–poly(ethylene glycol)microspheres. Journal of Controlled Release 68: 41–52.
15. Kostanski JW, Thanoo B, DeLuca PP (2000) Preparation, characterization, and *in vitro* evaluation of 1-and 4-month controlled release orntide PLA and PLGA microspheres. Pharmaceutical development and technology 5: 585–596.
16. Fischer D, Li Y, Ahlemeyer B, Krieglstein J, Kissel T (2003) *In vitro* cytotoxicity testing of polycations: influence of polymer structure on cell viability and hemolysis. Biomaterials 24: 1121–1131.

17. Wei Y, Wang Y-X, Wang W, Ho SV, Wei W, et al. (2011) mPEG-PLA microspheres with narrow size distribution increase the controlled release effect of recombinant human growth hormone. Journal of Materials Chemistry 21: 12691–12699.
18. Pan H, Soman NR, Schlesinger PH, Lanza GM, Wickline SA (2011) Cytolytic peptide nanoparticles ('NanoBees') for cancer therapy. Wiley Interdisciplinary Reviews: Nanomedicine and Nanobiotechnology 3: 318–327.
19. Shen J-M, Guan X-M, Liu X-Y, Lan J-F, Cheng T, et al. (2012) Luminescent/magnetic hybrid nanoparticles with folate-conjugated peptide composites for tumor-targeted drug delivery. Bioconjugate Chemistry 23: 1010–1021.
20. Zhang Z, Mao J, Feng X, Xiao J, Qiu J (2008) *In vitro* cytotoxicity of polyphosphoester as a novel injectable alveolar replacement material. Journal of Huazhong University of Science and Technology (Medical Sciences) 28: 604–607.
21. Kim K, Luu YK, Chang C, Fang D, Hsiao BS, et al. (2004) Incorporation and controlled release of a hydrophilic antibiotic using poly(lactide-co-glycolide)-based electrospun nanofibrous scaffolds. Journal of Controlled Release 98: 47–56.
22. Das TK (2012) Protein particulate detection issues in biotherapeutics development—Current status. AAPS PharmSciTech 13: 732–746.
23. Montalvo-Ortiz BL, Sosa B, Griebenow K (2012) Improved Enzyme Activity and Stability in Polymer Microspheres by Encapsulation of Protein Nanospheres. AAPS PharmSciTech: 1–5.
24. Panyam J, Dali MM, Sahoo SK, Ma W, Chakravarthi SS, et al. (2003) Polymer degradation and *in vitro* release of a model protein from poly(d,l-lactide-co-glycolide) nano- and microparticles. Journal of Controlled Release 92: 173–187.
25. Regnier-Delplace C, Thillaye du Boullay O, Siepmann F, Martin-Vaca B, Demonchaux P, et al. (2013) PLGAs bearing carboxylated side chains: Novel matrix formers with improved properties for controlled drug delivery. Journal of Controlled Release 166: 256–267.
26. Magenheim B, Levy MY, Benita S (1993) A new *in vitro* technique for the evaluation of drug release profile fromcolloidal carriers-ultrafiltration technique at low pressure. International Journal of Pharmaceutics. 94: 115–123.
27. Mohamed F, van der Walle CF (2008) Engineering Biodegradable Polyester Particles With Specific Drug Targeting and Drug Release Properties. Journal of pharmaceutical sciences. 97: 71–87.
28. Ghassemi AH, van Steenbergen MJ, Barendregt A, Talsma H, Kok RJ, et al. (2012) Controlled Release of Octreotide and Assessment of Peptide Acylation from Poly(D,L-lactide-co-hydroxymethyl glycolide) Compared to PLGA Microspheres. Pharmaceutical Research. 29: 110–120.
29. Crotts G, Park TG (1998) Protein delivery from poly (lactic-co-glycolic acid) biodegradable microspheres: release kinetics and stability issues. Journal of microencapsulation 15: 699–713.
30. Samadi N, van Nostrum C, Vermonden T, Amidi M, Hennink W (2013) Mechanistic Studies on the Degradation and Protein Release Characteristics of Poly (lactic-co-glycolic-co-hydroxymethylglycolic acid) Nanospheres. Biomacromolecules 14: 1044–1053.

3

Pharmacokinetics of Natural and Engineered Secreted Factors Delivered by Mesenchymal Stromal Cells

Jessica S. Elman[1,9], Ryan M. Murray[1,9], Fangjing Wang[1,9], Keyue Shen[1], Shan Gao[1], Kevin E. Conway[4], Martin L. Yarmush[1,2], Bakhos A. Tannous[4], Ralph Weissleder[3], Biju Parekkadan[1,5]*

1 Department of Surgery, Center for Engineering in Medicine and Surgical Services, Massachusetts General Hospital, Harvard Medical School and the Shriners Hospital for Children, Boston, Massachusetts, United States of America, **2** Department of Biomedical Engineering, Rutgers University, Piscataway, New Jersey, United States of America, **3** Center for Systems Biology, Massachusetts General Hospital, Harvard Medical School, Boston, Massachusetts, United States of America, **4** Department of Neurology, Experimental Therapeutics and Molecular Imaging Laboratory, Massachusetts General Hospital, Charlestown, Massachusetts, United States of America, **5** Harvard Stem Cell Institute, Boston, Massachusetts, United States of America

Abstract

Transient cell therapy is an emerging drug class that requires new approaches for pharmacological monitoring during use. Human mesenchymal stem cells (MSCs) are a clinically-tested transient cell therapeutic that naturally secrete anti-inflammatory factors to attenuate immune-mediated diseases. MSCs were used as a proof-of-concept with the hypothesis that measuring the release of secreted factors after cell transplantation, rather than the biodistribution of the cells alone, would be an alternative monitoring tool to understand the exposure of a subject to MSCs. By comparing cellular engraftment and the associated serum concentration of secreted factors released from the graft, we observed clear differences between the pharmacokinetics of MSCs and their secreted factors. Exploration of the effects of natural or engineered secreted proteins, active cellular secretion pathways, and clearance mechanisms revealed novel aspects that affect the systemic exposure of the host to secreted factors from a cellular therapeutic. We assert that a combined consideration of cell delivery strategies and molecular pharmacokinetics can provide a more predictive model for outcomes of MSC transplantation and potentially other transient cell therapeutics.

Editor: Eva Mezey, National Institutes of Health, United States of America

Funding: This work was supported of the National Institutes of Health (R01EB012521 and K01DK087770) and the Broad Medical Research Program of The Broad Foundation (BMRP498382) and Shriners Hospitals for Children. The funders had no role in study design, data collection and analysis, decision to publish, or preparation of the manuscript.

Competing Interests: The authors have declared that no competing interests exist.

* E-mail: biju_parekkadan@hms.harvard.edu

❾ These authors contributed equally to this work.

Introduction

Cell therapy is an exponentially growing field with >2,500 clinical trials in the world over the last 10 years [1]. Cell-based therapeutic products are positioned as a billion dollar per year industry with anticipated market growth [2,3]. The method of using cells as drugs is particularly advantageous when a higher-order approach to treatment is required. A fundamental issue, particularly for transient cell therapies which are the largest of the drug class (50%), is the lack of predictive measures of the body's response to the therapy and vice versa: traditionally known as a drug's pharmacokinetics (PK) and pharmacodynamics (PD). Without a rigorous PK/PD model of the mechanism of action of transient cell therapies, processes cannot be optimized to formulate a drug and physicians will be unable to effectively monitor and communicate the benefits and risks of a cell therapy to a patient.

Mesenchymal stem cells (MSCs) - an adult multipotent progenitor cell population initially derived from bone marrow [4] – have over a decade of clinical testing in thousands of patients worldwide. These cells have appealing manufacturing properties such as the ease of isolation, expansion, and cryopreservation, as well as the tolerability of allogeneic cell therapy. MSCs are widely being evaluated for the combinatorial treatment of a variety of diseases including myocardial infarction [5,6], bone marrow transplantation [7], stroke [8], autoimmune disease [9], and wound healing [10,11,12,13]. The predominant use of MSCs as an immunomodulatory agent is substantiated by the observation that MSCs can inhibit the activation and effector function of numerous immune cell types [14,15,16,17]. The mechanism of action of immune cell inhibition by MSCs is primarily due to the release of secreted factors by cells [18]. MSCs have proven effective in early stage clinical trials [19], yet, several Phase II and Phase III industry-led trials either have undergone early termination or have failed to meet primary endpoints [20]. New strategies to optimize this therapeutic are needed to help usher this promising cell population to the clinic.

A deep understanding of MSC pharmacology can provide insight on how to best deliver this therapeutic. A prevailing view of MSC trafficking is that, upon intravenous administration, cell homing, engraftment, proliferation, and/or differentiation are critical to induce a therapeutic effect. Sensitive monitoring techniques have demonstrated little, if any, long-term engraftment (>1 week) of MSCs upon systemic administration with the majority of administered MSCs (>90%) accumulating immediately in the lungs and then cleared with a half-life of 24 h [21,22,23]. Therefore, MSCs can be viewed conceptually as a transient cell therapy that delivers a "payload" of secreted factors to alter acute disease progression [20].

We put the concept of MSCs as a therapeutic delivery vehicle to the test with a focus on evaluating the systemic release of secreted factors. Investigators have studied the release of natural secreted proteins such as TSG-6 [22] and TRAIL [24] or engineered antibodies [25] from MSCs in the systemic circulation after transplantation, although a thorough pharmacological analysis was not performed nor compared to purified proteins. In this study, conventional cell biodistribution data was combined with serum profiles of natural or engineered secreted factors released by the cells to understand rate-limiting processes that alter exposure to intravenous MSC therapy, the most widely used administration method. Based on our combined PK analysis, we observed that molecular monitoring of serum secreted factors revealed interesting phenomena regarding the delivery of natural or engineered proteins, an active cell secretion mechanism, and the host immune response to the graft. This study can aid in designing an optimal cell delivery regimen to maximize MSC therapy.

Results

Comparison between the Bioavailability of Transplanted MSCs and Secreted Molecules

Secreted factors released by MSCs after transplantation have been a general phenomena that has been observed in several preclinical therapeutic studies [22,26]. It is reported that MSCs can secrete a wide range of cytokines and growth factors [18]. We designed a pharmacokinetic study to monitor both the viability and distribution of MSC transplants and overlay the serum profiles of a specific and detectable level of interleukin (IL)-6, a pleiotropic molecule secreted by MSCs [27]. Human MSCs were engineered with a luciferase reporter gene, injected via intravenous (IV) route (the convention used by the cell therapy community) and detected after injection using whole-body, bioluminescent imaging (BLI). By nearly 8 hours after IV cell injection the BLI signal was almost undetectable (**Figure 1A**). At the same imaging time points, using human MSCs that were not engineered, we also measured the serum levels of human IL-6. We observed that the release of human IL-6 by MSCs was short-lived and tracked accordingly to the cellular BLI signal of the graft (**Figure 1C**). Similar pharmacokinetics of two other protein secreted factors, monocyte chemoattrive protein (MCP)-1 and IL-8, were observed after IV injection in vivo further supporting our observation (**Figure S2A–B**). Future experiments continued to explore and evaluate the impact of these pharmacokinetic profiles, with a focus on molecular delivery of IL-6 by IV administration.

Cell Delivery of IL-6 Achieves Greater Exposure than Molecular Delivery of IL-6

Cells can be considered a "carrier" for their secreted factors. We used this perspective to understand the differences of delivering IL-6 in a purified form compared to a cell transplant. Conditioned medium from MSCs (referred to as MSC-CM) was generated in order to compare MSC-derived IL-6 without concerns of post-translational modifications that take place in other protein expression systems for recombinant forms of IL-6 that may affect bioavailability. Concentrated MSC-CM was prepared and a volume of 400 μL (containing 40 ng IL-6) was injected into mice. The content of soluble factors in this volume is equivalent to the secreted levels when 3×10^6 cells are cultured for

2 days in vitro and was normalized to 1×10^6 cells for comparison to cell transplants at the same cell dose. MSC-CM was administered by IV and the serum levels of IL-6 followed a classical bolus pharmacokinetic profile (**Figure 2A**). Pharmacokinetic parameters for serum IL-6 levels were calculated with the assumption that the clearance of IL-6 itself was a constant 218 ml/hr based on the literature [28]. The maximum serum IL-6 concentration was increased by ~400% when delivered by cell transplants (**Figure 2B**). This amounted to a greater than 7-fold increase in the exposure of the subject to IL-6 as measured by area under the curve (AUC) analysis (**Figure 2C**). The temporal kinetics of IL-6 was also artificially extended by way of cell transplantation. The time to reach maximum serum concentration, the half-life, and the elimination constant of IL-6 were all significantly modified for prolonged duration of IL-6 by the use of cell transplantation (**Figure 2D–F**). These data highlight the supplementary changes to molecular pharmacokinetic parameters by way of cellular delivery.

MSCs Utilize an Active, Golgi-Dependent Secretion Mechnaism to Release IL-6 *In Vivo*

The presence of human IL-6 in serum after cell transplantation could be due to passive mechanisms, such as cell rupture and cytokine release, or by active secretion pathways. Brefeldin A (BFA), a protein-transport inhibitor, was used to block IL-6 production by inhibiting Golgi apparatus-dependent vesicle secretion. A non-toxic concentration of 5 ug/ml BFA was chosen by evaluating a dose response of BFA to MSCs in vitro (**Figure 3A**). After incubating MSCs with BFA for one day, the in vitro secretion of IL-6 in the supernatant was significantly inhibited compared to the untreated controls (**Figure 3B**). The secretion of IL-6 was not restored after a day of incubation with BFA until 72 hrs later (**Figure 3B**). We were satisfied with blockade of IL-6 for >60 hours in vitro and advanced this cell formulation with impaired IL-6 secretion for in vivo PK studies. The PK profile of MSC-derived IL-6 was dramatically different, specifically a reduced maximal effective concentration (~5×) and AUC (~1000×) compared to the cells that were not treated with BFA (**Figure 3C–D**). This study highlights a powerful active mechanism that MSCs employ to deliver IL-6 to the bloodstream that requires the Golgi apparatus.

Exposure of MSC-derived IL-6 is a Function of Host Immune Cells

To study the natural process of protein release from non-engineered cells, we designed our PK model using human cell transplants in mice. This model afforded us the ability to detect human proteins in mouse serum with high specificity and sensitivity and correlate that to *in situ* cellular production. We were also interested in studying the immune response, albeit a xenogenic rejection response, and its ability to alter in vivo protein release. We transplanted human MSCs by IV administration in mice strains that are immunocompetent (C57Bl/6), less immunocompetent (Foxn1 −/−, thymic and peripheral loss of T cells), or severely immunodeficient (NOD-SCID-IL-2rg −/−, loss of B, T, and NK cells). The effect of the immune response on MSC-derived IL-6 serum kinetics was pronounced after IV administration. NOD-SCID-IL-2rg −/− mice treated with human MSCs had a delayed maximum effective concentration and a longer half-life of serum IL-6 than the same data gathered from Foxn1 −/−, or C57Bl/6 (**Figure 4A**). The exposure of the subject to MSC-derived IL-6 was quantifiably different amongst recipients (**Figure 4B**), suggesting that molecular monitoring of cell therapy

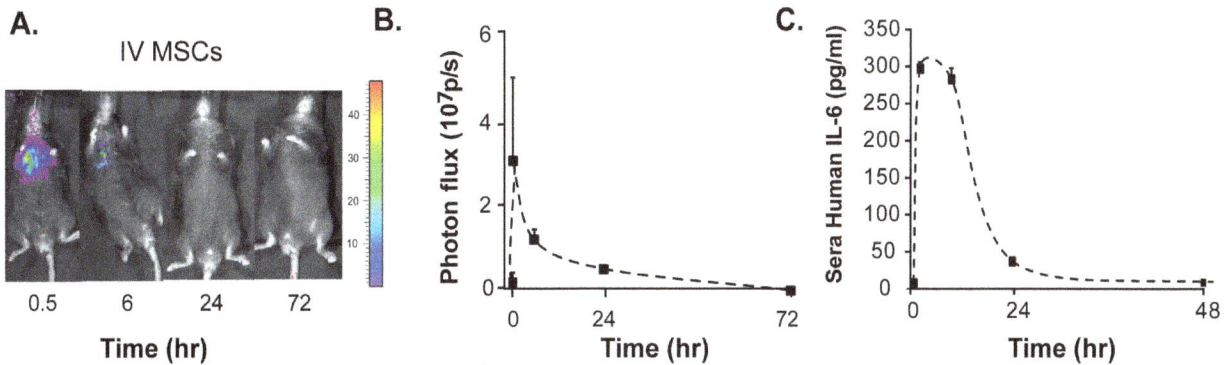

Figure 1. Combined pharmacokinetic monitoring of MSCs and MSC-secreted IL-6. (A) Bioluminescent images of C57Bl/6 mice over a period of three days after IV cell administration of one million luciferase-engineered human MSCs. (B) Photon flux of bioluminescent signal over time after IV cell administration. Durable BLI signals were detected up to 24 hours in mice that were injected IV with MSCs. (C) Serum ELISA measurements of human IL-6 released by IV cell transplants over time. Time points for serum and imaging analyses were 0.5, 8, 24, and 72 hours after cell injection. Pooled mouse serum was serially analyzed as batches of N = 5.

can distinguish clearance mechanisms of the MSC transplant and/or secreted factors, in particular a form of immune clearance.

Enhanced Systemic Exposure of Secreted Factors by Engineered MSCs

MSC-derived IL-6 is a natural and highly expressed secreted factor that enabled our molecular monitoring approach, however

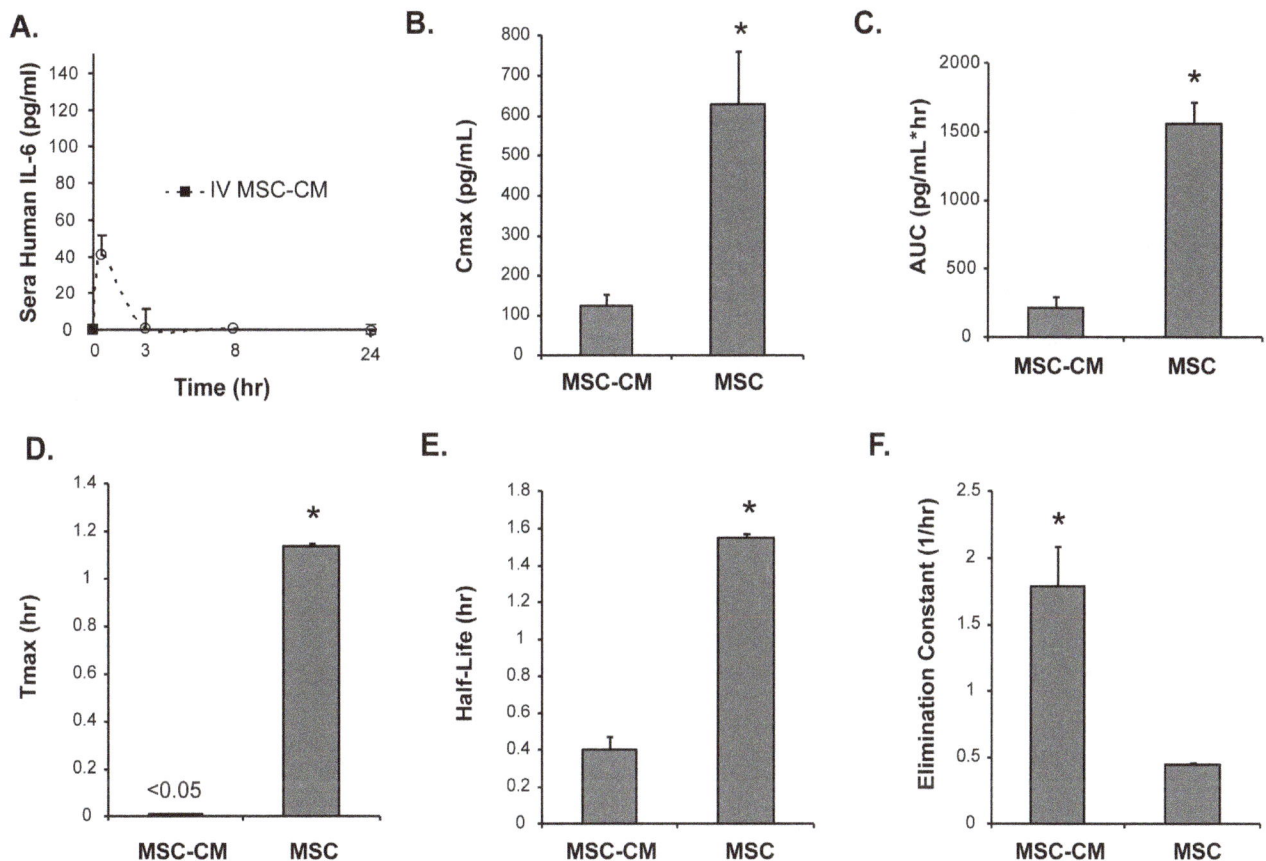

Figure 2. Enhanced delivery of IL-6 by MSC transplants compared to MSC conditioned medium. (A) Serum profiles of human IL-6 after IV administration of concentrated conditioned medium into C57Bl/6 mice. The plot was normalized to the dose of conditioned medium that was contributed by 1×10^6 cells. Pharmacokinetic parameters (B) Cmax, (C) AUC, (D) Tmax, (E) Half-life, and (F) Elimination constant were calculated for IL-6 exposure by cell transplants compared to CM administration. Significant differences between cell transplants compared to CM whereby higher levels of IL-6 and longer artificial duration was observed in plasma after cell transplantation. Time points for serum analyses were 0.5, 8, and 24 hours after cell or media injection. Mice were serially analyzed as batches of N = 5 per group. * denotes P>0.01.

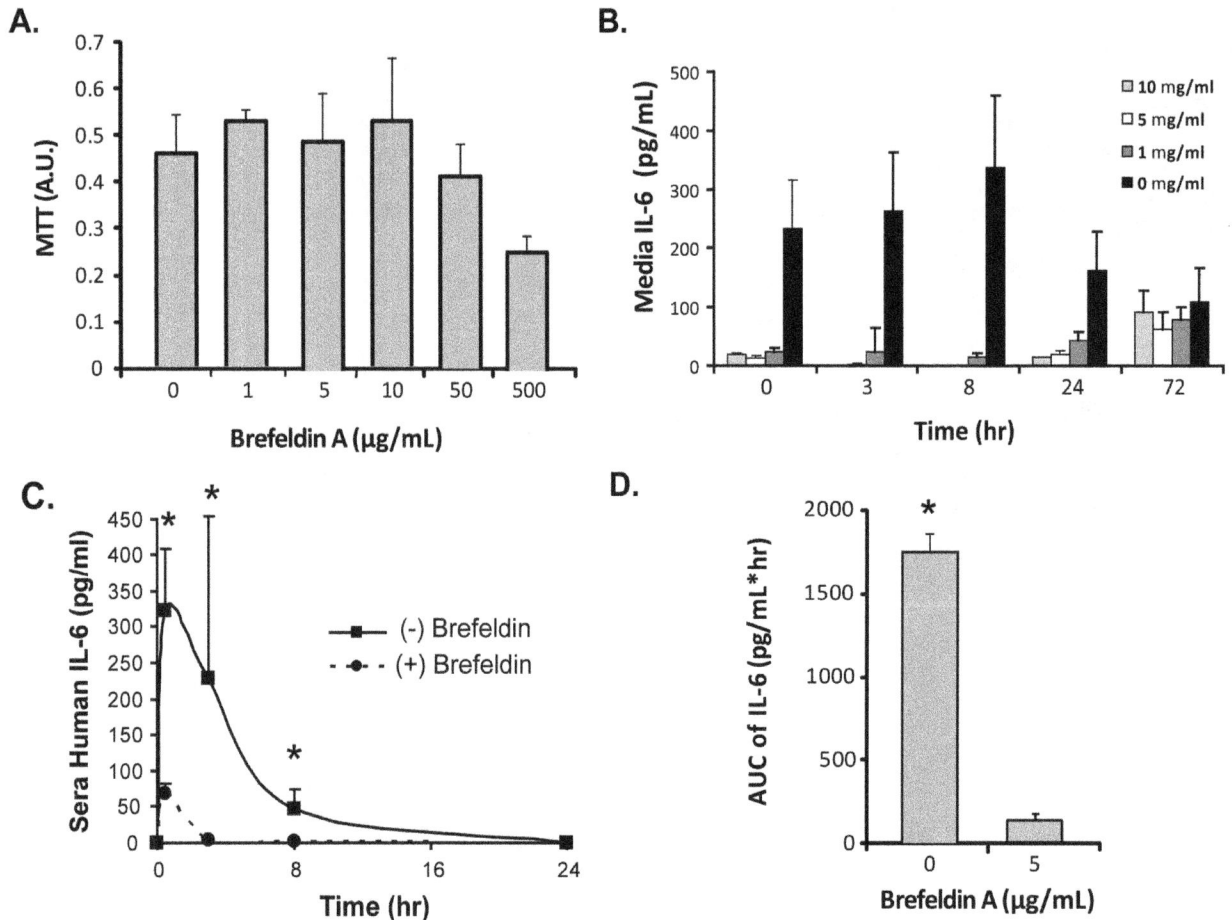

Figure 3. Golgi-dependent secretion mechanism of MSC-derived IL-6 in vivo. Brefeldin A pre-treatment of MSCs was used to evaluate blockade of IL-6 release in vitro and in vivo. (A) MTT assay of MSCs treated at different concentrations of brefeldin. A non-toxic dose of 5 ug/ml was used for functional studies. (B) Human IL-6 levels in vitro after brefeldin pre-treatment. Significant reduction in 24 hour release of IL-6 was observed across all doses. (C) Alteration in serum IL-6 delivery by MSCs pretreated with a Golgi-apparatus inhibitor, Brefeldin A. MSCs were incubated with 5 μg/ml of BFA for one day and then injected into C57Bl/6 mice and compared to untreated MSCs in terms of serum IL-6 delivery. Brefeldin treatment of MSCs led to diminished release of human IL-6 in vitro and in vivo. (D) Area-under-curve analysis of human IL-6 after MSC pre-treatment with brefeldin A and transplantation. Exposure to IL-6 was significantly reduced by inhibition of the Golgi apparatus. Time points for serum analyses were 0.5, 8, and 24 hours after cell injection. Mice were serially analyzed as batches of N = 5 per group. * denotes P>0.01.

IL-6 can be influenced by the *in vivo* microenvironment that MSCs encounter. In order to understand the maximal exposure of a subject to MSC secreted factor that was uninfluenced by host regulation, we developed genetically engineered MSCs with constitutive expression of the naturally secreted Gaussia luciferase (Gluc) reporter. Gluc has a circulation half-life of 5–10 minutes in mice, and has been used as a highly sensitive reporter (detection of ~1000 cells) for quantitative assessment of cells *in vivo* by measuring its level in the blood ex vivo [29]. GLuc activity can be easily quantified in blood by adding its substrate coelenterazine and measuring emitted photons using a luminometer. MSCs were first transduced with a lentivirus vector to stably express Gluc and GFP under the control of the constitutively active CMV promoter which yielded high transduction efficiency as monitored by fluorescent microscopy and flow cytometry for GFP (**Figure 5A–B**). Gluc expression and secretion was also readily detected in MSCs conditioned medium (**Figure 5C**). When infused into NOD-SCID mice, GLuc was detectable over a one week period with a time to peak concentration occurring at ~8 hours post-cells transplantation (**Figure 5D**). Engineering of MSCs with GLuc

revealed a longer exposure to cell therapy and suggests engineered cell formulations for therapeutic studies may be useful for minimizing cell dose and/or frequency to achieve durable responses.

Discussion

Pharmacology is a powerful discipline with many available methods to help understand and shape the characteristics of a drug to meet a therapeutic need. Monitoring a drug's PK is a necessary study of a drug formulation that has been modeled extensively by balancing the infusion, absorption, metabolism, and elimination of a drug, assuming the body is defined by a steady-state of discrete compartments that are permeable to a drug. Drug formulations that contain living cells are an ever-increasing class of therapeutics that can benefit from such pharmacological analysis. The classical monitoring strategy for a cell therapy is to define the trafficking and viability of a cellular formulation after introduction to the body. In this study, we coupled this strategy with molecular monitoring of secreted factors released by a cell transplant that became detectable in the systemic circulation. We identified that

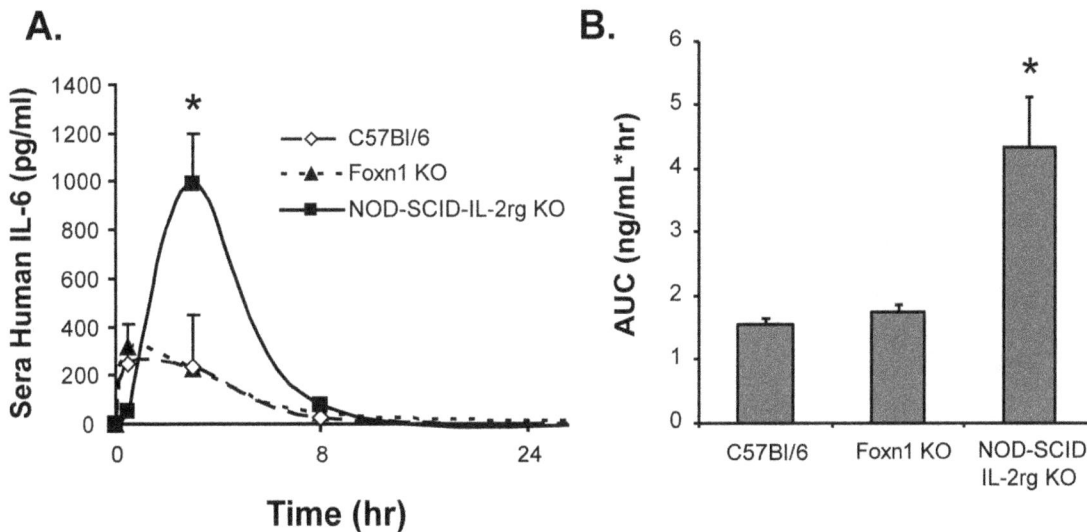

Figure 4. The immune system limits the bioavailability of MSC-derived IL-6. Pharmacokinetic profile of sera IL-6 after IV cell administration. Approximately 1×10^6 MSCs were injected into C57Bl/6, Foxn1 $-/-$, or NSG mice by IV injection. At different time points after cell injection, mice were sampled for blood plasma and serum human IL-6 levels were measured by ELISA. (B) AUC analysis of IL-6 exposure as a function of mouse strain. IV administration was significantly affected by mouse strain, particularly in severely immunodeficient mice, which had the highest exposure of IL-6 for a given cell mass. Data represent mean ± standard derivation of duplicate or triplicate experiments. Time points for serum analyses were 0.5, 8, and 24 hours after cell injection. Mice were serially analyzed as batches of N = 5 per study. * denotes P>0.01.

these two PK profiles - that is, the PK of an administered MSC population and MSC-secreted IL-6 - were discordant. This was dependent on the imaging modality used in this study (BLI), which has known limitations in whole-animal reporting due to tissue diffusion distance of light emission. BLI showed a prominent lung expression of the MSC graft for a period of several hours, which engineered MSC-Gluc releasing a secreted reporter could be detected for days. Exploration of the dynamics and rate-limiting aspects of MSC-derived secreted factors in blood serum, rather than the cells themselves, may provide more predictive power in their use as a therapeutic.

The PK of cell-derived molecules can be considered a lumped model of classical drug PK with additional complexity to consider due to cellular delivery. Cells as a delivery vehicle may be responsible for the difference in profiles compared to isolated molecules. Administration of a molecular drug bolus typically follows an exponentially decaying trajectory in terms of serum concentration of the drug. After cell administration, we observed that serum levels of secreted IL-6 followed an exponential decay independent of administration route. This may be attributed to limited engraftment MSCs entrapped in the lung. The diffusion of IL-6 from the cells would subsequently follow and be limited by tissue transport barriers before being detected in the bloodstream. In the systemic circulation secreted factors would likely follow their natural clearance pathways, which, in the case of IL-6, are very rapid (~minutes in half-life). We propose that traditional PK models can be modified to account for an active, cellular production term as well as the diffusion of material from an engrafted tissue bed.

The elimination, or clearance, of a drug compound can occur by metabolism or excretion of the drug in voided volume. In the case of a MSC transplant, we could detect the influence that the immune system has on the exposure of a subject to MSC secreted factors. The immune response we observed is likely a xenogenic rejection response that can be compartmentalized by arms of innate and adaptive immunity. Previous studies have shown that the immune competency of the host can have an impact on the cellular viability after transplantation [30]. There are a number of reports that describe the role of NK cells and other mechanisms that affect the viability of allogeneic MSCs after transplantation including the generation of immunological memory to the transplanted material over time [16,31,32]. The clearance of MSCs was substantial in IV transplanted MSCs, which were entrapped in lung tissue. NOD-SCID-IL-2rg $-/-$ mice had a much greater exposure to MSC-derived factors compared to Foxn1 $-/-$ mice or C57Bl/6 mice. The difference between the two immunocompromised strains lies in the absence of B cells, NK cells, and defects in cytokine signaling in NOD-SCID-IL-2rg $-/-$ mice suggesting that these cell populations and cytokines may be accountable for MSC clearance. This study, however, cannot distinguish immunologic elimination of the human cells versus elimination of the human secreted protein without further evaluation.

We, and others, have observed protection of acute liver injury by molecules derived from MSCs [33,34]. MSC molecules collectively had a dose-dependent effect on injured hepatocytes and stimulated a proliferation response in vitro and in vivo [33]. In this study, we used IL-6 as a model secreted factor to study the cellular release profile of this cytokine in vivo. Although specific mediators of therapy still remain elusive, there is considerable evidence that IL-6, itself, may be liver-protective. [35]. IL-6 is also shown to be important in improving acute inflammatory response [36,37]. We envision that other cytokine and growth factors released by MSCs will help broaden the overall PK profile of this transient cell therapy and begin to identify associations with relevant diseases that can be combated through the combination of factors released by MSCs. Cognate receptors for specific secreted factors will help clarify the pharmacodynamics of MSC action and if dosing is enough to activate downstream signaling of MSCs are amenable to *ex vivo* engineering to express therapeutic secreted factors such as IL-2 for cancer immunotherapy [38]. In this study, we first report the use of a non-specific GLuc reporter

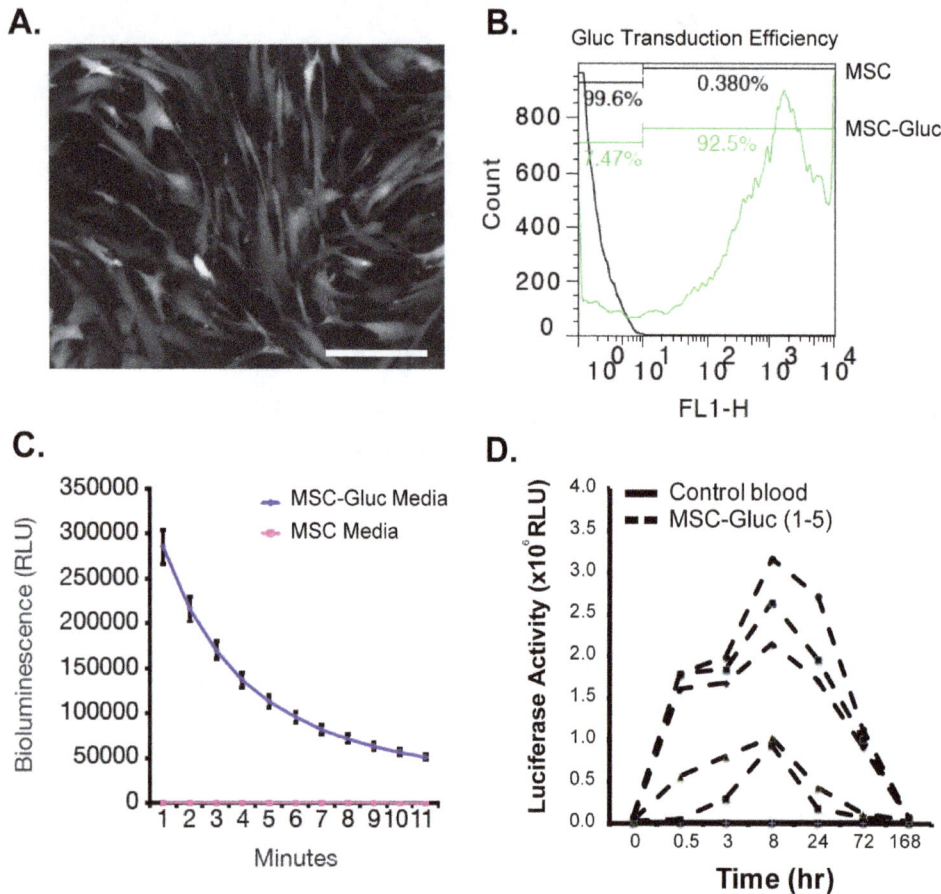

Figure 5. Blood Monitoring of Engineered Human MSCs with the Secreted Gaussia Luciferase Reporter. A lentivirus vector expressing GLuc and GFP was transduced into human MSCs at a confluence of 70% and multiplicity of infection of 4:1 in complex with 8 ug/ml of polybrene. (A) GFP micrograph and (B) flow cytometry showing high expression level and therefore transduction efficiency of construct. (C) The activity of GLuc was successfully measured in MSCs conditioned medium using a luminometer. (D) Five different engineered cell lines were infused into NOD-SCID mice and serum was individually collected at 0.5, 8, 24, 72, and 168 hours after cell injection in batches of N = 5 per study. MSCs constitutively expressing GLuc were detected in many cases over a week in duration.

that was engineered into MSCs for sensitive blood detection. MSC-Gluc revealed a longer exposure of the subject to a secreted factor implying that MSCs were persistent in the body although undetected by BLI. MSCs were genetically engineered ex vivo with a self-inactivating lentivirus vector which integrates the Gluc cDNA within the genome of the cells, leading to stable expression. This study cannot rule out the possibility that MSCs could fuse with a host cell (e.g. myeloid cells) after transplantation and thereby maintain a longer serum level. These data also suggest that constitutive secreted factors are necessary to reveal the true bioavailability of MSCs, as IL-6 and presumably other natural secreted factors may be regulated at the gene expression level by the host. The initial release dynamics of IL-6 were contributed by an active Golgi-dependent mechanism, which is presumed to be necessary for continued secretion of other protein factors such as GLuc. Non-protein secreted factors, such as nitric oxide or prostaglandin E2, may not be rate-limited by Golgi-secretion pathways but instead follow enzymatic reaction kinetics that require stimulation to generate these mediators *in vivo* [14,39]. MSC-Gluc can be an extremely useful tool for cell pharmacology studies that evaluate administration routes, initial dosage, and dosing frequency for optimizing the exposure of a cell therapy product.

This work serves as the first application of a combined cell biodistribution and molecular PK modeling approach to MSC therapeutics. By combined *in silico* modeling and empirical analysis, a functional PK/PD model can now begin to be developed to predict the nature of MSC therapy given a particular formulation and administration route. Allometric scaling laws that help predict the conversion of parameters from animal to human models may be applicable to guide clinical trials using MSC therapeutics. Although we focus on a few key mediators, a more comprehensive view of all bioactive MSC secreted factors can lead to second-generation models that better capture potential non-linearity in the data. In addition, this theoretical framework may serve as the foundation for other clinically used cell variants such as hematopoietic and embryonic stem cells, or T cells. Such predictive, *in silico* analysis of cell-based therapies may reduce experimental costs due to a systematic minimization of required testing, increase throughput of discovery, and ultimately lead to more efficacious treatment regimens.

Materials and Methods

Mice

Athymic Foxn1$-/-$ mice (nude, male, 6–8 weeks old), C57BL/6 mice (male, 8 weeks old), Balbc/J mice (female, 8 weeks old), and NOD.Cg-**Prkdc^{scid} Il2rg^{tm1Wjl}**/SzJ (NSG mice, male, 8–10 weeks old) were all purchased from Jackson Laboratories (Bar Harbor, ME) and housed at Massachusetts General Hospital Animal Facility following approved experimental protocols by the IACUC.

Human MSC Isolation and Expansion

Human MSCs were isolated and expanded following a previously established protocol [33,34]. Briefly, fresh human bone marrow aspirates were purchased from Lonza. Mononuclear cells were separated by Ficoll density gradient centrifugation (GE Healthcare) and plated on a T-175 flask (1×10^6 cells per flask). Mononuclear cells were cultured at 37°C with 10% CO_2 in MSC expansion medium. MSC expansion medium was composed of 15% fetal bovine serum, 2% penicillin and streptomycin, 0.2% gentamycin, 1 ng/L fibroblast growth factor, alpha-MEM with ribonucleosides and deoxyribonucleosides. Medium was changed 1 week later and unbound cells were washed away. The following week, colony-forming adherent cells were re-plated into a new flask for expansion. Medium was changed every 3–4 days. MSCs were subcultured when they reached 70–80% confluence. Only passage 2–5 MSCs were used for experiments. **Figure S1** outlines the immunophenotype of MSCs using antibodies purchased from BD Biosciences.

MSC Administration and Measurement of Human IL-6, MCP-1, and IL-8 Levels in Plasma

MSCs (1×10^6 MSCs in 200 µl FBS-free medium) were injected into mice by IV infusion. At 30 minutes, 3 hours, 8 hours, 24 hours and 72 hours, mice were anesthetized with 60 µl ketamine, 30 µl xylazine, and 60 µl saline per mouse and blood was withdrawn by cardiac puncture. After centrifugation at 14,000 rpm for 10 minutes at 4°C, plasma were collected and stored at -80°C before use. Human IL-6, MCP-1, and IL-8 levels were measured using an ELISA kit from BD Bioscience following the supplier's recommended procedures.

Preparation of Human MSCs Expressing a Firefly Luciferase Gene Reporter

The lentiviral vector pHR'MND-LRT containing a firefly luciferase reporter was constructed as previously described [40]. Infectious virus was produced by triple transient co-transduction of 293T/17 cells (ATCC) with pHR'MND-LRT, pCMVΔR8.91 i.e. packaging vector, and pMD.G i.e. VSVG pseudotyping vector. The titer of virus was determined by transduction of 293T cells followed by flow cytometry analysis of the mRFP reporter (Ex: 594 nm/Em: 620$\pm$15 nm). Cultures of 30–40% confluent human MSCs in a T-175 flask were incubated with the virus at a multiplicity of infection of 4 in a total of 20 ml expansion medium containing 8 µg/ml polybrene. This transduction protocol was repeated one more time. In each round, cells were incubated with the viral supernatant for 8 hours and then in MSC expansion medium for 16 hours. After the second round of infection, fresh medium was added to each flask and cultured for 3–4 days. Luciferase activity of transduced MSCs was confirmed with a luciferase activity assay before in vivo use.

Bioluminescence Imaging

A total of 1×10^6 luciferase-engineered MSCs were given to C57Bl/6 mice either IM or IV. At specific time points after cell injection, mice received an intraperitoneal injection of 4.5 mg of luciferase substrate solution (Molecular Imaging Products) and were imaged thereafter. The bioluminescent signal was measured in anesthetized mice on an IVIS-100 imaging system (Caliper LifeSciences) until a peak signal was reached. Data are expressed as photons/second/cm^2, encompassing a region of interest over the implanted cells, including lung, leg and whole body.

Preparation of Concentrated Conditioned Medium

MSCs were cultured to 70–80% confluency in T-175 culture flasks before 15 ml DMEM media consisted of 0.05% BSA and 2% penicillin and streptomycin were added. Cells were further cultured for 1–2 days and then the supernatants were collected and filtered. Cell number was quantified using a hemacytometer after trypsinization. Culture media were concentrated 20–50 folds using an Amicon filter (MWCO: 3,000 Da) by centrifuging at 3500 rpm for 2–3 hours. The human IL-6 levels were measured by ELISA by appropriate serial dilution before injection into mice. Concentrated conditioned medium (400 µl) were injected into C57Bl/6 mice by IV or IM routes.

Engineering and *In Vivo* Monitoring of MSCs with Secreted Gaussia Luciferase

MSCs were allowed to grow up to about 70% confluency before viral transduction. A lentivirus vector carrying the expression cassette for Gluc and GFP, separated by an internal ribosomal entry site, under the control of the CMV promoter was previously described [29] with a titer of 6.1×10^7 IU/ml. Polybrene was added to each T-175 flask diluted down to a final concentration of $1 \times$. Then 1 mL of virus was added to each flask. Cells were allowed to grow over night and then the virus-containing media was aspirated and replaced with fresh virus-free media. Transduction efficiency was confirmed by analyzing GFP expression using fluorescence microscopy and flow cytometry.

Fully confluent cells were trypsinized with $1 \times$ Trypsin (Fisher) and re-suspended in conditioning media at a density of 1×10^6 cells per 200 uL. 200 uL of cell suspension was injected into each mouse via tail vein. Blood was collected in Eppendorf tubes containing 4 µL of 20 mM EDTA via tail vein at 0.5 hour, 3 hour, 8 hour, 24 hour, 72 hour and 1 week post-MSCs injection. 10 uL blood was mixed with 100 uL 5 ug/ml coelenterazine substrate in a white, opaque 96-well plate and luminescence was detected using a BioTek microplate reader.

Brefeldin A Treatment of MSCs and Proliferation Assay

In a 6-well plate, MSCs were incubated with brefeldin A (Sigma-Aldrich) at a final concentration of 50, 10, 5, and 1 µg/ml for 24 hours. Supernatants were collected, and then MSCs were washed 3 times using PBS. Fresh medium was replaced, and cells continued to culture up to 3 days. Supernatants were collected at different time points for subsequent human IL-6 measurements. To measure the proliferation, BFA-treated cells were reseeded in a 96-well flat bottom plate and cultured with fresh medium for 72 hours. Cell proliferation was measured using a MTT assay kit (ATCC) following the supplier's recommended procedures.

Statistical Analysis

In all studies batches of 3–8 mice from 2–3 independent experiments are reported. Raw pharmacokinetic data were analyzed using a 1-tailed Mann-Whitney U test for nonparametric data with the mean ± SEM shown or using a two way ANOVA with Tukey's multiple comparison correction where pharmacokinetic parameters were calculated based on MATLAB software package models.

Supporting Information

Figure S1   Immunophenotyping of MSCs. Expanded cells were CD11b−, CD45−, CD45+, and CD73+ consistent with a bone marrow MSC identity.

Figure S2   Pharmacokinetics of MSC-derived IL-8 and MCP-1 after IV transplantation. ELISA measurements of mice injected with MSCs and analyzed for human (A) MCP-1 and

(B) IL-8 over time. Kinetics follow a similar trend compared to IL-6.
(TIF)

Acknowledgments

The authors are grateful for assistance from Ms. Jessica Sullivan and Mr. Peter Waterman in bioluminescence imaging.

Author Contributions

Conceived and designed the experiments: FW MLY BT BP. Performed the experiments: JE RM FW KS SG KC BP. Analyzed the data: JE RM FW BT BP. Contributed reagents/materials/analysis tools: KC RW BT. Wrote the paper: JE RM BT BP.

References

1. Culme-Seymour EJ, Davie NL, Brindley DA, Edwards-Parton S, Mason C (2012) A decade of cell therapy clinical trials (2000–2010). Regen Med 7: 455–462.
2. Mason C, Brindley DA, Culme-Seymour EJ, Davie NL (2011) Cell therapy industry: billion dollar global business with unlimited potential. Regen Med 6: 265–272.
3. Brindley DA, Davie NL, Sahlman WA, Bonfiglio GA, Culme-Seymour EJ, et al. (2012) Promising growth and investment in the cell therapy industry during the first quarter of 2012. Cell Stem Cell 10: 492–496.
4. Meirelles LDS, Chagastelles PC, Nardi NB (2006) Mesenchymal stem cells reside in virtually all post-natal organs and tissues. Journal Of Cell Science 119: 2204–2213.
5. Tang YL, Zhao Q, Zhang YC, Cheng LL, Liu MY, et al. (2004) Autologous mesenchymal stem cell transplantation induce VEGF and neovascularization in ischemic myocardium. Regulatory Peptides 117: 3–10.
6. Toma C, Pittenger MF, Cahill KS, Byrne BJ, Kessler PD (2002) Human mesenchymal stem cells differentiate to a cardiomyocyte phenotype in the adult murine heart. Circulation 105: 93–98.
7. Maitra B, Szekely E, Gjini K, Laughlin MJ, Dennis J, et al. (2004) Human mesenchymal stem cells support unrelated donor hematopoietic stem cells and suppress T-cell activation. Bone Marrow Transplantation 33: 597–604.
8. Honma T, Honmou O, Iihoshi S, Harada K, Houkin K, et al. (2006) Intravenous infusion of immortalized human mesenchymal stem cells protects against injury in a cerebral ischemia model in adult rat. Experimental Neurology 199: 56–66.
9. Parekkadan B, Tilles AW, Yarmush ML (2008) Bone marrow-derived mesenchymal stem cells ameliorate autoimmune enteropathy independently of regulatory T cells. Stem Cells 26: 1913–1919.
10. Wu Y, Chen L, Scott PG, Tredget EE (2007) Mesenchymal stem cells enhance wound healing through differentiation and angiogenesis. Stem Cells 25: 2648–2659.
11. Shumakov VI, Onishchenko NA, Rasulov MF, Krasheninnikov ME, Zaidenov VA (2003) Mesenchymal bone marrow stem cells more effectively stimulate regeneration of deep burn wounds than embryonic fibroblasts. Bull Exp Biol Med 136: 192–195.
12. McFarlin K, Gao X, Liu YB, Dulchavsky DS, Kwon D, et al. (2006) Bone marrow-derived mesenchymal stromal cells accelerate wound healing in the rat. Wound Repair Regen 14: 471–478.
13. Fu X, Li H (2009) Mesenchymal stem cells and skin wound repair and regeneration: possibilities and questions. Cell Tissue Res 335: 317–321.
14. Ren G, Zhang L, Zhao X, Xu G, Zhang Y, et al. (2008) Mesenchymal stem cell-mediated immunosuppression occurs via concerted action of chemokines and nitric oxide. Cell Stem Cell 2: 141–150.
15. Corcione A, Benvenuto F, Ferretti E, Giunti D, Cappiello V, et al. (2006) Human mesenchymal stem cells modulate B-cell functions. Blood 107: 367–372.
16. Spaggiari GM, Capobianco A, Becchetti S, Mingari MC, Moretta L (2006) Mesenchymal stem cell-natural killer cell interactions: evidence that activated NK cells are capable of killing MSCs, whereas MSCs can inhibit IL-2-induced NK-cell proliferation. Blood 107: 1484–1490.
17. Aggarwal S, Pittenger MF (2005) Human mesenchymal stem cells modulate allogeneic immune cell responses. Blood 105: 1815–1822.
18. Nasef A, Ashammakhi N, Fouillard L (2008) Immunomodulatory effect of mesenchymal stromal cells: possible mechanisms. Regen Med 3: 531–546.
19. Le Blanc K, Rasmusson I, Sundberg B, Gotherstrom C, Hassan M, et al. (2004) Treatment of severe acute graft-versus-host disease with third party haploidentical mesenchymal stem cells. Lancet 363: 1439–1441.
20. Parekkadan B, Milwid JM (2010) Mesenchymal Stem Cells as Therapeutics. In: Yarmush ML, Duncan JS, Gray ML, editors. Annual Review of Biomedical Engineering, Vol 12. 87–117.
21. Gao JZ, Dennis JE, Muzic RF, Lundberg M, Caplan AI (2001) The dynamic in vivo distribution of bone marrow-derived mesenchymal stent cells after infusion. Cells Tissues Organs 169: 12–20.
22. Lee RH, Pulin AA, Seo MJ, Kota DJ, Ylostalo J, et al. (2009) Intravenous hMSCs improve myocardial infarction in mice because cells embolized in lung are activated to secrete the anti-inflammatory protein TSG-6. Cell Stem Cell 5: 54–63.
23. Schrepfer S, Deuse T, Reichenspurner H, Fischbein MP, Robbins RC, et al. (2007) Stem cell transplantation: The lung barrier. Transplantation Proceedings 39: 573–576.
24. Sasportas LS, Kasmieh R, Wakimoto H, Hingtgen S, van de Water JA, et al. (2009) Assessment of therapeutic efficacy and fate of engineered human mesenchymal stem cells for cancer therapy. Proc Natl Acad Sci U S A 106: 4822–4827.
25. Balyasnikova IV, Ferguson SD, Sengupta S, Han Y, Lesniak MS Mesenchymal stem cells modified with a single-chain antibody against EGFRvIII successfully inhibit the growth of human xenograft malignant glioma. PLoS ONE 5: e9750.
26. Nemeth K, Keane-Myers A, Brown JM, Metcalfe DD, Gorham JD, et al. (2010) Bone marrow stromal cells use TGF-beta to suppress allergic responses in a mouse model of ragweed-induced asthma. Proceedings Of The National Academy Of Sciences Of The United States Of America 107: 5652–5657.
27. Majumdar MK, Thiede MA, Haynesworth SE, Bruder SP, Gerson SL (2000) Human marrow-derived mesenchymal stem cells (MSCs) express hematopoietic cytokines and support long-term hematopoiesis when differentiated toward stromal and osteogenic lineages. Journal of Hematotherapy & Stem Cell Research 9: 841–848.
28. Castell JV, Geiger T, Gross V, Andus T, Walter E, et al. (1988) Plasma clearance, organ distribution and target cells of interleukin-6/hepatocyte-stimulating factor in the rat. Eur J Biochem 177: 357–361.
29. Wurdinger T, Badr C, Pike L, de Kleine R, Weissleder R, et al. (2008) A secreted luciferase for ex vivo monitoring of in vivo processes. Nat Methods 5: 171–173.
30. Tolar J, O'Shaughnessy MJ, Panoskaltsis-Mortari A, McElmurry RT, Bell S, et al. (2006) Host factors that impact the biodistribution and persistence of multipotent adult progenitor cells. Blood 107: 4182–4188.
31. Sotiropoulou PA, Perez SA, Gritzapis AD, Baxevanis CN, Papamichail M (2006) Interactions between human mesenchymal stem cells and natural killer cells. Stem Cells 24: 74–85.
32. Zangi L, Margalit R, Reich-Zeliger S, Bachar-Lustig E, Beilhack A, et al. (2009) Direct imaging of immune rejection and memory induction by allogeneic mesenchymal stromal cells. Stem Cells 27: 2865–2874.
33. van Poll D, Parekkadan B, Cho CH, Berthiaume F, Nahmias Y, et al. (2008) Mesenchymal stem cell-derived molecules directly modulate hepatocellular death and regeneration in vitro and in vivo. Hepatology 47: 1634–1643.
34. Parekkadan B, van Poll D, Suganuma K, Carter EA, Berthiaume F, et al. (2007) Mesenchymal stem cell-derived molecules reverse fulminant hepatic failure. PLoS ONE 2: e941.
35. Bouffi C, Bony C, Courties G, Jorgensen C, Noel D (2010) IL-6-dependent PGE2 secretion by mesenchymal stem cells inhibits local inflammation in experimental arthritis. PLoS One 5: e14247.
36. Kopf M, Baumann H, Freer G, Freudenberg M, Lamers M, et al. (1994) IMPAIRED IMMUNE AND ACUTE-PHASE RESPONSES IN INTER-LEUKIN-6-DEFICIENT MICE. Nature 368: 339–342.
37. Klein C, Wustefeld T, Assmus U, Roskams T, Rose-John S, et al. (2005) The IL-6-gp130-STAT3 pathway in hepatocytes triggers liver protection in T cell-mediated liver injury. Journal of Clinical Investigation 115: 860–869.
38. Stagg J, Lejeune L, Paquin A, Galipeau J (2004) Marrow stromal cells for interleukin-2 delivery in cancer immunotherapy. Hum Gene Ther 15: 597–608.
39. Nemeth K, Leelahavanichkul A, Yuen PS, Mayer B, Parmelee A, et al. (2009) Bone marrow stromal cells attenuate sepsis via prostaglandin E(2)-dependent reprogramming of host macrophages to increase their interleukin-10 production. Nat Med 15: 42–49.
40. Love Z, Wang F, Dennis J, Awadallah A, Salem N, et al. (2007) Imaging of mesenchymal stem cell transplant by bioluminescence and PET. Journal Of Nuclear Medicine 48: 2011–2020.

4

Serotype-Specific Acquisition and Loss of Group B *Streptococcus* Recto-Vaginal Colonization in Late Pregnancy

Gaurav Kwatra[1,2], Peter V. Adrian[1,2]*, Tinevimbo Shiri[1,2], Eckhart J. Buchmann[4], Clare L. Cutland[1,2], Shabir A. Madhi[1,2,3]

1 Department of Science and Technology/National Research Foundation: Vaccine Preventable Diseases, University of the Witwatersrand, Johannesburg, South Africa, 2 MRC, Respiratory and Meningeal Pathogens Research Unit, University of the Witwatersrand, Johannesburg, South Africa, 3 National Institute for Communicable Diseases: a division of National Health Laboratory Service, Johannesburg, South Africa, 4 Department of Obstetrics and Gynaecology, University of the Witwatersrand, Johannesburg, South Africa

Abstract

Background: Maternal recto-vaginal colonization with Group B *Streptococcus* (GBS) and consequent vertical transmission to the newborn predisposes neonates to early-onset invasive GBS disease. This study aimed to determine the acquisition and loss of serotype-specific recto-vaginal GBS colonization from 20–37+ weeks of gestational age.

Methods: Vaginal and rectal swabs were collected from HIV-uninfected women at 20–25 weeks of gestation age and at 5–6 weekly intervals thereafter. Swabs were cultured for GBS and isolates were serotyped by latex agglutination. Serologically non-typable isolates and pilus islands were characterized by PCR.

Results: The prevalence of recto-vaginal GBS colonization was 33.0%, 32.7%, 28.7% and 28.4% at 20–25 weeks, 26–30 weeks, 31–35 weeks and 37+ weeks of gestational age, respectively. The most common identified serotypes were Ia (39.2%), III (32.8%) and V (12.4%). Of 507 participants who completed all four study visits, the cumulative overall recto-vaginal acquisition rate of new serotypes during the study was 27.9%, including 11.2%, 8.2% and 4.3% for serotypes Ia, III and V, respectively. Comparing the common colonizing serotypes, serotype III was more likely to be associated with persistent colonization throughout the study (29%) than Ia (18%; p = 0.045) or V (6%; p = 0.002). The median duration of recto-vaginal GBS colonization for serotype III was 6.35 weeks, which was longer than other serotypes. Pilus island proteins were detected in all GBS isolates and their subtype distribution was associated with specific serotypes.

Conclusion: South African pregnant women have a high prevalence of GBS recto-vaginal colonization from 20 weeks of gestational age onwards, including high GBS acquisition rates in the last pregnancy-trimesters. There are differences in specific-serotype colonization patterns during pregnancy.

Editor: Bernard Beall, Centers for Disease Control & Prevention, United States of America

Funding: This work was funded by research supported by the South African Research Chairs Initiative in Vaccine Preventable Diseases of the Department of Science and Technology and National Research Foundation. Part-funding was also granted by Novartis Vaccines, Italy. The funders had no role in study design, data collection, analysis, decision to publish, or preparation of the manuscript.

Competing Interests: RMPRU Laboratory has received partial funding for this study from a commercial source (Novartis Vaccines). However, Novartis vaccines did not play any role in the design of the study, data collection, analysis, decision to publish, or preparation of the manuscript.

* Email: adrianp@rmpru.co.za

Introduction

Maternal vaginal colonization with Group B *Streptococcus* (GBS) is the major risk factor for early onset invasive GBS disease (EOD) in newborns [1,2]. Screening of pregnant women for GBS colonization during the third trimester, coupled with targeted intrapartum antibiotic prophylaxis (IAP) of colonized women during labor, has reduced the incidence of invasive GBS disease in industrialized countries [3].

An alternate preventive strategy against EOD is vaccination of pregnant women, which could enhance transplacental transfer of anti-GBS antibody to the fetus. Studies have identified an association between high maternal serotype-specific anti-capsular polysaccharide (CPS) antibody concentrations with reduced risk of recto-vaginal colonization and reduced risk of newborns developing EOD [4,5]. Since GBS CPS-protein conjugate vaccines are serotype-specific, it is important to characterize the serotype distribution of GBS in different regions of the world as well as understand the changes which occur in GBS colonization during pregnancy [6]. Other potential vaccine candidates include GBS surface protein antigens such as pilus island (PI) proteins that are present in all GBS isolates [7]. Although it has been shown that maternal GBS colonization during pregnancy may fluctuate [8,9,10], there are limited longitudinal studies on the rate of serotype-specific GBS acquisition and duration of colonization during pregnancy.

We aimed to determine the acquisition and loss of GBS recto-vaginal colonization, including serotype-specific changes, among South African pregnant women from 20 weeks to at least 37 weeks of gestational age. We also studied the PI distribution of recto-vaginal colonizing GBS isolates and their association with capsular serotype.

Materials and Methods

Study Population

The study was conducted at prenatal community clinics in Soweto (Lillian Ngoyi, Diepkloof, Mofolo and Michael Maponya), Johannesburg from August 2010 to August 2011. Inclusion criteria were HIV-uninfected pregnant women confirmed by HIV ELISA test non-reactivity at enrolment, from 20–25 weeks of gestational age based on last menstrual cycle and who consented to study participation. Exclusion criteria at enrolment included antibiotic treatment in the previous two weeks, any acute illness, symptomatic vaginal discharge and a known or suspected condition in which clinical vaginal examinations were contradicted. If antibiotics were taken after the first visit, the collection of specimens was delayed for at least two weeks after the last antibiotic dose.

Swab collection and culture of GBS

Lower vaginal and rectal swabs were collected for GBS culture starting at 20–25 weeks (Visit-1), followed by three subsequent visits (Visits 2–4) at 5–6 weekly intervals, up to 37–40 weeks (Visit-4) of gestational age. Demographic and pregnancy-related data were collected at the first visit. All samples were collected by trained study nurses with rayon-tipped swabs that were placed into Amies transport medium without charcoal (cat #MW170, Transwab Amies, Medical wire, U.K.). Swabs were transported to the lab within 4 hours of collection, and processed within 2 hours. For GBS isolation, swabs were inoculated onto CHRO-Magar StrepB (CA; Media Mage, Johannesburg, South Africa) and the CA plates were incubated at 37°C for 18–24 hours in aerobic conditions [11]. If GBS-like colonies were not visible within 24 hours after incubation, the plates were incubated for a further 24 hours and re-examined for growth. Up to four GBS-like colonies were isolated and confirmed as GBS by testing for CAMP factor, inability to hydrolyze esculin, catalase negativity and group B antigen.

Capsular serotyping

Serotyping was performed by the latex agglutination method with specific antisera against types Ia, Ib and II to IX CPS antigens (Statens Serum Institute, SSI, Sweden) as described [12]. Isolates that tested negative by latex agglutination for all serotypes were further typed by a PCR method for serotypes Ia, Ib, II, III, IV and V using primer sequences described by Poyart et al [13]. The gene encoding dlts was used as a PCR positive control for GBS identification.

Pilus typing

Pilus island proteins of all GBS isolates were detected by PCR for PI-1, PI-2a and PI-2b, with primers that target the genomic regions coding for the ancillary protein (AP)-1 of each PI. Isolates that tested negative for all the AP1 genes, or isolates from which neither PI-2a or PI-2b could be detected, were amplified by a second set of primers representing conserved regions of AP-2 as described previously [7].

Statistical analysis

Data were analyzed using SAS version 9.2 software (SAS Institute, Inc., NC, USA). A visit sample pair of vaginal and rectal swabs was considered negative if no GBS growth was evident on either swab, and positive if GBS was grown from either swab. The pregnant women were grouped into transient, intermittent and persistent carriers according to the presence of GBS colonization and to individual serotypes at the four sampling time points. Transient carriers were defined as women who were colonized at only one of the four visits, intermittent carriers as those who were colonized at two or three of the visits and persistent carriers as those colonized at all four study visits.

Descriptive statistics included the prevalence of colonization at individual time points and changes of recto-vaginal colonization status. Analysis of the changes in recto-vaginal colonization over time was restricted to the 507 participants who completed all four study visits. New acquisition of GBS was defined as positive culture of a new serotype which was not previously present. The new acquisition rate was defined as the number of new serotype acquisitions divided by the number of participants who were at a risk of acquiring the new serotype. Thus, women who were already previously colonized by a particular serotype were excluded subsequently from the denominator for estimating acquisition rate for the homotypic serotype. The rate of new acquisitions by all GBS serotypes were calculated from the sum of acquisition rates for the individual serotypes, and by using the above methods for GBS acquisition rates in a serotype independent manner. Clearance of colonization was defined as a negative GBS culture for a specific serotype following a positive sample at the previous visit for the homotypic serotype. The rate of colonization clearance was defined as the number of GBS-negative participants at the analyzed time point divided by the number of participants at the previous visit who were positive for that serotype, and was also calculated in a serotype independent manner.

Survival analysis methods were used to estimate the duration of colonization of specific serotypes. A colonizing event was defined as the period of time between acquisition and clearance of a GBS serotype. Date of acquisition was calculated as the midpoint between the last visit without serotype-specific colonization and the first visit at which a positive sample was obtained for the homotypic serotype, while date for termination of serotype-specific colonization was calculated as the midpoint between the last visit with colonization and the subsequent negative visit for that serotype. In this analysis, if colonization occurred at the first visit, this was taken as the start of colonization, and if colonization occurred at the last visit, a right censoring approach was applied. We used the Kaplan-Meier method to estimate the duration of GBS colonization. The log-rank test was used to examine differences in duration of carriage between serotypes.

Positive predictive value (PPV) and negative predictive value (NPV) were calculated for the culture results at different sampling points with the 37–40 week visit as the reference standard. For participants who were colonized with same serotype on multiple visits, only one serotype specific isolate was used to study PI association with capsular serotype.

The chi-square test was used to compare proportions. Logistic regression analysis was used to determine the association between GBS colonization and demographic characteristics at enrolment. A p-value of <0.05 was considered significant.

Ethics statement

The study was approved by the Human Research Ethics Committee of the University of the Witwatersrand (IRB/Protocol-

M090937) and informed written consent was obtained from all participating mothers. The trial is registered with South African National Clinical Trials Register, number DOH-27-0210-3012.

Results

Demographic characteristics

Of the 661 enrolled participants, 621 (93.9%), 595 (90.0%) and 521 (78.8%) completed visits 2, 3 and 4, respectively. Five-hundred and seven (76.7%) women completed all four study visits. A detailed trial profile is indicated in figure 1. The main reason for women not attending all four visits was birth of the baby (13%; 86/661) before the final visit. The demographic characteristics are displayed in table 1. The mean age of the participants at enrolment was 25.9 (standard deviation; S.D$\pm$5.6) years. Only 5 (0.76%) pregnant women have taken antibiotic treatment during the study.

Prevalence of GBS colonization

The overall prevalence of recto-vaginal GBS colonization was 33.0% (218), 32.7% (203), 28.7% (171) and 28.4% (148) at 20–25 weeks, 26–30 weeks, 31–35 weeks and 37+ weeks of gestational age, respectively. The lower prevalence of colonization associated with 31–35 weeks and 37+ weeks compared to 20–25 weeks and 26–30 weeks was specifically associated with a decrease in prevalence of vaginal colonization, table 2 (23.3% to 19.0%). In the 86 women who gave birth before the final visit, vaginal GBS colonization was detected in 17(19.8%) at the last attended visit compared to 99/521 (19.0%) who gave birth after visit-4 (p = 0.867). The inclusion of rectal swab GBS-culture increased the overall detection of GBS colonization by approximately 10% across the four study time-points (p<0.0001) and the prevalence of rectal colonization remained similar at each study time-point.

Of several demographic characteristics evaluated at enrolment independently by univariate analysis, parity (OR: 1.22; 95% CI: 1.02–1.47; p = 0.030) and gravidity (OR: 1.17; 95% CI: 1.01–1.36; p = 0.046), (Table 3) were significantly associated with GBS recto-vaginal colonization, with the highest colonization prevalence observed among women with parity $\geq$3 (42.1%) and gravidity of $\geq$4 (41.7%), (Table 1). In a multivariate analysis, none of the demographic characteristics were found to be associated with GBS recto-vaginal colonization, (Table 3). In a serotype-specific univariate analysis at enrolment, multiparity was associated with a higher prevalence of serotype III colonization (OR: 1.37; 95% CI: 1.07–1.76; p = 0.012), gravidity also showed possible association with serotype III colonization (p = 0.068). In the multivariate analysis parity was found to be associated with serotype III colonization (Adjusted OR: 6.69; 95% CI: 1.47–30.4; P = 0.014). Gravidity (p = 0.053) and abortions (p = 0.057) also showed a possible association with serotype III colonization, (Table 3). None of the demographic characteristics were found to be associated with serotype Ia colonization in the univariate or multivariate analysis. There were no identifiable factors associated with a higher prevalence of colonization with GBS at visit-4 alone.

Serotype and pilus island distribution

The proportional representation of serotypes remained consistent at each of the consecutive sampling time-points. Of women colonized, the proportional representation of the major serotypes were 36.2% to 41.4% for Ia, 31.3% to 34.9% for III, 10.3% to 15.6% for V, 7.2% to 7.5% for II, 3.5% to 4.6% for Ib, 2.0% to 4.0% for IV and 0.0% to 3.3% for IX (Table S1 in file S1). The concordance of serotypes for GBS cultured concurrently from vaginal and rectal swabs was 91.3%, 89.5%, 94.1% and 94.1% for

the four consecutive visits, respectively. Only 1.6% of GBS isolates were serologically non-typable by latex agglutination and were serotyped by PCR.

All GBS isolates harbored one or more PIs, either PI-2a on its own or with a combination of PI-2a or PI-2b in combination with PI-1.The most common PI arrangement was PI-2a on its own, which occurred in 103/227 (45.4%), 92/211 (43.6%), 79/175 (45.1%) and 63/152 (41.5%) of isolates at visits 1–4, respectively, followed by PI combination PI-2b and PI-1, which occurred in 75/227 (33.0%), 69/211 (32.7%), 68/175 (38.9%) and 58/152 (38.2%) of isolates at visits 1–4, respectively. The least common PI arrangement was a combination of PI-2a and PI-1 which occurred in 49/227 (21.6%), 50/211 (23.7%), 29/175 (16.0%) and 31/152 (20.4%) of isolates at visits 1–4, respectively. There were no significant changes in the prevalence of PI distribution with respect to different visits, with the exception of PI-2a which was less common at visit-4 (18.0%, 94/521) compared to visit-1 (23.0%, 152/661; p = 0.007), and which was attributable to a lower prevalence of serotype Ia at visit-4 (10.6%, 55/521) compared to visit-1 (14.2%, 94/661).

There was a strong correlation between the presence of particular combinations of PI and the serotype; Figure 2. Most serotype Ia isolates were associated with PI-2a (94.9%; 148/156), whereas the majority of serotype III isolates were associated with the combination of PI-1 and PI-2b (88.2%; 105/119). The association between PIs and serotype V was more variable, with a PI-1+PI-2a combination occurring in 64.7% (33/51) and PI-2a alone occurring in 29.4% (15/51) of isolates.

Changes in GBS colonization overtime

Five hundred and seven participants who completed all four study visits were similar in their demographic characteristics compared to the 154 participants not included in this analysis (data not shown). In the analyzed subset, the prevalence of recto-vaginal GBS colonization was 32.1% (163), 30.4% (154), 29.0% (147) and 27.8% (141) at 20–25 weeks, 26–30 weeks, 31–35 weeks and 37+ weeks of gestational age, respectively. Two hundred and fifty-two (49.7%) women were colonized at least once during the study period, of whom 70 (27.8%) were persistent carriers, 83 (32.9%) transient carriers and 99 (39.3%) were intermittently colonized for any serotype (Table S2 in file S1).

The cumulative serotype-specific prevalence across the study period was 23.7% (120/507) for Ia, 18.3% (93/507) for III, 7.1% (36/507) for V, 4.3% (22/507) for II and 2.8% (14/507) for Ib. All GBS serotypes were variable in their colonization patterns. Comparing the three most common colonizing serotype carriers, 29% (27/93) of serotype III carriers were associated with persistent colonization compared to serotype Ia (18%; 21/120; p = 0.045) or V (6%; 2/36; p = 0.002). Serotype V was the most dynamic, with 94.4% (34/36) of colonized women either being transient or intermittent carriers compared to 82.5% (99/120; p = 0.106) for Ia and 71.0% (66/93; p = 0.004) for III. Only one serotype was detected in 83.3% (210/252) of GBS carriers during the study period, with 85.7% (60/70) of women persistently colonized being associated with the same serotype.

Of the 16.7% (42/252) women in whom multiple serotypes were detected over the study period, two serotypes were detected in 9.5% (24/252) and three serotypes in 7.1% (18/252) participants. Among women in whom multiple serotypes were detected, a new serotype was observed at the immediate next visit in 85.7% (36/42) of cases, while a new serotype was detected following a period of no colonization by the preceding serotype in six women.

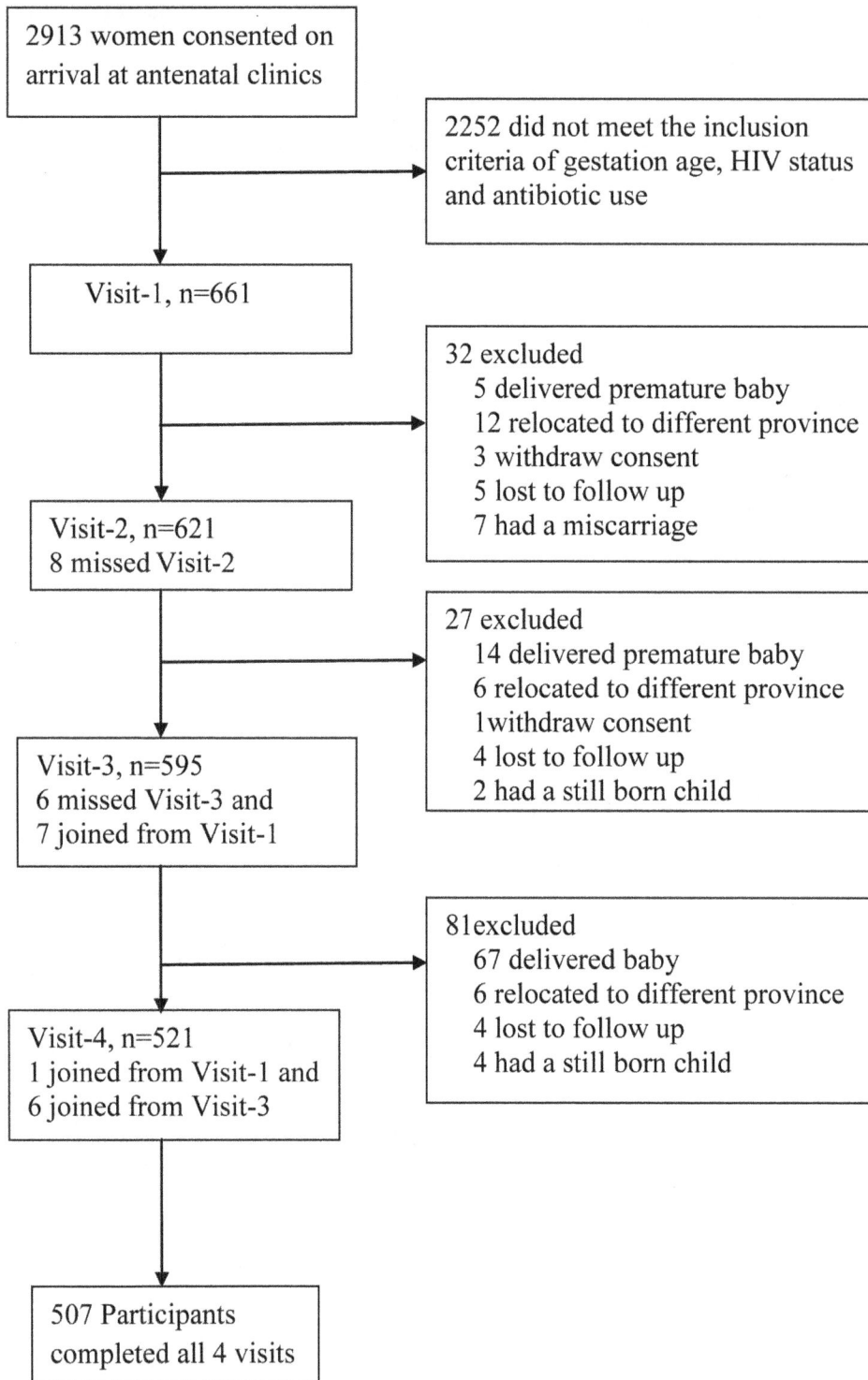

```
┌─────────────────────────────┐
│ 2913 women consented on     │
│ arrival at antenatal clinics│
└─────────────────────────────┘
              │
              │        ┌──────────────────────────────────┐
              │───────▶│ 2252 did not meet the inclusion   │
              │        │ criteria of gestation age, HIV    │
              │        │ status and antibiotic use         │
              ▼        └──────────────────────────────────┘
┌─────────────────────────────┐
│ Visit-1, n=661              │
└─────────────────────────────┘
              │
              │        ┌──────────────────────────────────┐
              │        │ 32 excluded                       │
              │        │   5 delivered premature baby      │
              │───────▶│   12 relocated to different prov. │
              │        │   3 withdraw consent              │
              │        │   5 lost to follow up             │
              ▼        │   7 had a miscarriage             │
┌─────────────────────────────┐ └────────────────────────┘
│ Visit-2, n=621              │
│ 8 missed Visit-2            │
└─────────────────────────────┘
```

Figure 1. Trial Profile.

New acquisition and clearance of colonization

Three hundred and forty-four participants who completed all four study visits were not colonized at visit-1, of whom 89 (25.9%) became colonized at one of the subsequent three visits. When including new serotype acquisition in those previously colonized by a heterotypic serotype (n = 39), the cumulative overall recto-vaginal acquisition rate of new serotypes during the study, calculated from the sum of acquisition rates for the individual serotypes was 27.9%. The number of new acquisitions was highest for serotypes Ia (11.2%, 49/436), III (8.2%, 37/451) and V (4.3%, 21/492); table S2 in file S1. The mean new acquisition rate of GBS was 11.4% (S.D ±0.5%) at 5–6 week visit intervals, including 11.6% between visit-1 and visit-2, and 10.8% and 11.7% in the

Table 1. Demographics of the study population at time of enrolment (n = 661).

Demographic characteristic		Overall (n = 661)	GBS Colonized	GBS Uncolonized
Age (years)	<20	92 (13.9%)[a]	27 (29.3%)[b]	65 (70.7%)[c]
Mean age: 25.9 (S.D±5.6)	20–24	234 (35.4%)	78 (33.3%)	156 (66.6%)
	25–28	161 (24.4%)	53 (32.9%)	108 (67.1%)
	29–32	95 (14.4%)	29 (30.5%)	66 (69.5%)
	33–35	40 (6.1%)	20 (50.0%)	20 (50.0%)
	36+	39 (5.9%)	11 (28.2%)	28 (71.8%)
Parity	0	338 (51.1%)	97 (28.7%)	241 (71.3%)
Median parity: 0 (range; 0–5)	1–2	304 (46.0%)	113 (37.2%)	191 (62.8%)
	3–5	19 (2.9%)	8 (42.1%)	11 (57.9%)
Gravidity	1	286 (43.3%)	80 (28.0%)	206 (72.0%)
Median gravidity: 2 (range; 1–8)	2	221 (33.4%)	80 (36.2%)	141 (63.8%)
	3	106 (16.0%)	38 (35.8%)	68 (64.2%)
	≥4	48 (7.3%)	20 (41.7%)	28 (58.3%)
Previous Abortion (spontaneous)	0	553 (83.7%)	176 (31.8%)	377 (68.2%)
Median abortion: 0 (range; 0–3)	1	88 (13.3%)	36 (40.9%)	52 (59.1%)
	2	19 (2.9%)	6 (31.6%)	13 (68.4%)
	3	1 (0.2%)	0 (0.0%)	1 (100%)
Stillborn	0	651 (98.5%)	214 (32.9%)	437 (67.1%)
Median stillbirths: 0 (range; 0–1)	1	10 (1.5%)	4 (40.0%)	6 (60.0%)

[a]Data are no (%) of total participants, [b,c]Data are row %.

intervals of subsequent consecutive visits. Of 163 participants who were colonized at visit-1, 76 (46.6%) were no longer colonized by visit-4. The rate of colonization-clearance was 75% (6/8) for serotype Ib, 73.3% (11/15) for V and 63.4% (45/71) for Ia. The overall clearance of any GBS colonization was 30.1% (49/163), 29.2% (45/154) and 32.7% (48/147) between visits-1 and -2, visits-2 and -3, and visits-3 and -4, respectively. No demographic characteristics were identified that were associated with either new acquisition or clearance of colonization.

Duration of GBS colonization

The median duration of recto-vaginal GBS colonization was 6.35 weeks for serotype III, which tended to be longer than other serotypes, including serotype Ia (median: 5.21 weeks; p = 0.02; table 4) which was the second most common colonizing serotype. The difference in duration of colonization between serotype III and less prevalent serotypes was not statistically significant.

Table 2. Prevalence of Group B *Streptococcus* colonization during the study visits.

Site of colonization	Visit-1	Visit-2	Visit-3	Visit-4
	(20–25 weeks)	(26–30 weeks)	(31–35 weeks)	37+weeks)
	n = 661	n = 621	n = 595	n = 521
	Mean gestation age: 22.7 weeks	Mean gestation age: 27.9 weeks	Mean gestation age: 32.5 weeks	Mean gestation age: 37.5 weeks
Vaginal only (%; 95% CI)	62	65	47	31
	(9.4%; 7.2–11.6)	(10.5%; 8.1–12.9)	(7.9%; 5.7–10.1)	(5.9%; 3.9–7.9)
Rectal only (%; 95% CI)	64	62	56	49
	(9.7%; 7.5–12.0)	(10%; 7.6–12.4)	(9.4%; 7.1–12.0)	(9.4%; 6.9–11.9)
Both vaginal and rectal (%; 95% CI)	92	76	68	68
	(13.9%; 11.3–16.5)	(12.2%; 9.63–14.8)	(11.4%; 8.9–14.0)	(13.1%; 10.2–16.0)
Vaginal and/or rectal (%; 95% CI)	218	203	171	148
	(33.0%; 29.4–36.6)	(32.7%; 29.0–36.4)	(28.7%; 25.1–32.3)	(28.4%; 24.5–32.3)

CI-Confidence interval, n = number of participants.

Table 3. Univariate and multivariate association between serotype-specific colonization and observed demographic characteristics at enrolment.

Characteristic	Overall GBS colonization at enrolment		Serotype III colonization at enrolment		Serotype Ia colonization at enrolment	
	Univariate	Multivariate	Univariate	Multivariate	Univariate	Multivariate
	OR (95% CI), p	AOR (95% CI), p	OR (95% CI), p	AOR (95% CI), p	OR (95% CI), p	AOR (95% CI), p
Age	0.98 (0.95–1.02),	1.01 (0.97–1.06),	0.98 (0.92–1.03),	1.00 (0.96–1.04),	0.99 (0.94–1.04),	
	0.536	0.527	0.45	0.96	0.656	
Parity	1.99 (0.83–4.79),	1.37 (1.07–1.76),	6.69 (1.47–30.4),	1.05 (0.82–1.34),	0.71 (0.27–1.90),	
	0.121	0.012	0.014	0.69	0.499	
Gravidity	0.63 (0.27–1.50),	1.22 (0.99–1.51),	0.22 (0.05–1.02),	1.11 (0.91–1.35),	1.48 (0.57–3.81),	
	0.296	0.068	0.053	0.317	0.422	
Abortion	1.77 (0.73–4.30),	1.10 (0.66–1.81),	4.14 (0.96–18.0),	1.25 (0.82–1.91),	0.86 (0.31–2.38),	
	0.207	0.721	0.057	0.298	0.774	
Stillborn	1.25 (0.32–4.94),	0.94 (0.12–7.51),	0.76 (0.08–7.30),	2.60 (0.66–10.3),	2.14 (0.49–9.29),	
	0.741	0.951	0.813	0.171	0.309	

OR: odds ratio; AOR: adjusted OR; CI: confidence interval.

Predictive values for each visit culture with respect culture status at visit-4

Positive and negative predictive values of serotype-specific culture at 20–25 weeks, 26–30 weeks and 31–35 weeks of gestational age compared to 37+ weeks colonization status are presented in table 5. The overall positive predictive values were 53.4%, 61.7% and 67.4% for GBS-positive cultures at 20–25 weeks, 26–30 weeks and 31–35 weeks, respectively, relative to positivity at 37+ weeks, while the negative predictive values for 20–25 weeks, 26–30 weeks and 31–35 weeks ranged from 84.3% to 88.3%. Serotypes Ia and V had lower PPVs compared with serotype III at each time-point. The observed PPVs at 31–35 weeks, were 55–70% for the three commonest serotypes.

Discussion

To our knowledge this is the first serotype-specific longitudinal study conducted of recto-vaginal GBS colonization in pregnant women, in whom we demonstrated a high prevalence and acquisition rate of GBS recto-vaginal colonization. The overall rate of new acquisition at 5–6 week interval is in agreement with a previous study of non-pregnant women, although, the serotype-specific rates differed [14]. All GBS serotypes were variable in their colonization patterns, possibly due to the complex interaction between immunity and specific GBS serotypes, which is still incompletely understood. It may be that the higher frequency of persistent colonization and longer overall duration of colonization by serotype III, is related to a weaker natural immune response

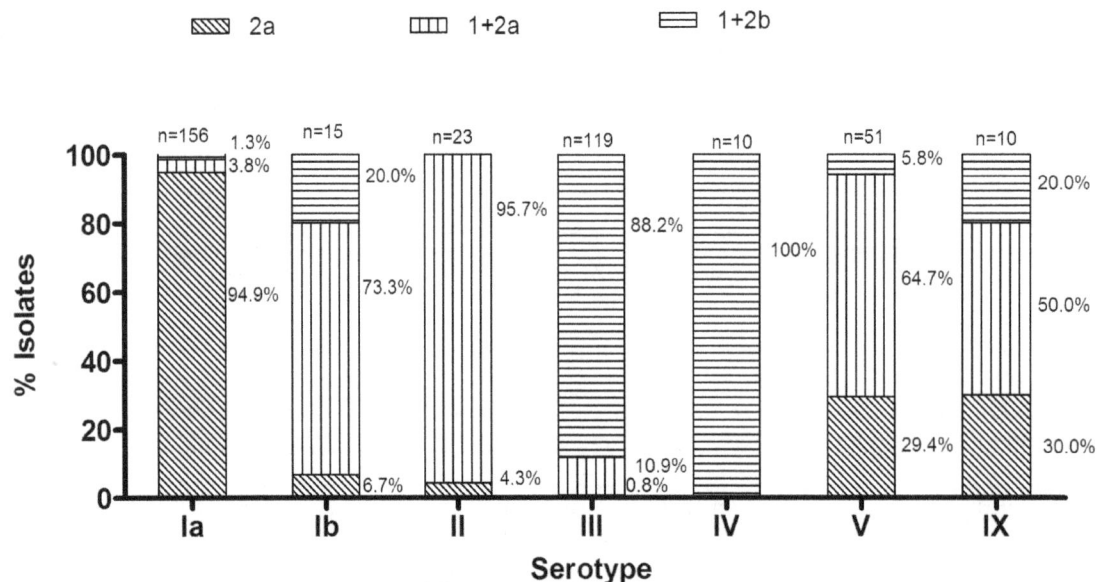

Figure 2. Association of pilus island proteins and serotypes among Group B *Streptococcus* isolates.

Table 4. Estimated duration of Group B *Streptococcus* recto-vaginal colonization.

Serotype	Colonization duration (weeks)*		
	Mean (95% CI)	Median	p-value[†]
Ia	7.52 (6.6–8.4)	5.21	0.026
Ib	5.22 (4.03–6.42)	3.62	0.358
II	6.11 (5.07–7.16)	4.24	0.736
III	9.15 (8.1–10.2)	6.35	Reference
IV	6.94 (3.8–10.0)	4.81	0.998
V	8.60 (6.80–10.39)	5.96	0.332
IX	6.21 (4.7–7.7)	4.31	0.651

*Time from enrolment, CI-Confidence interval,
[†]compared to serotype III.

associated with its colonization compared to other serotypes [15]. Consequently, there is a higher risk of exposure at birth to serotype III in our population, which corroborates with it being responsible for 49.2% to 57.7% of EOD in our setting [16,17]. The higher acquisition rate of serotype Ia may result in there being inadequate time for natural immunity to this serotype developing in the pregnant woman, which consequently increases the newborn's risk of developing EOD from serotype Ia, associated with 22.6% to 31% of EOD cases in our setting [16,17].

The high incidence of new acquisition and loss of colonization during pregnancy highlights why screening is required as late as 35–37 weeks' gestational age for the IAP strategy to be effective, which is concordant with another study in pregnant women [18]. In our study, if women had been screened at 31–35 weeks, 29.1% (42/141) of those who were colonized at 37+ would not have had IAP offered to them and a lesser proportion (13.3%; 48/366) may have unnecessarily received IAP as they were no longer colonized at 37+ weeks. Although we did not identify any demographic characteristics associated with new acquisition or clearance of GBS, additional risk factors such as sexual activity during pregnancy were not fully explored [19]. The PPV of GBS cultures obtained from 20–35 weeks varied in serotype distribution compared to that at 37+ weeks. The prevalence of different GBS serotypes in a particular population can affect the PPV of late antenatal GBS cultures.

The high cumulative prevalence of GBS colonization (49.7%) found in our study is comparable to longitudinal studies from Denmark and Zimbabwe [8,10]. Furthermore, the prevalence of colonization observed by us at 37+ weeks of gestational age was 28.4% (148/521), which was similar to that reported in cross-sectional studies from Europe [20] and USA [21]. The prevalence of GBS colonization from African countries ranges from 16.5% in Malawi, 21–23% in The Gambia, Ethiopia and Tanzania and 31.6% in Zimbabwe [22,23,24,25,26]. Our results also showed a decrease in the prevalence of GBS colonization with respect to increase in gestational age. This finding agrees with studies from the USA and Australia [9,27] but contrasts with others that reported an increase in colonization with increasing gestational age [28,29].

Our findings on the dominant serotypes are comparable with serotype distribution data of maternal colonizing isolates from industrialized countries, including 13% to 35% for serotype Ia and 15% to 44% for serotype III [6]. The identification of serotype IX in our study was notable in that it is rarely reported in colonizing studies and not previously described in Africa. To our knowledge, only 8 GBS colonizing isolates have been identified as serotype IX, including three from Denmark, two from Germany and one each from Canada, Hong Kong and Australia [30]. Our data on PI distribution is comparable to earlier published studies [7,31] showing that all GBS isolates carried at least one PI, and were

Table 5. Predictive value for 20–25, 26–30 and 31–35 weeks cultures in relation to culture status at 37+ weeks.

Serotype	20–25 weeks		26–30 weeks		31–35 weeks	
	PPV % (95% CI)	NPV % (95% CI)	PPV % (95% CI)	NPV % (95% CI)	PPV % (95% CI)	NPV % (95% CI)
Overall GBS	53.4 (45.4–61.2)	84.3 (80.0–88.0)	61.7 (53.5–69.4)	87.0 (83.0–90.3)	67.4 (59.1–74.9)	88.3 (84.6–91.5)
Ia	36.6 (25.5–48.9)	94.5 (91.9–96.4)	49.2 (36.1–62.3)	95.5 (93.2–97.2)	55.0 (41.7–67.9)	96.2 (94.0–97.8)
Ib	25.0 (3.9–65.0)	99.0 (97.7–99.7)	66.7 (22.7–94.7)	99.4 (98.3–99.9)	75.0 (20.3–95.9)	99.2 (98.0–99.8)
II	38.5 (14.0–68.4)	98.8 (97.4–99.6)	54.6 (23.5–83.1)	99.0 (97.7–99.7)	75.0 (42.8–94.2)	99.6 (98.5–99.9)
III	58.9 (45.0–71.9)	95.8 (93.5–97.4)	62.8 (48.1–75.9)	95.6 (93.3–97.3)	67.9 (53.7–80.1)	96.5 (94.3–98.0)
IV	50.0 (12.4–87.6)	100 (99.2–100)	60.0 (15.4–93.5)	100 (99.2–100)	75.0 (20.3–95.9)	100 (99.3–100)
V	26.7 (8.0–55.1)	97.2 (95.3–98.4)	47.6 (25.8–70.2)	98.4 (96.8–99.3)	57.1 (28.9–82.2)	98.0 (96.3–99.0)
IX	100 (19.3–100)	99.6 (98.6–99.9)	50.0 (12.4–87.6)	99.8 (98.9–100)	100 (30.5–100)	99.8 (98.9–100)

PPV: Positive predictive value, NPV: Negative predictive value, CI-Confidence interval.

associated with the presence of either PI-2a or PI-2b identified alone or in combination with PI-1.

Our study is limited by the sensitivity of detection of GBS on selective media which is estimated at 85% [11] and by the fact that in most cases only the dominant serotype was determined. This can lead to an underestimation of persistent colonization, an overestimation of new acquisitions, and an underestimation of the duration of carriage.

Recent developments in the clinical evaluation of a tri-valent GBS polysaccharide-protein conjugate vaccine has renewed interest in the potential of this vaccine to protect neonates against invasive GBS disease by reducing recto-vaginal colonization during pregnancy [32]. The findings of this study will be important in considering study design when evaluating the efficacy of maternal GBS vaccination protecting against GBS recto-vaginal acquisition and colonization during pregnancy as surrogate information on clinical vaccine efficacy may be gained by determining the immune responses that correlate with protection against serotype-specific GBS acquisition and colonization during pregnancy.

Acknowledgments

We acknowledge the contribution of the lab staff Bianca Smith and Makhosazana Sibeko.

We thank the antenatal staff of Lillian Ngoyi, Mofolo, Diepkloof and Michael Maponya community clinics in Soweto for all their help and support and the participating pregnant women for selflessly volunteering their participation.

Author Contributions

Conceived and designed the experiments: GK PVA EJB CLC SAM. Performed the experiments: GK PVA. Analyzed the data: GK PVA TS. Contributed reagents/materials/analysis tools: TS CLC. Wrote the paper: GK PVA EJB CLC SAM.

References

1. Verani JR, McGee L, Schrag SJ (2010) Prevention of perinatal group B streptococcal disease-revised guidelines from CDC, 2010. MMWR Recommendations and reports : Morbidity and mortality weekly report Recommendations and reports/Centers for Disease Control 59: 1–36.
2. Chan SHS WK, Lee WH (2000) Review on Group B Streptococcal Infection. HK J Paediatr (New Series) 5: 8.
3. Schrag SJ, Schuchat A (2004) Easing the burden: characterizing the disease burden of neonatal group B streptococcal disease to motivate prevention. Clinical infectious diseases: an official publication of the Infectious Diseases Society of America 38: 1209–1211.
4. Baker CJ, Kasper DL (1976) Correlation of maternal antibody deficiency with susceptibility to neonatal group B streptococcal infection. The New England journal of medicine 294: 753–756.
5. Baker CJ, Edwards MS, Kasper DL (1981) Role of antibody to native type III polysaccharide of group B Streptococcus in infant infection. Pediatrics 68: 544–549.
6. Ippolito DL, James WA, Tinnemore D, Huang RR, Dehart MJ, et al. (2010) Group B streptococcus serotype prevalence in reproductive-age women at a tertiary care military medical center relative to global serotype distribution. BMC infectious diseases 10: 336.
7. Madzivhandila M, Adrian PV, Cutland CL, Kuwanda L, Madhi SA (2013) Distribution of pilus islands of group B streptococcus associated with maternal colonization and invasive disease in South Africa. Journal of medical microbiology 62: 249–253.
8. Hansen SM, Uldbjerg N, Kilian M, Sorensen UB (2004) Dynamics of Streptococcus agalactiae colonization in women during and after pregnancy and in their infants. Journal of clinical microbiology 42: 83–89.
9. Goodman JR, Berg RL, Gribble RK, Meier PR, Fee SC, et al. (1997) Longitudinal study of group B streptococcus carriage in pregnancy. Infect Dis Obstet Gynecol 5: 237–243.
10. Mavenyengwa RT, Afset JE, Schei B, Berg S, Caspersen T, et al. (2010) Group B Streptococcus colonization during pregnancy and maternal-fetal transmission in Zimbabwe. Acta obstetricia et gynecologica Scandinavica 89: 250–255.
11. Kwatra G, Madhi SA, Cutland CL, Buchmann EJ, Adrian PV (2013) Evaluation of Trans-Vag broth, colistin-nalidixic agar, and CHROMagar StrepB for detection of group B Streptococcus in vaginal and rectal swabs from pregnant women in South Africa. J Clin Microbiol 51: 2515–2519.
12. Afshar B, Broughton K, Creti R, Decheva A, Hufnagel M, et al. (2011) International external quality assurance for laboratory identification and typing of Streptococcus agalactiae (Group B streptococci). Journal of clinical microbiology 49: 1475–1482.
13. Poyart C, Tazi A, Reglier-Poupet H, Billoet A, Tavares N, et al. (2007) Multiplex PCR assay for rapid and accurate capsular typing of group B streptococci. Journal of clinical microbiology 45: 1985–1988.
14. Foxman B, Gillespie B, Manning SD, Howard LJ, Tallman P, et al. (2006) Incidence and duration of group B Streptococcus by serotype among male and female college students living in a single dormitory. American journal of epidemiology 163: 544–551.
15. Davies HD, Adair C, McGeer A, Ma D, Robertson S, et al. (2001) Antibodies to capsular polysaccharides of group B Streptococcus in pregnant Canadian women: relationship to colonization status and infection in the neonate. The Journal of infectious diseases 184: 285–291.
16. Madzivhandila M, Adrian PV, Cutland CL, Kuwanda L, Schrag SJ, et al. (2011) Serotype distribution and invasive potential of group B streptococcus isolates causing disease in infants and colonizing maternal-newborn dyads. PloS one 6: e17861.
17. Madhi SA, Radebe K, Crewe-Brown H, Frasch CE, Arakere G, et al. (2003) High burden of invasive Streptococcus agalactiae disease in South African infants. Annals of tropical paediatrics 23: 15–23.
18. Manning SD, Lewis MA, Springman AC, Lehotzky E, Whittam TS, et al. (2008) Genotypic diversity and serotype distribution of group B streptococcus isolated from women before and after delivery. Clinical infectious diseases: an official publication of the Infectious Diseases Society of America 46: 1829–1837.
19. Meyn LA, Moore DM, Hillier SL, Krohn MA (2002) Association of sexual activity with colonization and vaginal acquisition of group B Streptococcus in nonpregnant women. American journal of epidemiology 155: 949–957.
20. Motlova J, Strakova L, Urbaskova P, Sak P, Sever T (2004) Vaginal & rectal carriage of Streptococcus agalactiae in the Czech Republic: incidence, serotypes distribution & susceptibility to antibiotics. The Indian journal of medical research 119 Suppl: 84–87.
21. Campbell JR, Hillier SL, Krohn MA, Ferrieri P, Zaleznik DF, et al. (2000) Group B streptococcal colonization and serotype-specific immunity in pregnant women at delivery. Obstet Gynecol 96: 498–503.
22. Suara RO, Adegbola RA, Baker CJ, Secka O, Mulholland EK, et al. (1994) Carriage of group B Streptococci in pregnant Gambian mothers and their infants. The Journal of infectious diseases 170: 1316–1319.
23. Joachim A, Matee MI, Massawe FA, Lyamuya EF (2009) Maternal and neonatal colonisation of group B streptococcus at Muhimbili National Hospital in Dar es Salaam, Tanzania: prevalence, risk factors and antimicrobial resistance. BMC Public Health 9: 437.
24. Musa Mohammed DA, Woldeamanuel Y, Demissie A (2012) Prevalence of group B Streptococcus colonization among pregnant women attending antenatal clinic of Hawassa Health Center, Hawassa, Ethiopia. Ethiop J Health Dev 26(1): 36–42.
25. Dzowela T KO, Lgbigbia A (2005) Prevalence of group B Streptococcus colonization in antenatal women at the Queen Elizabeth Central Hospital Blantyre-a preliminary study. Malawi Med J 17: 97–99.
26. Moyo SR, Mudzori J, Tswana SA, Maeland JA (2000) Prevalence, capsular type distribution, anthropometric and obstetric factors of group B Streptococcus (Streptococcus agalactiae) colonization in pregnancy. The Central African journal of medicine 46: 115–120.
27. Gilbert GL, Hewitt MC, Turner CM, Leeder SR (2002) Epidemiology and predictive values of risk factors for neonatal group B streptococcal sepsis. Aust N Z J Obstet Gynaecol 42: 497–503.
28. Zamzami TY, Marzouki AM, Nasrat HA (2011) Prevalence rate of group B streptococcal colonization among women in labor at King Abdul-Aziz University Hospital. Archives of gynecology and obstetrics 284: 677–679.
29. Baker CJ, Barrett FF, Yow MD (1975) The influence of advancing gestation on group B streptococcal colonization in pregnant women. American journal of obstetrics and gynecology 122: 820–823.
30. Slotved HC, Kong F, Lambertsen L, Sauer S, Gilbert GL (2007) Serotype IX, a Proposed New Streptococcus agalactiae Serotype. Journal of clinical microbiology 45: 2929–2936.
31. Margarit I, Rinaudo CD, Galeotti CL, Maione D, Ghezzo C, et al. (2009) Preventing bacterial infections with pilus-based vaccines: the group B streptococcus paradigm. The Journal of infectious diseases 199: 108–115.

32. Edwards MS, Gonik B (2013) Preventing the broad spectrum of perinatal morbidity and mortality through group B streptococcal vaccination. Vaccine 31 Suppl 4: D66–71.

5

Dual Extraction of Essential Oil and Podophyllotoxin from Creeping Juniper (*Juniperus horizontalis*)

Charles L. Cantrell[1]*, **Valtcho D. Zheljazkov**[2], **Camila R. Carvalho**[1,3], **Tess Astatkie**[4],
Ekaterina A. Jeliazkova[2], **Luiz H. Rosa**[3]

1 Natural Products Utilization Research Unit, Agricultural Research Service, United States Department of Agriculture, University, Mississippi, United States of America,
2 Sheridan Research and Extension Center, University of Wyoming, Sheridan, Wyoming, United States of America, 3 Laboratory of Systematic and Biomolecules of Fungi,
Microbiology Department, Institute of Biological, Sciences Federal University of Minas Gerais, Belo Horizonte, Minas Gerais, Brazil, 4 Faculty of Agriculture, Dalhousie
University, Truro, Nova Scotia, Canada

Abstract

Juniperus horizontalis Moench (Family Cupressaceae), commonly called creeping juniper, is a widely distributed species in the United States and much of Canada. It is potentially a source for two important chemical products, the anticancer drug synthetic precursor, podophyllotoxin and essential oils. The objectives of this study were to ascertain the likelihood of utilizing *J. horizontalis* needles for the simultaneous production of both (−)-podophyllotoxin and essential oil components and to determine the optimum distillation time (DT) needed for the production of essential oil containing a specific ratio of constituents. Eleven different distillation times were tested in this study: 20, 40, 80, 160, 180, 240, 480, 600, 720, 840, and 960 min. Total essential oil content increased with increasing distillation time from a minimum of 0.023% at 20 min to a maximum of 1.098% at 960 min. The major constituents present in the oil were alpha-pinene, sabinene, and limonene. The percent concentration of sabinene in the essential oil varied from a high of 46.6% at 80 min to a low of 30.2% at 960 min, that of limonene changed very little as a result of distillation time and remained near 30% for all distillation times, whereas the concentration of alpha-pinene was 9.6% at 20 min DT and decreased to 4.2% at 960 min. Post distillation analysis of needles revealed elevated amounts of (−)-podophyllotoxin remaining in the tissue varied in the amount of podophyllotoxin present, from a low of 0.281% to a high of 0.364% as compared to undistilled needles which gave 0.217% podophyllotoxin. As a result of this study, specific essential oil components can now be targeted in *J. horizontalis* by varying the distillation time. Furthermore, needles can be successfully utilized as a source of both essential oil and podophyllotoxin, consecutively.

Editor: Ing-Feng Chang, National Taiwan University, Taiwan

Funding: This research was partially funded by the University of Wyoming startup funding awarded to Dr. Zheljazkov. C.R. Carvalho was supported by Fundação de Apoio a Pesquisa de Minas Gerais (FAPEMIG) and L.H. Rosa by Conselho Nacional de Desenvolvimento Científico e Tecnológico (CNPq). The funders had no role in study design, data collection and analysis, decision to publish, or preparation of the manuscript.

Competing Interests: The authors have declared that no competing interests exist.

* Email: charles.cantrell@ars.usda.gov

Introduction

Juniperus species are cultivated worldwide and commonly found from sea level to above timberline. In many parts of North America *Juniperus* species have become almost weedy in nature and have invaded millions of acres of rangeland and farms [1]. The genus *Juniperus* consists of 67 species and recent reports have identified *Juniperus horizontalis* Moench as a possible source for the anticancer drug precursor, podophyllotoxin [2,3]. Creeping juniper (*J. horizontalis*) is commonly grown as an ornamental and its oil is useful in apothecary, fragrance, and pharmaceutical industries.

Podophyllum species such as the Himalayan mayapple (*Podophyllum hexandrum* Royle) are sources of (−)-podophyllotoxin, a lignan useful in the semi-synthesis of commercially used cancer treating drugs such as etoposide and teniposide [2,4,5,6]. These compounds have been used for the treatment of lung cancer, testicular cancer, neuroblastoma, hepatoma, and other tumors [7,8]. *P. hexandrum* is reportedly intensively collected and utilized for bulk extraction and production of (−)-podophyllotoxin. Some

reports have suggested it may become endangered due to overharvesting as the demand for (−)-podophyllotoxin derived drugs continues to increase [9]. Despite the reports on progress and improvements towards the total synthesis of (−)-podophyllotoxin, many fall short at becoming economically feasible in a commercial process. A more viable alternative domestic source of (−)-podophyllotoxin seems to be *Juniperus* species.

Essential oils and cedarwood oils from *Juniperus* species, primarily *J. virginiana*, are used in the fragrance and flavor industry [10]. While limited research has been done on extracts of the needles of *J. horizontalis* [11,12,13], the essential oil obtained from the wood of the plant (cedarwood oil) is used in a broad range of products and known for unique properties, such as aroma and toxicity that repel and kill many pests [14].

Previously, it was shown that podophyllotoxin does not degrade during a 90-min steam distillation of *J. virginiana* [15] and hence it may be possible to obtain intact podophyllotoxin following steam distillation. It was also reported that for maximum essential oil yield, female *J. scopulorum* needed to be distilled for at least

240 min [16], whereas male *J. scopulorum* needed to be distilled for 840 min [17]. Previous authors reported essential oil composition of *J. horizontalis*, however, the biomass was extracted for 90 min [2], or 120 min [11,12,13]. These shorter durations of DT may not have extracted the total oil, and secondly, the oil composition might have been different depending on the duration of the distillation time (DT).

The hypothesis of this study was that the duration of distillation time may affect essential oil yield and composition of *J. horizontalis*, and that podophyllotoxin may not degrade during extended distillation times of 12 or more hours. Furthermore, the duration of the distillation time may be used to obtain essential oil with specific chemical profile. Therefore, the objectives of this study were: (1) to ascertain the likelihood of utilizing *J. horizontalis* needles for the simultaneous production of both (−)-podophyllotoxin and essential oil components and (2) to determine the optimum distillation time needed for the production of essential oil containing the lowest/highest purity possible for a particular constituent(s).

Materials and Methods

2.1. Plant material and growing conditions

The plant material used in this study was collected in the Big Horn Mountains on 5 December, 2012. The plant material was obtained from a single creeping juniper plant, #131, which in a previous study, was identified to have relatively high concentration of podophyllotoxin [18]. This specific plant was found at elevation of 2,070 m above the sea level, with GPS coordinates N 440 37.108′ W 1070 05.072′. This juniper was identified as creeping juniper by Ms. Bonnie Heidel, a botanist at the Wyoming Natural Diversity Database, University of Wyoming [18]. Permission for sampling of junipers in the Big Horn Mountains National Forest was issued to Dr. Valtcho Jeliazkov by Mr. Clarke McClung, Tongue District Ranger on March 7, 2012 {authorization ID: TNG551, from U.S. Department of Agriculture, Forest Service, Temporary Special use permit with expiration date 12/31/2012 (FSH 2709.11 sec.54.6, Authority Organic Administration Act June 4, 1897)}.

2.2. Essential oil extraction

The essential oils were extracted via steam distillation, in 2-L steam distillation units as previously described [15,19]. Fresh samples (500 g) consisted of leaves (needles) and smaller than 2 mm in diameter branches. Prior to distillation, the samples were chopped into 2.5 cm long pieces. There were 11 different distillation times tested in this study as follows: 20, 40, 80, 160, 180, 240, 480, 600, 720, 840, and 960 min. These distillation times were selected based on previous trials with Rocky Mountain juniper, *J. socpulorum* [17]. The times were measured from the beginning of the distillation (when the first drop of essential oil was deposited in the Florentine); at the end of the distillation time the heating was cut off, the steam removed, the Florentine was also removed and the essential oil decanted. Each essential oil sample was weighed on analytical scale and kept in a freezer at minus 5°C until the gas chromatography analyses can be performed.

2.3. Gas chromatography-FID analysis of the essential oils

The essential oil samples of creeping juniper (all samples in three replicates) were analyzed on a gas chromatograph (GC, Hewlett Packard model 6890, Hewlett-Packard, Palo Alto, CA, USA). The carrier gas was helium at a flow rate of 40 cm/sec, 11.7 psi (60°C), 2.5 ml/min constant flow rate. The injection was split 60:1, 0.5 μL, the injector temperature was 220°C. The GC oven temperature program was as follows: 60°C for 1 min, 10°C/min to 250°C. The column was HP-INNOWAX (cross-linked PEG; 30 m × 0.32 mm × 0.5 μm), and the flame ionization detector (FID) temperature was set to 275°C. Individual constituents of the creeping juniper essential oils are expressed as percentage of the total oil. The identification of individual constituent peaks was done with the use of internal standards, by retention time and by mass-spectroscopy.

2.4 Quantitative analysis of podophyllotoxin

Podophyllotoxin analysis was performed essentially as described previously [2,20]. Briefly, 40 mg of each dry tissue sample was incubated at 20°C with 0.6 mL of 25 mM potassium phosphate buffer (pH of 7.0) on an Eppendorf Thermomixer R for 30 min at 750 rpm. Subsequently, 0.6 mL of ethyl acetate was added, and the incubation continued for an additional 5 min in the same manner. The aqueous and organic partitions were separated by centrifuge (Savant speed vac, svc 200). The organic layer was removed using a Pasteur pipette and evaporated under a stream of N_2, leaving the organic soluble material to be dissolved in methanol (100%) and analyzed by HPLC. Extracts were analyzed using an HPLC system (Agilent 1100 series consisting of a vacuum degasser, quaternary pump, ALS autosampler, a diode array detector, and an Agilent Eclipse XDB-C18, 4.6 mm × 150 mm, 5 μm column). The injection volume for all samples and for the podophyllotoxin standard was 10 μL and standards and samples were analyzed at 21°C. An analytical isocratic method was used (28% acetonitrile: 72% deionized water with 0.1% TFA) for 20 min followed by a 5 min column wash with methanol and a 10 minute re-equilibration. Analytes were detected at 220 nm.

Podophyllotoxin was purchased from Sigma-Aldrich (St. Louis, MO). Individual concentration gradients were prepared for podophyllotoxin to obtain a standard curve using five concentration points imposed by using response factors and regression coefficients independently. Response factors were calculated using the equation RF = DR/C, where DR was the detector response in peak area (PA) and C was the podophyllotoxin concentration. Confirmed integrated peaks were then used to determine the percentage of podophyllotoxin in the extract. The RF of the target chemical constituent was used to determine the "percent" for each sample using the equation: PA/RF/C × 100 = % (peak area/response factor/concentration) in the plant tissue.

2.5. Statistical analysis

The effect of distillation time on essential oil content, and the concentration of alpha-thujene, alpha-pinene, sabinene, myrcene, alpha-terpinene, limonene, gamma-terpinene, terpinolene, 4-terpineol, pregeijerene B, delta-cadinene, elemol, and podophyllotoxin was determined using a one-way analysis of variance. For each response, the validity of model assumptions was verified by examining the residuals as described in Montgomery [21]. Since the effect of distillation time was significant (p-value < 0.05) on all responses, multiple means comparison was completed using Duncan's multiple range test at the 5% level of significance, and letter groupings were generated. The analysis was completed using the GLM Procedure of SAS [22].

The relationship between distillation time and essential oil content, and the concentration of alpha-thujene, alpha-terpinene, gamma-terpinene, terpinolene, delta-cadinene, elemol, was adequately described by the Power – concave (Eq. 1, with $\theta_2 > 0$), the relationship between distillation time and the concentration of alpha-pinene was adequately described by the Power - convex (Eq. 1, with $\theta_2 < 0$), and that between distillation time and the concentration of sabinene, myrcene, limonene, 4-terpineol, and pregeijerene B was described by either a second order (Eq. 2) or a third order (Eq. 3) polynomial. While the Power model is nonlinear, the second and third order polynomial models are linear. The parameters of the nonlinear model were estimated iteratively using the NLIN Procedure of SAS [22].

$$Y = \theta_1 X^{\theta_2} + \varepsilon \tag{Eq.1}$$

$$Y = \beta_0 + \beta_1 X + \beta_2 X^2 + \varepsilon \tag{Eq.2}$$

$$Y = \beta_0 + \beta_1 X + \beta_2 X^2 + \beta_3 X^3 + \varepsilon \tag{Eq.3}$$

Where Y is the dependent (response) variable, X is the independent (distillation time) variable, and the error term ε is assumed to have normal distribution with constant variance.

Results and Discussion

Total essential oil content increased with increasing distillation time (Table 1) from a minimum of 0.023% at 20 min to a maximum of 1.098% at 960 min. A plot of distillation time versus essential oil content together with a fitted Power-concave model that described the relationship very well is shown in Figure 1. A steady and significant increase was observed from 20 min to 840 min. Overall, the effect of distillation time relative to each individual constituent was significant.

The percent concentration of alpha-thujene in the essential oil was also adequately described by a Power-concave model (Figure 1) and increased from around 1% at 20–160 min to a maximum of 1.5% at 720 min; further increase of the duration of the DT to 960 min did not affect the concentration of this oil constituent (Table 1). Similarly, alpha-terpinene (Figure 1), gamma-terpinene (Figure 1), terpinolene (Figure 1), delta-cadinene (Figure 1), elemol (Figure 2), all can be adequately described by the Power-concave model.

The percent concentration of alpha-terpinene in the essential oil increased from a low of 0.57% at 20 min to a maximum of 1.76% at 720 min (Table 1). The percent concentration of limonene in the essential oil changed very little as a result of distillation time (Table 1) and remained near 30% for all distillation times. The percent concentration of gamma-terpinene in the essential oil increased from a low of 0.91% at 20 min to a maximum of 2.91% at 720 min (Table 1). Terpinolene percent concentration in the essential oil increased from a low of 0.923% at 20 min to a maximum of 1.333% at 600 min (Table 1). Delta-cadinene percent concentration in the essential oil increased from a low of 0.273% at 20 min to a maximum of 1.440% at 960 min (Table 1). Elemol percent concentration in the essential oil increased from a low of 0.51% at 20 min to a maximum of 9.41% at 960 min (Table 1).

The percent concentration of alpha-pinene in the essential oil can be adequately described by a Power-convex model (Figure 2) and decreased from a high of 9.62% at 20 min to a 4.7% at 80 min; further increase of DT did not significantly change the concentration of this constituent (Table 1). Alpha-pinene was the only constituent to follow a declining (convex) pattern.

The percent concentration of sabinene in the essential oil can be adequately described by a third order polynomial model (Figure 2) and varied from a high of 46.6% at 80 min to a low of 30.2% at 960 min (Table 1). Pregeijerene B was the only other constituent

to adequately follow a third order polynomial model. Pregeijerene B percent concentration in the essential oil varied from a high of 2.78% at 240 min to a low of 1.60% at 20 min (Table 1).

Limonene (Figure 2) and 4-terpineol (Figure 2) can be adequately described by a second order polynomial model. Limonene percent concentration in the essential oil varied from a high of 30.6% at 240 min to a low of 29.5% at 40 min (Table 1). 4-terpineol percent concentration in the essential oil varied from a low of 0.83% at 20 min to a high of 2.38% at 600 min (Table 1).

The essential oil composition of the *J. horizontalis* in this study was dissimilar to the one reported previously [2], in which the plant material was distilled for 90 min. For example, the major oil constituents at 80 min DT in the present study were 4.7% alpha-pinene, 46.6% sabinene, 2.3% myrcene, 29.8% limonene, while the oil constituents in *J. horizontalis* in [2] were 0.47% beta-pinene, 1.82% myrcene, and 36.6% limonene. These differences might be due to different genetic material used in the two studies: wild collected *J. horizontalis* from the Big Horn Mountains in Wyoming was used in this study, whereas the *J. horizontalis* in [2] was the ornamental variety 'Plumosa compacta'.

Furthermore, reported [12] essential oil composition of *J. horizontalis* extracted for 120 min, contained 1.7% alpha-pinene, 37.2% sabinene, 2.8% myrcene, 3.5% limonene, 3.9% terpinen-4-ol, and was comparable to the essential oil composition obtained at 80 or 160 min DT in the present study (Table 1). The *J. horizontalis* analyzed by [12] was collected along the Saskatchewan River in Saskatoon, Canada (52.1333° N, 106.6833° W), which is approximately at the same western longitude as the Big Horn Mountains in Wyoming, USA (N 44°37.108′ N, W 107°05.072′).

Our study demonstrated the need for longer duration of the DT in order to extract the total oil from *J. horizontalis*. A study [11] reported 0.33 and 0.38% oil content in juvenile and adult leaves of *J. horizontalis* extracted for 2 hours, which corresponds to the 0.33% oil content at 160 min DT in our study. However, our study showed that the actual total oil content of *J. horizontalis* when extracted for 840 or 960 min was over 1.0%, which is 3 times higher than the one reported in previous studies [11,2].

Podophyllotoxin quantitative analysis was performed essentially as described previously [2,20] using HPLC methods. *J. horizontalis* needles that were not extracted using steam distillation gave 0.217% podophyllotoxin. The amount of podophyllotoxin in needles that had been used for steam distillation varied from a low of 0.281% at a 720 min distillation to a high of 0.364% for a 40 min distillation. Interestingly, the concentration of podophyllotoxin in the unextracted samples was significantly less than its concentration in the extracted samples from all DT. Perhaps this can be explained by the fact that much of the podophyllotoxin that exists in the plant is likely in the form of a glycoside and not an aglycone. The distillation may be converting much of the glycoside into its corresponding aglycone (and sugar) by hydrolysis. Canel et al. reported on this conversion; however, more research is needed to address this phenomenon [20].

Although collected from the same plant, podophylloxin concentration in this study was lower than the previously reported 0.457% [18]. These differences were most probably due to the different sampling time and seasonal variations in podophyllotoxin concentrations: the samples in [18] were collected in March 2012, while the samples in this study were collected in Dec, 2012. The podophylotoxin concentration in *J. horizontalis* in this study was higher than previously reported podophylotoxin concentration for two *J. horizontalis* ornamental varieties 'Wiltonii' (0.138%) and 'Plumosa Compacta' (0.351%) [2]. The results from this and

Table 1. Mean essential oil content (%)[b], and the concentrations (%)[c] of alpha-thujene, alpha-pinene, sabinene, myrcene, alpha-terpinene, limonene, gamma-terpinene, terpinolene, 4-terpineol, pregeijerene B, delta-cadinene, elemol, and podophyllotoxin content (%)[d] in extracted or unextracted samples.

DT (min)	Essent. oil content	Alpha-thujene	Alpha-pinene	Sabinene	Myrcene	Alpha-terpinene	Limonene	Gamma-terpinene	Terpinolene (%)	4-Terpineol	Pregeijerene B	Delta-cadinene	Elemol	Podophyllotoxin
					%[a]									
20	0.023 i	0.97 d	9.62 a	44.2 b	2.23 cd	0.57 f	29.6 abc	0.91 h	0.923 f	0.83 e	1.60 c	0.273 g	0.51 f	0.363 a
40	0.082 h	0.99 d	7.42 b	45.5 ab	2.30 abcd	0.68 f	29.5 bc	1.06 gh	0.943 ef	1.11 de	1.91 c	0.350 g	0.72 f	0.364 a
80	0.162 g	0.97 d	4.69 c	46.6 a	2.30 abcd	0.86 e	29.8 abc	1.35 fg	1.000 de	1.52 cd	2.40 b	0.387 g	1.31 e	0.344 abc
160	0.329 f	1.07 cd	4.31 c	43.8 bc	2.39 ab	1.05 d	30.2 abc	1.68 e	1.073 c	1.98 ab	2.62 ab	0.547 f	2.45 d	0.336abcd
180	0.460 e	1.15 c	4.41 c	44.5 b	2.41 a	0.95 de	30.5 ab	1.54 ef	1.047 cd	1.78 bc	2.65 ab	0.677 e	2.22 d	0.356 a
240	0.566 d	1.16 c	4.40 c	42.0 c	2.35 abc	1.01 d	30.6 a	1.64 e	1.060 cd	1.79 bc	2.78 a	0.883 d	3.40 c	0.353 ab
480	0.892 b	1.41 ab	4.31 c	37.9 d	2.22 cd	1.20 c	30.5 ab	1.96 d	1.093 c	1.76 bc	2.57 ab	1.200 b	5.56 b	0.329abcd
600	0.830 c	1.33 b	4.10 c	32.2 e	2.26 bcd	1.66 ab	30.3 ab	2.78 ab	1.333 a	2.38 a	2.63 ab	1.060 c	7.87 a	0.298 bcd
720	0.939 b	1.46 a	4.40 c	31.6 ef	2.22 cd	1.76 a	29.9 abc	2.91 a	1.330 a	2.22 a	2.48 ab	1.027 c	8.40 a	0.281 d
840	1.045 a	1.49 a	4.54 c	31.8 ef	2.20 d	1.57 b	30.0 abc	2.59 c	1.243 b	1.95 ab	2.48 ab	1.317 b	8.23 a	0.325abcd
960	1.098 a	1.49 a	4.19 c	30.2 f	2.19 d	1.58 b	29.1 c	2.66 bc	1.277 ab	1.71 bc	2.57 ab	1.440 a	9.41 a	0.290 cd
Unextracted														0.217 e

[a]Within each column, means followed by the same letter are not significantly different at the 5% level of significance.
[b]Percentage of essential oil by weight in fresh plant material.
[c]Percentage of each analyte in essential oil by weight.
[d]Percentage of podophyllotoxin by weight in dry needles.

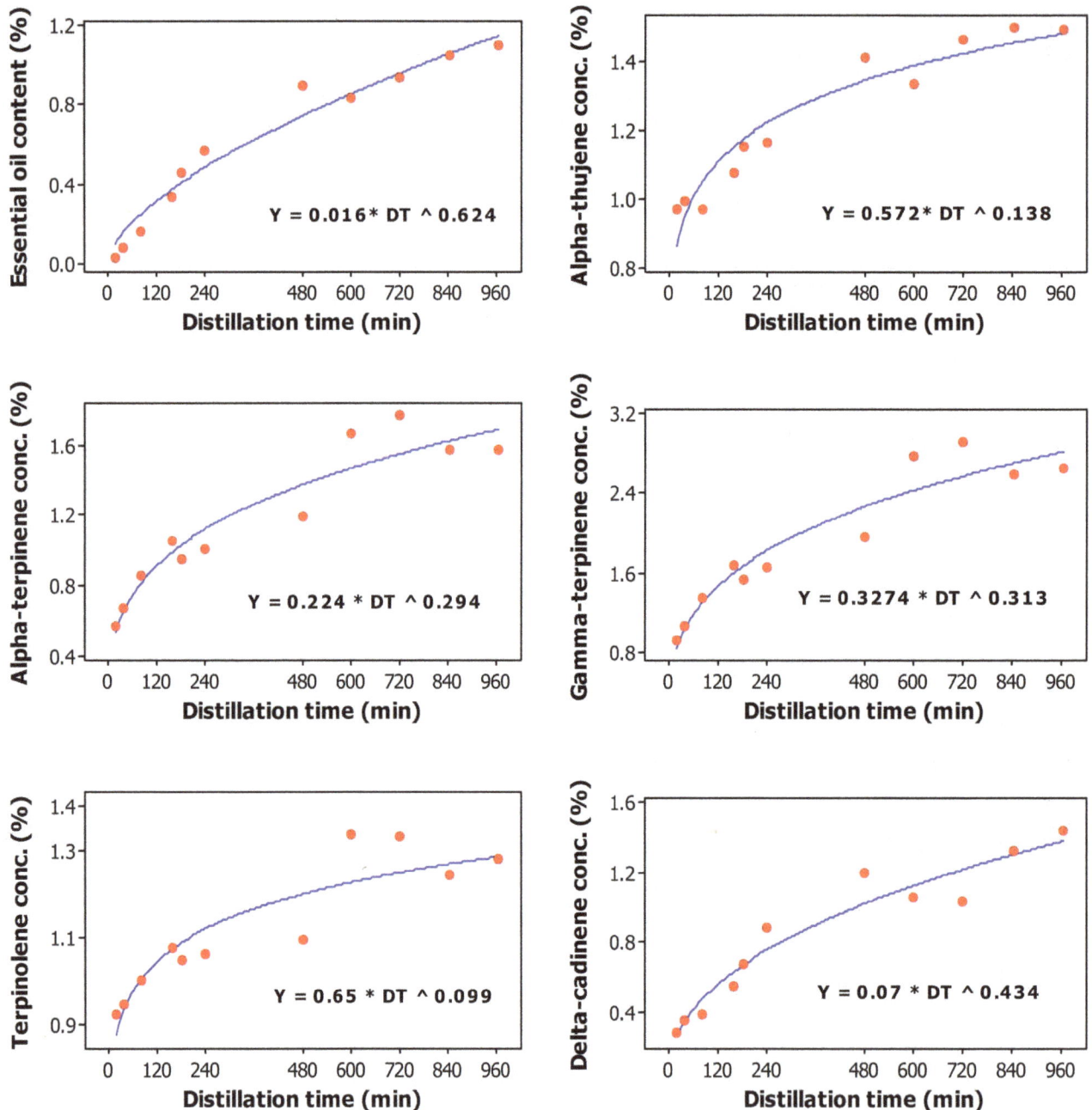

Figure 1. Plot of Distillation time versus essential oil content (wt/wt%) and the concentration in essential oil (%) of alpha-thujene, alpha-terpinene, gamma-terpinene, terpinolene, and delta-cadinene along with the fitted (solid line) Power–concave regression model.

previous studies indicate podophylotoxin may vary significantly due to the genetic material /collection site and collection time.

Conclusions

As a result of this study, it has been demonstrated that *J. horizontalis* needles can be successfully utilized as a source of essential oil and podophyllotoxin simultaneously. It was demonstrated that the total essential oil content of *J. horizontalis* was over 1%, which is approximately 3 times higher than that reported previously. In order to obtain the total amount of oil, *J. horizontalis* biomass must be steam distilled for at least 840 min.

It has also been shown that podophyllotoxin yield from needles may increase as a result of steam distillation. The length of steam distillation did not dramatically affect the podophyllotoxin yield. Furthermore, specific essential oil components can now be targeted in *J. horizontalis* by varying the DT, or an essential oil with a desirable composition can be generated. The findings of this study demonstrated the need for reporting the duration of DT when reporting oil content and composition of *J. horizontalis*.

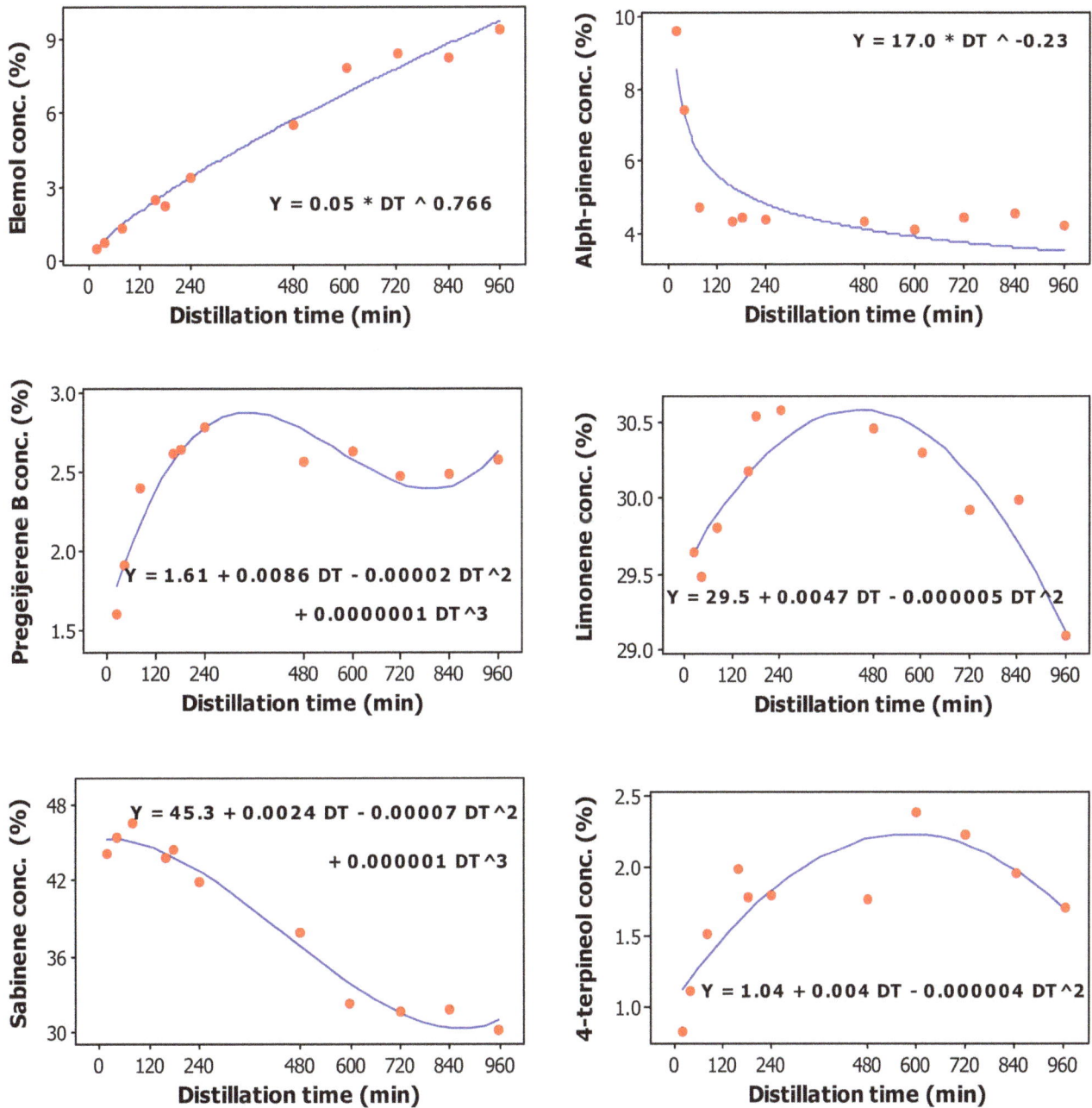

Figure 2. Plot of Distillation time versus the content (wt/wt%) in essential oil of elemol, alpha-pinene, pregeijerene B, limonene, sabinene, and 4-terpineol along with the fitted (solid line) Power–concave (elemol), Power-convex (alpha-pinene), third order polynomial (pregeijerene B, sabinene), and Second order polynomial (limonene, 4-terpineol) regression models.

Acknowledgments

Authors thank Amber Reichley and Solomon Green III for assistance with podophyllotoxin quantitative analysis. This research was partially funded by the University of Wyoming startup funding awarded to Dr. Zheljazkov. We thank the Forest Service of the U.S. Department of Agriculture for issuing us a permit to sample junipers in the Bighorn National Forest. We thank Mr. Travis Fack, Natural Resource Specialist, and Mr. Clarke McClung, Tongue District Ranger, for helping with the permit. We thank Mr. Lyn Ciampa for his help with the collections of junipers in the Big Horn Mountains. C.R. Carvalho was supported by Fundação de Apoio a Pesquisa de Minas Gerais (FAPEMIG) and L.H. Rosa by Conselho Nacional de Desenvolvimento Científico e Tecnológico (CNPq).

Author Contributions

Conceived and designed the experiments: CLC VDZ TA EAJ LR. Performed the experiments: CLC VDZ TA EAJ CC LR. Analyzed the data: CLC VDZ TA EAJ CC LR. Contributed reagents/materials/analysis tools: CLC VDZ TA EAJ CC LR. Contributed to the writing of the manuscript: CLC VDZ TA EAJ CC LR.

References

1. Adams RP (2008) Junipers of the World: The genus *Juniperus*. Trafford Publishing: 2nd ed. Victoria BC Canada.
2. Cantrell CL, Zheljazkov VD, Osbrink WA, Castro-Ruiz A, Maddox V, et al. (2013) Podophyllotoxin and essential oil profile of *Juniperus* and related species. Ind Crop Prod 43: 668–676.
3. Zheljazkov VD, Cantrell CL, Donega MA, Astatkie T (2013) Bioprospecting for podophyllotoxin in the Big Horn Mountains, Wyoming. Ind Crops Prod 43: 787–790.
4. Koulman A, Quax WJ, Pras N (2004) Biotechnology of medicinal plants: Vitalizer and therapeutic: podophyllotoxin and related lignans produced by plants; Ramawat, K. G., Ed.; Science Publishers: Enfield, NH.
5. Kusari S, Zeuhlke S, Spiteller M (2011) Chemometric evaluation of the anti-cancer pro-drug podophyllotoxin and potential therapeutic analogues in *Juniperus* and *Podophyllum* species. Phytochem Anal 22: 128–143.
6. Marques JV, Kim KW, Lee C, Costa MA, May GD, et al. (2013) Next generation sequencing in predicting gene function in podophyllotoxin biosynthesis. J Biol Chem 288(1): 466–479.
7. Stahelin HF, Wartburg AV (1991) The chemical and biological route from podophyllotoxin to etoposide. Cancer Res 51: 5–15.
8. Imbert F (1998) Discovery of podophyllotoxins. Biochimie 80: 207–222.
9. Nadeem M, Palni LMS, Purohit AN, Pandly H, Nandi SK (2000) Propagation and conservation of *Podophyllum hexandrum* Royle: An important medicinal herb. Biol Conserv 92: 121–129.
10. Panten J, Bertram HJ, Surburg H (2004) New woody and ambery notes from cedarwood and turpentine oil. Chem Biodivers 1(12): 1936–1948.
11. Adams RP, Palma MM, Moore WS (1981) Examination of the volatile oils of mature and juvenile leaves of *Juniperus horizontalis*: Chemosystematic significance. Phytochemistry 20: 2501–2502.
12. Adams RP (2009) The leaf essential oil of J. maritima R. P. Adams compared with *J. horizontalis*, *J. scopulorum* and *J. virginiana* oils. Phytologia 91(1): 31–39.
13. Palma-Otal M, Moore WS, Adams RP, Joswiak GR (1983) Genetic and biogeographical analyses of natural hybridization between *Juniperus virginiana* and *J. horizontalis* Moench. Can J Bot 61: 2733–2746.
14. Mourad AK, Zaghloul OA, El Kady MB, Nemat FM, Morsy ME (2005) A novel approach for the management of the chalkbrood disease infesting honeybee *Apis mellifera* L. (Hymenoptera: Apidae) colonies in Egypt. Commun Agric Appl Biol Sci 70(4): 601–611.
15. Gawde AJ, Cantrell CL, Zheljazkov VD (2009) Dual extraction of essential oil and podophyllotoxin from *Juniperus virginiana*. Ind Crops Prod 30: 276–280.
16. Zheljazkov VD, Astatkie T, Jeliazkova E, Tatman AO, Schlegel V (2012) Distillation time alters essential oil yield, composition and antioxidant activity of female *Juniperus scopulorum* trees. JEOR 25(1): 62–69.
17. Zheljazkov VD, Astatkie T, Jeliazkova EA, Schlegel V (2012) Distillation time alters essential oil yield, composition, and antioxidant activity of male *Juniperus scopulorum* trees. J Oleo Sci 61(10): 537–546.
18. Zheljazkov VD, Cantrell CL, Donega MA, Astatkie T, Heidela B (2012) Podophyllotoxin Concentration in Junipers in the Big Horn Mountains in Wyoming. HortScience 47(12): 1696–1697.
19. Gawde AJ, Zheljazkov VD, Maddox V, Cantrell CL (2009) Bioprospection of Eastern red cedar from nine physiographic regions in Mississippi. Ind Crop Prod 30: 59–64.
20. Canel C, Dayan FE, Ganzera M, Khan IA, Rimando A, et al. (2001) High yield of podophyllotoxin from leaves of *Podophyllum peltatum* by in situ conversion of podophyllotoxin-4-O-β-D-glucopyranoside. Planta Medica 67: 97–99.
21. Montgomery DC (2013) Design and analysis of experiments. 8th ed. Wiley: New York.
22. SAS Institute Inc (2010) SAS/STAT 9.3 User's Guide. SAS Institute Inc. Cary: NC.

6

High Throughput Micro-Well Generation of Hepatocyte Micro-Aggregates for Tissue Engineering

Elien Gevaert[1], Laurent Dollé[2], Thomas Billiet[3], Peter Dubruel[3], Leo van Grunsven[2], Aart van Apeldoorn[4], Ria Cornelissen[1]*

1 Tissue Engineering Group, Ghent University, Ghent, Belgium, 2 Liver cell biology laboratory, Vrije Universiteit Brussels (VUB), Brussels, Belgium, 3 Polymer Chemistry and Biomaterials Research Group, Ghent University, Ghent, Belgium, 4 Department of Developmental Bioengineering, University of Twente, Enschede, the Netherlands

Abstract

The main challenge in hepatic tissue engineering is the fast dedifferentiation of primary hepatocytes in vitro. One successful approach to maintain hepatocyte phenotype on the longer term is the cultivation of cells as aggregates. This paper demonstrates the use of an agarose micro-well chip for the high throughput generation of hepatocyte aggregates, uniform in size. In our study we observed that aggregation of hepatocytes had a beneficial effect on the expression of certain hepatocyte specific markers. Moreover we observed that the beneficial effect was dependent on the aggregate dimensions, indicating that aggregate parameters should be carefully considered. In a second part of the study, the selected aggregates were immobilized by encapsulation in methacrylamide-modified gelatin. Phenotype evaluations revealed that a stable hepatocyte phenotype could be maintained during 21 days when encapsulated in the hydrogel. In conclusion we have demonstrated the beneficial use of micro-well chips for hepatocyte aggregation and the size-dependent effects on hepatocyte phenotype. We also pointed out that methacrylamide-modified gelatin is suitable for the encapsulation of these aggregates.

Editor: Michiya Matsusaki, Osaka University, Japan

Funding: This work was supported by the IWT_SBO Grant 090066 HepStem from the 'Agentschap voor Innovatie door Wetenschap en Technologie'. LD and LvG: Interuniversity Attraction Poles (IAP) - phase VII - contract P7/47 (Federal Science Policy –BELSPO) (10/2012-09/2017); Brustem: Impulse program 2011-IP-LS-104 – Brustem (Brussels Government) (06/2011-05/2014). The funders had no role in study design, data collection and analysis, decision to publish, or preparation of the manuscript.port not to have conflicts of interest and the funders had no role in study design, data collection and analysis, decision to publish, or preparation of the manuscript.

Competing Interests: The authors have declared that no competing interests exist.

* Email: Ria.Cornelissen@UGent.be

Introduction

Upon isolation of their native micro-environment, hepatocytes rapidly lose their viability and metabolic functions. [1] This limits or prevents their use for clinical, engineering and research purposes. The prolonged maintenance of hepatocyte phenotype could e.g. lead to the development of an engineered donor tissue, bioartificial liver device, more efficient transplantation methods, the development of more reliable *in vitro* models thereby improving drug toxicity screening, liver disease research and many more. [2,3]

To improve hepatocyte performance many strategies have been addressed. One approach is the cultivation of hepatocytes as aggregates, allowing enhanced cell-cell contacts in a three dimensional context. Cell-aggregates can be considered as micro-tissues and are more representative for liver tissue than conventional two dimensional cell cultures. Different techniques such as static cell culture on non-adherent surfaces or micro patterned surfaces, hanging drop and rotary culture systems have been used for creating hepatocyte aggregates with variable dimensions. [4] These studies have demonstrated that the cultivation of hepatocytes as aggregates improves many of their metabolic functions such as cytochrome P450 activity, albumin secretion, urea production, glutathione S-transferase activity, etc. [5,6] [4,7]

Most living tissues, including the liver, are composed of repeating cellular units on a scale of hundreds of microns. Artificially generated three dimensional cell aggregates comprising hepatocytes could potentially serve as functional building blocks for the creation of larger constructs. [8] Assembly of these building blocks into larger constructs with more relevant dimensions, can be obtained by self-assembly or assembly in a more directed way using biomaterials to guide this process. [9,10] In this context, the immobilization and organization of the aggregates at high density, while allowing mass transport of nutrients and metabolites for hepatocyte survival and function, could be useful. [4],[8]

In this study, we used a microwell-based tissue culture platform to generate large quantities of hepatocyte aggregates of predefined dimensions and shapes. We observed that aggregate dimensions affect the overall performance of the hepatocytes and selected the most optimal aggregation parameters. Combining these well defined primary hepatocyte aggregates with a gelatin methacrylamide hydrogel allows the encapsulated aggregates to maintain a proper hepatocyte phenotype. The present work demonstrates the generation of large amounts of relatively small aggregates that can be organized into larger constructs by encapsulation in a gelatin hydrogel. [11,12]

Materials and Methods

The study protocol was approved by the Ethical committee for Animal Care and Use of Ghent University (permit number ECD 12/42). Institutes of Health principles of laboratory animal care (NIH) were followed.

2.1. Cell culture and isolation of primary hepatocytes

HepG2 cells were maintained in DMEM Glutamax supplemented with 10% v/v FBS, 50 U/ml penicillin and 50 µg/ml streptomycin, all provided by Life Technologies.

Primary mouse hepatocytes were isolated from adult mouse livers (ICR CD-1 mice, 8–14 weeks of age, Harlan Laboratories). The animals were anaesthetized with ketamin/xylazin and died during the perfusion procedure. The hepatocytes were isolated from the liver using a two-step collagenase perfusion method, followed by percoll gradient purification as described by Conçalves et al [13]. After isolation, cells were immediately seeded in microwells, or well plates coated with 0.1% collagen (BD Biscienses), in order to compare three dimensional with two-dimensional cell culture.

Primary hepatocytes were cultured in William's E medium (Life Technologies), supplemented with L-glutamine (292 mg/ml) (Life Technologies), glucagon (7 ng/ml) (sigma), insulin (0.5 µg/ml) (sigma), hydrocortisone (25 µg/ml), EGF (10 ng/ml), 10% v/v FBS (Life Technologies), 50 U/ml penicillin (Life Technologies) and 50 µg/ml streptomycin (Life Technologies).

Both the HepG2 cells and the primary hepatocytes were maintained in a humidified 5% CO_2-containing atmosphere at 37°C.

2.2. Micro-well synthesis and micro-aggregate formation

To produce the non-adherent agarose micro-wells, sterilized powder Ultrapure Agarose (Life Technologies) was dissolved (3% w/v) and heated in PBS. The liquid agarose solution was added to a tailor-made, negative polydimethylsiloxane mold (PDMS, as described previously [14,15]) and left to solidify at RT. After cooling, the gels were separated from the moulds and subsequently transferred into 12 well culture plates. Single cell suspensions of various densities (detailed information in table 1 and table 2) were seeded in the chip containing the micro-wells. After seeding, formation of micro-aggregates was supported by centrifugation for 1 min at 1500 rpm to let the cells settle into the bottom of the

micro-wells. Culture medium was replenished 24 h after seeding and cells were left in culture for 3 days to allow formation of stable micro-aggregates. The aggregates were harvested at different time points, as indicated in the results section.

Aggregate diameter, perimeter (p) and aggregate area (A) was determined using Xcellence image software. Subsequently circularity was calculated using the formula $f_{circ} = (4\pi A)/p^2$.

Aggregate volume was determined based on the diameter and the volume formula of a spherical object. The number of cells per aggregates was estimated, based on the number of microwells per chip and the amount of seeded cells per chips. All aggregate characteristics and parameters are represented in table 1 and table 2.

2.3. Aggregate encapsulation

Gelatin methacrylamide with a degree of substitution (DS) of 65% was used to encapsulate aggregates as described earlier.[16] Briefly, aggregates (2300 aggregates/ml) were mixed in dissolved gelatin (10% w/v in PBS) with 2 mol % Irgacure 2959 photo-initiator, as calculated relative to the (photo-sensitive) methacrylamide side groups. The aggregate-gelatin mixture was transferred (200 µl/well) into 48 well plates (Greiner Bio-one) and left for physical gelation during 30 min. Photocross-linking was carried out by exposure to UV-A light (365 nm, 2 mW/cm^2, UVP Inc.) for 10 min. After cross-linking, culture medium was added and refreshed every 24 h.

2.4. Cell viability

To assess the cell viability, aggregates were washed twice with PBS and incubated for 10 minutes with 2 µg/ml calcein-AM (AnaSpec) and 2 µg/ml propidium iodide (PI) (Sigma). After washing in PBS for 10 min, cell viability was evaluated by determining the ratio of green (live) versus red (dead) cells using an inverted fluorescence microscope (Olympus IX81) equipped with Xcellence software (Olympus).

2.5. Histology

Samples were fixed (4% paraformaldehyde) and embedded in paraffin. Five µm thick sections were stained with hematoxilin and eosin (HE), Periodic acid Schiff (PAS) or immunostained (IHC), all at room temperature.

For IHC staining, endogenous peroxidase was quenched using 3% v/v H_2O_2 for 1 h, and a 30 min treatment with blocking reagent (1% w/v BSA, 0.2% v/v Tween 20 in PBS) was performed. The samples were incubated with the primary antibody (dilution 1:100) for 2 h and subsequently with the

Table 1. Overview of the applied parameters for HepG2 cells and primary hepatocytes and their characteristics.

Seeded number of cells/chip	Mean aggregate diameter (µm)	Mean number of cells/aggregate	Mean aggregate volume (µm^3)	Diameter of micro-wells in the chip
1000000	307±13	629	15120449	400 µm
750 000	297±9	472	13745009	400 µm
500 000	261±15	314	9255967	400 µm
250 000	231±7	157	6479261	400 µm
1 000 000	166±11	87	2408105	200 µm
750 000	157±9	175	2010823	200 µm
500 000	142±7	262	1489732	200 µm
250 000	116±9	349	810959	200 µm

Table 2. Overview of the applied parameters for primary hepatocytes and their characteristics.

Seeded number of cells/chip	Mean aggregate diameter (µm)	Mean number of cells/aggregate	Mean aggregate volume (µm³)	Diameter of micro-wells in the chip
150 000	185±16	94	3336782	400 µm
75 000	90±13	47	385917	400 µm
150 000	95±13	52	452331	200 µm
75 000	60±8	26	111241	200 µm

secondary antibody (dilution 1:200) for 30 min. A goat anti-mouse albumin antibody (p20, Santa Cruz) and a rabbit anti-mouse HNF4α (H-171, Santa Cruz) was used as primary antibody for albumin and HNF4α respectively. A 3,3-diaminobenzidine tetrahydrochloride substrate was used to visualize the horse radish peroxidase coupled secondary antibody. After hematoxylin staining and mounting, the samples were visualized under the microscope. For HNF4α the whole staining procedure was preceded by antigen retrieval using citrate buffer (pH 6.00).

For PAS stain, the samples were treated with 1% v/v periodic acid for 15 min. After washing with PBS, samples were exposed to Schiff reagent (Sigma) for 30 minutes in the dark. After rinsing in water, the slides were stained with hematoxylin and mounted.

For transmission electron microscopy, aggregates were fixed with glutaraldehyde, postfixed with OsO_4 and embedded in epoxy resin. Sections (70 µm thick) were evaluated by a Jeol 1200 EX II electron microscope.

2.6. Cytochrome activity

Cyp3A4 activity of the primary hepatocyte aggregates was analyzed using a P450-Glo-CYP3A assay (Promega) according to the manufacturer's protocol for cell-based assays. After 72 h culture in the micro-wells, aggregates were exposed for 1 h to culture media containing luciferin-IPA (1:1000). After 1 h, an equal volume of the liquid was transferred to a 96 well plate and incubated with an equal volume of detection reagent. After 20 min, luciferase activity was detected using a Wallac 1420 Victor³ multilabel counter (Perkin Elmer). The detected luminescence was normalized for the amount of cells (MTT assay). Background subtraction was performed with culture medium considered as negative control.

2.7. Albumin secretion

To assess albumin secretion, media samples were collected at different time points. After omitting cross-reactivity for bovine albumin, the amount of secreted albumin was determined using a mouse albumin ELISA quantitation kit or a human albumin ELISA quantitation kit (Bethyl laboratories, Inc., UK) and normalized for the amount of cells using an MTT assay.

2.8. MTT assay

The hepatocytes were incubated with a 0.5 mg/ml solution of MTT (Calbiochem) in culture medium for four hours in the dark in a 5% CO_2 incubator at 37°C. After discarding the MTT solution, the formed formazan crystals were dissolved in isopropanol-0.04N HCl supplemented with 1% v/v Triton X100 (Sigma). Subsequently the absorbance was measured at 580 nm using an EL800 Universal microplate reader (BioTek instruments Inc.) and compared to a standard curve.

2.9. Real Time Polymerase chain reaction (RT-PCR)

Total RNA was extracted from hepatocyte aggregates using TRI Reagent (Sigma-aldrich) and treated with DNAse digestion kit (Invitrogen). RT Core Kit (Eurogentec) was used to synthesize cDNA, according to the manufacturer's protocol. A 7500 Fast Real-Time PCR system (Applied Biosystems) and a SYBR Green PCR kit (Eurogentec) were used according to the manufacturer's instructions and protocols. GAPDH expression was used as stable housekeeping marker for reference. The relative gene fold changes were determined by the $2^{-\Delta\Delta Ct}$ method. For comparative gene expression analysis of free floating aggregates gene expression was compared to expression levels of freshly isolated hepatocytes. Additionally, to assess the effect of hydrogel embedding, encapsulated hepatocyte aggregates were compared to aggregates before encapsulation (day 3). Primer sequences are depicted in table S1 and S2.

2.10. Statistical Analysis

Differences between groups were explored by one-way ANOVA, followed by a Student t-test using the statistical package GraphPad Prism 4 (San Diego California, USA).

Results

3.1. Development of micro-aggregates with controlled size

Tailor-made PDMS molds were used to generate agarose microwell-containing chips. Briefly, liquid agarose was poured on top of PDMS molds containing micro-sized cylindrical sticks. After solidifying, the PDMS molds were removed from the agarose resulting in agarose chips containing micro-sized wells. (illustrated fig. S1) The fabrication of these micro-well-containing chips resulted in micro-well array chips containing 2865 or 1585 wells with a diameter of 0.2 or 0.4 mm respectively in agarose. After fabrication, the chips were placed in a 12 well plate and used for controlled hepatocyte aggregation.

First, the micro-aggregation procedure was optimized using HepG2 cells. Although this human hepatocellular carcinoma cell line is less representative of the *in vivo* situation, these cells are user-friendly, robust and aggregate easily while maintaining some hepatocyte specific functions. Subsequently the procedure was adapted and performed using primary mouse hepatocytes. The micro-aggregation behavior of and its effect on these cells was evaluated and compared.

For both cell types, aggregate formation started from day 1 (fig. 1A). In addition, we observed that stable aggregates were formed within 3 days, which was accompanied by an increase in E-cadherin expression (fig. 1B). By varying parameters such as micro-well diameter, cell number and cell type, aggregates with different dimensions were obtained (fig. 1C–E). All applied parameters in relation to and affecting aggregate dimension are listed in tables 1 and 2. Aggregate diameters (φ) varied between 100 and 300 μm for HepG2 cells and between 50 to 200 μm for primary hepatocytes. The linear relation between aggregate volume and cell number observed in fig.1C–D, the constant circularity values starting from day 2 (fig. 1F) and microscopic observation indicate that the aggregates were spherical and uniform in size.

3.2. Hepatocyte specific performance is enhanced and is size dependent in micro-aggregates

For HepG2 aggregates, size dependent correlation of hepatocyte gene expression markers such as albumin, HNF4a and TTR was observed (fig. S6) and albumin secretion (fig. S7) was clearly enhanced for all conditions. It appeared that HepG2 cells are not very sensitive for variations in aggregate size shortly after aggregate formation (day 3, fig. S2), however 7 days after aggregate formation the smaller aggregates (φ≤231±7 μm) maintained higher hepatocyte-specific gene expression levels than the larger aggregates (φ≥261±15 μm). At this time point a

substantial amount of dead cells was observed in the center of the larger (φ≥261±15 μm diameter) aggregates (fig. S3).

The gene expression and protein secretion of albumin, an important serum protein produced by the liver, was evaluated and normalized using primary hepatocyte aggregates and compared to primary hepatocytes plated on collagen 1 coated tissue culture plates (TCP) 3 days after isolation (fig. 2 A–B). In some aggregates both gene expression as well as protein secretion was significantly (p<0.05) enhanced compared to the control culture. However, clear differences in both secretion (fig. 2B) and gene expression (fig. 2A) were observed between aggregates of different sizes with a significant enhancement of both secretion (p<0.01) and gene expression (p<0.001) for 95±13 μm diameter aggregates. Analysis of the albumin secretion at day 7 after isolation indicated a general drop in albumin secretion for all conditions. However the differences between aggregates of different sizes remained and the 95±13 μm aggregates maintained the highest albumin secretion levels. (fig. S4)

A significant (p<0.05) improvement, compared to cells cultured as monolayers, in both cyp3A enzyme activity (fig. 2D) and gene expression (fig. 2C) was noticed for the 95.2±12.5 μm and

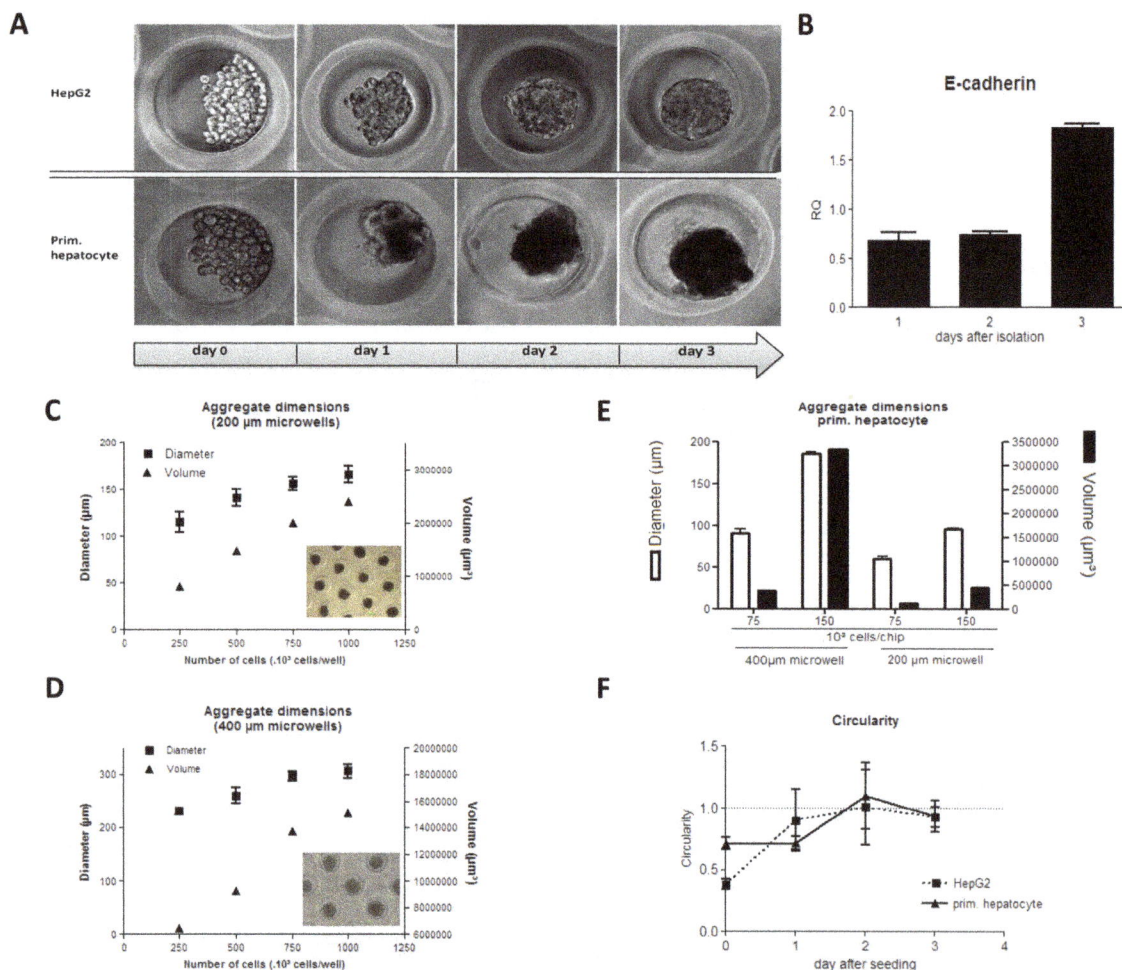

Figure 1. Formation of hepatocyte micro-aggregates in agarose microwells. (**A**) Aggregate formation over time for both HepG2 cells and primary hepatocytes. (**B**) E-cadherin gene expression in primary hepatocytes during aggregate formation (**C–D**) Correlation between number of cells, aggregate diameter (squares) and volume (triangles) for the formation of HepG2 cell aggregates in 200 (C) and 400 μm (D) microwells, n = 3. (**E**) Correlation between number of primary cells, aggregate diameter (solid line) and volume (dotted line) for the formation of primary hepatocyte aggregates in 200 (white squares) and 400 μm (black squares) microwells, n = 3. (**F**) circularity of aggregates during culture for HepG2 cells (squares) and primary hepatocytes (triangles), n = 3.

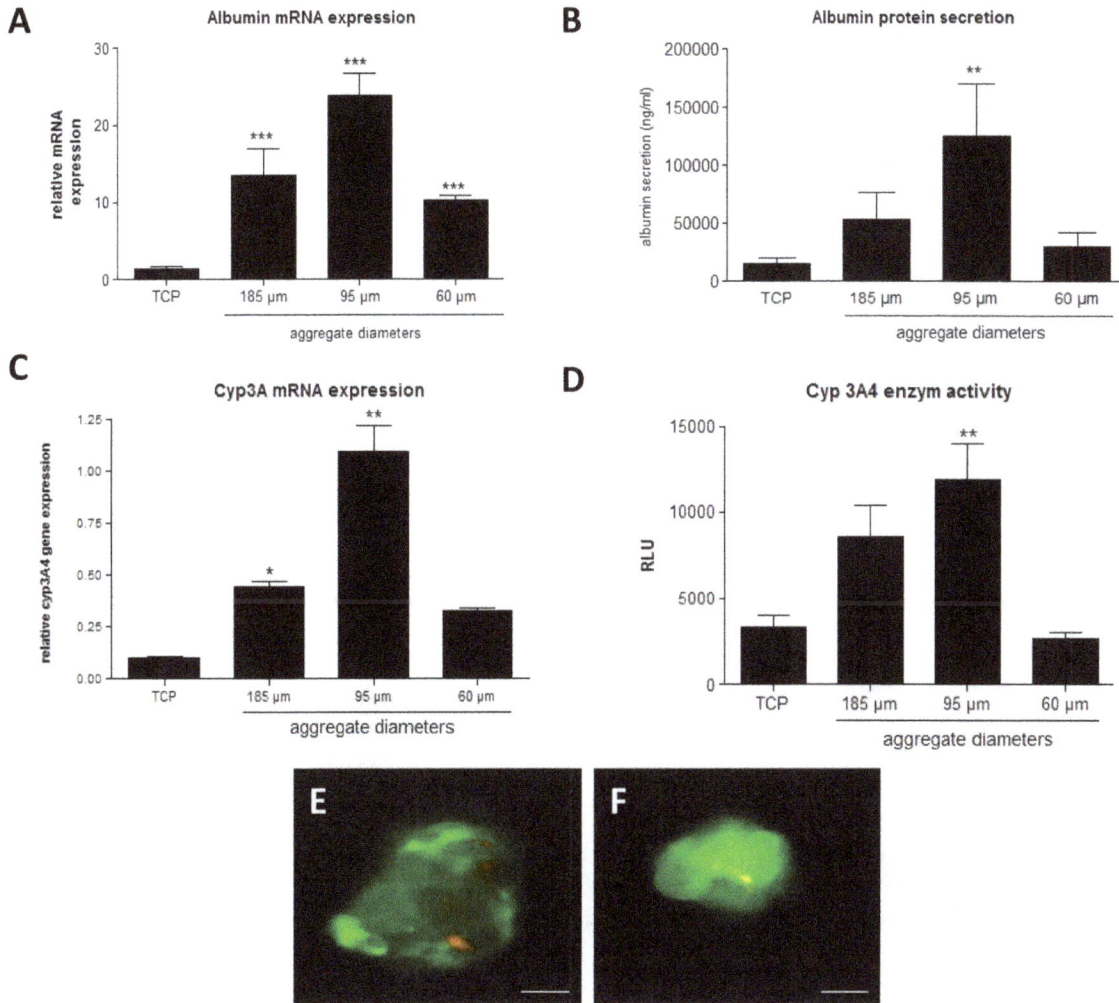

Figure 2. Evaluation of hepatocyte phenotype for different micro-aggregate sizes. (A) Gene expression of albumin. Gene expression levels of albumin were determined for different micro-aggregation conditions and compared to cells cultured on tissue culture plastic (TCP). **(B)** Albumin secretion at day 3 after isolation for different micro-aggregation conditions. *Data are mean ± SD, n = 3, **p<0,01; compared to cells cultivated as monolayers (TCP).* **(C)** Gene expression of CypA3. Gene expression levels of Cyp3A for different aggregate dimensions compared to cells cultured on tissue culture plates (TCP). Gene expression of Cyp3A was determined after 72 hours of cultivation in the micro-wells. *Data are mean RQ ± SD, n = 3. *p<0.05; **p<0.01* **(D)** Induced cytochrome 3A4 activity in aggregates of different diameter versus cells cultured on tissue culture plastic. Cyp3A4 activity was quantified after treatment with an inducing agent (hydrocortisone) using a luciferase based assay after 3 days of isolation. *Data are mean ± SEM, n = 3. *p<0,05; **p<0,01; ***p<0,001 compared to cells cultured as monolayers (TCP).* **(E–F)** Live/dead stain of micro-aggregates with diameters of 200 μm (E) and 100 μm (F). Dead cells are stained red, while viable cells are stained green. *scale bar = 50 μm.*

185±16 μm aggregates, while this improvement is less clear for the 60±8 μm aggregate, 3 days after isolation. Different aggregate sizes lead to different cyp3A performance with the medium sized aggregates (φ 95±13 μm, obtained by seeding 150 000 cells in the 200 μm micro-well) displaying the highest activity and the smallest aggregates (φ 60±8 μm) showing the lowest activity 3 days after isolation. The cyp3A4 enzyme activity at day 7 (fig. S5) showed a decrease for all conditions and for cells cultivated as monolayers the activity was not detectable. For the aggregates, the 95±13 μm aggregates displayed the highest cyp3A4 activity when compared to the 185±16 μm and 60±8 μm aggregates.

It was clear that hepatocyte phenotype depends on aggregate parameters and increasing aggregate dimensions did not necessarily lead to better performance. Live/dead staining of the different aggregates indicated excellent cell viability in the aggregates, however more dead cells were observed in the largest aggregates (φ≥185±16 μm, fig. 2E) when compared to the other

aggregates (fig. 2F). This observation could indicate nutritional/waste diffusion limitations and explain why no clear relation between hepatocyte performance and aggregate size was observed.

3.3. Long term hepatocyte function is affected by aggregate dimensions

Since aforementioned results indicated that 95±13 μm diameter primary hepatocyte aggregates performed most optimal, these were further evaluated. The hepatocyte specific function (fig. 3A) of two-dimensional cultured hepatocytes and hepatocyte aggregates were compared to freshly isolated non-cultured hepatocytes over time. At day 10 and 15, no expression of the genes of interest was detected for two-dimensional cultured cells (fig. 3A, TCP N.D.). For all examined genes, aggregates displayed a clear and significant upregulation of albumin, connexin32 (Cx32), hepatocyte nuclear factor 4α (HNF4α), E-cadherin, cyp3A, cytochrome

1A2 (cyp1A2) compared to cells in monolayers. The gene expression of HNF4α, an important transcription factor for the expression of hepatocyte specific genes, was maintained at a similar level in the aggregate as in freshly isolated hepatocytes, and increased over time. Gene expression of Cx32, indicative of gap junctions between cells, and cyp3A, indicative of active phase I metabolism, had decreased. Gene expression of E-cadherin, important for cell-cell adhesion and required for aggregate formation and stability, was upregulated in aggregates when compared to freshly isolated cells and remained stable during 15 days of culture.

The synthesis of albumin and HNF4α protein in the 100 μm aggregate was visualized using IHC staining and storage of glycogen was determined by PAS staining. Albumin secretion was significantly enhanced (2-fold increase) as compared to the plated cells at all time points.

Transmission electron microscopy (fig. S8) showed the presence of narrow contacts (desmosomes and gap junctions) between the cells and normal cell morphology with numerous mitochondria, abundant RER within the cytoplasm of hepatocytes cultured for 10 days in aggregates.

3.4. Micro-aggregates remain viable and functional upon encapsulation in gelatin

For tissue engineering purposes, the creation of larger constructs might be desirable (i.e. for the creation of bio-artificial liver devices, incorporation in a bioreactor). To organize these micro-aggregates at a larger scale, encapsulation and immobilization in a hydrogel could be a useful approach.

Therefore aggregates (φ 95±13 μm) were encapsulated and cultured in a methacrylamide-gelatin hydrogel and gene expression and cell metabolism were compared with non-encapsulated aggregates. The viability of the immobilized aggregates compared to the non-encapsulated aggregates indicated that primary hepatocytes were not affected by the encapsulation procedure. Most of the aggregates maintained their rounded morphology while some cellular outgrowth was observed at day 10 of culture (fig. 4A and B).

Similar gene expression profiles (fig 4D) between encapsulated and non-encapsulated aggregates were found, suggesting that gelatin encapsulation did not affect hepatocyte functions.

Immunohistochemistry on encapsulated aggregates demonstrate that expression of albumin and HNF4α protein was maintained during 10 days of culture. Fig. 4C depicts the cumulative albumin

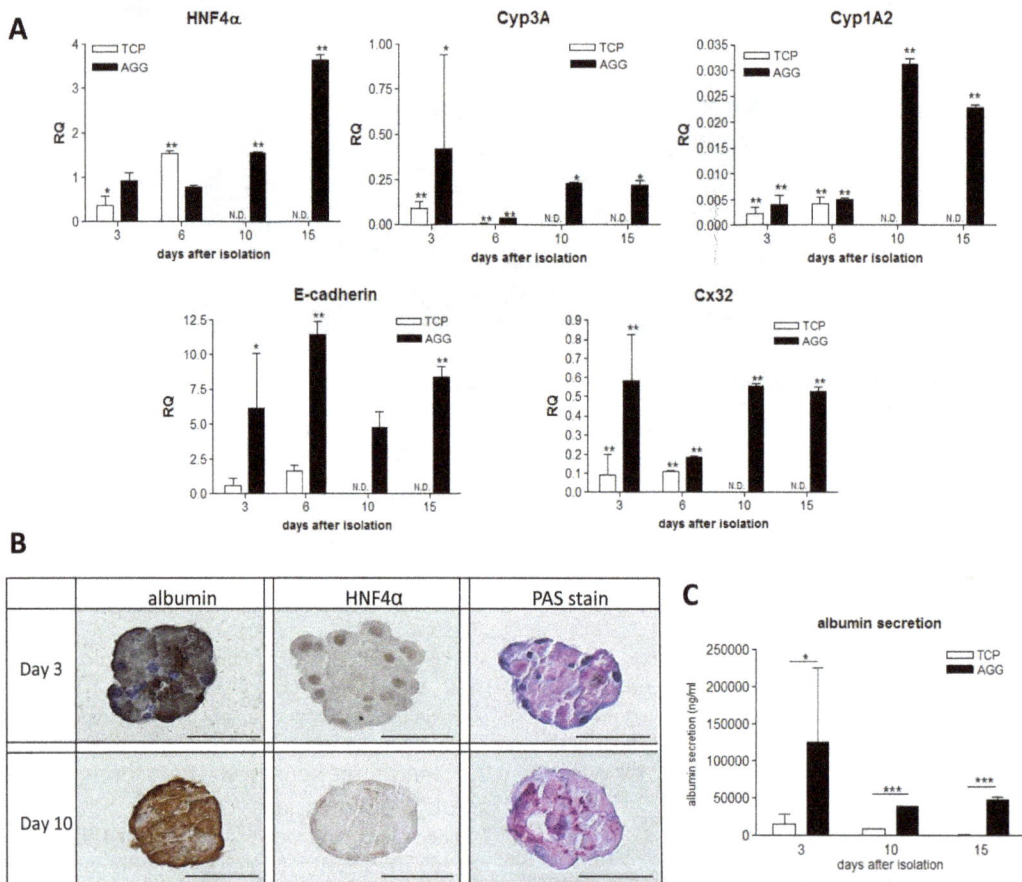

Figure 3. Evaluation of hepatocyte phenotype maintenance in micro-aggregates. (A) Gene expression analysis using real-time PCR. Gene expression of HNF4α, Cyp3A, Cyp1A2, E-cadherin and connexin 32 (Cx32) were determined for cells cultured on tissue culture plastic (white bars, TCP) and aggregates (black bars, AGG) at day 3, 6, 10 and 15 after isolation. The gene expression was normalized using GAPDH as stable housekeeping gene and related to freshly isolated hepatocytes (value = 1). *Data are mean RQ ± SD, compared to freshly isolated, non cultured hepatocytes, n = 3. *p< 0.05; **p<0.01.* **(B)** Albumin, HNF4α, and PAS staining to visualize glycogen storage day 3 and day 10. *scale bar = 50 μm.* **(C)** Albumin secretion of plated cells and microaggregates determined by ELISA. Albumin secretion during 24 hours at day 3, 10 and 15 was evaluated for cells cultured on tissue culture plastic (white bars, TCP) and aggregates (black bars, AGG). * p<0.05, ***p<0.001

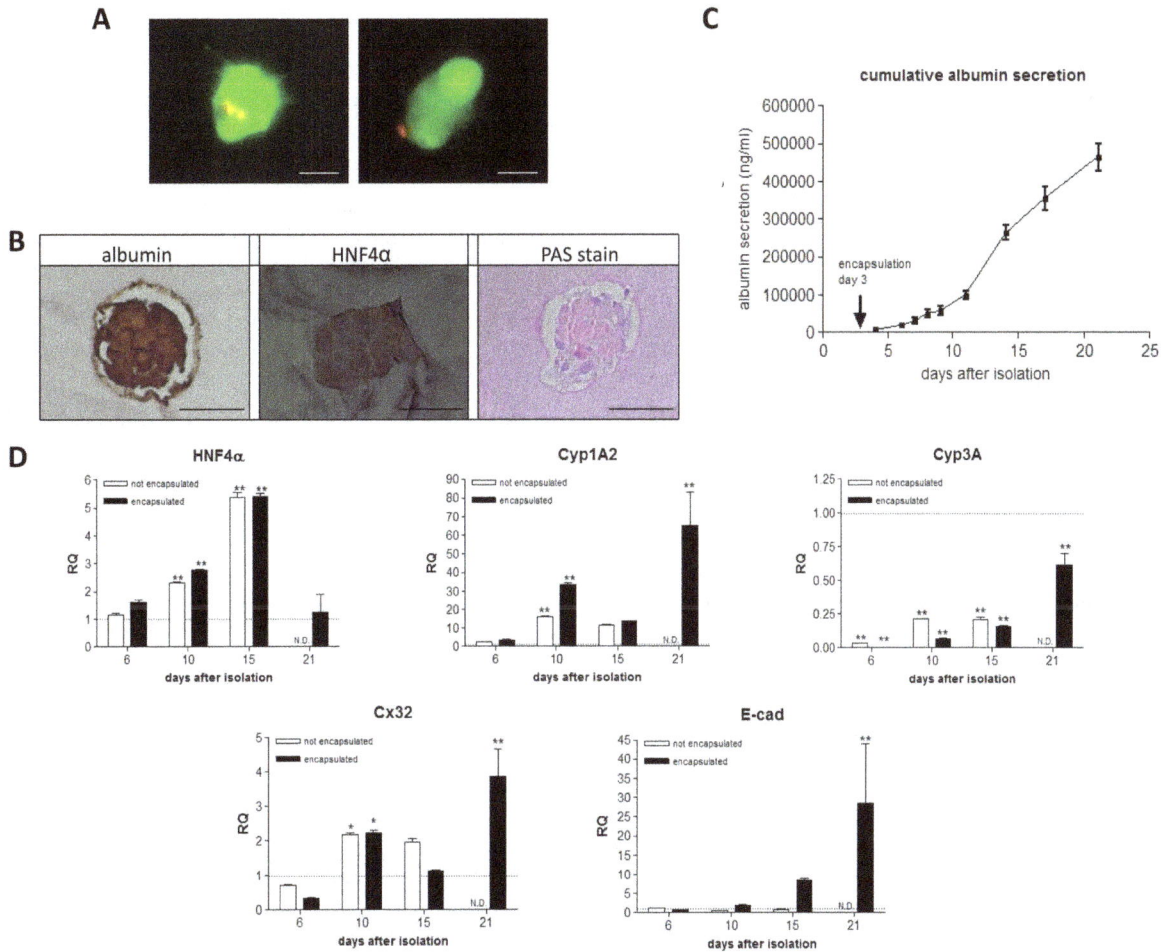

Figure 4. Evaluation of micro-aggregates after encapsulation in a gelatin hydrogel. (**A**) Live/dead stain of aggregates encapsulated in gelatin hydrogel at day 10. *scale bar = 50 μm* (**B**) Stainings of the immobilized micro-aggregates at day 10 after isolation. The pictures represent stainings for albumin and HNF4α and PAS staining to visualize glycogen storage. *Pictures were recorded at 20 x magnification at day 10, scale bar = 50 μm.* (**C**) Cummulative albumin secretion deterimend by ELISA. Albumin secretion of the immobilized cells was evaluated during 21 days of cultivation by ELISA. *Data are mean ± SD, n = 3.* (**D**) Real-time PCR for gene expression analysis after immobilization in the hydrogel. Gene expression levels of HNF4α, Cyp3A4, Cyp1A2, E-cadherin and connexin 32 (Cx32) were determined for not immobilized (white bars, not encapsulated) and immobilized micro-aggregates (black bars, encapsulated) at day 3, 6, 10 and 15 after isolation. The expression values were normalized using GAPDH as stable housekeeping gene and compared to aggregate values before encapsulation (day 3, value = 1). *Data are mean RQ ± SD, n = 3. *$p < 0.05$; **$p < 0.01$*

secretion profile of the immobilized aggregates and suggests that albumin is secreted 21 days during cell culture.

Discussion

Currently, several cell aggregation methods have been described in literature e.g. static cell culture on non-adherent surfaces, hanging drop and rotary culture systems leading to variable aggregate dimensions mostly involving cumbersome technical handling of cells and culture media.[5,6] The creation of large amounts of aggregates with predefined, controlled and uniform sizes in a reproducible and accurate manner is hard to control with the above-mentioned culture techniques and limits further development of aggregate based, or modular tissue engineered constructs. In this study, the potential of an agarose micro-well system has been investigated which allows controlled aggregation of primary hepatocytes into a large number of uniform cell aggregates with predefined dimensions (±50–100–180 μm) within 3 days after cell seeding and isolation from mouse livers. In

addition, we confirm that HepG2 cells, a commonly used hepatocyte cell line, benefit from aggregation and three dimensional cell culture and that their function is increased in the larger aggregates used in this study. This is in line and complementary with studies reporting differentiation and increased expression of several hepatocyte specific markers (such as increased albumin secretion, urea, …) in HepG2 spheroids.[7,17]

For the practice of aggregate based tissue engineering (e.g. the directed assembly of aggregates into larger constructs using bioprinting applications), aggregate uniformity might be important. In these approaches, the use of aggregates with predefined sizes might be desirable as well. Some papers report the improved functional performance of uniform hepatocyte aggregates, formed in PDMS or polystyrene micro-wells. However, the success of these systems was dependent on rotary culture systems and in both papers only aggregates with variable dimensions (ranging from 100–300 μm) have been used for further functional evaluation, assuming that all aggregates perform in the same way.[4,18]

In contrast to the aforementioned studies we demonstrate that hepatocyte performance is directly affected by aggregate size and the number of cells/aggregate. While aggregates of about 200 μm diameter showed enhanced expression of hepatocyte specific markers as compared to cells cultured in monolayers, we found that hepatocyte function was further improved in 95±13 μm diameter aggregates. We observed more dead cells in the centre of the 185±16 μm diameter aggregates, as compared to the 95±13 μm aggregates. This is in contrast to others who observed no cell death in 180 μm diameter aggregates.[4] HepG2 cells were found to be less prone to cell viability effects related to the aggregate size. However, a substantial amount of dead cells was observed in aggregates with diameters exceeding 200 μm. This is in line with the knowledge that spheroids above 200 μm become hypoxic at the core. [19] For HepG2 cells, a substantial amount of dead cells was observed in the centre of the largest aggregates and this was more pronounced at day 7 as compared to day 3. Nevertheless no significant increase in aggregate diameter was observed between these time points (fig. S2). This made us suggest that the HepG2 cells did not proliferate, however we can not completely exclude this possibility since the aggregates might experience a further compactation between day 3 and day 7 while proliferating. The observation that more dead cells were present at day 7 when compared to day 3 for the larger aggregates can be explained as follows: It takes 48–72 hours to form stable aggregates, during that time the cells are more exposed to nutrients and oxygen than after compactation of the spheroid (taking place at 48–72 hours). During the next few days the oxygen and nutrient limitations become more important/limited in the larger spheroids, as a consequence more cells die within the larger aggregates at the later time point.

We postulate that differences in functional performance between 100 μm and 200 μm aggregates can be attributed to an impaired nutrient and oxygen diffusion in the largest aggregates. Our findings are in line with studies modeling mass transfer in hepatocytes indicating 100 μm diameter aggregates as 'ideal'.[20,21] Further decreasing the aggregate diameter to 50 μm did not improve the functional performance of hepatocytes. The dimensions of these aggregates might be too limited to create a functional three dimensional organization with sufficient cells in close contact with each other.

Gene expression of the 95±13 μm aggregate was further evaluated and compared to the gene expression of freshly isolated hepatocytes, reflecting the gene expression in vivo. The expression of HNF4α, an important hepatocyte specific transcription factor, remained unchanged and increased at day 10 and 15 after isolation. The expression of Cx32 and Cyp3A had decreased to 50–75%, indicating some loss of function, but significantly less than in two-dimensional cultured cells. A clear upregulation of E-cadherin, a cell adhesion molecule, expression was observed in the aggregates. This enabled cell aggregation by increasing cell-cell contacts and allowing compactation and is in line with data in literature reporting this increase as necessary for cell aggregation.[22] [23]

To use aggregates as building blocks for modular tissue engineering one needs to organize and immobilize these small aggregate structures into a larger construct while cells remain viable and maintain their appropriate function. Others have described directed assembly of cell-laden microgels for the creation of larger functional pseudo-tissues. [24,25] Here we demonstrate that aggregates can be efficiently encapsulated in cross-linked methacrylamide-gelatin hydrogel, without interfering with cell viability and hepatocyte specific function. We found that encapsulating multiple well defined primary hepatocyte aggregates

into methacrylamide gelatin hydrogel in bulk can already lead to a viable and functional construct without the need for microencapsulating each individual aggregate to form a large functional tissue. Another more practical application of predefined and controlled cell aggregation could be the use of organ specific aggregates for cell printing of large tissue constructs. Our group and others showed that by using gelatin to print hepatocytes such tissue engineered scaffolds can be made without impeding cell viability and function. Printing, or plotting, of hepatocyte aggregates as building blocks in predefined structures with high accuracy, resolution and control over pore dimensions leads to further improvement in mass transport of nutrients and metabolites.[26,27] Our results clearly show that aggregate dimensions need to be carefully considered since aggregate size and cell number affect cell function and survival in a direct manner and that primary hepatocytes seem to function best in aggregates between 90–120 micrometer diameter.

In conclusion our findings show that the suggested agarose microwells are well suited for the large scale production of uniform hepatocyte aggregates. Moreover the results suggest that a selection of aggregate parameters might influence the outcome of the experiment. Our results also demonstrate that a modified gelatin hydrogel might be well suited for the (directed) immobilization of these aggregates in order to generate larger scale constructs for a tissue engineering approach.

Supporting Information

Figure S1   Schematic overview of microwell fabrication.

Figure S2   live/dead fluorescence staining of aggregates in the 400 μm agarose chip. Pictures, recorded at 10x magnification, represent HepG2 aggregates after 3 days (a–d) and 7 days (e–h) of cultivation in the 400 μm agarose chip at variable cell densities yielding aggregates with a diameter of 231 μm (a,e), 261 μm (b,f), 297 μm (c,g) and 307 μm (d,h).

Figure S3   live/dead fluorescence staining of aggregates in the 200 μm agarose chip. Pictures, recorded at 20x magnification, represent HepG2 aggregates after 3 days (a–d) and 7 days (e–h) of cultivation in the 200 μm agarose chip at variable cell densities yielding aggregates with diameters of 116 μm (a,e), 142 μm (b,f), 157 μm (c,g) and 166 μm (d,h).

Figure S4   Albumin secretion of primary hepatocyte aggregates with diverse dimensions 7 days after isolation. Albumin secretion in the cultivation medium during 24 hours is determined by ELISA and normalized using MTT assay. Data are means ± SD (n = 2).

Figure S5   Induced cytochrome 3A4 activity in aggregates of different diameter versus cells cultured on tissue culture plastic. Cyp3A4 activity was quantified after treatment with an inducing agent (hydrocortisone) using a luciferase based assay after 7 days of isolation. Data are mean ± SD, n = 2.

Figure S6   Real-time PCR analysis of HepG2 cell aggregates with diverse dimensions. Gene expression levels of albumin, TTR and HNF4α determined after 3 or 7 days of cultivation in the agarose chip. RNA levels were normalized using GAPDH as a stable housekeeping marker and the relative gene fold changes, compared to the gene expression of the control culture (TCP plated cells), were determined using the $2^{-\Delta\Delta Ct}$ method. Data are mean RQ $\pm$ SD, n = 3.

Figure S7 Albumin secretion of HepG2 cell aggregates with diverse dimensions. Albumin secretion in the cultivation medium during 24 hours is determined by ELISA and normalized using MTT assay. Data are means $\pm$ SEM (n = 3).

Figure S8 Transmission electron micrographs of primary hepatocytes cultured for 10 days as aggregates. The cytoplasm of the cells displays numerous mitochondria and an abundant RER (A). Adjoining cells show narrow contacts between the cells and the presence of junctional structures as desmosomes (B) and gap junctions (C).

Author Contributions

Conceived and designed the experiments: EG RC AVA. Performed the experiments: EG LD. Analyzed the data: EG RC. Contributed reagents/materials/analysis tools: AVA TB PD LD LVG. Contributed to the writing of the manuscript: EG LD TB PD LVG AVA RC.

References

1. Shulman M, Nahmias Y (2013) Long-term culture and coculture of primary rat and human hepatocytes. Methods Mol Biol 945: 287–302.
2. Uygun BE, Yarmush ML (2013) Engineered liver for transplantation. Curr Opin Biotechnol 24: 893–899.
3. Jindal R, Patel SJ, Yarmush ML (2010) Tissue-Engineered Model for Real-Time Monitoring of Liver Inflammation. Tissue Eng Part C Methods.
4. Wong SF, No da Y, Choi YY, Kim DS, Chung BG, et al. (2011) Concave microwell based size-controllable hepatosphere as a three-dimensional liver tissue model. Biomaterials 32: 8087–8096.
5. van Zijl F, Mikulits W (2010) Hepatospheres: Three dimensional cell cultures resemble physiological conditions of the liver. World J Hepatol 2: 1–7.
6. Miranda JP, Rodrigues A, Tostoes RM, Leite S, Zimmerman H, et al. (2010) Extending Hepatocyte Functionality for Drug-Testing Applications Using High-Viscosity Alginate-Encapsulated Three-Dimensional Cultures in Bioreactors. Tissue Engineering Part C-Methods 16: 1223–1232.
7. Ramaiahgari SC, den Braver MW, Herpers B, Terpstra V, Commandeur JN, et al. (2014) A 3D in vitro model of differentiated HepG2 cell spheroids with improved liver-like properties for repeated dose high-throughput toxicity studies. Arch Toxicol.
8. Pang Y, Montagne K, Shinohara M, Komori K, Sakai Y (2012) Liver tissue engineering based on aggregate assembly: efficient formation of endothelialized rat hepatocyte aggregates and their immobilization with biodegradable fibres. Biofabrication 4: 045004.
9. Mei Y, Luo H, Tang Q, Ye Z, Zhou Y, et al. Modulating and modeling aggregation of cell-seeded microcarriers in stirred culture system for macrotissue engineering. J Biotechnol 150: 438–446.
10. Mironov V, Visconti RP, Kasyanov V, Forgacs G, Drake CJ, et al. (2009) Organ printing: tissue spheroids as building blocks. Biomaterials 30: 2164–2174.
11. Nichol JW, Khademhosseini A (2009) Modular Tissue Engineering: Engineering Biological Tissues from the Bottom Up. Soft Matter 5: 1312–1319.
12. Rivron NC, Rouwkema J, Truckenmuller R, Karperien M, De Boer J, et al. (2009) Tissue assembly and organization: developmental mechanisms in microfabricated tissues. Biomaterials 30: 4851–4858.
13. Goncalves LA, Vigario AM, Penha-Goncalves C (2007) Improved isolation of murine hepatocytes for in vitro malaria liver stage studies. Malar J 6: 169.
14. Rivron NC, Vrij EJ, Rouwkema J, Le Gac S, van den Berg A, et al. (2012) Tissue deformation spatially modulates VEGF signaling and angiogenesis. Proc Natl Acad Sci U S A 109: 6886–6891.
15. Spijker HS, Ravelli RBG, Mommaas-Kienhuis AM, van Apeldoorn AA, Engelse MA, et al. (2013) Conversion of Mature Human beta-Cells Into Glucagon-Producing alpha-Cells. Diabetes 62: 2471–2480.
16. Billiet T, Gasse BV, Gevaert E, Cornelissen M, Martins JC, et al. (2013) Quantitative Contrasts in the Photopolymerization of Acrylamide and Methacrylamide-Functionalized Gelatin Hydrogel Building Blocks. Macromol Biosci.
17. Taguchi T, Rao Z, Ito M, Matsuda M (2011) Induced albumin secretion from HepG2 spheroids prepared using poly(ethylene glycol) derivative with oleyl groups. Journal of Materials Science-Materials in Medicine 22: 2357–2363.
18. Fukuda J, Nakazawa K (2005) Orderly arrangement of hepatocyte spheroids on a microfabricated chip. Tissue Eng 11: 1254–1262.
19. Asthana A, Kisaalita WS (2012) Microtissue size and hypoxia in HTS with 3D cultures. Drug Discov Today 17: 810–817.
20. Glicklis R, Merchuk JC, Cohen S (2004) Modeling mass transfer in hepatocyte spheroids via cell viability, spheroid size, and hepatocellular functions. Biotechnol Bioeng 86: 672–680.
21. Brophy CM, Luebke-Wheeler JL, Amiot BP, Khan H, Remmel RP, et al. (2009) Rat hepatocyte spheroids formed by rocked technique maintain differentiated hepatocyte gene expression and function. Hepatology 49: 578–586.
22. Lin RZ, Chou LF, Chien CC, Chang HY (2006) Dynamic analysis of hepatoma spheroid formation: roles of E-cadherin and beta1-integrin. Cell Tissue Res 324: 411–422.
23. Luebke-Wheeler JL, Nedredal G, Yee L, Amiot BP, Nyberg SL (2009) E-cadherin protects primary hepatocyte spheroids from cell death by a caspase-independent mechanism. Cell Transplant 18: 1281–1287.
24. Du Y, Lo E, Ali S, Khademhosseini A (2008) Directed assembly of cell-laden microgels for fabrication of 3D tissue constructs. Proc Natl Acad Sci U S A 105: 9522–9527.
25. Du Y, Lo E, Vidula MK, Khabiry M, Khademhosseini A (2008) Method of Bottom-Up Directed Assembly of Cell-Laden Microgels. Cell Mol Bioeng 1: 157–162.
26. Wang X, Yan Y, Pan Y, Xiong Z, Liu H, et al. (2006) Generation of three-dimensional hepatocyte/gelatin structures with rapid prototyping system. Tissue Eng 12: 83–90.
27. Billiet T, Gevaert E, De Schryver T, Cornelissen M, Dubruel P (2014) The 3D printing of gelatin methacrylamide cell-laden tissue-engineered constructs with high cell viability. Biomaterials 35: 49–62.

7

Decreased Circulating Visfatin Is Associated with Improved Disease Activity in Early Rheumatoid Arthritis: Data from the PERAC Cohort

Ondřej Sglunda[1], Heřman Mann[1,2], Hana Hulejová[1], Markéta Kuklová[1], Ondřej Pecha[3], Lenka Pleštilová[1], Mária Filková[1], Karel Pavelka[1,2], Jiří Vencovský[1,2], Ladislav Šenolt[1,2]*

1 Institute of Rheumatology, Prague, Czech Republic, 2 Department of Rheumatology, First Faculty of Medicine, Charles University in Prague, Prague, Czech Republic, 3 Technology Centre ASCR, Prague, Czech Republic

Abstract

Objective: To evaluate circulating visfatin and its relationship with disease activity and serum lipids in patients with early, treatment-naïve rheumatoid arthritis (RA).

Methods: Serum visfatin was measured in 40 patients with early RA before and after three months of treatment and in 30 age- and sex-matched healthy individuals. Disease activity was assessed using the Disease Activity Score for 28 joints (DAS28) at baseline and at three and 12 months. Multivariate linear regression analysis was performed to evaluate whether improved disease activity is related to serum visfatin or a change in visfatin level.

Results: Serum visfatin was significantly elevated in early RA patients compared to healthy controls (1.92 ± 1.17 vs. 1.36 ± 0.93 ng/ml; $p=0.034$) and significantly decreased after three months of treatment (to 0.99 ± 0.67 ng/ml; $p<0.001$). Circulating visfatin and a change in visfatin level correlated with disease activity and improved disease activity over time, respectively. A decrease in visfatin after three months predicted a DAS28 improvement after 12 months. In addition, decreased serum visfatin was not associated with an improved atherogenic index but was associated with an increase in total cholesterol level.

Conclusion: A short-term decrease in circulating visfatin may represent an independent predictor of long-term disease activity improvement in patients with early RA.

Editor: Oreste Gualillo, SERGAS, Santiago University Clinical Hospital, IDIS Research Laboratory 9, NEIRID Lab, Spain

Funding: This work was supported by a Ministry of Health of the Czech Republic (MHCR) grant (NT-13696-4), SVV project (264 511) and project of MHCR for conceptual development of a research organization (023728). The funders had no role in study design, data collection and analysis, decision to publish, or preparation of the manuscript.

Competing Interests: The authors have declared that no competing interests exist.

* Email: senolt@revma.cz

Introduction

Visfatin was originally discovered and named pre-B-colony enhancing factor [1] but was later renamed visfatin, reflecting its predominant secretion by visceral adipose tissue [2]. However, visfatin is also produced by several types of immune cells and synovial fibroblasts [3,4]. Recent studies have demonstrated the involvement of visfatin in innate immunity and inflammation [5], particularly in rheumatoid arthritis (RA). Visfatin is strongly up-regulated in the RA synovial lining layer and at sites of joint invasion, promoting synovial fibroblast motility and increasing the production of pro-inflammatory cytokines and matrix degrading enzymes by synovial fibroblasts and monocytes [3,6,7].

In RA, persistent synovial inflammation and invasive behaviour by activated synovial fibroblasts contribute to joint damage, leading to disability [8]. The discovery of novel molecules has contributed to a better understanding of RA pathogenesis and may lead to the identification of biomarkers that would allow for the monitoring of disease activity and individualising prognosis in RA patients [9]. Visfatin may represent a novel biomarker for disease severity. Some data indicate that visfatin is elevated in RA and may be associated with the degree of inflammation, clinical disease activity and radiographic joint damage [3,10,11]. However, these findings are not consistent throughout all studies [12–14].

The objective of the present study was to characterise 1) the association between serum visfatin level and disease activity in early RA, 2) the effect of treatment with conventional synthetic disease modifying drugs (csDMARDs) on the visfatin level and 3) the relationship between visfatin level and serum lipids.

Methods

Patients

A total of 40 patients (28 women) with early RA were included in the study. The inclusion criteria were as follows: 1) age >18 years, 2) fulfilment of the ACR/EULAR 2010 classification criteria for RA at baseline [15], 3) symptom duration of ≤6 months and 4) no or only symptomatic therapy with nonsteroidal antirheumatic drugs at baseline. Patients were prospectively followed in the Prague Early RA Clinic (PERAC) at the Institute of Rheumatology in the Czech Republic. The disease activity was assessed using the 28-joint count Disease Activity Score (DAS28-ESR). The control group consisted of 30 age- and sex-matched healthy individuals. Consent procedure was approved by the Ethics Committee of the Institute of Rheumatology. Each participant provided written informed consents prior to entering the study. Both original consents were given to the patients and documented in the patient's files.

Laboratory analysis

Fasting blood samples were collected from all patients at baseline and after three months. The samples were immediately centrifuged and stored at −20°C. The serum concentration of visfatin was measured using a commercially available enzyme-linked immunosorbent assay (ELISA) (Biovision, Milpitas, California, USA) as described previously [14]. The levels of serum anti-cyclic citrullinated peptide antibodies (anti-CCP) and IgM rheumatoid factor (IgM-RF) were measured using a standard ELISA assay (Test Line S.R.O., Czech Republic). CRP and total and HDL-cholesterol were determined using routine laboratory techniques.

Statistical analysis

Pearson's and Spearman's rank correlations were used in cases of normal and non-normal distributions. The T-test was used for normal variables, and the Mann-Whitney test was used for non-parametric variables. Multivariate linear regression analysis was performed to assess the influence of visfatin (its change) on disease activity and blood lipids. P values of less than 0.05 were considered to be statistically significant. Statistical analyses were performed using SPSS 17 (SPSS Inc., Chicago, IL, USA) and GraphPad Prism 5.0 (GraphPad Software, Inc., San Diego, CA, USA). The data are presented as the median [range] or mean and standard deviation (SD) in the case of abnormal or normal distribution.

Results

Patients and demographic data

Table 1 shows the baseline characteristics of patients and healthy controls included in the study. Twenty patients met the criteria for highly active disease (DAS28>5.1), 18 patients had moderate disease activity (3.2<DAS28≤5.1), and two patients had low disease activity (2.6<DAS28≤3.2) at baseline. Treatment with csDMARDS was initiated in 38 patients at baseline: 31 patients on methotrexate (mean weekly dose at month three was 15 mg; range, 10–20 mg), six on sulphasalazine and one on leflunomide. Additionally, 34 patients were receiving glucocorticoids (mean daily dose at month three was 5 mg; range, 1.25–15.0 mg of prednisone or equivalent per day). Two patients were initially only on glucocorticoids either due to planned pregnancy or elevated aminotransferases. After three months of treatment, a significant reduction in disease activity was observed (DAS28: from 5.3±1.5 to 2.8±1.3; CRP: from 7.7 [0.6–77.8] to 2.3 [0.2–14.3]; p<0.001 for all comparisons).

Visfatin is elevated in early RA and correlates with disease activity

The baseline visfatin level in early RA patients was significantly higher compared to that in healthy controls (1.92±1.17 vs. 1.36±0.93 ng/ml; p = 0.034) (Fig. 1A). Using bivariate analysis, the visfatin level correlated positively with DAS28 (r = 0.383, p = 0.015) and CRP level (r = 0.456, p = 0.003) at baseline (Fig. 1B). The serum visfatin level was not related to age, gender or body mass index (BMI), but there was a negative association between visfatin and anti-CCP level (r = −0.400, p = 0.011) albeit not with IgM-RF (r = −0.045, p = 0.787).

A decreased visfatin level is associated with disease activity improvement

The serum visfatin level significantly decreased after three months compared to baseline (1.92±1.17 vs. 0.99±0.67 ng/ml; p<0.0001) (Fig. 1A). Similar to baseline, after three months of treatment, the visfatin level correlated with DAS28 (r = 0.338, p = 0.035) and CRP (r = 0.588, p = 0.001).

A decrease in visfatin level correlated with a decrease in DAS28 (r = 0.378, p = 0.018) and CRP (r = 0.386, p = 0.015) after three months (Fig. 2A). Furthermore, a decrease in visfatin level after three months correlated with a decrease in DAS28 (r = 0.354, p = 0.027) and CRP (r = 0.365, p = 0.022) after 12 months (Fig. 2B). Using multiple linear regression analysis, a visfatin decrease after three months predicted DAS28 improvement between baseline and month three (p = 0.021, adjusted $R^2 = 11.9\%$) and between baseline and month 12 (p = 0.031, adjusted $R^2 = 10.1\%$).

Visfatin level and lipid profile

The visfatin level did not correlate with serum lipids or atherogenic index at baseline in early RA patients (data not shown). While the mean total cholesterol (5.17±1.20 to 5.73±1.40 mmol/l; p<0.001) and HDL-cholesterol (1.07±0.25 to 1.32±0.29 mmol/l; p<0.001) significantly increased from baseline to month three, there was an improvement in the atherogenic index (4.02±1.35 to 3.50±1.29; p<0.01). Although a decrease in serum visfatin was not associated with an improved atherogenic index (r = 0.095, p = 0.567), the decrease was associated with an increase in total cholesterol (r = −0.328, p = 0.041). A decrease in visfatin significantly and independently predicted an increase in total cholesterol in all RA patients (p = 0.015). Another independent significant predictor in this model (adjusted $R^2 = 34.1\%$) was a decrease in CRP between baseline and month three (p = 0.007).

Discussion

In this study, we have shown that an elevated visfatin level correlates with disease activity and that a decrease in visfatin level during the first three months of treatment independently predicts further disease activity improvement after 12 months in patients with treatment naïve early RA. The atherogenic index improved but was not related to visfatin reduction.

Consistent with previous studies demonstrating an increased visfatin level in patients with RA [3,10,14], we have shown that an elevated circulating visfatin in the early phase of the disease significantly decreased after three months of treatment. Because visfatin is up-regulated in several immune cells [3] and improvement in disease activity is associated with a decrease in macrophages in RA synovial tissue [16], a decrease in circulating visfatin may reflect a decrease in synovial immune cells following effective treatment. In addition, the visfatin level correlated with

Table 1. Baseline characteristics of patients with early rheumatoid arthritis (RA) and healthy controls.

Characteristics	Early RA (n = 40)	Healthy controls (n = 30)
Gender (F/M)	22/18	19/11
Age (years)	52±17	48±16
BMI	24±4.0	25±3.1
CRP (mg/l)	7.7 [0.6–77.8]	-
DAS28 score	5.25±1.50	-
RF positivity, n (%)	24 (60)	-
Anti-CCP positivity, n (%)	21 (53)	-
Drugs (csDMARDs/GC)	38/31	-

Anti-CCP, anti-cyclic citrullinated peptide antibody; RF, rheumatoid factor; CRP, C-reactive protein; DAS, disease activity score; csDMARDs, conventional synthetic disease modifying antirheumatic drugs; GC, glucocorticoids; RA, rheumatoid arthritis; F, female; M, male; MTX, methotrexate. The data are expressed as a mean (SD) or median [range].

clinical and laboratory measures of disease activity at baseline and during treatment, which has been reported in some [3,17], but not all, studies [12,14]. This inconsistency may be explained by differences in populations and treatments because in patients with long-term and active RA on biological therapy, an association between visfatin and disease activity was not observed [12,14].

Adipokines represent large group of highly bioactive substances secreted by adipocytes and immune cells that are involved in both metabolic and immunomodulatory functions. In addition to visfatin, Gonzalez-Gay et al demonstrated rapid reduction of serum resistin [18], but not adiponectin [19] levels in patients with long-term and active RA during anti-TNF-alpha therapy with infliximab. Resistin levels were positively associated with inflammatory markers of RA [18], whereas adiponectin levels were inversely associated with disease activity and low adiponectin levels clustered with metabolic syndrome features that reportedly contribute to atherogenesis in RA patients with severe disease [19].

We have found that a decrease in circulating visfatin correlates with disease activity improvement over the first three months of treatment. Furthermore, although baseline visfatin was not

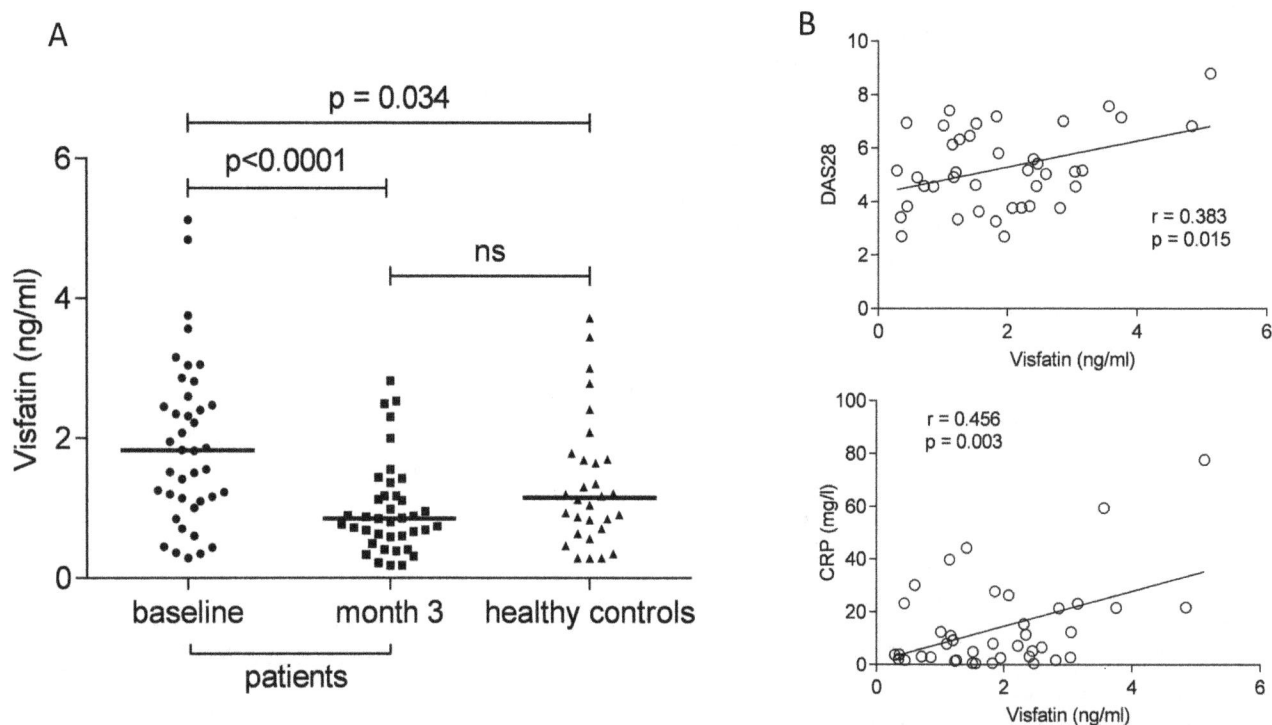

Figure 1. Comparison of serum visfatin levels between patients with early, treatment-naïve rheumatoid arthritis and healthy controls and change in serum visfatin after three months of treatment with conventional synthetic disease modifying antirheumatic drugs. (A). Association between baseline serum visfatin level and disease activity (B). CRP, C-reactive protein; DAS, disease activity score.

A

B

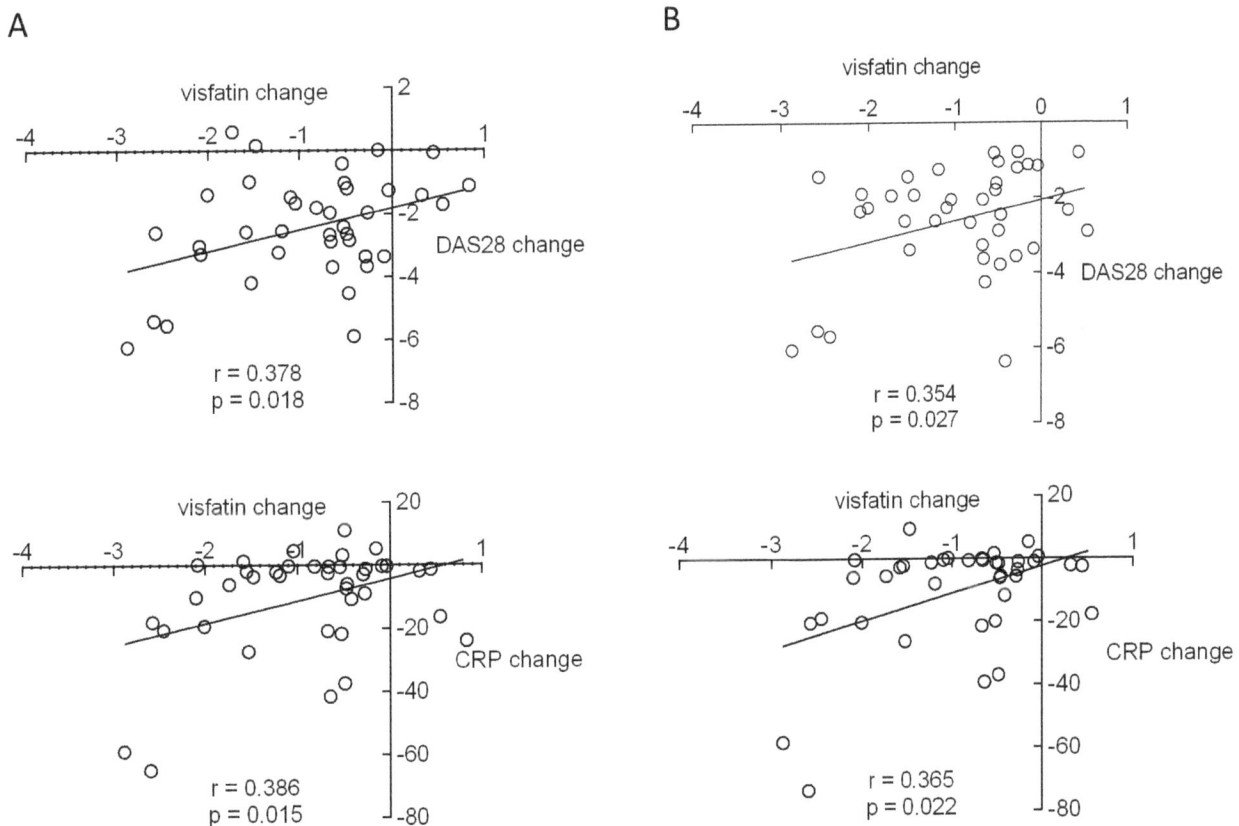

Figure 2. Correlations between visfatin reduction and disease activity improvement after three months (A) and between visfatin reduction after three months and disease activity improvement after 12 months (B). CRP, C-reactive protein; DAS, disease activity score.

predictive, the change of visfatin level over the first three months predicted disease activity improvement after 12 months of treatment. Thus, a higher visfatin level in treated RA patients may be associated with more severe disease and thus higher risk of structural progression as demonstrated previously [11,13]. These data further support a significant role for visfatin in the pathogenesis of RA.

There is evidence that a high visfatin level is associated with an increased risk of cardiovascular disease [20]. Klaasen et al. reported a relationship between a high visfatin level and an increased atherogenic index in adalimumab-treated RA patients and suggested that visfatin reduction can lead to decreased cardiovascular risk independent of disease activity [6]. However, in our study, the visfatin level correlated inversely with baseline total-cholesterol and its increase but not with atherogenic index. This finding may be explained by a different patient population and is consistent with a recent study by El-Hini et al. [20]. Because our patients had an improvement in atherogenic index during treatment [21], we suggest that the association between visfatin and total cholesterol level may be caused by dyslipidaemia, which

occurs in early RA [21]. However, this hypothesis requires further investigation.

In conclusion, our study demonstrates an association between an elevated visfatin level and disease activity, and short-term reduction of visfatin is an independent predictor of long-term disease activity improvement in early, treatment-naïve RA patients. These results however need to be validated in larger and independent cohorts of patients with RA.

Acknowledgments

We thank all of the patients and healthy volunteers for blood donation.

Author Contributions

Conceived and designed the experiments: LS JV KP HM. Performed the experiments: HH MF. Analyzed the data: MK HH LP OP. Contributed reagents/materials/analysis tools: HH MF MK. Contributed to the writing of the manuscript: OS LS JV KP HM. Statistical analysis: OP. Enrolled patients to the study: LS HM.

References

1. Samal B, Sun Y, Stearns G, Xie C, Suggs S, et al. (1994) Cloning and characterization of the cDNA encoding a novel human pre-B cell colony-enhancing factor. Mol Cell Biol 14: 1431–7.
2. Fukuhara A, Matsuda M, Nishizawa M, Segawa K, Tanaka M, et al. (2005) Visfatin: a protein secreted by visceral fat that mimics the effects of insulin. Science 307: 426–30.
3. Brentano F, Schorr O, Ospelt C, Stanczyk J, Gay RE, et al. (2007) Pre-B cell colony-enhancing factor/visfatin, a new marker of inflammation in rheumatoid arthritis with proinflammatory and matrix-degrading activities. Arthritis Rheum 56: 2829–39.
4. Nowell MA, Richards PJ, Fielding CA, Ognjanovic S, Topley N, et al. (2006) Regulation of pre-B cell colony-enhancing factor by STAT-3-dependent interleukin-6 trans-signaling: implications in the pathogenesis of rheumatoid arthritis. Arthritis Rheum 54: 2084–95.
5. Luk T, Malam Z, Marshall JC (2008) Pre-B cell colony-enhancing factor (PBEF)/visfatin: a novel mediator of innate immunity. J Leukoc Biol 83: 804–16.

6. Klaasen R, Herenius MM, Wijbrandts CA, de Jager W, van Tuyl LH, et al. (2012) Treatment-specific changes in circulating adipocytokines: a comparison between tumour necrosis factor blockade and glucocorticoid treatment for rheumatoid arthritis. Ann Rheum Dis 71: 1510–6.

7. Présumey J, Courties G, Louis-Plence P, Escriou V, Scherman D, et al. (2013) Nicotinamide phosphoribosyltransferase/visfatin expression by inflammatory monocytes mediates arthritis pathogenesis. Ann Rheum Dis 72: 1717–24.

8. Ospelt C, Gay S (2008) The role of resident synovial cells in destructive arthritis. Best Pract Res Clin Rheumatol 22: 239–52.

9. Smolen JS, Aletaha D, Grisar J, Redlich K, Steiner G, et al. (2008) The need for prognosticators in rheumatoid arthritis. Biological and clinical markers: where are we now? Arthritis Res Ther 10: 208.

10. Otero M, Lago R, Gomez R, Lago F, Dieguez C, et al. (2006) Changes in plasma levels of fat-derived hormones adiponectin, leptin, resistin and visfatin in patients with rheumatoid arthritis. Ann Rheum Dis 65: 1198–201.

11. Rho YH, Solus J, Sokka T, Oeser A, Chung CP, et al. (2009) Adipocytokines are associated with radiographic joint damage in rheumatoid arthritis. Arthritis Rheum 60: 1906–14.

12. Gonzalez-Gay MA, Vazquez-Rodriguez TR, Garcia-Unzueta MT, Berja A, Miranda-Filloy JA, et al. (2010) Visfatin is not associated with inflammation or metabolic syndrome in patients with severe rheumatoid arthritis undergoing anti-TNF-alpha therapy. Clin Exp Rheumatol 28: 56–62.

13. Klein-Wieringa IR, van der Linden MP, Knevel R, Kwekkeboom JC, van Beelen E, et al. (2011) Baseline serum adipokine levels predict radiographic progression in early rheumatoid arthritis. Arthritis Rheum 63: 2567–74.

14. Senolt L, Krystufkova O, Hulejova H, Kuklova M, Filkova M, et al. (2011) The level of serum visfatin (PBEF) is associated with total number of B cells in patients with rheumatoid arthritis and decreases following B cell depletion therapy. Cytokine 55: 116–21.

15. Aletaha D, Neogi T, Silman AJ, Funovits J, Felson DT, et al. (2010) Rheumatoid arthritis classification criteria: an American College of Rheumatology/European League Against Rheumatism collaborative initiative. Ann Rheum Dis 69: 1580–8.

16. Haringman JJ, Gerlag DM, Zwinderman AH, Smeets TJ, Kraan MC, et al. (2005) Synovial tissue macrophages: a sensitive biomarker for response to treatment in patients with rheumatoid arthritis. Ann Rheum Dis 64: 834–8.

17. El-Hini SH, Mohamed FI, Hassan AA, Ali F, Mahmoud A, et al. (2013) Visfatin and adiponectin as novel markers for evaluation of metabolic disturbance in recently diagnosed rheumatoid arthritis patients. Rheumatol Int 33: 2283–9.

18. Gonzalez-Gay MA, Garcia-Unzueta MT, Gonzalez-Juanatey C, Miranda-Filloy JA, Vazquez-Rodriguez TR, et al. (2008) Anti-TNF-alpha therapy modulates resistin in patients with rheumatoid arthritis. Clin Exp Rheumatol 26: 311–6.

19. Gonzalez-Gay MA, Llorca J, Garcia-Unzueta MT, Gonzalez-Juanatey C, De Matias JM, et al. (2008) High-grade inflammation, circulating adiponectin concentrations and cardiovascular risk factors in severe rheumatoid arthritis. Clin Exp Rheumatol 26: 596–603.

20. Chang YH, Chang DM, Lin KC, Shin SJ, Lee YJ (2011) Visfatin in overweight/obesity, type 2 diabetes mellitus, insulin resistance, metabolic syndrome and cardiovascular diseases: a meta-analysis and systemic review. Diabetes Metab Res Rev 27: 515–27.

21. Boers M, Nurmohamed MT, Doelman CJ, Lard LR, Verhoeven AC, et al. (2003) Influence of glucocorticoids and disease activity on total and high density lipoprotein cholesterol in patients with rheumatoid arthritis. Ann Rheum Dis 62: 842–5.

8

Differentiation of Human Umbilical Cord Mesenchymal Stem Cells into Prostate-Like Epithelial Cells *In Vivo*

Wang Li[1]9, Bo Ye[2]9, Xiao-Yan Cai[1], Jian-Hua Lin[3], Wei-Qiang Gao[1,4]*

1 State Key Laboratory of Oncogenes and Related Genes, Renji-Med X Clinical Stem Cell Research Center, Ren Ji Hospital, School of Medicine, Shanghai Jiao Tong University, Shanghai, China, 2 Department of Thoracic Surgery, Shanghai Chest Hospital, Shanghai Jiao Tong University, Shanghai, China, 3 Department of Obstetrics and Gynecology, Ren Ji Hospital, School of Medicine, Shanghai Jiao Tong University, Shanghai, China, 4 School of Biomedical Engineering & Med-X Research Institute, Shanghai Jiao Tong University, Shanghai, China

Abstract

Although human umbilical cord mesenchymal stem cells (hUC-MSCs) have been identified as a new source of MSCs for potential application in regenerative medicine, their full potential of differentiation has not been determined. In particular, whether they have the capability to differentiate into epithelial cells of endodermal origin such as the prostate epithelial cells is unknown. Here we report that when hUC-MSCs were combined with rat urogenital sinus stromal cells (rUGSSs) and transplanted into the renal capsule in vivo, they could differentiate into prostate epithelial-like cells that could be verified by prostate epithelial cell-specific markers including the prostate specific antigen. The prostatic glandular structures formed in vivo displayed similar cellular architecture with lumens and branching features as seen for a normal prostate. In addition, the human origin of the hUC-MSCs was confirmed by immunocytochemistry for human nuclear antigen. These findings together indicate that hUC-MSCs have the capability to differentiate into epithelial-like cells that are normally derived from the endoderm, implicating their potential applications in tissue repair and regeneration of many endoderm-derived internal organs.

Editor: Pranela Rameshwar, Rutgers - New Jersey Medical School, United States of America

Funding: The study is supported by funds to WQG from the Chinese Ministry of Science and Technology (2012CB966800 and 2013CB945600), the National Natural Science Foundation of China (81130038 and 81372189), Science and Technology Commission of Shanghai Municipality (Pujiang program), Shanghai Education Committee Key Disciplines and Specialties Foundation (J50208), Shanghai Health Bureau Key Disciplines and Specialties Foundation and KC Wong foundation. The funders had no role in study design, data collection and analysis, decision to publish, or preparation of the manuscript.

Competing Interests: The authors have declared that no competing interests exist.

* Email: gao.weiqiang@sjtu.edu.cn

9 These authors contributed equally to this work.

Introduction

Human mesenchymal stem cells (MSCs) are multipotent stem cells found in several adult tissues [1]. These cells are reported to be capable of differentiating into various cell types, particularly the mesoderm-derived tissues including the bone, cartilage, muscle, ligament, tendon, and adipose [2–4]. Currently, the most common source of adult MSCs which have a great therapeutic potential is from the bone marrow (BM) because of their capacity of self-renewal and multi-lineage differentiation [5–9]. However, there is a great need to identify alternative MSCs sources due to the limited number of BM-MSCs available for autologous uses, the invasive procedures of aspiration of BM, and a significant decrease of frequency and differentiation potential of BM-MSCs as age proceeds [10]. Recent studies have reported an attractive, alternative tissue source of MSCs from human umbilical cord (hUC) [11].

Human UC-MSCs have generated a great deal of interest for their potential use in regenerative medicine and tissue engineering due to their superior advantages compared to the MSCs from BM. The hUC contains two arteries and one vein, which are surrounded by mucoid connective tissues called Wharton's jelly (WJ) [12]. WJ possesses desirable characteristics such as a large, rapidly available MSCs pool, a non-invasive and painless collection procedure, and ethically non-controversial source of MSCs [13]. In addition, it is believed that the hUC-MSCs are more primitive or less immunogenic than the MSCs derived from other tissue sources, and are endowed with more superior plasticity and a greater expansion capability [14].

Although hUC-MSCs have been shown, as MSCs from the bone marrow, to be able to differentiate into mesodermal tissues such as the bone, cartilage, muscle, ligament, tendon, and adipose, whether they have the capability to differentiate into epithelial cells of endodermal origin such as the prostate epithelial cells is not determined. The prostate is formed through epithelial budding from the urogenital sinus (UGS) derived from the endoderm around days 17–18 of gestation in the mouse [15,16]. The gland undergoes extensive ductal outgrowth and branching, which continue for several weeks after birth [16]. In humans, budding of the prostatic epithelium is seen at 10 weeks of gestation [17]. The prostate is an important male accessory sex gland found only in mammals that functions to produce a major fraction of seminal fluid, which contains secretory protein prostate specific antigen (PSA).

In the present study, we isolated hUC-MSCs and rat urogenital sinus stromal cells (rUGSSs) and co-transplanted them into renal capsules in vivo. We demonstrated clearly that hUC-MSCs have the capability to differentiate into prostate epithelial-like structures. These structures display similar epithelial lumen, branching patterns as seen for normal prostates, which express prostate-specific markers including PSA. Thus, the hUC-MSCs may have important implications for repair/regeneration of epithelial tissues of endoderm-derived organs.

Materials and Methods

Animals

Eighteen-day-pregnant SD rats and male BALB/c nude mice (postnatal day 5 weeks-old) were purchased from Shanghai SLAC Laboratory Animal Co., Ltd. All experiments were approved by the Animal Research Ethics Committee of Renji Hospital, Shanghai Jiao Tong University School of Medicine.

Antibodies

Antibodies were purchased from the following sources: PE conjugated CD105, FITC conjugated CD29, APC conjugated CD31, PerCP-Cy5.5 conjugated CD45, and PE-Cy7 conjugated CD34 were from eBioscience. p63, AR, CK8, CK5, PSA and vimentin antibodies were from Santa Cruz Biotechnology. Testosterone and collagenase IV were from Sigma and human nuclei antibody was from Millipore.

Preparation of Dissociated urogenital sinus stromal cells

The rUGSSs isolation procedure was done as previously described [18]. Briefly, E18 embryos from pregnant SD rats were sacrificed and urogenital sinuses were collected. After separation of the UGS from the urogenital sinus epithelium, the cells were digested with 1 mg/ml collagenase IV combined with 0.125% Trypsin for 30 min at 37°C, washed twice and triturated in the culture medium (DMEM supplemented with 10% FBS, 2 mM glutamine, 100 U/ml penicillin and 100 mg/ml streptomycin) and cultured in the same medium in plates. rUGSSs were passaged at confluency by trypsin digestion and cultured in vitro for up to 2 weeks before they were used for tissue recombination with hUC-MSCs prior to transplantation into the renal capsules in the nude mice.

Isolation and preparation of hUC-MSCs

Fresh hUC were collected from abdominal delivery operation of Renji hospital with the consent of the parents and stored in normal saline. The study protocol was approved by the ethics review board of Renji hospital (protocol #2012-01). We have obtained written informed consent from all study participants. All of the procedures were done in accordance with the Declaration of Helsinki and relevant policies in China. The tissue was disinfected with 70% alcohol for 30 s and cleared extensively with normal saline. The washing was repeated until they were cleaned from blood or blood clots. In order to avoid any contamination of the cultures by the endothelial cells, the vein was flushed with saline prior to the openning at the external surface of the umbilical cord with a sterile scalpel. The cord vessels (arteries and vein) were removed from cord segments, and the exposed WJ tissue was cut into small pieces [19]. After having been minced into 1–2 mm^3 fragments, WJ tissues were incubated with 1 mg/ml collagenase type IV combined with 0.125% Trypsin for 30 min at 37°C. Following digestion, the mixture was then centrifuged at 400 g for 8 min, washed twice in PBS. WJ cells were placed in plates and cultured in DMEM supplemented with 8% (v/v) fetal bovine serum (FBS), 2 mM L-glutamine, 100 U/ml penicillin, 100 mg/ml streptomycin. The culture plate was placed in an incubator with saturated humidity at about 37°C containing 5% (v/v) CO_2.

Human UC-MSCs were passaged at confluency by trypsin digestion and cultured in vitro for up to 2 weeks.

Flow cytometry

Once 80% confluence had been reached, adherent cells were analyzed using standard flow cytometry. Compensation adjustments were performed with single color positive controls. Briefly, P0-P8 hUC-MSCs were stained with several antibodies (CD105, CD29, CD45, CD34, CD31) and analyzed on a BD FACSAria II cytometer.

rUGSSs and hUC-MSCs cultures and immunostaining analyses

rUGSSs and hUC-MSCs were grown on glass coverslips and fixed in 4% paraformaldehyde (for CK8, p63, CK5, AR, PSA, vimentin, human nuclear antigen immunostaining). The cells were then incubated with primary antibody in a humidified chamber overnight at 4°C, processed with secondary antibodies for 1 hr at room temperature in dark. The immunostaining were observed and images were acquired on a Nikon microscope with a digital camera.

Prostate regeneration assays *in vivo*

The prostate regeneration was performed as previously described [18]. hUC-MSCs (100,000 cells per graft) were mixed with rUGSSs (250,000 cells per graft) in 3 mg/ml collagen type I (20 μl per graft), incubated at 37°C for 1 h to allow collagen gelation, and overlaid with culture medium. After incubation overnight at 37°C, collagen gel was grafted under the renal capsule in 6-8-week-old BALB/c nude mice, along with a subcutaneous slow-release testosterone pellet (12.5 mg per pellet per mouse). Grafts were harvested and analyzed 2 months after implantation. All animal studies were approved by and conducted according to the guidelines of the Renji Hospital Animal Care and Ethics Review Committee.

Immunohistochemistry

BALB/c nude mouse bearing prostate grafts under the kidney capsule were sacrificed 2 months after surgery. Optimal cutting temperature (OCT) compound-frozen tissues were sectioned at 8 μm, fixed in 4% paraformaldehyde. Sections were stained with hematoxylin/eosin [20]. For immunohistochemistry, sections were incubated with the primary antibody in a humidified chamber overnight at 4°C and secondary antibodies for 1 hr at room temperature in dark. Images were acquired on a Nikon microscope with a digital camera.

Results

Isolation and Characterization of hUC-MSCs and rUGSSs

By enzyme digestion method, cells from human UC fragments were seeded at a density of 1000 cells/cm^2. As early as 24 h following plating, adherent cells with fibroblastic morphology could be observed and they were hUC-MSCs (Fig. 1A). Rat rUGSSs were prepared from E17-E18 rat embryos as previously described [18]. As compared to the hUV-MSCs, rUGSSs are smaller in size (Fig. 1B). While immunofluorescent staining for human nuclei antibody which recognizes nuclei of all the human cell types labeled all hUC-MSCs (Fig. 1C), all rUGSSs were negative for as expected (data not shown). In addition, the rUGSSs expressed vimentin (Fig. 1D), confirming the stromal cell identity of the rUGSSs.

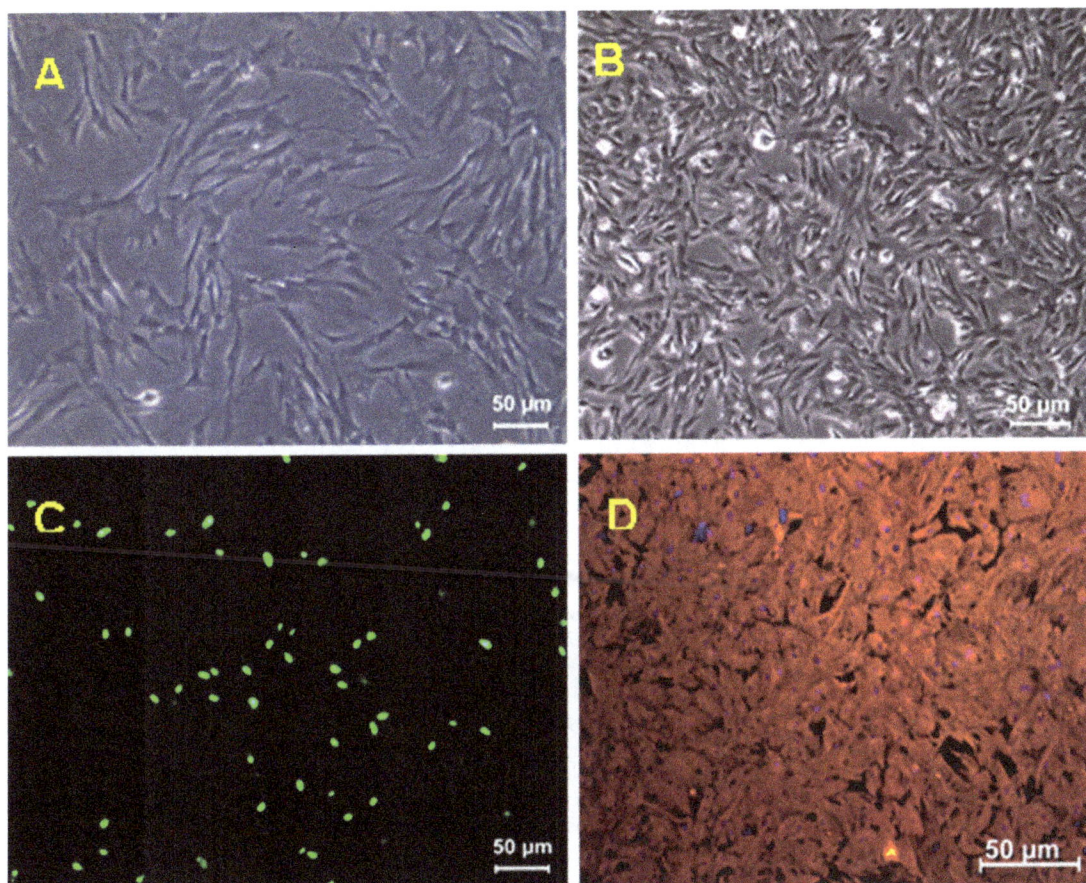

Figure 1. The morphology and characterization of hUC-MSCs and rUGSSs. (A), Seven days after the initial plating, adherent cells derived from hUC displayed a fibroblastic morphology. (B), rUGSSs were small and fibrous in appearance. (C), hUC-MSCs were immunostained by an anti-human nuclei monoclonal antibody (green). (D), rUGSSs were immunostained by vimentin antibody (red). Scale bar: 50 μm.

To further characterize the hUC-MSCs that we prepared, we analyzed the cells by flow cytometry at P0-P8. As shown in Figure 2, hUC-MSCs exhibited positive surface expression of integrin marker (CD29) (Fig. 2A), MSCs marker (CD105) (Fig. 2B), but were negative for hematopoietic lineage markers (CD45, CD34) (Fig. 2C, D) nor the platelet/endothelial cell adhesion molecule (CD31) (Fig. 2E). The CD29+CD105+ hUC-MSCs population accounted for 85%–99.9% of the total cells.

Prostate Generation Assays

To determine whether they have the capability to differentiate into epithelial cells of endodermal origin such as the prostate epithelial cells, we performed renal capsule cell recombination prostate generation assays. Cells tend to have more robust growth under the kidney capsule, most likely due to the rich blood supply and inductive microenvironment in that area [21,22]. rUGSSs provide the critical paracrine factors needed for induction of hUC-MSCs growth and development into prostatic epithelial cells. We co-transplanted the hUC-MSCs and rUGSSs into the sub-renal region in nude mice. Grafts were allowed to develop for a period of 2 months before harvest and analysis. We also transplanted solely rUGSSs and solely hUC-MSCs as control experiments. We found that these grafts from sole rUGSSs or hUC-MSCs were small and fibrous in appearance (Fig. 3A, B) and microscopically, they showed a cluster of cells without obvious epithelial glandular structures (Fig. 3D, E). However, in sharp contrast, when the

hUC-MSCs were combined with rUGSSs and co-transplanted under the kidney capsule, the grafts formed large translucent epithelial-like glandular structures (Fig. 3C), resembling closely the prostate epithelial acini. These tubular epithelial-like structures in the grafts also displayed lumen filled with fluid (Fig. 3F).

Detailed immunohistochemical characterization revealed that the grafts expressed prostate luminal cell marker CK8 (Fig. 4A, B, F and Fig. 5A, B), basal cell marker p63 (Fig. 4C, D) and androgen receptor (Fig. 4G, H). Figure 4E shows single staining for the basal cell marker CK5 (green) and Figure 4F shows triple-staining for the basal cell marker CK5 (green), luminal marker CK8 (red) and DAPI counter staining (blue). In addition, the human origin and functionality of the regenerated grafts were confirmed by expression of anti-human nuclear antigen. As shown in Figure 5, some human nuclear antigen positive cells(Fig. 5C, D) in the graft were double labeled by CK8 antibody (Fig. 5E, F), Furthermore, the epithelial-like cells derived from the grafted hUC-MSCs displayed secretory function as they were specifically labeled by the prostate specific antigen (PSA) antibody (Fig. 5G, H). Of 30 renal capsule grafts with co-transplanted hUC-MSCs and rUGSSs, four showed the formation of prostate epithelial glandular structures. In sharp contrast, in 30 control mice in which sole rUGSSs (15 mice) or sole hUC-MSCs were transplanted (15 mice), none of them displayed any prostate epithelial glandular structures even though some grafted cells survived (Figure 3D, E). Taken together, these

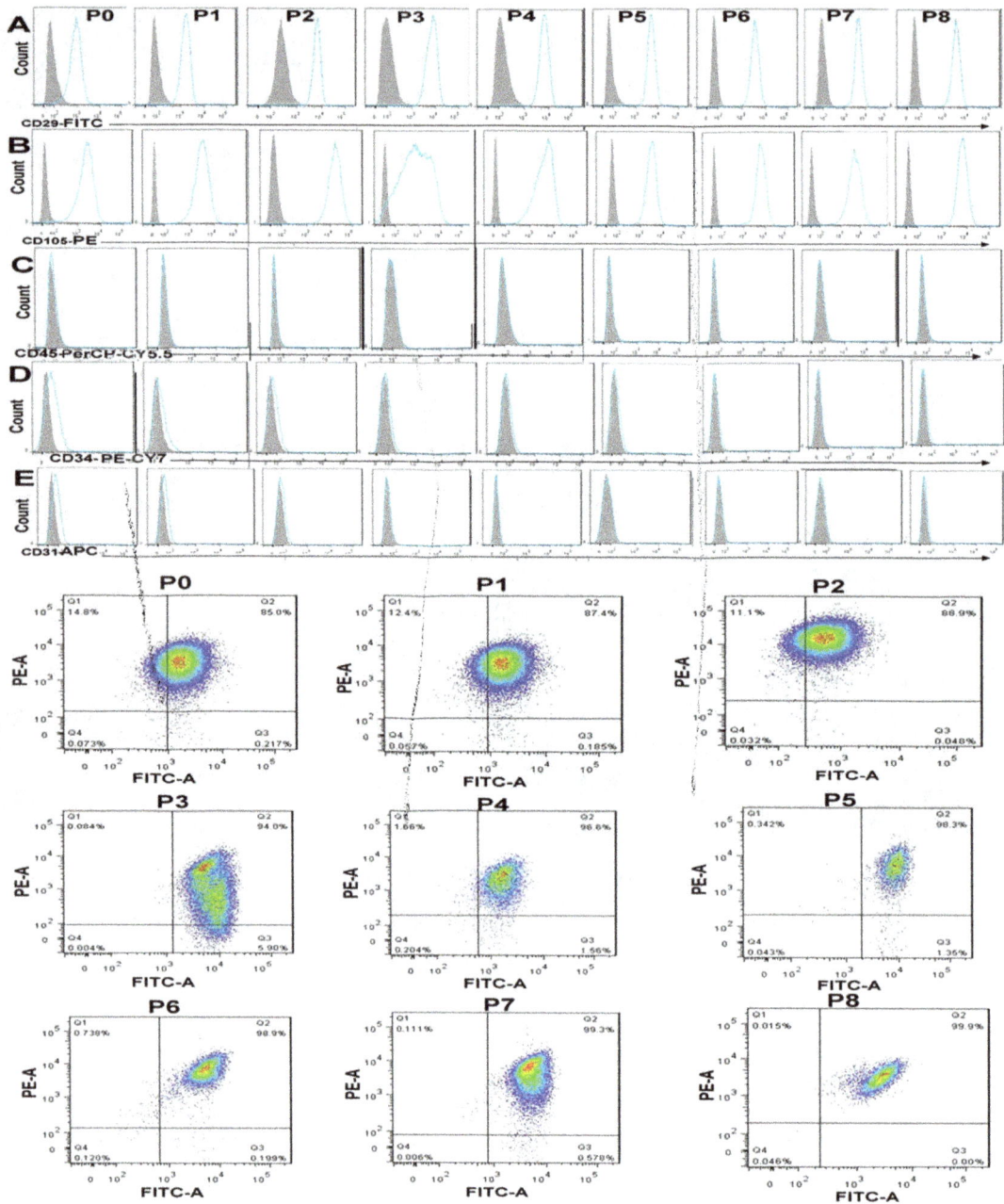

Figure 2. Immunophenotype analysis of P0-P8 hUC-MSCs by FACS. Cells were from P0-P8 hUC-MSCs and stained with CD29, CD105, CD34, CD45, and CD31 antibodies. The upper half of the figure is the flow histogram of single antibody staining. The shaded area shows the profile of the negative control. The lower half of the figure is CD29-FITC and CD105-PE expression of P0-P8 hUC-MSCs. (A) hUC-MSCs exhibit positive surface expression of integrin marker (CD29), (B) MSC marker (CD105), (C-E) but are negative for hematopoietic lineage markers (CD34, CD45) nor the platelet/endothelial cell adhesion molecule (CD31). The CD29+CD105+ hUC-MSC population accounts for 85%~99.9% of all cells.

findings indicate that the hUC-MSCs had differentiated into prostate epithelial-like cells under these experimental conditions.

Discussion

Using a cell recombination procedure previously developed by Cunha and Lung [23] or Li et al [18]. We have shown in the present study that a prostate branching structure (Fig. 3F) with epithelial-like tubules composed of basal (p63, CK5; Fig. 4C, E) and luminal (CK8; Fig. 4A, F) cell lineages is formed after co-

transplantation of hUC-MSCs together with rUGSSs under renal capsule. The grafts express the prostate specific antigen (PSA) (Fig. 5G) and androgen receptor (AR) (Fig. 4G), indicating generation of a functional prostate. Using a human nuclear antigen antibody, we have verified that the newly generated prostate epithelial-like cells in the grafts were of human origin and not due to contaminating rat epithelial cells from the rUGSSs preparations. We have shown in the present study that hUC-MSCs have the potential to differentiate into prostate epithelial-

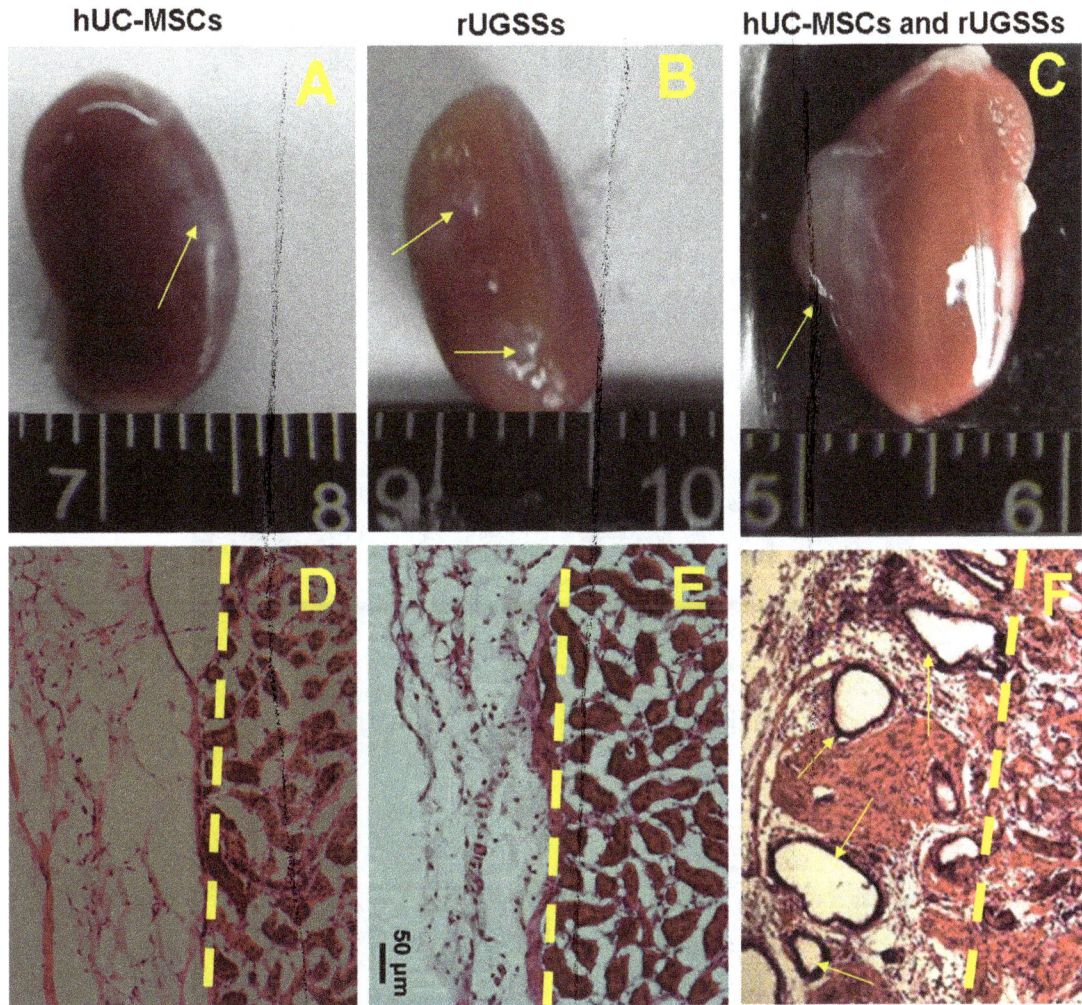

Figure 3. Human UC-MSCs combined with rUGSSs can generate prostate glands. Mice were sacrificed 2 months after co-transplantation surgery, and the kidneys from the cell implanted nude mice were collected. (A) Graft initiated with hUC-MSCs alone and (B) rUGSSs alone were used as negative control, respectively. (C) Graft derived with hUC-MSCs and rUGSSs. (D–F) Histological analyses of the sections of the graft stained for haematoxylin and eosin (H&E). (D) Note that while hUC-MSCs alone and (E) rUGSSs single cell type transplantation fail to regenerate prostate glandular structures. (F) co-transplantation of hUC-MSCs and rUGSSs gives rise to prostate glandular structures. Scale bar 50 μm.

like cells in vivo. The prostate generation rate from the hUC-MSCs is about 13%. While hUC-MSCs are originated from mesoderm [24], the prostate epithelial cells are derived from the endoderm [25]. Although previous studies have reported that hUC-MSCs can differentiate into mesodermal tissue such as the bone, cartilage, muscle, ligament, tendon, and adipose, to our knowledge, the present work is the first report to clearly demonstrate the capability of hUC-MSCs to differentiate into the endoderm-related prostate epithelium.

Consistent with previous findings, the rUGSSs appear to provide a stem cell niche, which provides necessary signals for the development and generation of prostate structures [23]. During normal embryogenesis, the prostate develops from the urogenital sinus (UGS), a structure derived from bifurcation of the cloaca. The UGS is a midline structure with an endodermally derived epithelial layer (UGE) surrounded by a mesodermally derived stromal cell layer [25]. As with many other tissue, prostate formation is initiated as a consequence of interactions between epithelial and surrounding stromal tissues [16,20,26–31]. Such

rUGSSs appear to provide a stem cell niche that promotes the hUC-MSCs to differentiate into prostate epithelial-like cells. The nature and signaling molecules involved in this process remain to be determined.

Our histological and immunnocytochemical characterization of the grafts provide strong evidence that the glandular structures formed following co-transplantation of hUC-MSCs and rUGSSs are composed of prostatic epithelial-like cells. The generated prostate tissues show the branching epithelial-like morphology and expression pattern of specific marker genes similar to that of normal prostate tissues. The cells in the graft express specific markers for the phenotypically distinct populations of differentiated epithelial cells within the normal prostate. The secretory luminal cells express PSA and cytokeratins 8 [32–35] while the basal cells express p63 and CK5 and are located in the basal layer [36]. In addition, the epithelial-like cells also express androgen receptor, an important marker for prostate epithelial cells. Although there is a third, minor population of prostate epithelial cells, called neuroendocrine cells that express synaptophysin, we

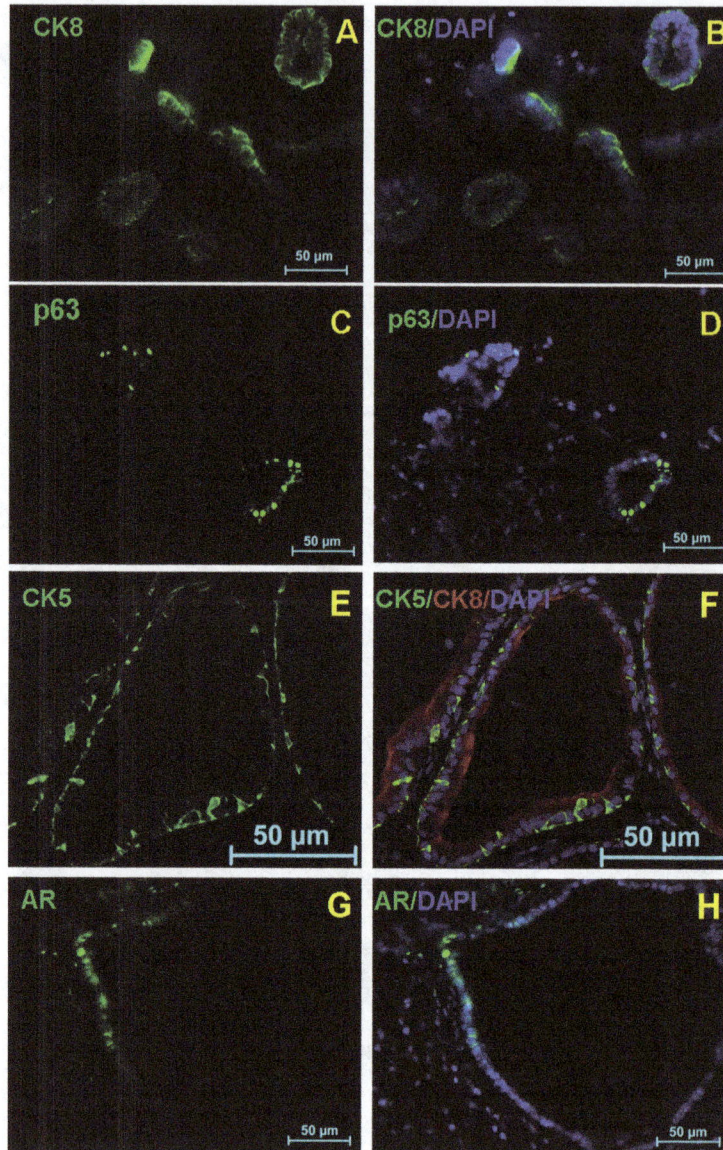

Figure 4. Regenerated prostates resemble the phenotypes of normal prostates. (A, C, E, G) Immunofluorescence analysis of the expression of CK8, p63, CK5 and androgen receptor (AR) in regenerated prostate tissue. (F) shows triple-staining for the basal cell marker CK5 (green), luminal marker CK8 (red) and DAPI counter staining (blue). (B, D, F, H) The tissue sections were counterstained with 4, 6-diamidino-2-phenylindole (DAPI; blue). Scale bar 50 μm.

failed to observe synaptophysin positive cells in the grafts formed, suggesting that either hUC-MSCs do not have to potential to differentiate into this population or the number of this population is too small for us to detect.

It is important to note that not only the cells in the grafts express prostate luminal and basal epithelial cells markers, they also express AR and produce PSA. These findings indicate that the prostate structures formed in the renal capsule are functional. In addition, using an antibody that recognizes specifically the nuclear antigen of human cells, we confirmed that the prostate structures formed are indeed from the hUC-MSCs, rather than from the recipient nude mouse cells. Double immunohistochemical analyses show that human nuclear antigen positive cells in the graft are co-labeled with CK8 antibody, indicating that the CK8 positive

luminal cells are derived from hUC-MSCs. Interestingly, we also found that some hUC-MSCs can differentiate into only luminal cell type, suggesting a possibility that some of the hUC-MSCs may follow an unipotent luminal cell lineage while others take a bipotential or multipotential route [37–40]. However, the mechanisms controlling the unipotency and bi- or multi-potency of stem cells during prostate development and regeneration require more studies.

Taken together, this study adds to the advancement demonstrating that a functional organ can be generated from a given type of stem cells. Our study clearly demonstrates that stem cells of the mesodermal origin can generate cells/tissue of the endodermal origin. Thus hUC-MSCs might potentially be useful for repair/regeneration of a broader type of tissues.

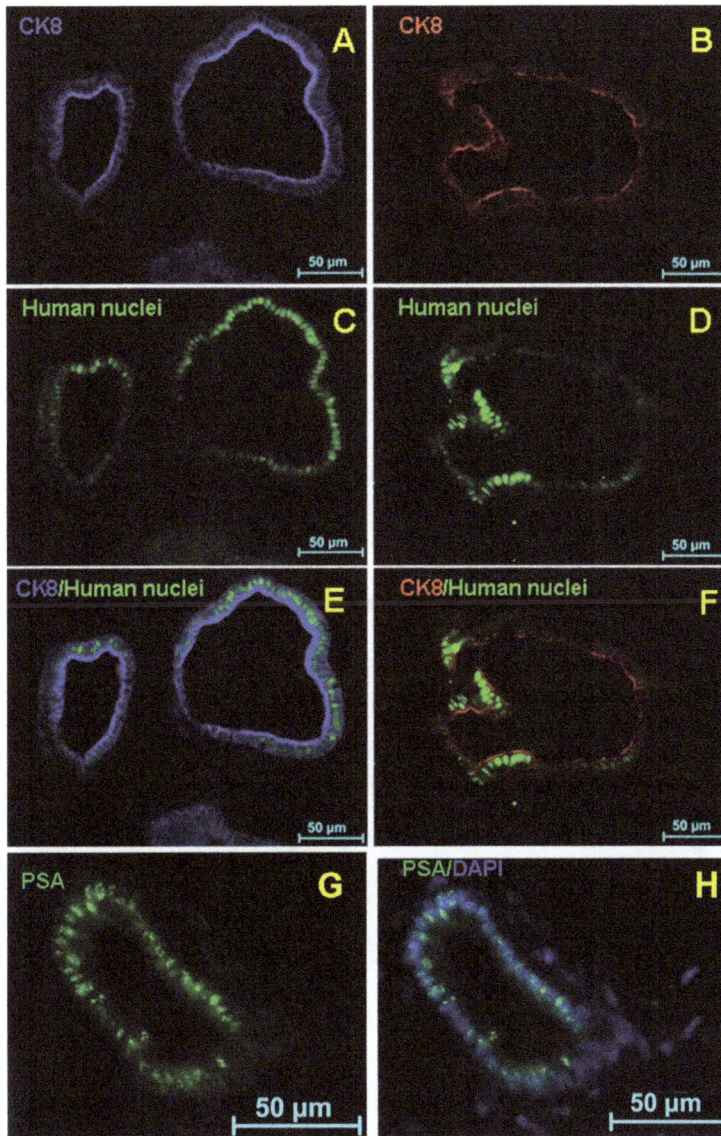

Figure 5. Detection of human cells in the regeneration of prostate. The field of prostate epithelial regeneration can be seen within the graft transplanted with hUC-MSCs and rUGSSs. (A, B) Immunofluorescent staining for CK8 in the new graft. (C, D) Detection of human cells in the new graft (green). (E, F) Note that the human nuclear antigen+ cells (green) in the graft can be co-stained with CK8. (G, H) The grafts express the prostate specific antigen (PSA). Scale bar 50 μm.

Author Contributions

Conceived and designed the experiments: WQG. Performed the experiments: WL BY. Wrote the paper: WL WQG. Conducted hUC-MSCs cultures: XYC. Collected and contributed clinical tissue samples: JHL.

References

1. Pittenger MF, Mackay AM, Beck SC, Jaiswal RK, Douglas R, et al. (1999) Multilineage potential of adult human mesenchymal stem cells. Science 284: 143–147.
2. Barry FP, Murphy JM (2004) Mesenchymal stem cells: clinical applications and biological characterization. Int J Biochem Cell Biol 36: 568–584.
3. Kastrinaki MC, Papadaki HA (2009) Mesenchymal stromal cells in rheumatoid arthritis: biological properties and clinical applications. Curr Stem Cell Res Ther 4: 61–69.
4. Pittenger MF, Martin BJ (2004) Mesenchymal stem cells and their potential as cardiac therapeutics. Circ Res 95: 9–20.
5. Burdon TJ, Paul A, Noiseux N, Prakash S, Shum-Tim D (2011) Bone marrow stem cell derived paracrine factors for regenerative medicine: current perspectives and therapeutic potential. Bone Marrow Res 2011: 207326.
6. Ikehara A, Maeda H, Kimura T, Saito S, Ochiai A (2012) Bone marrow-derived macrophages are associated with androgen modulated prostate regeneration. Prostate 72: 1–11.
7. Krause DS, Theise ND, Collector MI, Henegariu O, Hwang S, et al. (2001) Multi-organ, multi-lineage engraftment by a single bone marrow-derived stem cell. Cell 105: 369–377.
8. Placencio VR, Li X, Sherrill TP, Fritz G, Bhowmick NA (2010) Bone marrow derived mesenchymal stem cells incorporate into the prostate during regrowth. PLoS One 5: e12920.
9. Stamm C, Westphal B, Kleine HD, Petzsch M, Kittner C, et al. (2003) Autologous bone-marrow stem-cell transplantation for myocardial regeneration. Lancet 361: 45–46.

10. Rao MS, Mattson MP (2001) Stem cells and aging: expanding the possibilities. Mech Ageing Dev 122: 713–734.

11. Romanov YA, Svintsitskaya VA, Smirnov VN (2003) Searching for alternative sources of postnatal human mesenchymal stem cells: candidate MSC-like cells from umbilical cord. Stem Cells 21: 105–110.

12. Wang HS, Hung SC, Peng ST, Huang CC, Wei HM, et al. (2004) Mesenchymal stem cells in the Wharton's jelly of the human umbilical cord. Stem Cells 22: 1330–1337.

13. Lu LL, Liu YJ, Yang SG, Zhao QJ, Wang X, et al. (2006) Isolation and characterization of human umbilical cord mesenchymal stem cells with hematopoiesis-supportive function and other potentials. Haematologica 91: 1017–1026.

14. Arufe MC, De la Fuente A, Fuentes I, Toro FJ, Blanco FJ (2011) Umbilical cord as a mesenchymal stem cell source for treating joint pathologies. World J Orthop 2: 43–50.

15. Sciavolino PJ, Abrams EW, Yang L, Austenberg LP, Shen MM, et al. (1997) Tissue-specific expression of murine Nkx3.1 in the male urogenital system. Dev Dyn 209: 127–138.

16. Sugimura Y, Cunha GR, Donjacour AA (1986) Morphogenesis of ductal networks in the mouse prostate. Biol Reprod 34: 961–971.

17. Kellokumpu-Lehtinen P, Santti R, Pelliniemi LJ (1980) Correlation of early cytodifferentiation of the human fetal prostate and Leydig cells. Anat Rec 196: 263–273.

18. Xin L, Ide H, Kim Y, Dubey P, Witte ON (2003) In vivo regeneration of murine prostate from dissociated cell populations of postnatal epithelia and urogenital sinus mesenchyme. Proc Natl Acad Sci U S A 100 Suppl 1: 11896–11903.

19. Margossian T, Reppel L, Makdissy N, Stoltz JF, Bensoussan D, et al. (2012) Mesenchymal stem cells derived from Wharton's jelly: comparative phenotype analysis between tissue and in vitro expansion. Biomed Mater Eng 22: 243–254.

20. Sugimura Y, Cunha GR, Donjacour AA (1986) Morphological and histological study of castration-induced degeneration and androgen-induced regeneration in the mouse prostate. Biol Reprod 34: 973–983.

21. Lukacs RU, Goldstein AS, Lawson DA, Cheng D, Witte ON (2010) Isolation, cultivation and characterization of adult murine prostate stem cells. Nat Protoc 5: 702–713.

22. Scott MA, Levi B, Askarinam A, Nguyen A, Rackohn T, et al. (2012) Brief review of models of ectopic bone formation. Stem Cells Dev 21: 655–667.

23. Cunha GR, Lung B (1978) The possible influence of temporal factors in androgenic responsiveness of urogenital tissue recombinants from wild-type and androgen-insensitive (Tfm) mice. J Exp Zool 205: 181–193.

24. Can A, Karahuseyinoglu S (2007) Concise review: human umbilical cord stroma with regard to the source of fetus-derived stem cells. Stem Cells 25: 2886–2895.

25. Marker PC, Donjacour AA, Dahiya R, Cunha GR (2003) Hormonal, cellular, and molecular control of prostatic development. Dev Biol 253: 165–174.

26. Abate-Shen C, Shen MM (2000) Molecular genetics of prostate cancer. Genes Dev 14: 2410–2434.

27. Cunha GR (1994) Role of mesenchymal-epithelial interactions in normal and abnormal development of the mammary gland and prostate. Cancer 74: 1030–1044.

28. Cunha GR, Fujii H, Neubauer BL, Shannon JM, Sawyer L, et al. (1983) Epithelial-mesenchymal interactions in prostatic development. I. morphological observations of prostatic induction by urogenital sinus mesenchyme in epithelium of the adult rodent urinary bladder. J Cell Biol 96: 1662–1670.

29. Hayward SW, Rosen MA, Cunha GR (1997) Stromal-epithelial interactions in the normal and neoplastic prostate. Br J Urol 79 Suppl 2: 18–26.

30. Parrinello S, Coppe JP, Krtolica A, Campisi J (2005) Stromal-epithelial interactions in aging and cancer: senescent fibroblasts alter epithelial cell differentiation. J Cell Sci 118: 485–496.

31. Sugimura Y, Foster BA, Hom YK, Lipschutz JH, Rubin JS, et al. (1996) Keratinocyte growth factor (KGF) can replace testosterone in the ductal branching morphogenesis of the rat ventral prostate. Int J Dev Biol 40: 941–951.

32. Bello D, Webber MM, Kleinman HK, Wartinger DD, Rhim JS (1997) Androgen responsive adult human prostatic epithelial cell lines immortalized by human papillomavirus 18. Carcinogenesis 18: 1215–1223.

33. Lang SH, Sharrard RM, Stark M, Villette JM, Maitland NJ (2001) Prostate epithelial cell lines form spheroids with evidence of glandular differentiation in three-dimensional Matrigel cultures. Br J Cancer 85: 590–599.

34. Nagle RB, Brawer MK, Kittelson J, Clark V (1991) Phenotypic relationships of prostatic intraepithelial neoplasia to invasive prostatic carcinoma. Am J Pathol 138: 119–128.

35. Xue Y, Smedts F, Debruyne FM, de la Rosette JJ, Schalken JA (1998) Identification of intermediate cell types by keratin expression in the developing human prostate. Prostate 34: 292–301.

36. Kurita T, Medina RT, Mills AA, Cunha GR (2004) Role of p63 and basal cells in the prostate. Development 131: 4955–4964.

37. Shackleton M, Vaillant F, Simpson KJ, Stingl J, Smyth GK, et al. (2006) Generation of a functional mammary gland from a single stem cell. Nature 439: 84–88.

38. Leong KG, Wang BE, Johnson L, Gao WQ (2008) Generation of a prostate from a single adult stem cell. Nature 456: 804–808.

39. Keller G (2005) Embryonic stem cell differentiation: emergence of a new era in biology and medicine. Genes Dev 19: 1129–1155.

40. Xin L, Lukacs RU, Lawson DA, Cheng D, Witte ON (2007) Self-renewal and multilineage differentiation in vitro from murine prostate stem cells. Stem Cells 25: 2760–2769.

9

In-Vitro Study of the Effect of Anti-Hypertensive Drugs on Placental Hormones and Angiogenic Proteins Synthesis in Pre-Eclampsia

Subrata Gangooly[1], Shanthi Muttukrishna[†1,2], Eric Jauniaux[1]*

1 Institute for Women's Health, University College London, London, United Kingdom, 2 Anu Research Centre, Department of Obstetrics and Gynaecology, University College Cork, Cork University Maternity Hospital, Cork, Republic of Ireland

Abstract

Introduction: Antihypertensive drugs lower the maternal blood pressure in pre-eclampsia (PE) by direct or central vasodilatory mechanisms but little is known about the direct effects of these drugs on placental functions.

Objective: The aim of our study is to evaluate the effect of labetolol, hydralazine, α-methyldopa and pravastatin on the synthesis of placental hormonal and angiogenic proteins know to be altered in PE.

Design: Placental villous explants from late onset PE (n = 3) and normotensive controls (n = 6) were cultured for 3 days at 10 and 20% oxygen (O_2) with variable doses anti-hypertensive drugs. The levels of activin A, inhibin A, human Chorionic Gonadotrophin (hCG), soluble fms-like tyrosine kinase-1 (sFlt-1) and soluble endoglin (sEng) were measured in explant culture media on day 1, 2 and 3 using standard immunoassays. Data at day 1 and day 3 were compared.

Results: Spontaneous secretion of sEndoglin and sFlt-1 were higher ($p < 0.05$) in villous explants from PE pregnancies compared to controls. There was a significant time dependant decrease in the secretion of sFlt-1 and sEndoglin in PE cases, which was seen only for sFlt-1 in controls. In both PE cases and controls the placental protein secretions were not affected by varying doses of anti-hypertensive drugs or the different O_2 concentration cultures, except for Activin, A which was significantly ($p < 0.05$) higher in controls at 10% O_2.

Interpretation: Our findings suggest that the changes previously observed in maternal serum hormones and angiogenic proteins level after anti-hypertensive treatment in PE could be due to a systemic effect of the drugs on maternal blood pressure and circulation rather than a direct effect of these drugs on placental biosynthesis and/or secretion.

Editor: Rudolf Kirchmair, Medical University Innsbruck, Austria

Funding: Private donations managed by UCLH special trustees. The funders had no role in study design, data collection and analysis, decision to publish, or preparation of the manuscript.

Competing Interests: The authors have declared that no competing interests exist.

* Email: e.jauniaux@ucl.ac.uk

† Deceased.

Introduction

Normal placentation in human pregnancy is characterized by deep invasion of the placental bed by the extravillous trophoblast through the decidua down to the inner or junctional zone of the uterine myometrium [1]. Placental-related diseases of pregnancy are almost unique to the human species and affect around a third of human pregnancies [2]. These diseases include mainly miscarriages and pre-eclampsia (PE), which are respectively at the opposite end of a spectrum of major disorders of the development of the utero-placental interface. In miscarriage, placentation is severely impaired from an early stage leading to complete degeneration and rapid collapse of the placental structure before the end of the first trimester [2]. In PE, placentation is sufficient to allow partial development of the placenta but too shallow for complete development of the utero-

placental circulation and normal fetal growth during the second half of pregnancy [3,4].

The incomplete conversion of the end branches of the uterine circulation in PE results in retention of smooth muscle cells within their walls [5,6]. As a consequence, some vaso-reactivity persists in the utero-placental vascular bed leading not only to reduced perfusion of the intervillous chamber of the definitive placenta but also to intermittent perfusion exposing the placental tissue to low grade ischemia-reperfusion and chronic oxidative stress [7,8]. Chronic oxidative stress inside the placenta leads to progressive damage of the villous tissue, fetal growth restriction and finally to diffuse maternal endothelial cell dysfunction and clinical PE [2,6,9,10].

The exact pathogenic molecular mechanisms leading to the systemic endothelial dysfunction of PE remain to be determined [11]. The endothelial dysfunction associated with PE involves multiple maternal organ systems including the placental tissue itself resulting in major functional changes and progressive "placental insufficiency" [12]. Intra-placental oxygen (O_2) distribution is likely to be an important regulator of trophoblast function in PE [6,10] but other factors such as immune maladaption, excessive shedding of trophoblast debris, oxidative stress and genetic factors have been found to contribute to the pathogenesis of the abnormal placentation [2,11,13]. Production of placental anti-angiogenic factors and in particular, soluble fms-like tyrosine kinase-1 (sFlt-1) and soluble endoglin (sEng), have been shown to be up-regulated in PE and their levels are found to be increased in maternal circulation, weeks before the onset of the disease [14,15]. Placental anti-angiogenic factors are released into the maternal circulation and are known to disrupt the maternal endothelium functions resulting in hypertension, proteinuria and the other systemic manifestations of PE [11,12].

Anti-platelet agents, alpha- and beta-blockers, calcium channel blockers, diuretics vasodilators (NO agents) and magnesium sulphate are the main drugs used in the management of PE [11]. Recent research using animal models to evaluate the different secondary effects of the disease has revealed some of the underlying mechanisms of PE [4]. However, PE is a disorder of deep invasive placentation, limiting the study of pharmacologic interventions to humans and a few other higher primates. We have previously shown the anti-hypertensive drug α-methyldopa (Mdopa) has an effect on maternal serum levels of angiogenic proteins and placental hormones in pregnancies complicated by PE [16,17]. This effect may be independent of Mdopa known antihypertensive central action and we have suggested that Mdopa may directly influence trophoblastic protein synthesis and/or release and thus some of the main placental biological functions. The aim of this study was to further investigate the possible effect of Mdopa and the other drugs, routinely used in the management and prevention of PE, on the placental secretion of hormones and angiogenic protein known to be altered in pregnancies complicated by PE.

Materials and Methods

Women booked for elective delivery by caesarean section at term at University College London Hospital (UCLH) were recruited for this study. Women with a multiple pregnancy, with a history of smoking, assisted reproductive treatment or with any pre-existing medical disorders such as chronic hypertension, diabetes, renal disease or immune disorders were excluded from the study.

In the PE group (n = 3), the diagnosis of late onset PE was confirmed using clinical and biochemical parameters [18]. The maternal blood pressure (BP) was measured in duplicate using a standard mercury sphygmomanometer and the average of two readings taken. Korotkoff sounds 1 and 5 were used to define systolic and diastolic BP respectively. The mean BP was calculated as diastolic BP+1/3 pulse pressure. PE was defined according to the guidelines of the International Society for the Study of Hypertension in Pregnancy [19]. The diagnosis of PE was based on two recordings of diastolic blood pressure 90 mm Hg, at least four hours apart; or one recording of diastolic BP≥120 mm Hg, in a previously normotensive woman; and urine protein excretion ≥ 300 mg in 24 hours, or two readings of ++ or more on dipstick analysis of a midstream or catheter specimen of urine, if no 24 hour collection was available. In all 3 cases, the average resistance and pulsatility indices were above the 95th centile of the normal ranges.

The control group (n = 6) included only uncomplicated single-ton spontaneous conceptions booked for elective caesarean section at term. The indication for caesarean section in the controls was a previous caesarean section in five cases and a fibroid in lower segment with fetal transverse presentation in one case.

The study was approved by the Joint UCL/UCLH Committees on the Ethics of Human Research (Reference Number: 05/ Q0505/82). All women received information about the study and written consent was obtained prior to the caesarean section.

Samples

In both groups the placenta was collected immediately from the operating theatre during a caesarean section. The placenta was kept on a sterile tray and sterile forceps and scissors were used to obtain five placental samples from central part. The samples were then rinsed thoroughly between 5 to 7 times with sterile HBSS (Hanks balanced salt solution, GIBCO, UK) to remove all blood and blood clots. The villous samples were immediately transferred to the laboratory, placed under the laminar flow hood and cut into smaller placental biopsies of maximum 1 cm in diameter. Each villous biopsy was weighed in a sterile Bijou bottle (Sterilin Ltd, Staffordshire, UK) before transfer to the culture well containing the medium.

In vitro cultures

Villous samples were cultured in sterile 12 well culture plates (Nunc-immunoplate, SIGMA-Aldrich Co, UK). The culture media contained Dulbecco's modified eagle medium (DMEM, GIBCO, UK) with glutamate and 10% fetal calf serum (SIGMA-Aldrich Co, UK); 100 U/ml penicillin and 100 µg/ml strepto-mycin. Each culture well-contained 1.5 ml of culture media and were cultured in a humidified 5% CO_2 incubator at 37°C, for 3 days.

We tested the following drugs at 3 different dosages as previously described by Xu et al., [20,21]: labetolol (LABE) (low dose 15.6 µgm/ml; medium dose 250 µg/ml; high dose 4000 µg/ ml), hydralazine (HDZ) (low dose 5 µg/ml; medium dose 125 µg/ ml; high dose 1000 µg/ml;), Mdopa (low dose 39 µg/ml; medium dose 625 µg/ml; high dose 10000 µg/ml) and pravastatin sodium (low dose 0.039 µg/ml; medium dose 1.25 µg/ml; high dose 20 µg/ml). Control medium included 75 µl of HBSS (GIBCO, UK) for LABE, HDZ and pravastatin and 75 µl of 0.05 M of HCL for Mdopa.

For each experiment, two sets of culture plates/drug from both groups were incubated in 2 different CO_2 incubators at ambient atmospheric O_2 concentration (20%) and 10% O_2 concentration as previously described [5].

After 24 hours of incubation (day 1), the culture supernatant from all culture experiment was collected and frozen at −80 c until assayed. The villous explants were washed three times with HBSS (GIBCO, UK) and 1.5 ml of fresh culture medium and 75 µl of the different drug concentration solutions was added. The same procedure was repeated on day 2 and day 3. For each sample, after 24 h and 48 h, the media was removed and the villous explants were washed and replaced with fresh culture media and drug solutions.

All our experiments were carried out in triplicate wells and minimum repeated 3 times totalling 540 samples analyzed for the entire experiment.

Immunoassays

Total activin A (follistatin bound and unbound) was measured using a two-site enzyme linked immunosorbent assays ELISA [22,23]. Affinity purified human activin A was used as the assay standard. The detection limit of the assay for purified human Activin A was 50 ng/ml. Intra- and inter assay coefficients of variation were 9% and 10%, respectively.

Dimeric inhibin A was measured using a two-site ELISA [25,26]. The sensitivity of the assay was 2 pg/ml and the intra- and inter- assay variations were 5.2% and 6.5%, respectively.

hCG was measured using a commercially available kit from IBL with standards at concentrations of 0 miu/ml, 5 miu/ml, 25 miu/ml, 100 miu/ml, 200 miu/ml.

Human sFlt-1 and sEng were measured using a two-site (ELISAs) from R & D Systems (Minneapolis, Minnesota, USA). Measurements were conducted in duplicate according to the manufacturer's protocol. The assay was validated in our laboratory and dilution curves created to get the correct dilution for each assay. The minimum detectable levels for sFlt-1, and sEng were 5 pg/ml and 7 pg/ml respectively. Intra- and inter-assay coefficients of variation respectively in our laboratory were as follows: sFlt-1 7%, 9%; and sEng 6%, 8%, as previously described [17].

All measured concentrations were normalised against the gram (g) weight of the tissue sample.

Statistical Analysis

The data were analyzed using the Pad Prism 5 statistical data analysis and statistical software package (GraphPad Software, La Jolla, CA, USA). Standard Kurtosis analysis indicated that some values were not normally distributed and the results are presented as median and standard deviation (SD). A non-parametric analysis Mann-Whitney (Wilcoxon) W test was used to compared cases and controls. A Kruskal-Wallis test with Dunns post hoc tests was performed to evaluate statistical differences when more than 2 variables were tested. A P value of <0.05 was considered statistically significant.

Results

There was no significant difference in the median maternal age, parity, body mass index (BMI) and gestation at delivery between the PE and controls. The systolic and diastolic BP, levels of proteinuria and of all hepatic enzymes were significantly (P< 0.001) higher in the PE compared to controls.

Baseline secretion

After 1 day in culture at ambient O_2 (20%), the median levels of sFlt-1 and sEng were significantly (P<0.05) higher in villous explants from pregnancies presenting with PE than in normal controls (figure 1). There was no difference in the levels of activin A, inhibin A and hCG after 1 day in culture between the PE and control group.

Effect of Time

There was a significant (P<0.001) decrease in all protein median levels over the 3 days in culture at ambient O_2 in both PE samples and controls (figure 1). The most pronounced changes were found in PE explants, which showed a 10-fold decrease for Sflt1 and a 3-fold decrease for sEng, between day 1 and day 3 in culture.

Effect of O_2 concentrations

There was no difference in the placental hormones and angiogenic protein secretion at different O_2 concentrations, except for the secretion of activin A which was significantly (P<0.05) increased in the controls at 10% O_2 during the first day in culture and second day. This effect was not observed after 3 days in culture.

Dose dependant effect of anti-hypertensive drugs

No significant difference was found in villous explants secretion in both controls and PE cases when cultured for up to 3 days with no drug (control media zero concentration) compared with increasing doses of LABE (15.6, 250 and 4000 μg/ml), HDZ (5, 125 and 1000 μg/ml), Mdopa (39, 625 and 10,000 μg/ml) or Pravastatin (0.039, 1.25 and 20 μg/ml) at ambient or 10% O_2 concentration. Figures 1A and 1B illustrates the effect of no drug compared with maximum dose for each drug tested after 1 day in culture at ambient O_2 on the median levels of placental hormones and angiogenic protein.

Discussion

Our study shows that in vitro secretion of angiogenic proteins sEng and sFlt-1 is higher in villous tissue obtained at the time of elective caesarean section performed at term in women presenting with late PE compared to normal controls obtained under the same experimental condition. By contrast, in vitro secretion of placental hormones inhibin A, activin A and hCG is not different in PE than in controls although these proteins have been found in higher concentrations in the circulation of women with PE, months before they present with the clinical symptoms of the disease. In both cases and controls, the secretion of all proteins tested was time-dependent in vitro but not affected by the addition of anti-hypertensive drugs or statins to the culture medium.

Tissue culture experiments have been previously used In PE to evaluate the synthesis of various proteins and to test for the effect of different O_2 concentrations [24,25]. We found only two previous studies on the effect of clonidine, diazoxide, frusemide and hydralazine (HDZ) on placental production of sFlt-1, sEng cytokines over 24 hours in placental explants from term pregnancies complicated by PE [20,21]. With the exception of frusemide, none of the other drugs tested in culture over 24 hours had any effect on sFlt-1 and sEng production in placental explants from both PE and normal controls. Furthermore, except for HDZ, the other drugs studied are now rarely used in clinical practice for the treatment of PE and other hypertensive disorders of pregnancy [26,27]. Intravenous HDZ or LABE are both considered first-line drugs for the management of acute and severe hypertension during pregnancy whereas oral Mdopa or LABE are used most commonly in the management of non-severe hypertension [27].

The pharmacokinetic, pharmacological effects and pharmacogenetic of these drugs are very different. HDZ acts by dilating resistance arterioles, thus reducing peripheral resistance and has a direct catecholamine-mediated positive inotropic and chronotropic stimulation of the heart, resulting in an increase in cardiac output [28]. Mdopa is a DOPA analogue, which is converted to α methyl-norepinephrine an agonist of presynaptic central nervous system α2-adrenergic receptors [29]. Activation of these receptors inhibits sympathetic nervous system output and lowers blood pressure [30]. LABE is a β-blockers with antagonistic properties at both α- and β-adrenergic receptors, with direct vasodilator activity [31]. HDZ appears to activate guanylatecyclase, leading to increase cyclic GMP in arterial vascular smooth muscle and causing vasorelaxation [32]. The data of the present study indicate that the anti-hypertensive drugs do not modify the trophoblastic secretions of placental hormones and angiogenic proteins and up to 3 days in culture suggesting that these drugs do not have a direct effect on placental biosynthesis.

Clinical PE is associated with deficient intravascular production of prostacyclin and excessive production of thromboxane, which is a vasoconstrictor and stimulant of platelet aggregation. This observation has led to the concept two decades ago that anti-

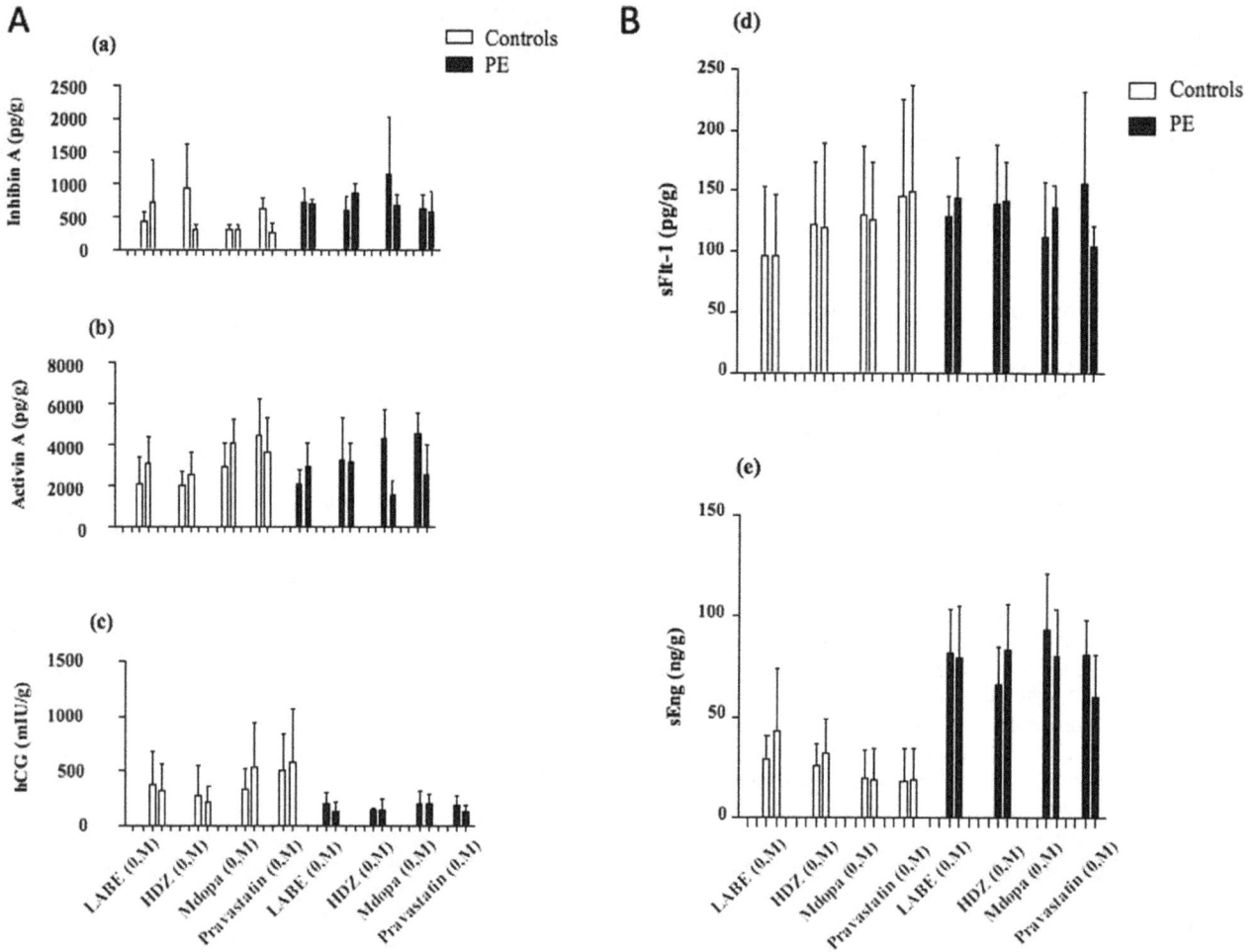

Figure 1. Comparison of the effect of no drug (0) compared with maximum (M) dose for LABE (4000 mg/ml), HDZ (1000 mg/ml), Mdopa (10,000 mg/ml) and Pravastatin (20 mg/ml) after 1 day in culture at ambient O_2 on the median (SD) levels of placental hormones (Fig. 1A) and angiogenic protein (Fig. 1B). The beta errors for no drug versus max dose of Mdopa are: 0.0465 & 02451 on Inhibin A; 0.0001 & 0.9761 on Activin A; 0.0019 & 0.0367 for hCG; 0.0655 & 0.0054 for sFlt-1 and 0.0559 & 0.1977 for sEng, respectively.

platelet agents, mainly aspirin can be used from early in pregnancy to prevent the development of PE [33]. 3-Hydroxy-3-methylglu-taryl-coenzyme A (HMG-CoA) reductase is the key enzyme of cholesterol synthesis and statins which are HMG-CoA reductase inhibitors have been increasingly used in patients with hypercholesterolemia and/or at risk of vascular diseases [34]. Pravastatin and other statins have also been shown to reverse various pathophysiologic pathways associated with PE, such as angiogenic imbalance, endothelial injury, inflammation, and oxidative stress [35]. Pravastatin has been shown to induce the VEGF-like angiogenic factor placental growth factor (PGF) in a mouse model but there are no data on its possible pharmacological effects on the human placenta. The results of the present study indicate that similarly to anti-hypertensive drugs, pravastatin does not have a direct effect on placental biosynthesis of placental hormones and angiogenic proteins.

Inhibin A, activin A and hCG are all produced by the villous trophoblast and known to be increased in the second trimester serum samples from women presenting with clinical PE later in pregnancy [36]. There is mounting evidence that oxidative stress or an imbalance in the oxidant/antioxidant activity in utero-placental tissues plays a pivotal role in the development of PE [2].

Uterine contractions during labor are known to be associated with intermittent utero-placental perfusion and placentas subjected to prolonged active labor shown biological changes similar to those observed in PE [37]. This is further demonstrated by the increase in activin A and sFlt-1 maternal serum levels during labor compared to pre-labor in PE [36]. We have previously shown that the first trimester human placenta syncytiotrophoblast is acutely sensitive to O_2-mediated damage [38] and that the changes in intra-placental O_2 concentration during the first half of pregnancy are essential for trophoblast differentiation and placental development [39,40]. Furthermore, we recently found a direct relationship in the early intrauterine PaO_2 in vivo and inhibin A and sFLT-1 concentrations in placental bed blood confirming our hypothesis by intrauterine O_2 tension play a role in the placental proteins synthesis [41]. It has also been recently suggested that the oxidative status of the trophoblast may regulate glycosylation of proteins and thereby modulate major trophoblast cell functions [42]. In the present study, we found a significant increase in-vitro of activin A synthesis during the first two days in culture at 10% O_2 in normal controls suggesting that intra-placental O_2 tension may have an effect on some placental synthesis during all three trimesters in normal pregnancy. However, compared to the first trimester trophoblast, which develops in 8–10 O_2 [2,5], the third trimester villous tissue biological activities are less likely to affected by changes in O_2 tension in culture.

Activin A is know to promote the invasion of first-trimester cytotrophoblast until 10 weeks gestation [43] may play a role in the pathogenesis of PE by inducing excessive apoptosis in placenta indirectly through enhancing Nodal expression [44,45]. It has been recently suggested that the increase in placental secretion of inhibin A, activin A and hCG results from premature accelerated differentiation of the villous cytotrophoblasts and could be linked to chronic intra-placental oxidative stress.

PE is almost exclusively a disorder of human deep placentation, in-vitro cultures of human placental explants are essential to better understand the pathophysiology of PE but also the impact of anti-hypertensive drugs on placental biology. As shown in the present study, the biosynthesis of these placental hormones does not seem to be influenced by the presence of anti-hypertensive drugs or Pravastatin in the culture medium. Our study is limited to late-onset PE and included only three cases but we assume that the samples represent the same process and are therefore justified in repetitive sampling of three placenta specimens. The effects of anti-hypertensive drugs are not restricted to the placenta but a better understanding the impact of these drugs on placental functions in PE is essential to the development of more selectively targeted drugs ensuring swift introduction of optimal treatment whilst minimizing the use of inappropriate or ineffective drugs.

Author Contributions

Conceived and designed the experiments: SG SM EJ. Performed the experiments: SG. Analyzed the data: SG SM. Contributed reagents/materials/analysis tools: SM EJ. Wrote the paper: SG SM EJ.

References

1. Pijnenborg R, Vercruysse L, Brosens I (2011) Deep placentation. Best Pract Res Clin Obstet Gynaecol 25: 273–285.
2. Jauniaux E, Poston L, Burton GJ (2006) Placental-related diseases of pregnancy: Involvement of oxidative stress and implications in human evolution. Hum Reprod Update 12: 747–755.
3. Khong Y, Brosens I (2011) Defective deep placentation. Best Pract Res ClinObstetGynaecol. 25: 301–311.
4. Brosens I, Pijnenborg R, Vercruysse L, Romero R (2011) The "Great Obstetrical Syndromes" are associated with disorders of deep placentation. Am J Obstet Gynecol. 204: 193–201.
5. Burton GJ, Charnock-Jones DS, Jauniaux E (2006) Working with oxygen and oxidative stress in vitro. Methods Mol Med 122: 413–25.
6. Kimura C, Watanabe K, Iwasaki A, Mori T, Matsushita H, et al. (2012) The severity of hypoxic changes and oxidative DNA damage in the placenta of early-onset preeclamptic women and fetal growth restriction. J Matern Fetal Neonatal Med 26: 491–496.
7. Hung TH, Skepper JN, Burton GJ (2001) In vitro ischemia-reperfusion injury in term human placenta as a model for oxidative stress in pathological pregnancies. Am J Pathol 159: 1031–1043.
8. Hung T, Charnock-Jones D, Skepper J, Burton G (2004) Secretion of tumour necrosis factor alpha from human placental tissues induced by hypoxia-reoxygenation causes endothelial cell activation in vitro: a potential mediator of inflammatory response in pre-eclampsia. Am J Pathol 164: 1049–1061.
9. Vanderlie J, Venardos K, Clifton VL, Gude NM, Clarke FM, et al. (2005) Increased biological oxidation and reduced anti-oxidant enzyme activity in pre-eclamptic placentae. Placenta 26: 53–58.
10. Lee SM, Romero R, Lee YJ, Park IS, Park CW, et al. (2012) Systemic inflammatory stimulation by microparticles derived from hypoxic trophoblast as a model for inflammatory response in preeclampsia. Am J Obstet Gynecol 207: 337. e1–8.
11. Williams PJ, Morgan L (2012) The role of genetics in pre-eclampsia and potential pharmacogenomic interventions. Pharmgenomics Pers Med 5: 37–51.
12. Vatten LJ, Asvold BO, Eskild A (2012) Angiogenic factors in maternal circulation and preeclampsia with or without fetal growth restriction. Acta Obstet Gynecol Scand 91: 1388–1394.
13. Redman CW, Tannetta DS, Dragovic RA, Gardiner C, Southcombe JH, et al. (2012) Review: Does size matter? Placental debris and the pathophysiology of pre-eclampsia. Placenta 33: S48–54.
14. Anderson UD, Olsson MG, Kristensen KH, Åkerström B, Hansson SR (2012) Biochemical markers to predict preeclampsia. Placenta 33: S42–47.
15. Kleinrouweler CE, Wiegerinck MM, Ris-Stalpers C, Bossuyt PM, van der Post JA, et al. (2012) Accuracy of circulating placental growth factor, vascular endothelial growth factor, soluble fms-like tyrosine kinase 1 and soluble endoglin in the prediction of pre-eclampsia: a systematic review and meta-analysis. BJOG 119: 778–787.
16. Khalil A, Muttukrishna S, Harrington K, Jauniaux E (2008) Effect of Antihypertensive Therapy with Alpha Methyldopa on Levels of Angiogenic Factors in Pregnancies with Hypertensive Disorders. PLoS ONE 3: e2766.
17. Khalil A, Jauniaux E, Harrington K, Muttukrishna S (2009) Placental production and maternal serum and urine levels of inhibin A and activin A are modified by antihypertensive therapy in hypertensive disorders of pregnancy. Clin Endocrinol 70: 924–391.
18. Kucukgoz Gulec U, Ozgunen FT, Buyukkurt S, Guzel AB, Urunsak IF, et al. (2013) Comparison of Clinical and Laboratory Findings in Early- and Late-Onset Preeclampsia. J Matern Fetal Neonatal Med 26: 1228–1233.
19. Brown MA, Lindheimer MD, de Swiet M, Van Assche A, Moutquin JM (2001) The classification and diagnosis of the hypertensive disorders of pregnancy: statement from the International Society for the Study of Hypertension in Pregnancy (ISSHP) Hypertens Pregnancy 20: IX–XIV.
20. Xu B, Makris A, Thornton C, Ogle R, Horvath JS, et al. (2006) Antihypertensive drugs clonidine, diazpxide, hydralazine and furosemide regulate the production of cytokines by placenta and peripheral blood mononuclear cells in normal pregnancy. J Hypertension 24: 915–922.
21. Xu B, Thornton C, Tooher J, Ogle R, Lim S, et al. (2009) Effects of anti-hypertensive drugs on production of soluble fms-like tyrosine kinase 1 and soluble endoglin from human normal and pre-eclamptic placentas in vitro. Clin Exp Pharmacol Physiol 36: 839–842.
22. Muttukrishna S, Fowler PA, George L, Groome NP, Knight PG (1996) Changes in peripheral serum levels of total activin A during the human menstrual cycle and pregnancy. J Clin Endocrinol Metab 81: 3328–3334.
23. Muttukrishna S, Jauniaux E, McGarrigle H, Groome N, Rodeck CH (2004) In-vivo concentrations of inhibins, activin A and follistatin in human early pregnancy. Reprod Biomed Online 8: 712–719.
24. Royle C, Lim S, Xu B, Tooher J, Ogle R, et al. (2009) Effect of hypoxia and exogenous IL-10 on the pro-inflammatory cytokine TNF-alpha and the anti-angiogenic molecule soluble Flt-1 in placental villous explants. Cytokine 47: 56–60.
25. Orendi K, Kivity V, Sammar M, Grimpel Y, Gonen R, et al. (2011) Placental and trophoblastic in vitro models to study preventive and therapeutic agents for preeclampsia. Placenta 32: S49–54.
26. Vest AR, Cho LS (2012) Hypertension in pregnancy. Cardiol Clin 30: 407–423.
27. Kattah AG, Garovic VD (2013) The management of hypertension in pregnancy. Adv Chronic Kidney Dis 20: 229–239.
28. Cohn JN, McInnes GT, Shepherd AM (2011) Direct-acting vasodilators. J Clin Hypertens13: 690–692.
29. Head GA, Chan CK, Burke SL (1998) Relationship between imidazoline and alpha2-adrenoceptors involved in the sympatho-inhibitory actions of centrally acting antihypertensive agents. J Auton Nerv Syst 72: 163–169.
30. Head GA (1999) Central imidazoline- and alpha 2-receptors involved in the cardiovascular actions of centrally acting antihypertensive agents. Ann N Y A-cad Sci 881: 279–286.
31. Falkay G, Melis K, Kovacs L (1994) Correlation between beta- and alpha-adrenergic receptor concentrations in human placenta. J Recept Res 14: 187–195.
32. Leitch IM, Read MA, Boura AL, Walters WA (1994) Effect of inhibition of nitric oxide synthase and guanylatecyclase on hydralazine-induced vasodilatation of the human fetal placental circulation. Clin Exp Pharmacol Physiol 2: 615–622.
33. Sibai BM, Caritis SN, Thom E, Klebanoff M, McNellis D, et al. (1993) Prevention of preeclampsia with low-dose aspirin in healthy, nulliparous pregnant women. The National Institute of Child Health and Human Development Network of Maternal-Fetal Medicine Units. N Engl J Med 329: 1213–1218.
34. Duggan ST (2012) Pitavastatin: a review of its use in the management of hypercholesterolaemia or mixed dyslipidaemia. Drugs 72: 565–584.
35. Costantine MM, Cleary K (2013) Eunice Kennedy Shriver National Institute of Child Health and Human Development Obstetric-Fetal Pharmacology Research Units Network. Pravastatin for the prevention of preeclampsia in high-risk pregnant women. Obstet Gynecol 121: 349–353.
36. Reddy A, Suri S, Sargent IL, Redman CW, Muttukrishna S (2009) Maternal circulating levels of activin A, inhibin A, sFlt-1 and endoglin at parturition in normal pregnancy and pre-eclampsia. PLoS One 4:e4453.
37. Cindrova-Davies T, Yung HW, Johns J, Spasic-Boskovic O, Korolchuk S, et al. (2007) Oxidative stress, gene expression, and protein changes induced in the human placenta during labor. Am J Pathol 171: 1168–1179.
38. Watson AL, Skepper JN, Jauniaux E, Burton GJ (1998) Susceptibility of human placental syncytiotrophoblastic mitochondria to oxygen-mediated damage in relation to gestational age. J Clin Endocrinol Metab 83: 1697–1705.

39. Jauniaux E, Watson AL, Hempstock J, Bao YP, Skepper JN, et al. (2000) Onset of maternal arterial blood flow and placental oxidative stress. A possible factor in human early pregnancy failure. Am J Pathol 2000; 157: 2111–2122.

40. Jauniaux E, Hempstock J, Greenwold N, Burton GJ (2003) Trophoblastic oxidative stress in relation to temporal and regional differences in maternal placental blood flow in normal and abnormal early pregnancies. Am J Pathol 162: 115–125.

41. Muttukrishna S, Suri S, Groome N, Jauniaux E (2008) Relationships between TGF-beta proteins and oxygen concentrations inside the first trimester human gestational sac. PLoS One 3:e2302.

42. Pidoux G, Gerbaud P, Cocquebert M, Segond N, Badet J, et al. (2012) Human trophoblast fusion and differentiation: lessons from trisomy 21 placenta. Placenta 33: S81–86.

43. Bearfield C, Jauniaux E, Groome N, Sargent IL, Muttukrishna S (2005) The secretion and effect of inhibin A, activin A and follistatin on first-trimester trophoblasts in vitro. Eur J Endocrinol 152: 909–916.

44. Nadeem L, Munir S, Fu G, Dunk C, Baczyk D, et al. (2011) Nodal signals through activin receptor-like kinase 7 to inhibit trophoblast migration and invasion: implication in the pathogenesis of preeclampsia. Am J Pathol 178: 1177–89.

45. Yu L, Li D, Liao QP, Yang HX, Cao B, et al. (2012) High levels of activin a detected in preeclamptic placenta induce trophoblast cell apoptosis by promoting nodal signalling. J Clin Endocrinol Metab 97: 1370–1379.

10

Structure Driven Design of Novel Human Ether-A-Go-Go-Related-Gene Channel (hERG1) Activators

Jiqing Guo[1,9], Serdar Durdagi[2,3,9], Mohamed Changalov[4,9], Laura L. Perissinotti[2], Jason M. Hargreaves[4], Thomas G. Back[4]*, Sergei Y. Noskov[2]*, Henry J. Duff[1]*

1 Libin Cardiovascular Institute of Alberta, University of Calgary, Calgary, Alberta, Canada, 2 Centre for Molecular Simulation, Biochemistry Research Cluster, Department of Biological Sciences, University of Calgary, Calgary, Alberta, Canada, 3 Department of Biophysics, School of Medicine, Bahcesehir University, Istanbul, Turkey, 4 Department of Chemistry, University of Calgary, Calgary, Alberta, Canada

Abstract

One of the main culprits in modern drug discovery is apparent cardiotoxicity of many lead-candidates via inadvertent pharmacologic blockade of K^+, Ca^{2+} and Na^+ currents. Many drugs inadvertently block hERG1 leading to an acquired form of the Long QT syndrome and potentially lethal polymorphic ventricular tachycardia. An emerging strategy is to rely on interventions with a drug that may proactively activate hERG1 channels reducing cardiovascular risks. Small molecules-activators have a great potential for co-therapies where the risk of hERG-related QT prolongation is significant and rehabilitation of the drug is impractical. Although a number of hERG1 activators have been identified in the last decade, their binding sites, functional moieties responsible for channel activation and thus mechanism of action, have yet to be established. Here, we present a proof-of-principle study that combines de-novo drug design, molecular modeling, chemical synthesis with whole cell electrophysiology and Action Potential (AP) recordings in fetal mouse ventricular myocytes to establish basic chemical principles required for efficient activator of hERG1 channel. In order to minimize the likelihood that these molecules would also block the hERG1 channel they were computationally engineered to minimize interactions with known intra-cavitary drug binding sites. The combination of experimental and theoretical studies led to identification of functional elements (functional groups, flexibility) underlying efficiency of hERG1 activators targeting binding pocket located in the S4–S5 linker, as well as identified potential side-effects in this promising line of drugs, which was associated with multi-channel targeting of the developed drugs.

Editor: Steven Barnes, Dalhousie University, Canada

Funding: This work was supported by the Canadian Institutes of Health Research [Grant 201103MOP-CSA-244888] (to S.Y.N. and H.J.D.); and the Heart and Stroke Foundation of Alberta [Grants 2010HSF-2013DUFF; 2011HSF-2014NOSKOV] (to H.J.D. and S.Y.N.). S.Y.N. is an Alberta Heritage Foundation for Medical Research Scholar. H.J.D. is an Alberta Heritage Foundation for Medical Research Medical Scientist. S.D. is supported by postdoctoral fellowships from the Canadian Institutes of Health Research and Alberta Innovates Health Solutions. The computational support for this work was provided by West-Grid Canada through a resource allocation award to S.Y.N. S.D. was supported in part by The Scientific and Technological Research Council of Turkey (TUBITAK) and EU 7th Framework Marie Curie Actions under Co-Funded Brain Circulation Scheme (TUBITAK2236 112C017). S.D. also acknowledges support from Bilim Akademisi - The Science Academy, Turkey, under the BAGEP program. The funders had no role in study design, data collection and analysis, decision to publish, or preparation of the manuscript.

Competing Interests: The authors have declared that no competing interests exist.

* Email: tgback@ucalgary.ca (TGB); snoskov@ucalgary.ca (SYN); hduff@ucalgary.ca (HJD)

9 These authors contributed equally to this work.

Introduction

Novel therapeutic interventions are required to control heart rhythm disturbances. One promising strategies is to increase the magnitude of potassium currents which underlie normal cardiac repolarization. Pharmacologic binding of small molecule "activators" to the hERG1 (*KCNH2* or Kv11.1) potassium channel is such an example. These activators might be useful in suppressing drug-induced, disease-induced or mutation- induced Long QT Syndromes. Remediating components of the cardio-toxicity observed in retro-viral, anti-cancer, anti-fungal, antibiotic and antipsychotic drugs by multi-pharmacology interventions containing specific channel activators may be essential for recovery of cardiac function [1,2]. In addition, it was originally proposed that the endogenous hERG1 tail current, resulting from recovery from C-type inactivation, could reinforce phase-3 repolarization and thus may protect from spurious depolarizing forces associated with depolarization-mediated arrhythmias [3]. Thus enhancing the hERG-related tail current could be intrinsically anti-arrhythmic [4]. NS1643 is one of the best-characterized and potent activators of hERG1 [5–8]. The molecular mechanism(s) by which activators mediates its pharmacologic effects remains controversial [7–12]. Low concentrations of NS1643 (10 μM) increase the magnitude of the tail current whereas higher concentrations (20–30 μM) pharmacologically block the channel [13]. In addition, progressive increase in concentration above 10 μM produced near-linear increases in the leftward shift in the $V_{1/2}$ of activation. In contrast, the effect of NS1643 to shift the voltage-dependence of C-type inactivation of the hERG1 channel developed at 3 μM; with no further increment at higher concentrations. While location of the unique binding site for hERG1 openers is debatable, previous structural and functional studies indicate the possibility of multiple binding sites for activator in the hERG1 channel [7,12,13]. The additional evidence for multiple binding sites relates to biphasic concentration-response relationship in response to NS1643.

Recent docking studies combined with electrophysiological studies led to identification of three potential binding sites: one near the selectivity filter; one at the S4 and S4–S5 linker and another in the inner cavity of the hERG1 pore domain [7], which is an obvious culprit for agonist design. Numerous experimental studies indicate that binding to the inner pore of the channel results in the pharmacologic block of hERG1 [14,15], while binding to the site at the S4–S5 linker appears to contribute substantially to channel activation [7]. The mutations at the E544, within the S4–S5 linker region, increased the NS1643-induced shift in the $V_{1/2}$ of activation and exaggerated slowing of deactivation [7]. Therefore, we have at least one established activator site and a swarm of structural models enabling rational design of specific channel activators with NS1643 as a template. For the first time, it is possible to assess whether molecules designed to bind selectively to the proposed activator-specific site would have unique pharmacologic effects. The hypothesis tested in this study is that designer drugs that interact in the neighborhood of the activation gate would change $V_{1/2}$ of activation and deactivation without substantial pharmacologic block of hERG1. Accordingly this study focuses on design of molecules that interact with hERG1 in the neighborhood of E544 within the S4–S5 linker. We propose that the neighborhood of E544 is an attractive potential binding site for the following reasons:

1) Previous studies indicate that the S4–S5 linker is fundamentally involved in the activation process [16].

2) The E544L mutation substantially increased pharmacologic response to NS1643. Specifically the NS1643 -induced shift in the $V_{1/2}$ of activation was -18 ± 3 mV in wild type (WT) versus -24 ± 3 in E544L [7–12].

The NS1643- induced slowing of deactivation was 1.9 fold for WT but 3.5 fold for E544L. In addition the NS1643-induced increase in tail current amplitude was 13% for WT and 398% for E544L. Therefore we reasoned that a drug designed to interface with the neighborhood of E544 might selectively affect activation and deactivation of hERG1. We focus on mechanism(s) of action of NS1643, by designing modifications of its structure to selectively target domains of the hERG1 channel. A combined simulation/experiment strategy was used to design a molecule that selectively binds to a site in the neighborhood of E544 within the S4–S5 linker. Here we find that a drug designed to interface with the neighborhood of E544 selectively affects activation and deactivation of hERG1. Our combined simulation/experiment strategy to design a molecule that selectively binds to a site in the neighborhood of E544 within the S4–S5 linker suggests that this is a potential "druggable" site for activators that can be used to manipulate channel gating.

Experimental and Computational Methods

Ligand-Based and Receptor-Based Models on the Designing of Novel Compounds

Several available small molecule databases (i.e., PUBCHEM, ZINC, Asinex) have been screened using our previously developed atomistic receptor based hERG1 model. (Figure 1, and Figures S1–S5 in File S1). The summary of all computational results for ligand screening and optimization is provided in Tables S1 to S4 in File S2. Together with available structure databases a combined ligand- and receptor-based model for the *in silico* design of novel compounds was also used. The fragment database of Schrodinger (~4000 small-compound database) was used for construction of novel structures to be used for molecular docking. Together with different binding combinations of the fragments with 10 enumeration sites for the chosen template e.g. NS1643, the total number of derivatives was ~40000. (Figure S1 in File S1) The relevance of the NS-derivative and therefore consideration for the future design were evaluated by assessing intra-cavitary binding (QSAR model developed previously) and statistical model for activity developed from available literature data on hERG1 activators. The rationale for derivatives design and details on 5-site QSAR model AADHR.4 can be found in Tables S3 and S4 in File S2 and Figures S1–S6 in File S1.

Molecular Docking

The docking studies were performed using open and closed states of the target structure [17,18]. Glide-XP (Grid-based Ligand Docking with Energetics, extra precision) [19] and Induced Fit Docking (IFD) together with Generalized Optimized ligand Docking (GOLD) [20] were used. SiteMap utility from Schrödinger software package [21] was used to obtain information on the location and character of the potential binding sites. The site maps generated were then used to define the different grids for each binding site found, and were used to do the docking with Glide/XP and GOLD. The docking results for all derivatives considered in this study is summarized in Table S1 in File S2. Example of binding pose and site definition can be found in Figure 2. The details of the used docking algorithms, quantum-mechanical (QM) computations used to evaluate ionization energies and stable conformations along with protocols are provided in Methods S1. Table S2 in File S2 summarizes all of the results of QM computations for selections of stable ionization states and conformers for the synthesized compounds. Table S5 in File S2 provides comparison to available experimental data on fragment-homologs. The QM-optimized geometries for synthesized compounds are shown in Figures S7 to S9 in File S1 for substitutions in the positions R1 to R3, respectively. The corresponding energy iso-contours, dipole moments and electron density distributions are shown in Figures S9 to S12 in File S1.

Synthesis of NS1643 Analogs

The synthesis of NS1643 analogs is shown in Figures 3 and 4, respectively. All tested compounds for which elemental analyses were not provided were of >95% purity, as determined by HPLC analysis, except for **2**, **10**, **14**, **17**, **18**, **23** and **24**, for which NMR spectra are provided in the Supporting Information. HPLC analyses were performed under the following conditions: Novapak C_{18} reversed-phase column, 3.9×150 mm; solvent: acetonitrile-water, 70:30, 0.8 mL/min; UV detector: 254 nm. ^{1}H NMR spectra were obtained at 300, 400 or 600 MHz. ^{13}C NMR spectra were obtained at 75, 101 or 151 MHz. ^{19}F NMR spectra were obtained at 376 MHz with hexafluorobenzene (-164 ppm) as the external standard, relative to trichlorofluoromethane (0.00 ppm). The syntheses of compounds **3–15** and **17** were performed by minor variations of the methods employed for the preparation of compounds **25** and **2**. The full disclosure on the preparation and characterization data for **3–15** and **17** are provided in Synthesis S1.

Electrophysiology

Transfected HEK cells on glass cover slips were placed in a chamber mounted on a modified stage of an inverted microscope. The chamber was superfused at a rate of 2 mL/min with a normal

LIGAND DATABASE SCREENING BASED ON 3D SIMILARITY TO THE 5-SITE BEST PHARMACOPHORE MODEL AADHR.4

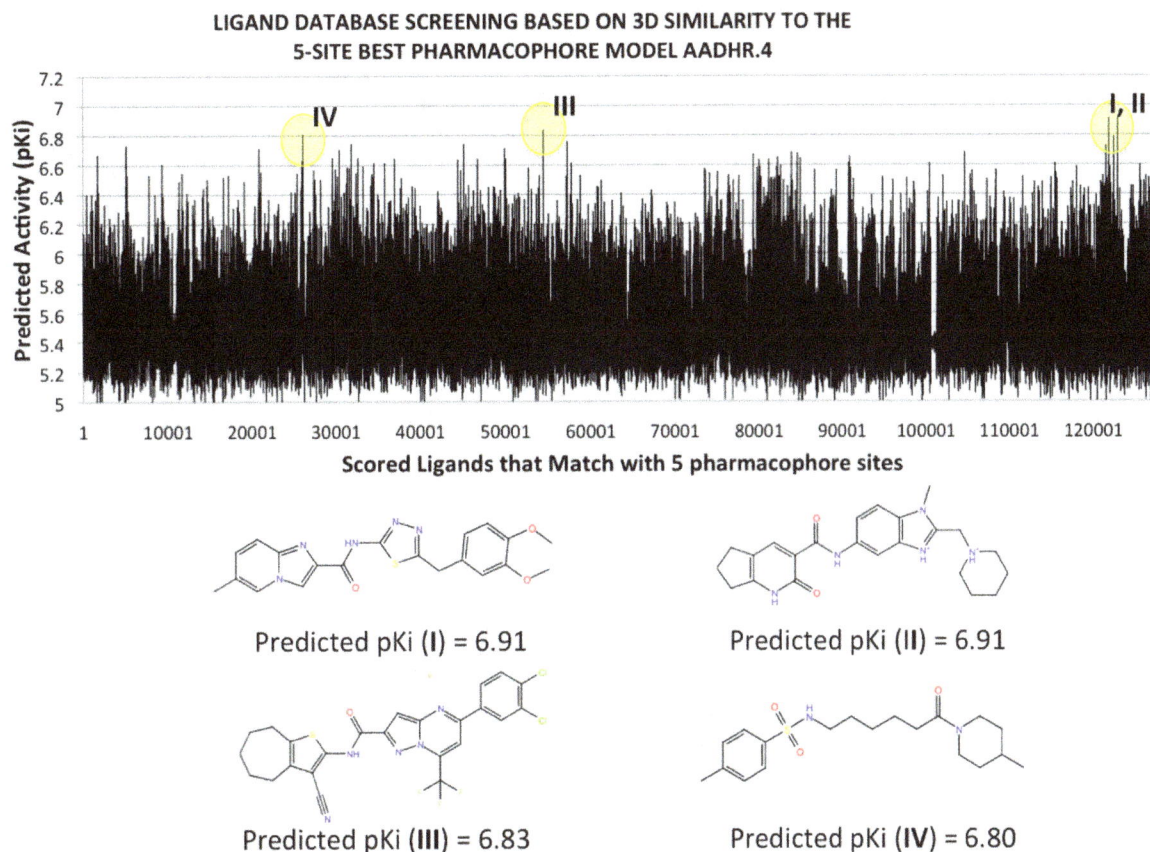

Predicted pKi (I) = 6.91

Predicted pKi (II) = 6.91

Predicted pKi (III) = 6.83

Predicted pKi (IV) = 6.80

Figure 1. Combined computational approach to opener's design. (Top) Example of 500000 ligands screening from Asinex Small Molecule library. Their activities are assessed with developed 5-site pharmacophore model AADHR.4. (Compounds with low predicted pKi values, i.e., pKi<5.0 are not shown). (Bottom) Selected top-scored compounds are shown together with predicted pKi values.

external solution. The extracellular solution contained (in mM) NaCl 140, KCl 5.4, $CaCl_2$ 1, $MgCl_2$ 1, HEPES 5, glucose 5.5, pH 7.4, with NaOH. Micropipettes were pulled from borosilicate glass capillary tubes on a programmable horizontal puller (Sutter Instruments, Novato, CA). Standard patch-clamp methods were used to measure the whole cell currents of hERG1 mutants expressed in HEK 293 cells using the AXOPATCH 200B amplifier (Axon Instruments) [22]. Unless otherwise indicated, tail currents were recorded when the voltage was returned to −50 mV from +50 mV. Further details on electrophysiological methods are collected in Methods S1.

Action potentials were recorded from neonatal (day 1) mouse ventricular myocytes as previously reported [23]. Although I_{Kr} has little physiologic importance to the action potential of the adult rodent heart, we previously reported that I_{Kr} is the dominant repolarizing current in day 1 neonatal myocytes, with little or no I_{Ks} [23]. Thus, these neonatal cells are well suited to assess the physiologic relevance of blockade of I_{Kr} to the action potential characteristics. In contrast, to address the possibility that compounds inadvertently interact with other channels, action potentials were recorded from adult cardiac myocytes. Myocytes on glass coverslips were placed in a chamber mounted on a modified stage of an inverted microscope.

Statistical Analysis

Statsview (Abacus Concepts, Berkeley, CA) was used to analyze the data. The data are presented as the mean ± SE. An unpaired

Student's t-test was used to compare the data. A two-tailed p-value of 0.05 was designated as being significant.

Because of limited space, detailed information of methods for chemical synthesis, electrophysiology, generation of 3D QSAR models, selection criteria for generated ligand databases and available ligand libraries, approaches to molecular docking, and a short summary of QM computations can be found in Methods S1.

Results

Development of Non-Blocking hERG1 Activators

The development of non-blocking ligands for hERG1 with improved ability to target tentative opener's site is viable route to structure-inspired opener's design. In the previous study we suggested the possibility of multiple binding sites for NS1643 [7,13]. Binding of NS1643 to the central cavity site appears to mediate pharmacologic block of hERG1 [13]. In the present study we focus primarily on a binding site in the neighborhood of E544, which appears to be involved in slowing of deactivation and shifts in the voltage-dependence of activation. To generate the initial statistical model for QSAR analysis and rational drug design of channel openers we investigated key interactions between ligands from the small-molecular database (i.e., Asinex, ZINC) and the receptor using previously identified binding pockets in hERG1 [7]. A two-steps drug docking performed with blind docking (i.e., a whole receptor is used as the active site) on a coarse grid covering the entire region of S4–S5 linker of hERG1 in open state [24].

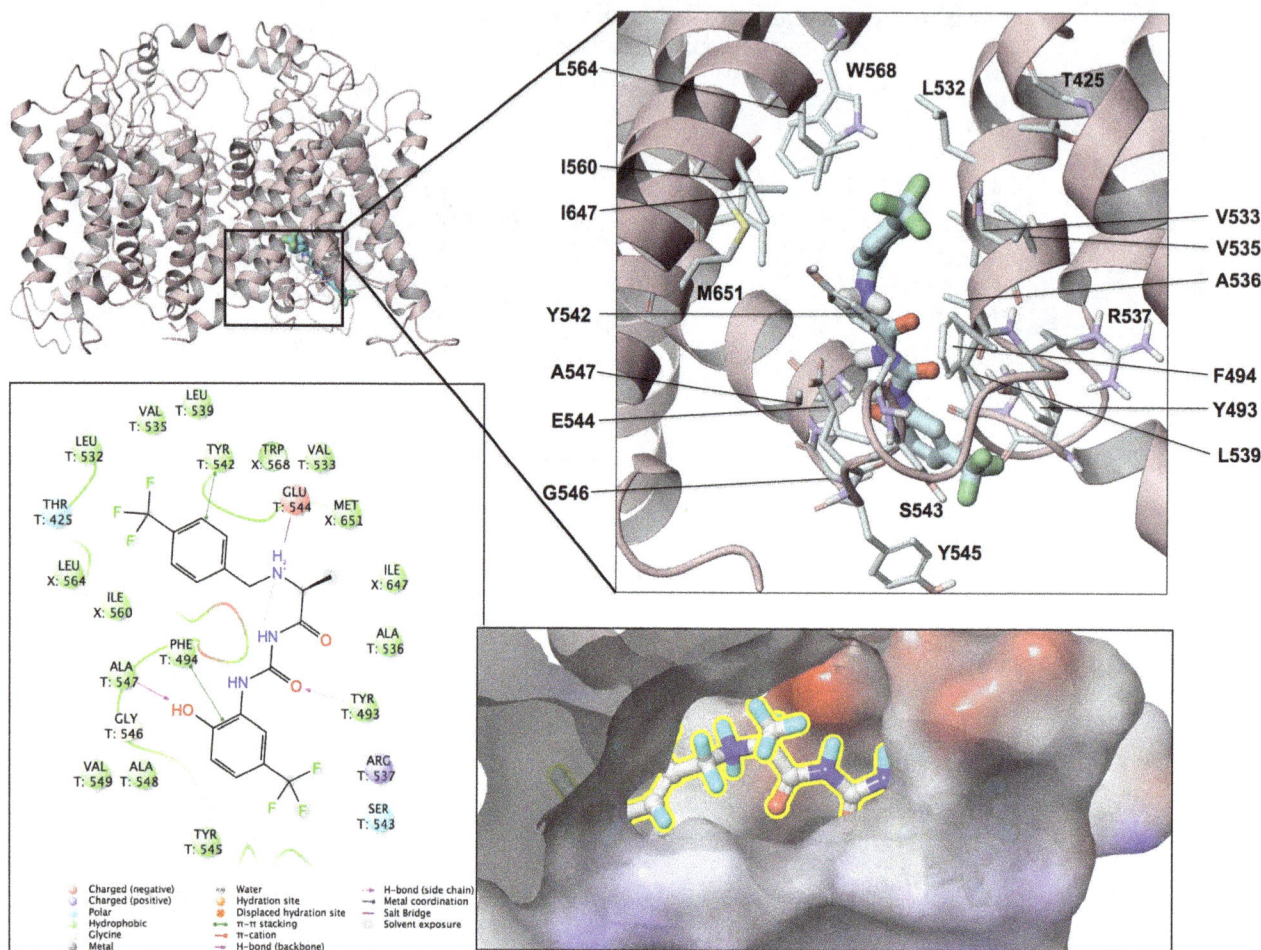

Figure 2. Mapping of the bound conformations for MC-II-157c at the S4–S5 domain of the receptor. 2D ligand interactions diagram (left-bottom panel) and surface representation of docked pose (right-bottom panel) are also shown at the figure.

The regions with high-density of bound states identified in docking were analyzed and further refined with high-precision and fine-grid docking simulations. A combined ligand- and receptor-based model for *in-silico* design of novel compounds is considered to develop pharmacophore model for a range of NS1643 derivatives. The Schrodinger's molecular modeling packages fragment database was used to generate of modifications of selected template starting compounds (i.e., NS1643, MC-I-159b, MC-II-43c). (Figure S1 to S6 in File S1). All compounds were then screened in silico for their predicted ability to block hERG1 using a previously build pharmacophore model by our group [25] and a receptor-based model (Glide/XP docking scores to the central cavity of hERG) developed [17,18]. Compounds that have low-affinity were selected for synthesis and are collected in Table 1. Electrophysiological measurement results of these novel compounds are listed at Table 2. Table 3 shows comparison of the best poses found with Glide/XP and GOLD docking programs for selected drugs binding to the binding pockets at different regions of hERG1 (i.e., S4–S5 linker site close to E544, outer mouth of selectivity filter site, EC domains, and pore domain). The subset of candidates was chosen for chemical synthesis based on the docking studies and a targeted modifications of the functional moieties responsible for channel blockade and binding to established activator site, respectively. Several substitutions in the

positions labeled R1 to R3 in Figure 5 were found to produce desired effect *in silico* screening. The ideal (desired effect) target for synthesis from *in silico* modeling entails lowered intra-cavitary affinity compared to original NS1643 and enhanced ability to target previously identified binding pocket around E544. The use of fragment-based approach in the design of the improved activators allows for blinded drug-development thus offering foot-printing of the activator binding pocket in hERG1. The details of the synthesis of the various molecules are provided in File S1/Synthesis S1 and in Figures 3 and 4. The list of substitution groups selected on the basis of in-silico screening and collection of synthesis intermediates is shown in Figure 5 together with definition of compound groups.

Electrophysiological Evaluation of Designed Molecules

The pharmacologic-responses to the molecules designed and synthesized for this study are shown in Table 2 and Figures 6 to 8. Of all the compounds developed, the *bromo-* substitution (i.e., MC-II-159c) and the *trifluoro-* substitution (i.e., MC-II-157c) produced the greatest decrease in deactivation rate (Figures 6–8). Importantly, both MC-II-159c and MC-II-157c slowed the rate of deactivation substantially more than NS1643. The extent of prolongation of deactivation was greatest for MC-II-159c. At 2 μM, MC-II-159c minimally blocked the channel (I/Icon = 0.76)

Scheme 1

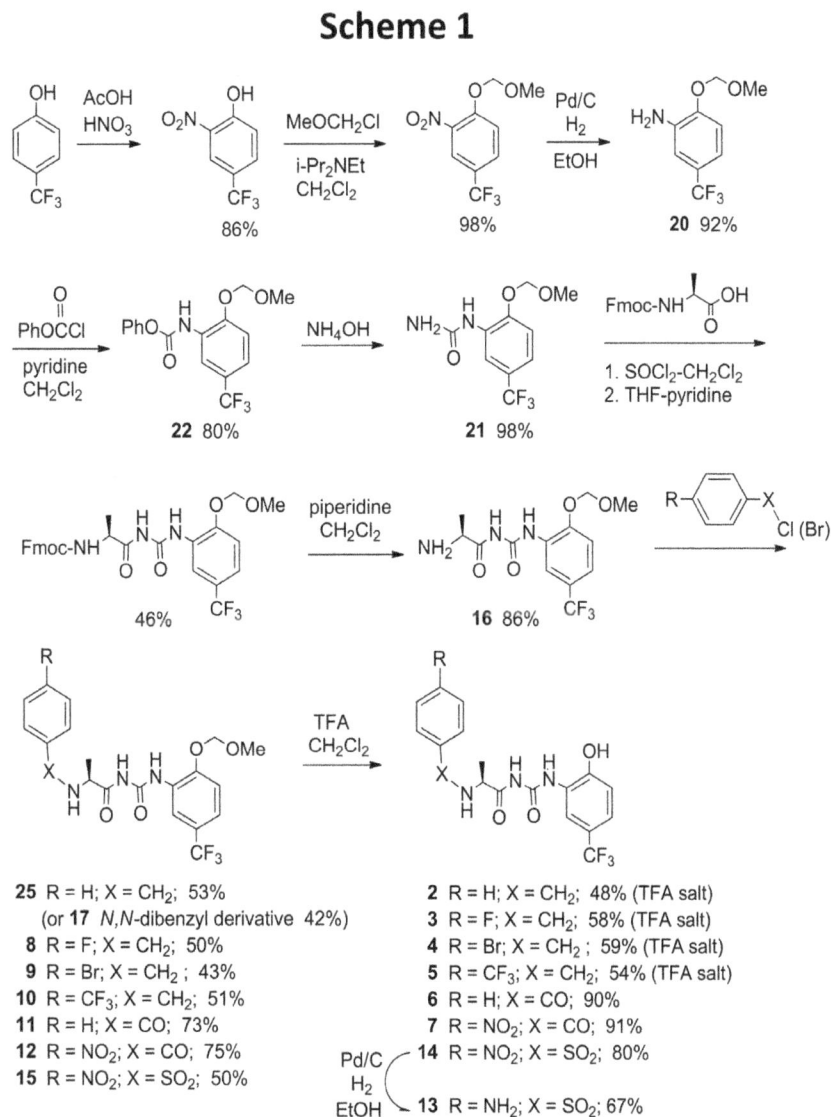

Figure 3. Synthesis of NS1643 Analogs and Intermediates (Scheme 1).

significantly prolonged deactivation but minimally left shifted the $V_{1/2}$ of activation by -5 ± 2 mV. However at 20 µM it blocked the hERG1 tail current ($I/I_{con} = 0.6$). For MC-II-157c there is

little evidence for concentration-dependent pharmacologic block at the µM range of concentrations. Importantly, at 3 µM, MC-II-157c significantly increased the tail-current amplitude to an extent similar to that seen with NS1643. At 10 µM the normalized current ($I/Icon$) was 0.88; at 20 µM the $I/Icon$ was 0.86 and at 50 µM the $I/Icon$ was 0.83. Indeed these values are comparable to that seen during prolonged placebo treatment ($I/Icon = 0.89$). Prolonged whole-cell dialysis of cells can result in run-down of the hERG1 current. Moreover, we never observed increase in current during drug washout. Interestingly MC-II-157c produced monotonic concentration-dependent shifts in the $V_{1/2}$ of activation and slowing of deactivation. The magnitude of the effects on activation and deactivation are approximately 6-10 fold greater than that previously reported with NS1643 signifying relevance of the proposed binding site at the S4–S5 linker and viability of the rational design for openers.

Scheme 2

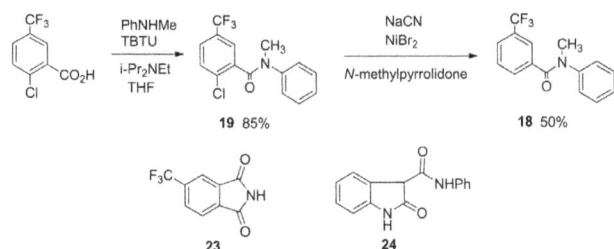

Figure 4. Synthesis of NS1643 Analogs and Intermediates (Scheme 2).

Table 1. NS1643 and its synthesized derivatives are used in the construction of PHASE Pharmacophore Model.

Comp. No	Name	2D structure	Dock. Score (kcal/mol)	Glide pKi	Phase pKi	# of Confs.
1	NS1643		−9.01	6.56	6.17	30
Group 1						
2	MC-II-43c	R_1: -H, R_2: -H, R_3: -H	−8.56	6.24	6.27	164
3	MC-II-163c	R_1: -H, R_2: -H, R_3: -F	−8.00	5.83	6.25	176
4	MC-II-159c	R_1: -H, R_2: -H, R_3: -Br	−10.64	7.75	7.79	166
5	MC-II-157c	R_1: -H, R_2: -H, R_3: -CF$_3$	−11.41	8.31	7.92	144
6	MC-II-61c	R_1: -H, R_2: =O, R_3: -H	−10.14	7.39	7.13	48
7	MC-II-63c	R_1: -H, R_2: =O, R_3: -NO$_2$	−9.68	7.05	7.12	48
8	MC-II-161b	R_1: -CH2OCH3, R_2: -H, R_3: -F	−9.02	6.57	7.17	142
9	MC-II-155b	R_1:-CH$_2$OCH3, R_2: -H, R_3: -Br	−9.38	6.83	7.24	69
10	MC-II-153b	R_1:-CH$_2$OCH$_3$, R_2: -H, R_3: -CF$_3$	−10.19	7.42	7.28	129
11	MC-II-57c	R_1: -CH$_2$OCH$_3$, R_2: =O, R_3: -H	−9.17	6.68	6.57	173
12	MC-II-59c	R_1: -CH$_2$OCH$_3$, R_2: =O, R_3: -NO$_2$	−8.69	6.33	6.35	39
Group 2						
13	MC-I-159b	R_1: -H, R_2: -NH$_2$	−9.73	7.09	7.38	165
14	MC-I-169b	R_1: -H, R_2: -NO$_2$	−9.59	6.99	7.29	125
15	MC-I-155b	R_1: -CH$_2$OCH$_3$, R_2: -NO$_2$	−7.64	5.57	6.22	86
Group 3						
16	MC-I-153b	R_1: -CH$_2$OCH$_3$, R_2: -H	−9.12	6.64	6.44	12
17	MC-II-67b	R_1: -CH$_2$OCH$_3$, R_2: -(CH$_2$C$_6$H$_5$)$_2$	−8.74	6.37	6.51	177
Group 4						
18	MC-I-165b	R_1: -H, R_2: -CO-(NCH$_3$)C$_6$H$_5$	−7.15	5.21	-	10
19	MC-I-163b	R_1: -Cl, R_2: -CO-(NCH$_3$)C$_6$H$_5$	−6.51	4.74	-	7
20	MC-I-89b	R_1: -OCH$_2$OCH$_3$, R_2: -NH$_2$	−7.41	5.40	5.21	4
21	MC-I-93b	R_1: -OCH$_2$OCH$_3$, R_2: -NH-CO-NH$_2$	−7.73	5.63	5.66	7
22	MC-I-167b	R_1: -OCH$_2$OCH$_3$, R_2: -NH-CO$_2$-C$_6$H$_5$	−6.95	5.06	5.20	15
Group 5						
23	MC-I-161b	R_1: -CF$_3$, R_2: CO, R_3: -NH, R_4: CO	−7.20	5.25	5.42	3
24	MC-II-17c	R_1: -H, R_2: NH, R_3: CO, R_4: CH-CO-NH-C$_6$H$_5$	−8.03	5.85	5.65	4

Table includes calculated (from Glide/XP) and predicted pKi values of compounds as well as number of conformers of each compound used in the construction of models. 2D structures for compound groups are shown in Figure 5.

Pharmacologic Responses to MC-II-157c and MC-II-159c Are Significantly Less in E544L

Figure 9 compares the pharmacologic responses to NS1643, MC-II-157c and MC-II-159c in hERG1 WT versus E544L. In WT hERG1, MC-II-157c and MC-II-159c like NS1643 slows deactivation and shifts voltage-dependence of activation to hyperpolarized potentials. In E544L, NS1643 produces exaggerated pharmacologic responses with significantly greater magnitudes of shifts in voltage-dependence of activation and slowing of deactivation. However in E544L, MC-II-157c and MC-II-159c produces significantly and substantially less pharmacologic responses. These data provide evidence that MC-II-157c and MC-II-159c are effectively targeting the neighborhood surrounding E544, and that interaction with this neighborhood mediates shifts in voltage-dependence of activation and deactivation. Moreover, these data provide evidence that the neighborhood surrounding E544 appears to be a true binding site. The measurements of voltage-dependence of inactivation for E544L are considered estimates only. For E544L the rate of deactivation is very rapid, with its tau being similar to that of inactivation.

Moreover, for E544L, the voltage–dependence of deactivation and inactivation overlap substantially. These elements may confound the accuracy of measurement of inactivation.

Contribution of the Peptide-Like Side-Chain Linker between the Benzene Rings to Channel Blockade

Several recent studies emphasized importance of drug rigidity for efficient binding to channel with a reduced blockade [26,27]. We investigated the effect of the peptide-like chain linker between benzene rings. The length of the linker can be used to control flexibility of the designed molecules. This varying length and flexibility of the linker was implemented in the structures of MC-I-153b to MC-II-67b listed in Table 1. The compound MC-I-153b has a single benzene ring with an intact peptide-linker. Interestingly this compound still left shifted the $V_{1/2}$ of activation at 50 μM but produces pharmacologic block at that concentration ($I/I_{con} = 0.3$). At lower concentration such as 10 μM, the compound still shifts $V_{1/2}$ of activation to hyperpolarized potentials but also had modest capacity to block hERG1 currents ($I/I_{con} = 0.6$). Compounds **18–24** (Table 1) manifest little or no

Table 2. Summary of electrophysiologic effects for the novel molecules studied.

Comp No.	Name	Conc. μM	Amplitude I/I_{con}	Activation $V_{1/2}$ (mV)	Inactivation $\Delta V_{0.3}$	Deactivation $\Delta\lambda/\lambda_{con}$
1	NS1643	10	1±0.04	−21±2.3	+6±0.6	1±0.4
2	MC-II-151c	20	0.4±0.02	−14.5±5.5	−21±0.0	0.6±0.4
3	MC-II-163c	20	0.6±0.14	−17.3±0.3	−7.5±4.5	1.7±0.3
		2	0.6±0.14	−17.3±0.3	−7.5±4.5	1.7±0.3
4	MC-II-159c	20	0.6±0.07	−33±14	−4.5±1.5	3.1±1.6
		2	0.76±0.14	−5±2	−0.5±0.5	0.25±0.02
5	MC-II-157c	50	0.83±0.1	−27.5±3.5	26±1	4.5±0.1
		20	0.86±0.1	−15.3±4.1	+9.3±2.0	3.5±0.2
		10	0.88±0.1	−14±3.6	14.0±2.7	3.3±1.3
		3	1.1±0.04	−6.5±0.5	1±1	0.8±0.1
		1	0.95±0.02	−2±0.0	1.3±0.9	0.2±0.1
6	MC-II-61c	20	0.7±0.02	−3.7±0.7	−2.5±1.5	0.8±0.1
7	MC-II-63c	20	0.6±0.1	−7±1.1	−3.5±4.5	0.6±0.3
8	MC-II-161b	20	0.1±0.0	−12.5±2.5	−4±8	−0.1±0.04
9	MC-II-155b	20	0.5±0.1	−9.1±2.1	−3.5±1.5	−0.1±0.1
10	MC-II-153b	20	0.4±0.02	−13.7±3.2	−12.3±3.4	0.5±0.03
11	MC-II-57c	20	0.6±0.04	−12.7±2.7	−1.5±1.5	−0.1±0.2
12	MC-II-59c	20	0.6±0.19	−6.3±2.7	−7.3±1.9	−0.1±0.1
13	MC-I-159b	50	1±0.03	−2.5±3.0	+10±0.6	0.5±0.1
		20	1.0	−5±3	+8±0.4	0.3±0.1
		2	1.0	−2±3	n/a	
14	MC-I-169b	50	0.39±0.04	−7.7±3.0	2.5±3.5	0.6±0.3
		2	0.93±0.01	−3±0.02	n/a	0.4±
15	MC-I-155b	30	0.5±0.04	0±0	−10±0	−0.01±0.07
		10	0.7±0.12	−3±3	−11±2	−0.1±0.1
16	MC-I-153b	50	0.3±0.02	−19±3	−27±2	0.003±0.14
		10	0.6±0.06	−7±2	n/a	−0.07±0.1
17	MC-II-67b	50	0.95±0.03	−2±0	+4±0	0.25±0.18
		10	±0.01	−5±0.6	−1±0.6	0.07±0.08
18	MC-I-165b	50	0.8±0.07	3.3±0.3	−11.7±7.3	−0.2±0.05
19	MC-I-163b	50	0.7±0.06	1±3	−2±1	−0.2±0.08
		5	0.9±0.1	0	n/a	
20	MC-I-89b	100	0.9±0.04	−3.3±1.3	−1±0	−0.06±0.2
		5	0.02	−2.5±0.5	0±1	0.03±0.01
21	MC-I-93b	50	0.9±0.04	−1.3±2.4	0.7±3.7	0.02±0.1
22	MC-I-167b	50	0.9±0.04	−1.7±2.3	0±0	−0.2±0.09
23	MC-I-161b	50	1.0±0.01	−2.3±1.3	−2±1.2	0.2±0.1
24	MC-II-17c	50	0.8±0.03	−2.3±0.9	8±0	0.2±0.2

pharmacologic activity even at concentrations of 50 μM. Therefore, it can be concluded that the binding site in the receptor imposes tight dimensional requirements for the size of the peptide linker and additional flexibility in the linker may lead to pronounce intra-cavitary blockade. Similar conclusions were reached in in-silico designs of minimally structured hERG1 blockers, as well as re-designed analogs of high-affinity blocker dofetilide [26,27].

Review of Key Features of the Designed Molecules

The pharmacologic responses to the new activators designed herein were compared to the parent compound, NS1643. For the NS1643 molecule, the ratio of the concentration producing channel blockade (30 μM) to the concentration increasing current density (10 μM) is approximately 3:1. In a previous study, the tail current was increased upon application of 10 μM of the activator [7]. The pharmacologic blockade becomes apparent at 30 μM of NS1643. Such a small therapeutic ratio may not provide a huge safety factor for that compound. Two of the newly synthesized molecules (MC-II-157c and MC-II-159c) had novel and interesting pharmacologic effects. The drugs both slowed deactivation of hERG1 and left-shifted voltage-dependence of activation. Thus for the hERG1 channel MC-II-157c appears to have a reasonable therapeutic ratio with minimal blockade signifying possibility of

Table 3. Comparison of the best poses found with Glide/XP and GOLD for selected drugs binding to open hERG1 channel.

Site\Drug	NS1643	MC-II-159c	MC-II-157c	MC-II-153b	MC-I-169b
IC1 (S4–S5 linker)	XPScore (Glide) kcal/mol				
	−7.25	−7.61	−8.61	−6.76	−6.62
	ChemScore (GOLD) kcal/mol				
	−7.13 (64)	−8.90 (83)	−7.24 (53)	−7.12 (100)	−7.69 (100)
SF (outer mouth)	XPScore (Glide) kcal/mol				
	−5.8	−5.13	−6.54	−6.48	−4.28
	ChemScore (GOLD) kcal/mol				
	−6.32(38)	−6.52(69)	−7.68(61)	−6.80(35)	−6.06(57)
EC2	XPScore (Glide) kcal/mol				
S3–S4	−4.72	−5.34	−6.47	−6.39	−4.25
	ChemScore (GOLD) kcal/mol				
S2–S1	−7.14(98)	−6.75(74)	−7.43(87)	−8.46(83)	−8.11(72)
Pore Domain (PD)	XPScore (Glide) kcal/mol				
S5–S6	**−7.46**	**−4.92**	**−4.70**	**−5.83**	**−6.31**

In parentheses is the population of the cluster from which the best pose comes from (always most populated one). In the case of Glide/XP, the output is only giving the selected best poses using a selection criteria explained in the methods. For definitions of the binding pockets see Durdagi et al. [7].

the rational design of channel's openers. In context, many supposed agonists (increasing tail current density) such as NS1643 also block the channel but do so at higher concentrations[22]. Interestingly the effects on deactivation of MC-II-159c and MC-II-157c were still manifest at lower drug concentrations ~2 µM. Unlike NS1643, MC-II-159c slows deactivation and shifts voltage-dependence of activation to hyperpolarized potentials but does not shift voltage-dependence of inactivation to depolarized potentials.

The potential dangers of hERG1 channel agonists may relate to off-target binding to other cardiac channels [28,29]. To address whether these drugs have a specific effect on the hERG1 channel or whether they may target other cardiac channels, we recorded action potentials and examined the effects MC-II-157c and MC-II-159c had on fetal mouse ventricular myocytes. Both MC-II-157c and MC-II-159c affected the upstroke of the action potential, the overshoot potential and the excitability threshold but only at the highest studied concentrations (i.e., 20 µM) as illustrated in Figure 9. At the low concentrations there was no impact of these

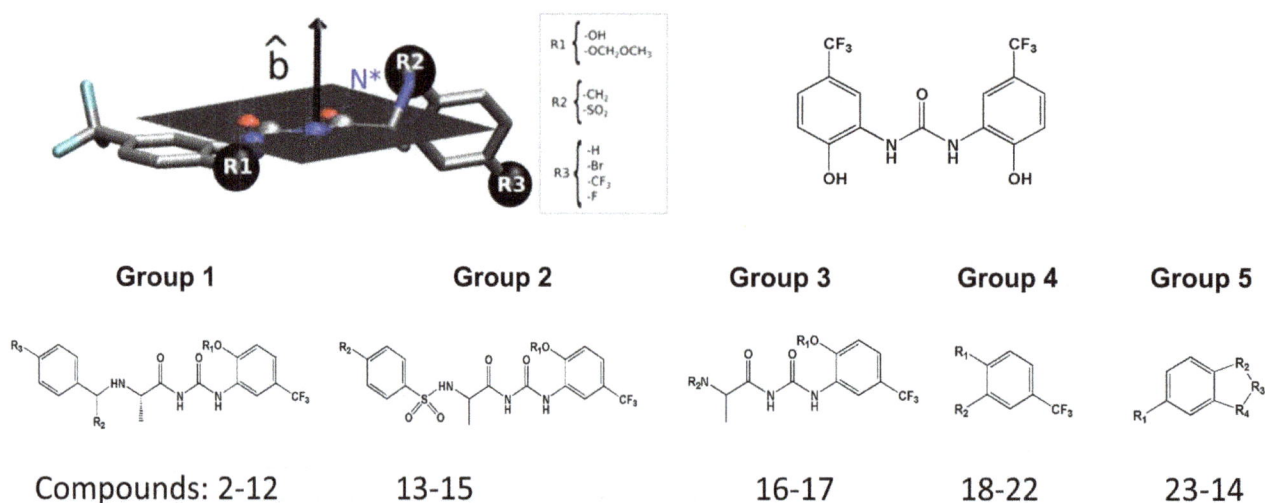

Figure 5. Schematic representation of the studied compounds topology showing the different R1, R2 and R3. The groups were identified to be critical determinants of high-affinity/high-specificity binding of activator to site located in S4–S5 linker of the hERG1 channel. Atom N* depicted in blue represents tentative protonation site. The black arrow represents the versor (^b) perpendicular to the plane defined by atoms N, C, O, N, C and O of the polyamide moiety, common structure element present in all molecules structure. Top panel shows NS-1643 and chemical group identification. Bottom panel illustrates compound groups synthesized.

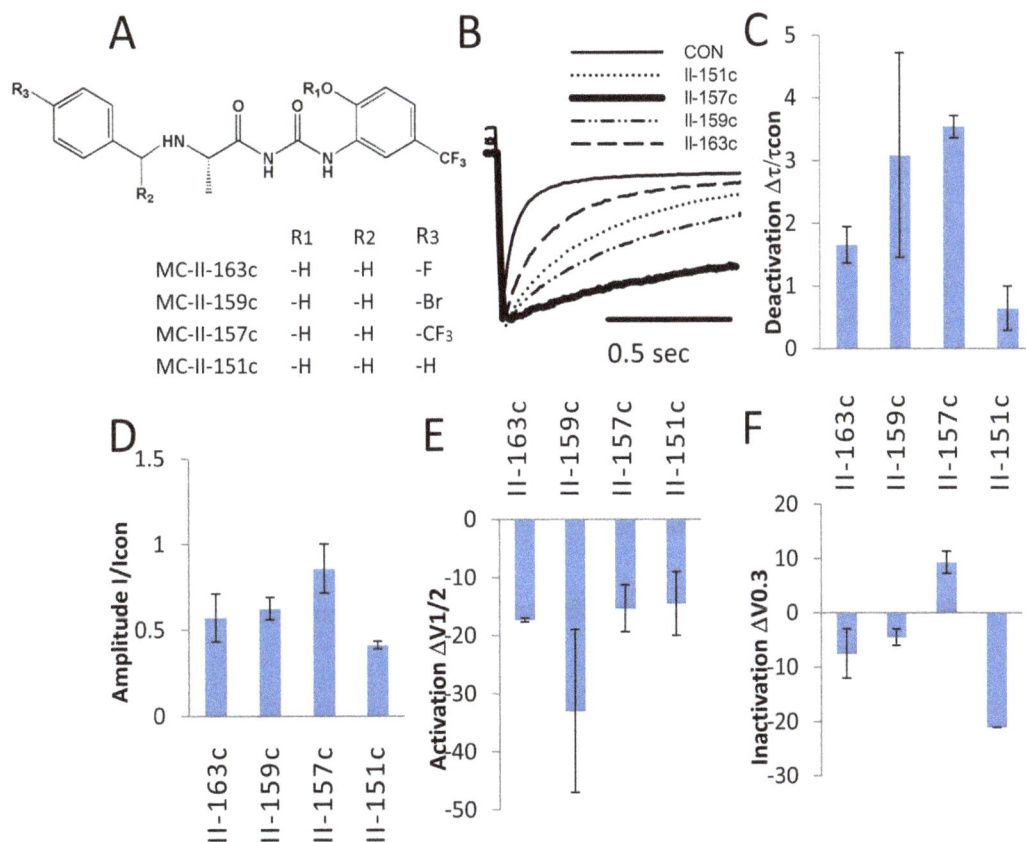

Figure 6. Substitutions in benzene ring (position R3) are determinants of prolongation of deactivation. Electrophysiologic responses to four molecules, MC-II-163c, MC-II-159C, MC-II-157b, and MC-II-43c are compared. Panel A shows the structures. All four molecules are similar except for the substituents on benzene ring #2. MC-II-43c is unsubstituted, whereas MC-II-163c, MC-II-159C, MC-II-157b are *para* substituted with fluoro, bromo and tri-fluoro groups respectively. Panel B shows raw examples of the slowing in the deactivation rate. Panel C shows the deactivation time constants relative to the base lines. Panel D shows the magnitude of the tail current relative to baseline. Panel E shows the shift in the voltage-dependence of activation and Panel F shows the shift in the voltage-dependent of inactivation. Panels C-F show no significant differences between the molecules except for their effects on deactivation. All 4 molecules shifted voltage dependence of activation to hyperpolarized potentials.

molecules on the action potential. However at 20 μM, there were clear changes in excitability and the overshoot potential decreased significantly. This manifested a blockade of the sodium current (I_{Na}). Therefore MC-II-157c is a hERG1 activation gate modifier with off-site interactions. It does not block hERG1 at 20 μM, but blocks a cardiac sodium channel. It would be difficult to predict this off-target problem if action potentials had not been recorded in this study. Even so, MC-II-157c still does shift voltage dependence of activation at 3 μM, increases tail current amplitude and slows deactivation. Thus the ratio of the concentration modify activation appears to be roughly 6-fold lower than the concentration blocking the sodium current. Such a small ratio does not provide a huge safety factor for specificity of effect, but still considerably better than original safety factor (3-fold) for NS1643. Even so, modification of its design is absolutely necessary to obviate interaction with the sodium channel, as an off-target site.

Discussion

hERG1 Activators as New Antiarrhythmic Drugs

There have been few new antiarrhythmic drugs developed in the past 20 years, even fewer if drugs with novel mechanisms are considered. Moreover, the strategy of blocking ion channels has been tested extensively and has universally failed (CAST) [30]. One potentially new approach is the development of hERG

activators that increase hERG currents to oppose congenital and acquired Long QT Syndromes (LQTS). Acquired Long QT Syndromes include those induced by pharmacologic block of hERG1 and those induced by heart failure. There are gaps in our knowledge. How can we design drugs that activate the hERG1 channel with minimized propensity to pharmacologic blockade? In addition, some studies report that drugs that shift the voltage-dependence of C-type inactivation to depolarized potentials could increase the time-dependent current at the expense of increasing the tail current. Increasing the time-dependent current could potentially truncate the action potential and create a pharmacologically-induced Short QT Syndrome. Such a prodysrhythmic potential has been reported by Patel et al for PD-118057 [31]. A second question is: -how do we design drugs that modify the hERG1 function without this prodysrhythmic potential? These are complex issues. This study just begins to address some of these issues. In this study we design drugs that shift $V_{1/2}$ of activation and slow deactivation with less propensity to pharmacologically block hERG1 and with less rightward shift in the voltage-dependence of C-type inactivation. However, an unforeseen limitation of our design is that these molecules also block I_{Na} in cardiac myocytes. Further refinements must consider multi-target models, specifically including SCN5a, to obviate off-target activity.

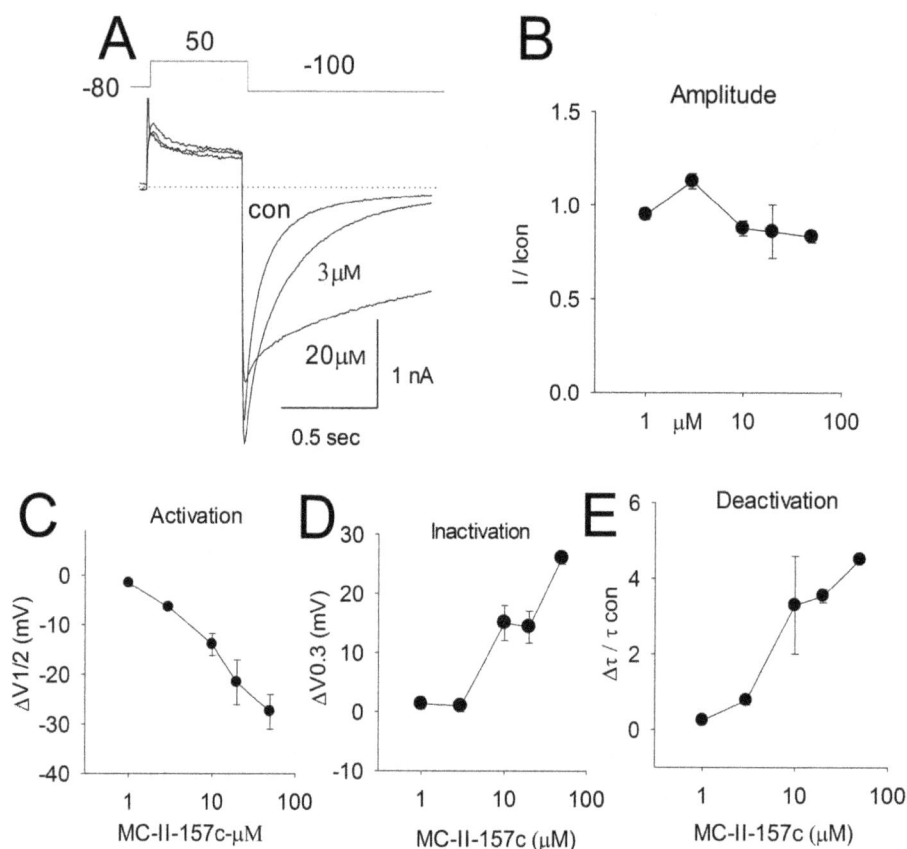

Figure 7. The concentration-response relationship of MC-II-157c. Panel A shows the raw currents elicited by the protocol shown in the inset. Panels B-E show the concentration-response relationships for mean tail current amplitude (Panel B), mean Δ shift in $V_{1/2}$ of activation (Panel C), mean Δ shift in $V_{1/2}$ of inactivation in Panel D and mean prolongation of the deactivation in Panel E.

Chemical Structure of Designed Molecules and Channel Blockade/Activation

It is instrumental to analyze key chemical properties of molecules designed in our work and to relate them to the observed effects on the hERG1 function. The electronic structure computations (Methods S1) suggest that introduction of a sulfonamide moiety has a dramatic effect on the distribution between charged and neutral forms of the drug by stabilizing the neutral form of the drug. This leads to a weaker intra-cavitary blocking ability and therefore represent a desired effect for development of non-blocking molecules. To test whether or not this feature manifests itself *in vitro*, we performed electrophysiological measurements on two synthesized molecules (MC-I-159b and MC-I-169b) from Table 1 containing a sulfonamide moiety between the R3 benzene ring and the peptide- like linker (Figure 8). The compound MC-I-159b, like NS1643 shifted the voltage-dependence of inactivation to depolarized potentials. Importantly at this same concentration (50 μM), the compound did not produce pharmacological block of hERG1 tail current in keeping with predictions from QM computations. At lower concentration (i.e., 20 μM), the drug still significantly shifted voltage-dependence of inactivation to depolarized potentials but at 1 μM it had no pharmacologic activity. The congener MC-I-169b produced significantly more pharmacologic block at 50 μM than seen with MC-I-159b (Figure 8). These data indicate that the exact substituents on the R3 benzene ring (see Figure 5) and the character of the linker to the peptide-like chain are important modulators of electrophysiological activity

and support the prediction from QM computations regarding ionization state. An introduction of a different functional group (ester-) suggested by fragment-based design and molecular docking abolish any physiological activity of the designed compounds (#2 to #18 in Table 1). This finding is in keeping with the prediction from QM computations that an ether group changes the compound considerably and, probably, leads to a different mode of binding.

Molecular Organization of the Binding Pocket for Openers

Current study provides substantial insights on critical interactions responsible for specific interactions with activators. While key-amino acid residues at the binding site for MC-II-157c are Y493, E544, and A547, stabilizing interactions for MC-II-159c involve Y542, E544, A547, and T548 side-chains (Figure 2). The decomposition analysis of binding energies emphasizes importance of π-π stacking interactions between F494 and Y542 side-chains and MC-II-157c. MC-II-159c is stabilized by π -π stacking interactions with Y542. The docked conformations of two high affinity ligands are very similar. (Figures S13 and S14 in File S1). Superimposition of top docking poses of MC-II-157c and MC-II-159c has been given in Figure S14 in File S1. E544 is found to forms multiple polar contacts and stabilizing hydrogen-bonding with high affinity ligands, while not involved in stabilizing low-affinity substrates in the identified binding site (S4-S5 helices). To illustrate interactions responsible for high-affinity binding, we are

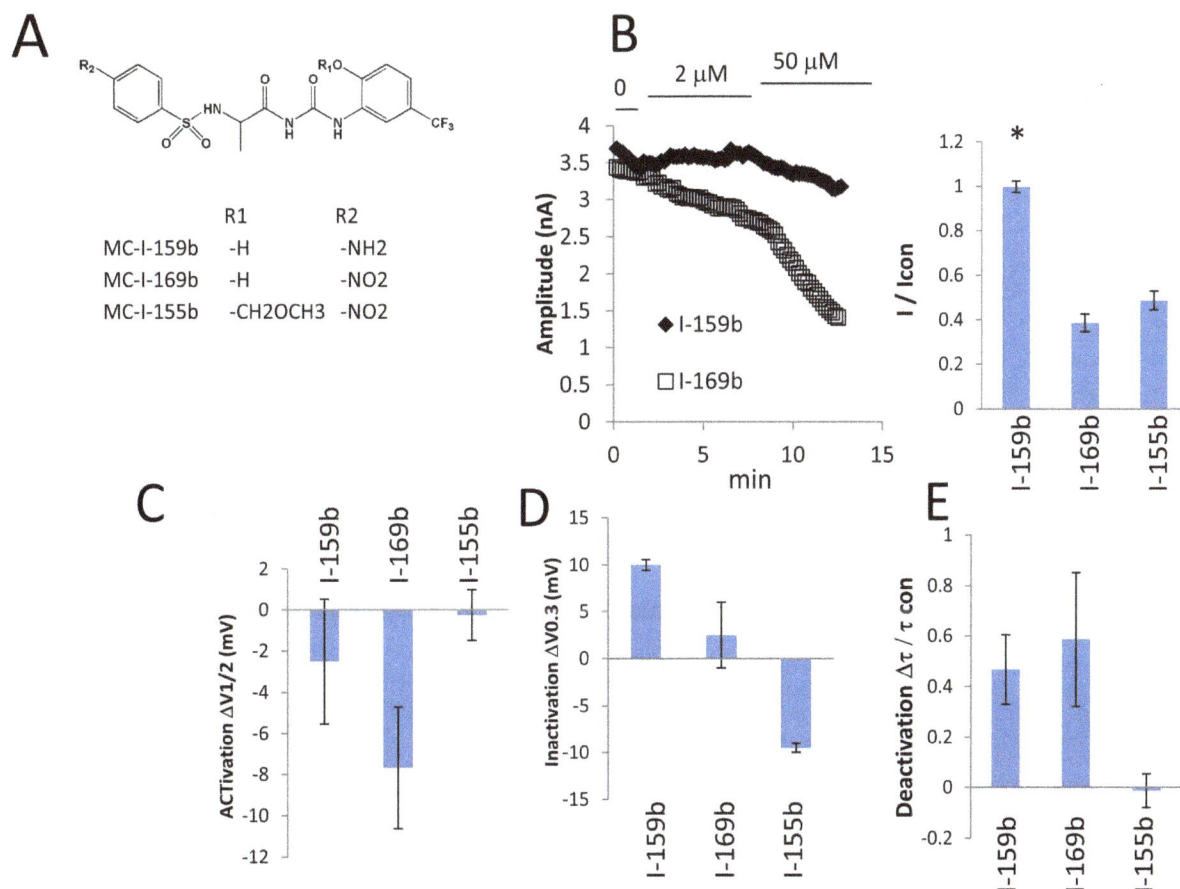

Figure 8. Concentration dependence of compounds MC-I-159b, MC-I-169b and MC-I-155b. Panel A: Chemical structures of compounds are shown. Panel B: Time dependent changes of tail current magnitudes in response to different drug concentrations. Panel C: The magnitude of the tail current relative to baseline. Panel D: The shifts in the voltage-dependence of activation and in the voltage-dependent of inactivation. The deactivation time constants relative to base lines is represented at bottom-right Panel E.

showing 2D and 3D ligand interactions diagram for one of the low-affinity compounds (MC-I-167b shown in Figure S14 in File S1 and electrophysiological evaluation of its binding effects are shown in Figure S15 in File S1). There are no π-π stacking interactions with the ligand and E544 forms only one hydrogen bond. (Figure S14 in File S1, top-left panel). To provide further evidence that the pharmacologic response to MC-II-157c and MC-II-159c relates to a true interaction with hERG1 in the neighborhood of E544 we assessed whether their pharmacologic responses were disrupted in the E544L mutation. Indeed we found that the pharmacologic responses to MC-II-157c and MC-II-159c were significantly and substantially reduced in E544L hERG. This contrasts with the response to the parent compound, NS1643, which manifests an exaggerated response in E544L. Accordingly, these data provide evidence that the neighborhood surrounding E544 appears to be a true binding site and that binding of MC-II-157c and MC-II-159c to this site mediates slowing of deactivation and the shifts in the voltage-dependence of activation.

Proposed Mechanism of Action

In this study, we were able to dissociate the pharmacologic effects on activation/deactivation from effects on inactivation by rationally designing opener molecules. The fact that *in silico* modeling can design a congener of NS1643 that selectively affects activation/deactivation but not inactivation suggests that the

putative drug pocket in the neighborhood of E544 maybe a genuine binding site for activators. It seems reasonable to assume that another binding site mediates the pharmacologic effects on inactivation. Earlier we had reported another putative binding pocket in the neighborhood of the selectivity filter [7]. It may be reasonable to assume that binding in the neighborhood of the selectivity filter might mediate rightward shift in the voltage-dependence of inactivation. These data are in keeping with our previous study, which had suggested multiple binding sites for NS1643 in the hERG1 potassium channel. Binding of activators in the neighborhood of E544 appears to alter movement of the S4 or the S4–S5 linker mediating changes in activation/deactivation process. This supposition is in keeping with the study of Tristani-Firouzi *et al.* [16] which provide evidence that interactions between the S4–S5 linker and the S6 helix are critically involved in activation/deactivation.

Classification of Drugs as Activators *versus* Blockers

Any classification of a drug as an activator versus a blocker probably needs to take into consideration the therapeutic ratio e.g. the ratio of the concentration producing hERG1 blockade versus the concentration producing a potentially therapeutic effect [4]. Most activators have a low therapeutic ratio. For example, NS1643 increases the tail current magnitude at 10 μM but produces substantial block at 30 μM. Therefore the therapeutic

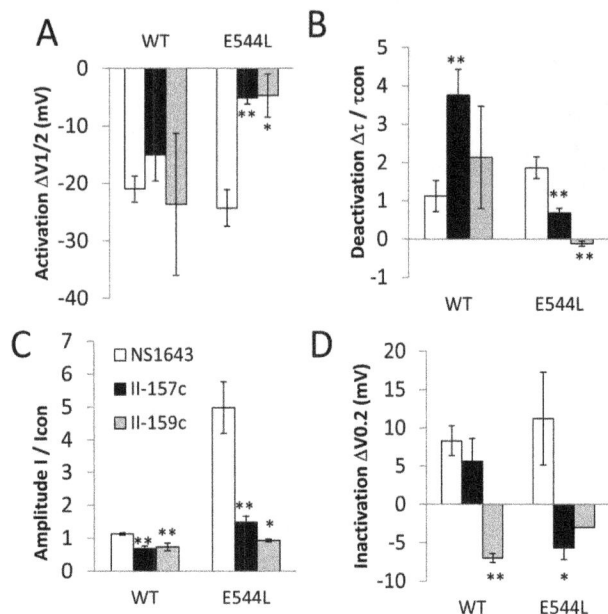

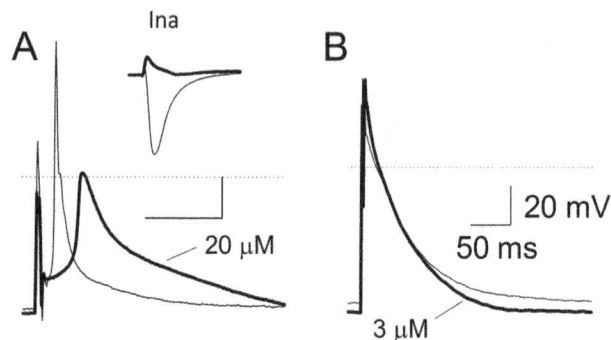

Figure 10. Drug effect on action potential in cardiomyocytes. Panel A. The effect of 20 μM and 3 μM Panel B. MC-II-157c on action potentials neonatal cardiomyocytes. The inset in Panel A shows the effect of 20 μM MC-II-157c on I_{Na} of same kind of cells. In patch clamp studies, the I_{Na} was induced by depolarizations to −30 mV from holding potentials of −100 mV. The light traces are baseline and bold traces were recorded with MC-II-157c.

Figure 9. Pharmacologic response (Δ) to NS1643 (open white bars at 10 μM), MC-II-157c (black bars at 10 μM) and MC-II-159C (grey bars at 10 μM) are compared in wild type (WT) versus E544L. Panel A: In WT, NS1643 MC-II-157c and MC-II-159c, all shift voltage-dependence of activation and Panel B: slow deactivation. (top) In E544L, pharmacologic response to NS1643 is exaggerated whereas Δ response to MC-II-157c and Δ MC-II-159c were markedly diminished. (bottom-left) Panel C: In terms of amplitude of the tail current, in E544L response to NS1643 is exaggerated whereas response to MC-II-157c and MC-II-159C is markedly diminished. Pharmacologic response in terms of inactivation is complex. Panel D: In WT, MC-II-157c shifts voltage-dependence of inactivation to depolarized potentials whereas MC-II-159C shifts voltage dependence to hyperpolarized potentials. Pharmacologic response to NS1643 is exaggerated in E544L whereas for MC-II-157c and MC-II-159C responses are diminished. (bottom-right) * evaluates the statistical significance of the Δ response to NS1643 compared to Δ response to MC-II-157c or Δ response MC-II-159c. * designates p<0.05; ** designates p<0.01. n values were: For Activation panel in WT n=10,8 and 3; for E544L n=9,6 and 3. For deactivation in WT n=8,8,3 respectively and for E544L n=4,6,3. For tail current amplitude, in WT n=9,8,3 and in E544L n=8,6,2. For inactivation, n=9,8,3 and for E544L n=5,6,2.

ratio of that molecule is very approximately 3:1. For the sake of safety one might hope for a therapeutic ratio of >10:1 in order to have some confidence that pharmacologic blockade would not occur leading to a myocardial disease and electrolyte disturbance. MC-II-157c produced a modest slowing of deactivation, shifting $V_{1/2}$ of activation to hyperpolarized potentials and a modest increase in tail current amplitude at 3 μM and did not show a concentration-dependent block of hERG1 even at 50 μM. To assess the potential impact of MC-II-157c on the heart, cardiac action potentials were recorded. At 3 μM MC-II-157c shortened action potential duration and its Phase III shape. However, at 20 μM, MC-II-157c substantially blocks I_{Na} an unforeseen off-target effect (Figure 10). Even so, the therapeutic ratio of MC-II-157c as defined as the ratio of concentrations affecting I_{hERG}/I_{Na} is approximately 6:1. Many of the developed hERG1 activators exhibit concentration-dependent channel blockade at higher concentrations [32]. While developed activators show minimal ability to block hERG1 currents at low μM concentrations, it is worthwhile to understand its molecular mechanism. For two potent activators (MC-II-159c and MC-II-157c) we observed

minimal blockade at high drug concentrations. High-precision docking for these two compounds was used to better understand molecular determinants of observed blockade (Table 3). The intra-cavitary binding pocket for developed compounds is predominantly formed by T623, S624, S649, Y652 and F656. The hydroxyl groups (i.e., S624 and S649 for MC-II-159c) are predicted to be important for the formation of stable H-bonds with the drug [33] [26]. However, the aromatic moiety F656 is important construct π-π stacking interactions for drug stabilization in the cavity. (Figure S16 in File S1) Mutations in the S6 region, such as F656X, often inhibit the blocking ability of some of the activators (such as RPR260243 and ICA-105574) [4,6]. Importantly, as molecular analysis of high-affinity binding for activator suggest, very same interactions with a binding site located at the interface S4–S5 are responsible for channel's activation. A strategy that may work the best to increase binding to an "activators" site involves optimization of interactions with charges moieties in the channel (E544) exposed to aqueous solutions.

Off-Target Interactions by the Existing and Novel Activators

We prospectively designed molecules to avoid substantial blockade of the central cavity of hERG1. Importantly, none of the molecules designed herein substantially blocked the hERG1 current at <10 μM. This suggests that computational models combining QSAR/docking with atomistic models of hERG1 reliably design drugs that avoid high affinity blockade of the hERG1 current. Even so, blockade of this current was observed at concentrations in the range of ~50 μM. To address whether lead molecule MC-II-157c produces other unpredictable off-target effects we recorded fetal mouse ventricular action potentials before and after treatment with MC-II-157c and MC-II-159c (Figure 10). At high concentrations (20 μM), MC-II-157c decreased the upstroke dV/dt of the action potential, the overshoot potential and excitability threshold. The inset of Figure 10 shows that these effects results from blockade of the cardiac sodium current (I_{Na}). Even so, MC-II-157c, at low concentration (3 μM), significantly shortened action potential duration (Figure 10, right panel). Thus the ratio of the concentrations that modify deactivation of the hERG1 current is 6-fold lower than the concentration required to block the cardiac sodium current. Further modifications of MC-II-157c are required to ablate its interaction with the cardiac sodium channel. Therefore, our work raises awareness of this unforeseen issue when designing hERG1 activators. Further studies may need to take into consideration alternative ion channels as targets. The crystal structure for the bacterial homo-tetrameric voltage-gated Na$^+$ channel from *Arcobacter butzleri* (NavAb) has been reported however, the structure for SCN5a has yet to be described and is expected to be very different from that of NavAb [34]. It is important to mention that issue of multiple receptors for existing drugs, while often ignored, is well known and represent significant challenge in targeted drug development [35].

Conclusions

The study had two prospectively defined goals: 1) To use *De Novo* drug design-assisted synthesized NS1643 analogues based on 3D QSAR design and molecular docking or available NS-like drugs from available drug databases to the neighborhood of E544 to identify molecules that shifted voltage- dependence of activation to hyperpolarized potentials and slowed deactivation without shifting the voltage dependence of inactivation. 2) To avoid pharmacological block of the hERG1 current at low micromolar concentrations. These goals were successfully achieved in this study. The therapeutic ratio between amplification of current density and hERG1 blockade was improved from 3:1 to almost 10:1. Therefore, our study showed that it is possible to selectively target activation/inactivation of hERG1 channel with small molecule. One of the designed molecules, MC-II-157c, substantially shifted the voltage-dependence of activation and slowed deactivation greater than that observed with NS1643. However, at concentrations of (>20 μM) it blocked I_{Na}. The side effect, reported for the first time in our study, may be common to other activators. It would be difficult to predict or even to observe this

off-target problem if action potentials had not been recorded in this study in fetal mouse ventricular myocytes. Inadvertent blockade of off-target ion channels not considered in the design represents a challenge for *in silico* design of drugs. Multi-ion channel targets will need to be considered in future designs.

Author Contributions

Conceived and designed the experiments: JG SD MC LLP TGB SYN HJD. Performed the experiments: JG SD MC LLP JMH. Analyzed the data: JG SD MC LLP TGB SYN HJD. Contributed reagents/materials/analysis tools: TGB SYN HJD. Contributed to the writing of the manuscript: JG SD LLP TGB SYN HJD.

References

1. Seebohm G (2005) Activators of cation channels: potential in treatment of channelopathies. Mol Pharmacol 67: 585–588.
2. Fernandez D, Sargent J, Sachse FB, Sanguinetti MC (2008) Structural basis for ether-a-go-go-related gene K+ channel subtype-dependent activation by niflumic acid. Mol Pharmacol 73: 1159–1167.
3. Smith PL, Baukrowitz T, Yellen G (1996) The inward rectification mechanism of the HERG cardiac potassium channel. Nature 379: 833–836.
4. Sanguinetti M (2014) HERG1 channel agonists and cardiac arrhythmia. Curr Opin Pharmacol 15: 22–27.
5. Asayama M, Kurokawa J, Shirakawa K, Okuyama H, Kagawa T, et al. (2013) Effects of an hERG Activator, ICA-105574, on Electrophysiological Properties of Canine Hearts. Journal of Pharmacological Sciences 121: 1–8.
6. Casis O, Olesen SP, Sanguinetti MC (2006) Mechanism of action of a novel human ether-a-go-go-related gene channel activator. Molecular Pharmacology 69: 658–665.
7. Durdagi S, Guo JQ, Lees-Miller JP, Noskov SY, Duff HJ (2012) Structure-Guided Topographic Mapping and Mutagenesis to Elucidate Binding Sites for the Human Ether-a-Go-Go-Related Gene 1 Potassium Channel (KCNH2) Activator NS1643. Journal of Pharmacology and Experimental Therapeutics 342: 441–452.
8. Hansen RS, Diness TG, Demnitz J, Olesen SP, Grunnet M (2005) NS1643 is a new activator of HERG potassium channels. Circulation 112: U87–U87.
9. Garg V, Stary-Weinzinger A, Sachse F, Sanguinetti MC (2011) Molecular Determinants for Activation of Human Ether-a-go-go-related Gene 1 Potassium Channels by 3-Nitro-N-(4-phenoxyphenyl) Benzamide. Molecular Pharmacology 80: 630–637.
10. Kang JS, Chen XL, Wang HG, Ji JZ, Cheng H, et al. (2005) Discovery of a small molecule activator of the human ether-a-go-go-related gene (HERG) cardiac K+ channel. Molecular Pharmacology 67: 827–836.
11. Perry M, Sachse FB, Sanguinetti MC (2007) Structural basis of action for a human ether-a-go-go-related gene 1 potassium channel activator. Proceedings of the National Academy of Sciences of the United States of America 104: 13827–13832.
12. Grunnet M, Abbruzzese J, Sachse FB, Sanguinetti MC (2011) Molecular Determinants of Human Ether-a-go-go-Related Gene 1 (hERG1) K+ Channel Activation by NS1643. Molecular Pharmacology 79: 1–9.
13. Bilet A, Bauer CK (2012) Effects of the Small Molecule HERG Activator NS1643 on Kv11.3 Channels. PloS One 7: e50886.
14. Vandenberg JI, Perry MD, Perrin MJ, Mann SA, Ke Y, et al. (2012) hERG K+ Channels: Structure, Function and Clinical Significance. Physiological Reviews 92: 1393–1478.
15. Sanguinetti MC, Tristani-Firouzi M (2006) hERG potassium channels and cardiac arrhythmia. Nature 440: 463–469.
16. Tristani-Firouzi M, Chen J, Sanguinetti MC (2002) Interactions between S4–S5 linker and S6 transmembrane domain modulate gating of HERG K+ channels. Journal of Biological Chemistry 277: 18994–19000.
17. Durdagi S, Deshpande S, Duff HJ, Noskov SY (2012) Modeling of Open, Closed, and Open-Inactivated States of the hERG1 Channel: Structural Mechanisms of the State-Dependent Drug Binding. J Chem Inf Model 52: 2760–2774.
18. Subbotina J, Yarov-Yarovoy V, Lees-Miller J, Durdagi S, Guo JQ, et al. (2010) Structural refinement of the hERG1 pore and voltage-sensing domains with ROSETTA-membrane and molecular dynamics simulations. Proteins-Structure Function and Bioinformatics 78: 2922–2934.
19. Friesner RA, Murphy RB, Repasky MP, Frye LL, Greenwood JR, et al. (2006) Extra precision glide: Docking and scoring incorporating a model of hydrophobic enclosure for protein-ligand complexes. J Med Chem 49: 6177–6196.
20. Jones G, Willett P, Glen RC, Leach AR, Taylor R (1997) Development and validation of a genetic algorithm for flexible ligand docking. Abstracts of Papers of the American Chemical Society 214: 154-COMP.
21. Maestro v (2007). Portland, OR: Schrodinger.
22. Lees-Miller JP, Subbotina JO, Guo JQ, Yarov-Yarovoy V, Noskov SY, et al. (2009) Interactions of H562 in the S5 Helix with T618 and S621 in the Pore Helix Are Important Determinants of hERG1 Potassium Channel Structure and Function. Biophys J 96: 3600–3610.
23. Guo JQ, Zhan S, Lees-Miller JP, Teng GQ, Duff HJ (2005) Exaggerated block of hERG (KCNH2) and prolongation of action potential duration by erythromycin at temperatures between 37 degrees C and 42 degrees C. Heart Rhythm 2: 860–866.
24. Durdagi S, Deshpande S, Duff HJ, Noskov SY (2012) Modeling of Open, Closed, and Open-Inactivated States of the hERG1 Channel: Structural Mechanisms of the State-Dependent Drug Binding. Journal of Chemical Information and Modeling 52: 2760–2774.
25. Durdagi S, Duff HJ, Noskov SY (2011) Combined Receptor and Ligand-Based Approach to the Universal Pharmacophore Model Development for Studies of Drug Blockade to the hERG1 Pore Domain. J Chem Inf Model 51: 463–474.

26. Zachariae U, Giordanetto F, Leach AG (2009) Side Chain Flexibilities in the Human Ether-a-go-go Related Gene Potassium Channel (hERG) Together with Matched-Pair Binding Studies Suggest a New Binding Mode for Channel Blockers. Journal of Medicinal Chemistry 52: 4266–4276.

27. Carvalho JFS, Louvel J, Doornbos MLJ, Klaasse E, Yu ZY, et al. (2013) Strategies To Reduce hERG K+ Channel Blockade. Exploring Heteroaromaticity and Rigidity in Novel Pyridine Analogues of Dofetilide. Journal of Medicinal Chemistry 56: 2828–2840.

28. Bentzen BH, Bahrke S, Wu K, Larsen AP, Odening KE, et al. (2011) Pharmacological Activation of Kv11.1 in Transgenic Long QT-1 Rabbits. Journal of Cardiovascular Pharmacology 57: 223–230.

29. Kramer J, Obejero-Paz CA, Myatt G, Kuryshev YA, Bruening-Wright A, et al. (2013) MICE Models: Superior to the HERG Model in Predicting Torsade de Pointes. Scientific Reports 3: Artn 2100.

30. CAST (1989) Preliminary report: effect of encainide and flecainide on mortality in a randomized trial of arrhythmia suppression after myocardial infarction. The Cardiac Arrhythmia Suppression Trial (CAST) Investigators. New England Journal of Medicine 321: 406–412.

31. Patel C, Antzelevitch C (2008) Cellular basis for arrhythmogenesis in an experimental model of the SQT1 form of the short QT syndrome. Heart Rhythm 5: 585–590.

32. Casis O, Olesen SP, Sanguinetti MC (2006) Mechanism of action of a novel human ether-a-go-go-related gene channel activator. Mol Pharmacol 69: 658–665.

33. Durdagi S, Randall T, Chamberlin AC, Duff HJ, Noskov SY (2014) Rehabilitating drug-induced long-QT promoters: In-silico design of hERG-neutral cisapride analogues with retained pharmacological activity. BMC Pharmacol Toxicol 15: 14.

34. Payandeh J, Scheuer T, Zheng N, Catterall WA (2011) The crystal structure of a voltage-gated sodium channel. Nature 475: 353–358.

35. Kell DB, Dobson PD, Bilsland E, Oliver SG (2013) The promiscuous binding of pharmaceutical drugs and their transporter-mediated uptake into cells: what we (need to) know and how we can do so. Drug Discovery Today 18: 218–239.

11

Highly Sensitive Quantitative Imaging for Monitoring Single Cancer Cell Growth Kinetics and Drug Response

Mustafa Mir[1¤], Anna Bergamaschi[2], Benita S. Katzenellenbogen[2], Gabriel Popescu[1*]

1 Quantitative Light Imaging Laboratory, Department of Electrical and Computer Engineering, Beckman Institute for Advanced Science and Technology, University of Illinois at Urbana-Champaign, Urbana, Illinois, United States of America, 2 Department of Molecular and Integrative Physiology, University of Illinois at Urbana-Champaign, Urbana, Illinois, United States of America

Abstract

The detection and treatment of cancer has advanced significantly in the past several decades, with important improvements in our understanding of the fundamental molecular and genetic basis of the disease. Despite these advancements, drug-screening methodologies have remained essentially unchanged since the introduction of the *in vitro* human cell line screen in 1990. Although the existing methods provide information on the overall effects of compounds on cell viability, they are restricted by bulk measurements, large sample sizes, and lack capability to measure proliferation kinetics at the individual cell level. To truly understand the nature of cancer cell proliferation and to develop personalized adjuvant therapies, there is a need for new methodologies that provide quantitative information to monitor the effect of drugs on cell growth as well as morphological and phenotypic changes at the single cell level. Here we show that a quantitative phase imaging modality known as spatial light interference microscopy (SLIM) addresses these needs and provides additional advantages over existing proliferation assays. We demonstrate these capabilities through measurements on the effects of the hormone estradiol and the antiestrogen ICI182,780 (Faslodex) on the growth of MCF-7 breast cancer cells. Along with providing information on changes in the overall growth, SLIM provides additional biologically relevant information. For example, we find that exposure to estradiol results in rapidly growing cells with lower dry mass than the control population. Subsequently blocking the estrogen receptor with ICI results in slower growing cells, with lower dry masses than the control. This ability to measure changes in growth kinetics in response to environmental conditions provides new insight on growth regulation mechanisms. Our results establish the capabilities of SLIM as an advanced drug screening technology that provides information on changes in proliferation kinetics at the cellular level with greater sensitivity than any existing method.

Editor: Aamir Ahmad, Wayne State University School of Medicine, United States of America

Funding: This work was supported by the National Science Foundation (NSF) Grants: Science and Technology Center on Emergent Behaviors of Integrated Cellular Systems CBET 0939511 (to G.P.), NSF CAREER 08-46660 (to G.P.), CBET-1040461 MRI (to G.P.), Breast Cancer Research Foundation (to B.S.K.), National Institutes of Health (NIH) P50 AT006268 (to B.S.K.), and a Postdoctoral Fellowship from the Department of Defense, W81XWH-09-1-0398 (to A.B.). The funders had no role in study design, data collection and analysis, decision to publish, or preparation of the manuscript.

Competing Interests: The authors have read the journal's policy and have the following conflicts: G. Popescu has financial interests in Phi Optics, Inc., a company developing quantitative phase microscopes, which, however, did not sponsor this research.

* E-mail: gpopescu@illinois.edu

¤ Current address: California Institute for Regenerative Medicine, University of California Berkeley, Berkeley, California, United States of America

Introduction

Cell growth and mass homeostasis have been described as fundamental to biology, yet they are insufficiently understood [1]. This shortcoming can be traced back to the lack of methods capable of quantifying single cell mass with the required sensitivity. As a result, recently, significant progress has been made toward developing new technology for studying cell growth. These methods can be divided into *micromechanical* [2–4], translating resonant frequency shifts of microstructures into cell buoyancy mass, and *optical* [5–8], converting quantitative phase images into dry mass density maps. Optical methods are ideally suited for studying growth of adherent single cells as well as cell clusters. This capability opens up new opportunities in cancer cell biology, where sensitive measurements of cell proliferation can lead to improved understanding of the disease as well as quantitative monitoring of drug efficacy. Here we demonstrate that *quantitative phase imaging (QPI)* provides a highly sensitive method for studying cancer cell growth and for testing drugs. We use breast cancer cell lines as a model for proving the principle of our method.

Breast cancer accounts for 30% of all diagnosed cancer cases and for 14% of all cancer related deaths in women [9]. A significant decrease (7%) in incidence has been observed since 2002 that can be directly attributed to a better understanding of the link between estrogen and the growth of breast cancer[10–16]. This knowledge has led to the development of a class of agents that directly modulate the estrogen receptor (ER) and are now the cornerstone of treatment and prevention in ER positive patients (70% of all cases) [17]. With the realization that it is possible to exercise control over cancer growth through anti-hormones and chemotherapeutic agents came the need for large scale testing of possibly useful compounds. By 1974, over 40,000 compounds were being tested annually using murine models [18,19]. In 1990, NCI established the primary screen of 59 human cell lines, which remains in use today [20,21]. This new primary screen required methods to assess growth *in vitro*. Several metabolic assays were developed to measure cell growth and viability –which, to date, have remained largely unchanged [20,22–26].

A widely used approach is based on the reduction of a colorless tetrazolium salt to yield a colored formozan proportional to the number of viable cells. Although such assays are useful for measuring the overall cytotoxic effectiveness of a compound, large number of cells (10^3–10^5) [27] have to be used to avoid incorrect conclusions from effects such as variable doubling times [20]. Furthermore, since many drugs have effects on cell cycle arrest that do not result in metabolic changes, in some cases a false readout may be made[28]. Non-tetrazolium based assays have also been developed. These assays utilize dyes that bind electrostatically to basic amino acids [25] and the measured signal is thus linear with the cell count. Despite the practical difficulties involved, one such reagent known as sulforhodamine B (SRB) was eventually adopted for routine screenings. Both assay types provide indirect measurements of growth: the tetrazolium based assays measure metabolic activity whereas the SRB assay essentially measures total protein concentration. Both methods rely on using large numbers of cells, only provide bulk measurements on the entire collection of cells, and are unable to measure time dependent responses to drugs at the cellular level. Typically, growth assay data are supplemented with fluorescence-activated cell sorting (FACS) experiments to provide additional statistical information, and study gene expression and cell cycle progression. Although very informative, FACS analyses require cells to be removed from their normal culture conditions, cell clusters to be separated, causing alterations in phenotype and morphology.

Therefore, it is becoming increasingly clear that to truly understand the nature of cancer cell proliferation and to develop personalized adjuvant therapies, there is a need for new methodologies that provide quantitative information to monitor the drug effects on cell growth and the accompanying morphological and phenotypic changes at the single cell level. The ideal drug screen should be sensitive enough to rapidly assess the response of a small number of cells to a variety of potential therapies in order to directly evaluate the response of a patient or the efficacy of a particular drug. Here we show that QPI [29] addresses this technological gap. Spatial light interference microscopy (SLIM) [30] is a QPI approach that has femtogram level sensitivity to changes in dry mass and can simultaneously provide this information at both the single cell and population level [31]. SLIM can be combined with fluorescence microscopy to measure cell cycle dependent growth [31]. In this work, we use the Estrogen Receptor (ER)-positive MCF-7 breast cancer cell line [32,33] as a model system to demonstrate that SLIM can be used as a highly sensitive drug proliferation assay.

The MCF-7 cell line has been a widely used model for studying hormonal influence on breast cancer growth, particularly, in response to estrogens that plays a key role in promoting the growth and progression of cancer cells. We measured the growth of MCF-7 cell clusters in standard cell culture media (Veh) and under the influence of estradiol (E2), the predominant form of estrogen during reproductive years, and ICI, 182, 780 – also known as Faslodex–[34], a complete antagonist of the ER used to treat metastatic breast cancer in postmenopausal women. The results shown here establish that, in addition to being a valuable proliferation assay, quantitative phase imaging also provides biologically relevant information at the individual cell and cell cluster population level that is not accessible through other

methods. Such measurements, in combination with existing molecular assays have the potential to improve drug design and characterization and to bridge the connection between our molecular understanding of cancer and drug treatment effects on cell growth and phenotypic properties such as cell size/mass.

Results

MCF-7 cells were seeded in a two well slide chamber and measurements were performed in three cell culture conditions (see *Materials and Methods* for more details on cell culture and treatment). First, typical cell growth media as the control vehicle (Veh), second cell growth media containing 10 nM Estradiol (E2), and finally cell growth media with the antiestrogen 1 μM ICI182,780 +10 nM E2 (E2+ICI). For the E2+ICI treatment, cells were grown under E2 conditions for 10 hours before ICI was added. The 10-hour point was chosen to administer the drug since this is the earliest point at which a significant difference between the growth rates of Veh and E2-treated populations was observed (Fig. S1). A 1.55×1.16 mm^2 area of each well was scanned every 30 minutes using a commercial phase contrast microscope equipped with a SLIM add-on module. For each experiment, one well contained an untreated control population (Veh) and the second well contained the E2 or E2 + ICI treated population. Two measurements were performed in such a manner for each condition. All data will be made freely available on request.

A schematic of the instrument and representative SLIM images from one well are shown in Fig. 1 A and B respectively. SLIM maintains subcellular resolution (Fig. 1B) over a large area by scanning each chamber in a mosaic pattern (for more details on the measurement refer to *Materials and Methods*). From the large mosaic images, the edges of individual clusters (composed of 2–3 cells at t = 0 hours) were traced at each time point and the surface area and total dry mass were measured (see Movie S1 for a time lapse of the field of view for all groups). In this manner, we can analyze both the overall growth trends of each group and the heterogeneity at the cluster level within each population. It should be noted that this type of measurement is currently impossible to perform with any existing proliferation assay.

Temporal Changes in Mass and Area

First, we establish the capabilities of SLIM as a proliferation assay by measuring the effects of Estradiol on the relative changes in growth, which is qualitatively similar to the information provided by conventional assays. The quantities of interest here are the relative amounts of growth in size and mass, not the absolute values. To perform this analysis, the mass and surface area of each cluster is normalized relative to its initial size, M(t)/M(t = 0) and Area(t)/Area(t = 0), respectively. The normalized area and mass for all analyzed clusters (at least 5 per group) were separated into 15-hour bins as shown in Figs. 1C and 1D. There is no significant difference in the normalized area at every time point. By contrast, the differences in the normalized mass are detectable throughout the measurement period (Fig. 1 C–D). This highlights the importance of measuring mass rather than simply the area of a cluster. Moreover, ICI treatment takes effect rapidly as the E2 group exhibits greater relative growth in the mass within 30 hours. A difference between the E2+ICI and control group can be detected by 60 hours. It should be noted that while current proliferation assays rely on using a large number of cells, SLIM measurements were performed at the individual cluster level.

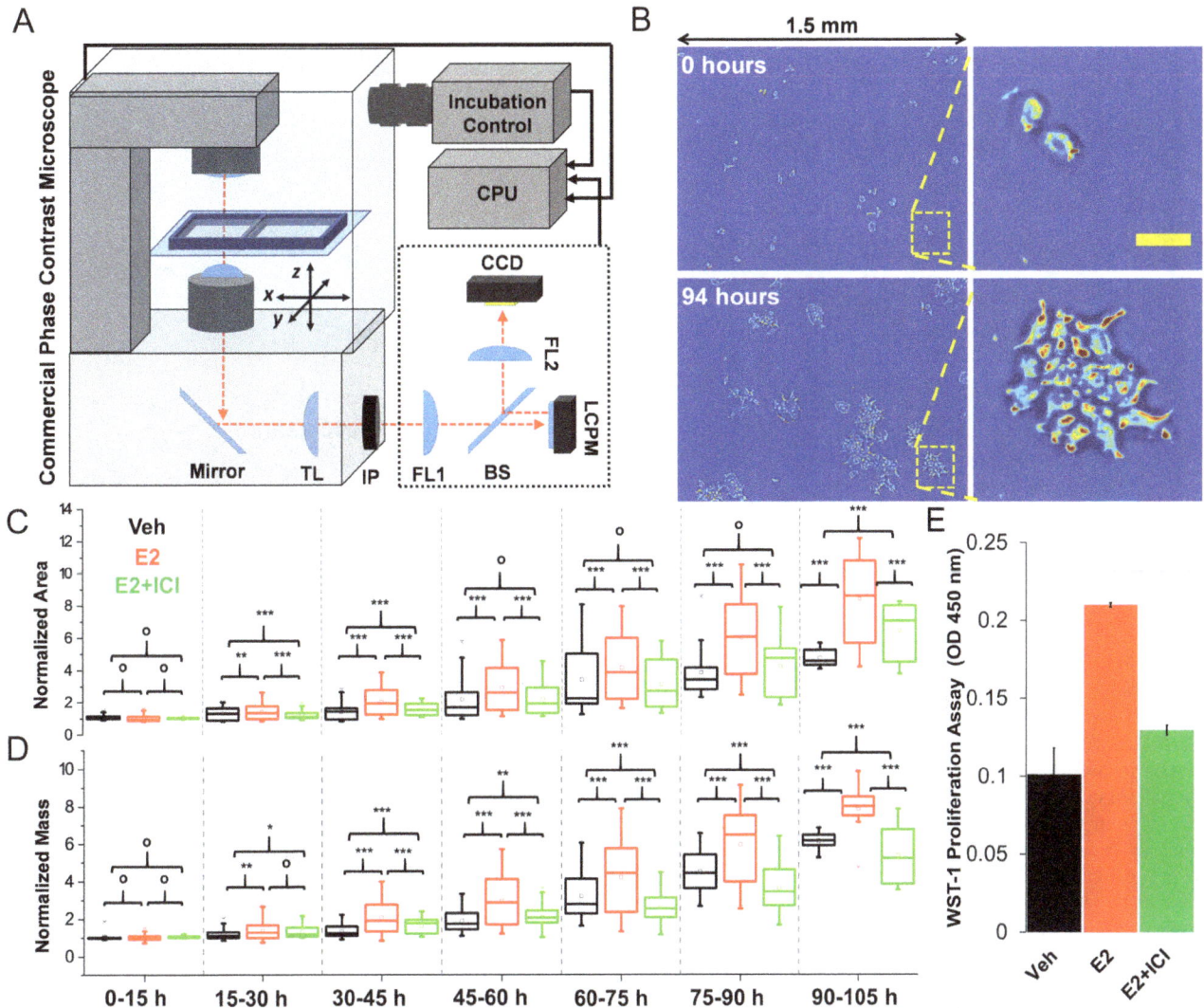

Figure 1. Measurement of cancer cell proliferation using SLIM dry mass measurements. (A) Schematic of experimental setup. A fully automated commercial phase contrast microscope equipped with stage top incubation control and x, y, z-scanning capabilities was used to scan a 1.5 mm ×1.2 mm area in each well of a 2-well slide every 30 minutes. The components in the dotted line comprise the SLIM add-on module: Fourier Lens 1 (FL1) projects the pupil plane of the phase contrast microscope onto a Liquid Crystal Phase Modulator (LCPM), which provides control over the phase delay between the scattered and un-scattered light; Fourier Lens 2 projects the phase-modulated image onto a CCD. All components of the instrument were synchronized using the CPU. (B) Representative images of a scanned field of view in one of the chambers at 0 hours and 94 hours, the area in the dashed yellow line is enlarged and shown at each time point (yellow scale bar is 50 microns). (C) Average normalized surface area for clusters in each group in the labelled time periods. (D) Average normalized mass for clusters in each group in the labelled time periods. (C–D) Square markers indicate mean, centerline is median, top of box is 25th percentile line, bottom is 75th percentile line, whiskers indicate 5th and 95th percentiles, significance was tested using an un-paired t-test, o: p>0.05, *: p<0.05, **: p<0.01, ***: p<0.001. (E) WST-1 proliferation assay measurement at 72 hours.

Comparison with Colorimetric Assay

For comparison, measurements from a WST-1 assay taken after 72 hours of treatment are shown in Fig. 1E. It can be seen that there is a good qualitative agreement between the WST-1 data, which indirectly indicate proliferation rate, and the normalized area measurements after 75 hours. However, the normalized mass is higher in the control than the E2+ICI group after 60 hours. These differences are likely because the WST-1 assay simply measures the reduction of a tetrazolium dye outside the cell. Although the level of this reduction is related to the metabolic activity of the cells and reflects the number of viable cells in the population, it is not a direct measurement of cellular mass or size. Furthermore, such assays are restricted to providing one number

for a bulk population and provide no practical way to study the heterogeneity in the population. In order to better illustrate the measured variability in the data the normalized mass and area for individual clusters are shown in Fig. 2.

Temporal Changes in Mass Growth Rate

In addition to providing a quantitative understanding of how various treatments affect relative changes in size and mass, SLIM can also measure changes in the growth rate of small cell clusters as a function of time or size. Measuring the growth rate with high sensitivity is more informative than simply measuring relative changes in mass as it provides an understanding of when treatments begin to take effect and how long the effect persists.

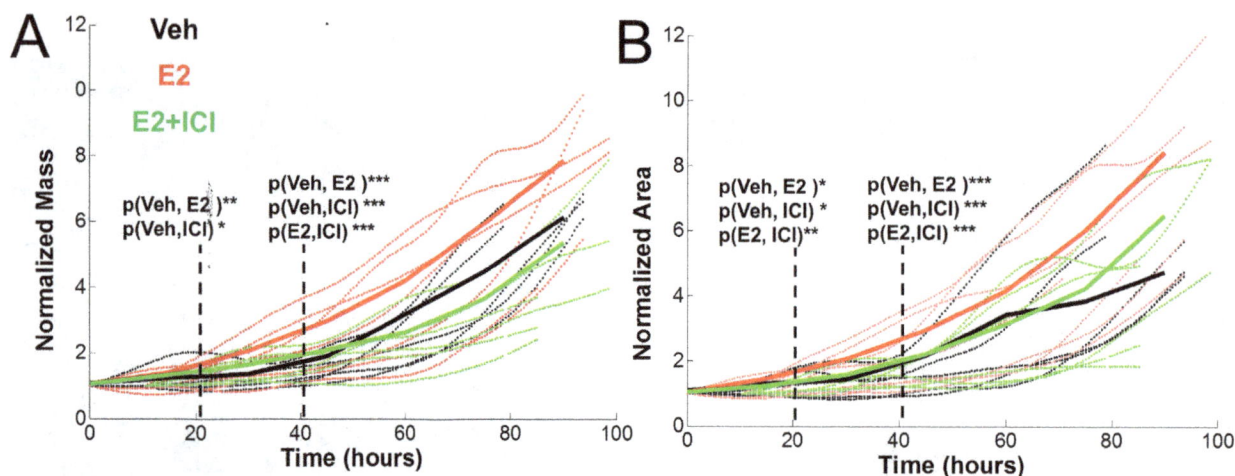

Figure 2. Growth data for all clusters. (A) Normalized mass vs. Time for all clusters that were analyzed. (B) Normalized area vs. time for all clusters. (A–B) Dotted lines show individual cluster data and solid lines show averaged data. Dashed lines indicate where the difference between groups becomes significant.

Dry mass density maps of typical clusters from each group over time are shown in Fig. 3A (see Movie S2 for). Fig. 3B shows the growth rate of clusters in each group vs. time. A significant difference in the growth rate between all three groups can be detected as early as 15 hours (5 hours after ICI treatment was administered), which is 15 hours earlier than the detectable change in both the area and mass. Furthermore, although the normalized mass is greater for the E2+ICI group than the control up to 60 hours, the growth rate of the control exceeds the E2+ICI group by 45 hours. It can also be seen that although clusters in the E2 group achieve much larger relative masses and areas than the control, there is no significant difference in the growth rates between the two groups after 90 hours.

By plotting the growth rate as a function of the normalized mass (Fig. 3C) the growth trend (exponential or linear) of the groups can be determined. It can be seen that the mean growth rate of clusters in the E2 and Veh groups continues to increase until a 4-fold increase in mass is achieved, after which the growth rate is either stable or decreases. This trend implies that for approximately two mass doublings both groups exhibit exponential growth, after which the growth is linear. In contrast, the E2+ICI group exhibits exponential growth (linear trend in Fig. 3C) until a 2-fold increase in mass is achieved, after which the growth is linear (constant curve in Fig. 3C). It is important to note here that a doubling in the mass does not necessarily correspond to a complete cell cycle as both estrogen and ICI are known to result in changes in how a cell progresses through the cell cycle, i.e., the doubling time and size and division both may be affected.

Effects of Estradiol on Cell Size and Doubling Time

To determine how changes at the single cell level contribute to the measurable changes in relative size, mass, and growth rates, we measured the doubling time and percent change in mean cell size for individual cells that compose the clusters (Fig. 4). The doubling time is calculated simply as $t_f / \log_2 [N_{cell}(t_f)/N_{cell}(0)]$, where t_f is the last time point, t_0 is the initial time point, and $N_{cell}(t)$ is the cell count at time t. The doubling times for the E2 group were found to be significantly lower than both the Veh and E2+ICI groups (Fig. 4A). These data show that estradiol induces cells to divide at almost twice the rate of the control group and that treatment with ICI almost completely reverses this effect. In line with previously

reported studies, we find that estrogens accelerate cells through the cell cycle, resulting in an increase in cell proliferation. Of note is that the effect of ICI in increasing cell-doubling time does not imply that the cell cycle is returned to normal conditions but more likely is a result of the cells spending a larger amount of time in a specific phase of the cell cycle.

The change in mean cell mass over time was calculated by dividing the total mass of each cluster by the number of cells in the cluster. Figure 4B shows the percent change in the mean cell mass between the initial and final time points for each cluster. The results indicate a significant decrease in the mean cell mass over time in the E2 and E2+ICI cells as compared to the control. This decrease in cell mass and doubling time show that compared to the control, estrogen results in smaller, faster dividing cells, and that adding ICI results in longer doubling times along with smaller cells. The smaller cells in the E2+ICI groups imply that although the doubling time has returned to control levels, ICI is affecting the cells' metabolic activity and ability to grow normally. As shown in Fig 4C, the doubling time and change in mean cell mass provide a reliable "growth signature" for each group and suggest that the levels of expression of the estrogen receptor or presence of an ER modulator may be assessed simply by examining these two parameters. Since current assays do not provide a direct measurement of cellular growth, these are the first measurements, performed continuously on a population, which elucidate how estrogen affects MCF-7 growth kinetics at the individual cell level.

Discussion

The results shown here establish that SLIM measurements of dry mass density can be used as highly sensitive proliferation assays. The main advantages over existing methods are that SLIM can detect changes in growth kinetics on fewer number of cells, in less time, and can be used to study differences within a population rather than just providing a number for the bulk growth of a culture. As a comparison, the WST-1 assay works with cell numbers in 10^3–10^5 range [27] whereas SLIM is sensitive to changes in the proliferation of even a single cell. Furthermore, SLIM provides the capability to analyze the growth rate of individual cells and clusters as a function of their mass, providing insight on the mechanism of growth regulation (e.g. whether a cell

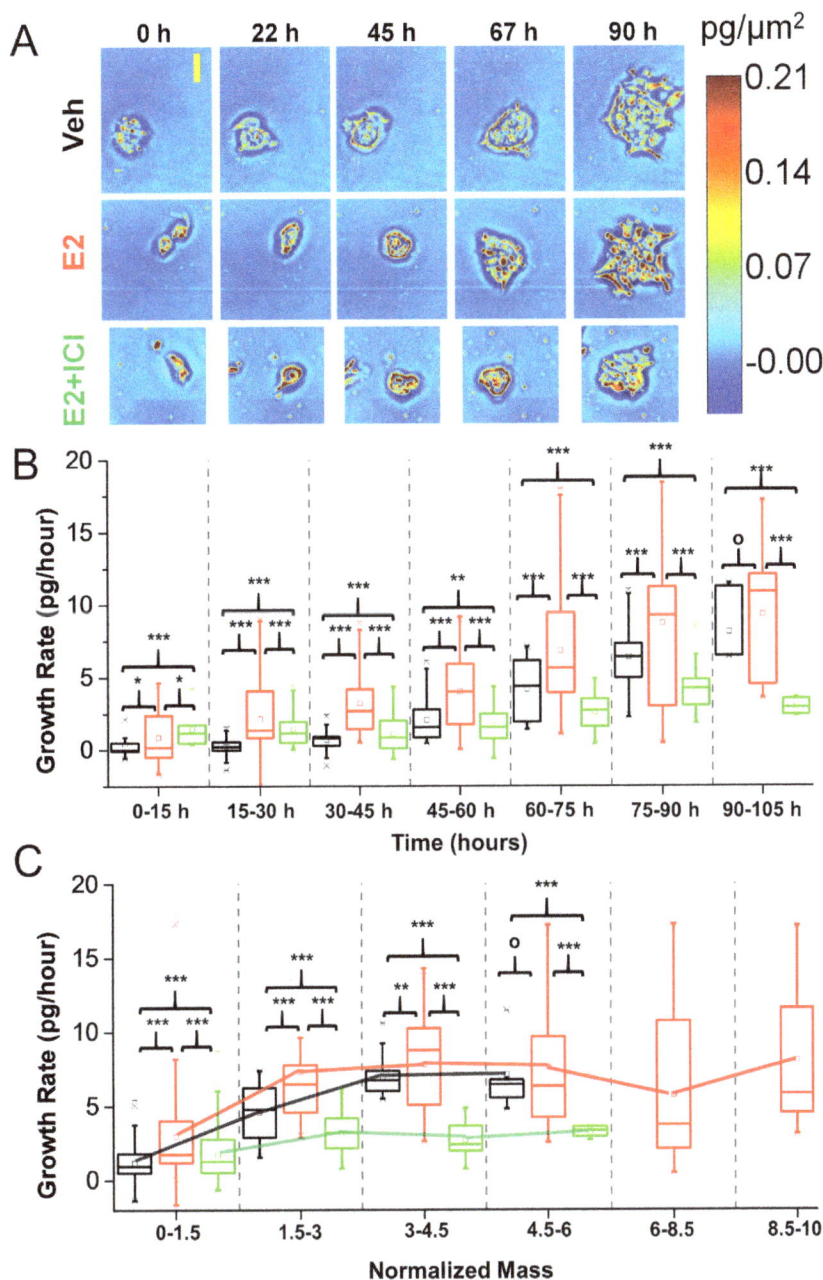

Figure 3. Cluster growth rate analysis. (A) Dry mass density maps of representative clusters from each group of MCF-7 breast cancer cells at every 22 hours. The colors indicate the dry mass density at each pixel as shown on the color bar. The yellow scale bar is 50 microns. Note that in the E2 + ICI group, ICI was added to each sample at 10 hours. (B) Cluster growth rate in each group in the shown time period. (C) Cluster growth rate in each group as a function of normalized mass. Solid lines are shown as a guide to the eye to determine how the growth rate is changing as a function of mass growth. (B–C) Square markers indicate mean, centerline is median, top of box is 25th percentile line, bottom is 75th percentile line, whiskers indicate 5th and 95th percentiles, significance was tested using an un-paired t-test, o: p>0.05, *: p<0.05, **: p<0.01, ***: p<0.001.

size or age checkpoint is being utilized)[35]. This information is inaccessible to any existing proliferation assay. This system can be readily used to measure growth kinetics and phenotypic effects for any cell type and treatment.

Our results also demonstrate that measuring growth at the cellular and cluster level not only provides advantages in terms of improved sensitivity and reduced sample sizes, but also yields additional information that is not accessible by existing methods. In particular, we show the kinetics and modality of action of E2 in MCF-7. Indeed MCF-7 under the influence of E2, divide faster

and achieve lower masses, resulting in an increased number of cells that are on average smaller. Due to the reduced doubling time, this still results in an overall increase in total mass for E2 when compared to the control group. For cells grown in E2 and subsequently treated with ICI the doubling times returned to those found in the control, however the reduction in cell size was still greater than in the control group.

The effects of E2 and anti-estrogens on cell-cycle progression have previously been studied in detail[11,15,36,37]. Both rapid and transient effects have been observed due to functional activity

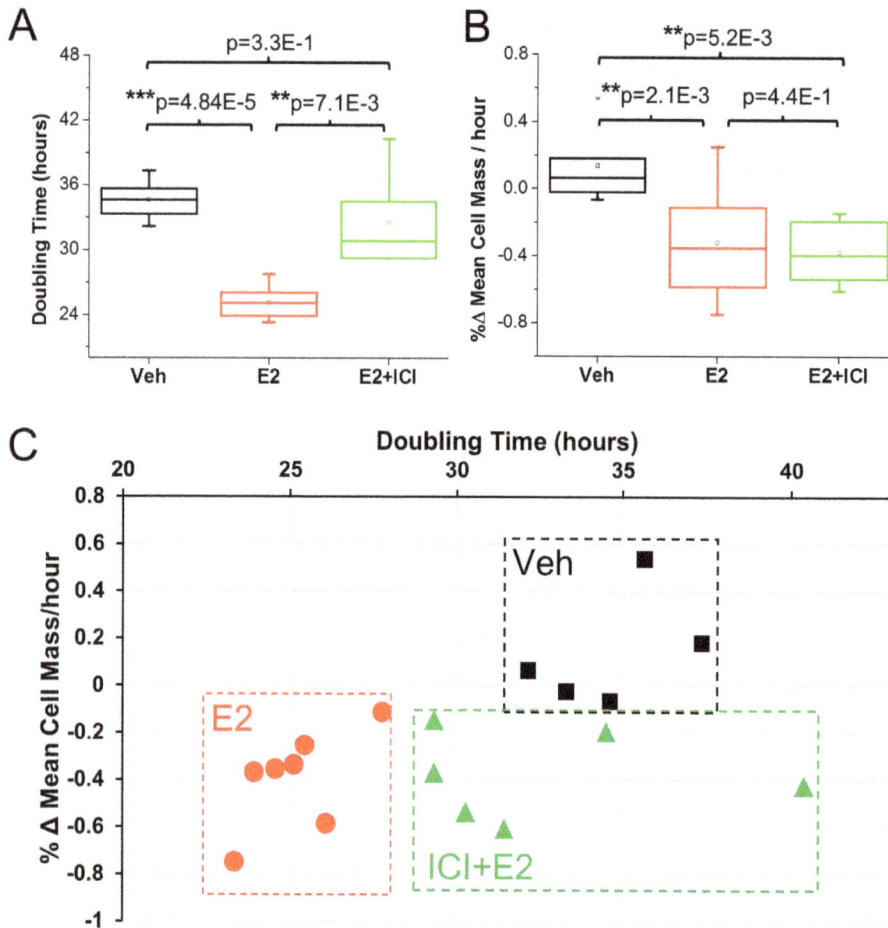

Figure 4. Estrogen modulated changes in proliferation kinetics. (A) Doubling time in each group, the mean doubling time is reduced by 12 hours in the E2 group compared to the Veh and E2 + ICI groups, indicating that adding ICI returns the doubling time to control levels. (B) Percent change in the mean cell mass over the measurement period for each group. A significant decrease in the cell mass is observed in both the E2 and E2+ICI groups compared to the control. (C) Measured doubling time vs. change in mean cell mass for each cluster that was measured, these two parameters can be used to separate the three groups completely and can serve as a growth signature.

in both the nucleus (genomic effects) and extranuclear compartment (non-genomic effects) [38]. The rapid effects on growth are clearly observable in our data as the differences in the growth rate between the E2 and Veh exposed cells are observable after 10 hours (Fig. S1) and can be attributed to the early activation of metabolism-related genes[39]. Upon the addition of ICI, a pure ER antagonist, differences in the growth rate between the E2 and E2+ICI groups begin to appear over time (Fig. 3B). The transient effects of E2+ICI are also manifested in how the growth rate changes as a function of increase in cell size (Fig. 3C), a clear break in the growth rate can be observed when the ICI clusters approximately double in size.

Estrogens are known to activate transduction cascades that regulate many genes –both positively and negatively—that play key roles in cell proliferation and metabolism[10–15,39]. It has also been shown that estrogens cause non-cycling cells (G_0 phase) to enter the cell cycle and to rapidly progress through the G_1 to the S phase[11,15,37]. This rapid progression through the cell cycle accounts for both the decreased doubling time and reduction in average cell mass observed in the E2 group (Fig. 4). On the other hand, ICI has been shown to block MCF-7 cells in the G0-G_1 phase[15,28,37]. This inhibitory action on the progression through G1 is manifested in the increased doubling time of the

E2+ICI group when compared to the E2 group. ICI also affects transcription of several genes responsible for growth regulation in all phases of the cell cycle. The down regulation of genes known to be responsible for proliferation in combination with the increased time spent in G1 are likely responsible for the reduction in the cell size observed in the E2+ICI group[15].

As in the case of the estrogen receptor, cell proliferation is also controlled through the activation and modulation of regulatory signaling cascades by growth factors; measuring growth at the cellular level has the potential to bridge the gap between the molecular understanding of cancer growth and actual tumor growth. Thus, it is of great interest to combine these growth measurements with fluorescence markers for cell cycle phase (as was done previously for U2OS cells [31]) or for other proteins known to play key roles in regulating proliferation. Measurement of changes in the growth kinetics as a function of the cell cycle or more specifically gene activations, will allow for better understanding of the particular action of a compound/drug on cell cycle progression.

In sum, we have demonstrated a new highly sensitive proliferation assay for drug screening applications. Although we have focused on a specific model cell system here, the experimental setup applies without alteration to other cell types and treatments. In addition to measuring growth kinetics, our method also simultaneously provides information on cellular morphology and motility [40], and can also be readily combined with other microscopy modalities. A subject of future study will be to understand and characterize the morphological differences that arise as a result of modulating the ER (see Movies S1 and S2). The biological insights provided by SLIM measurements in combination with other molecular assays will undoubtedly improve our understanding of cancer cell growth in general, and have the potential to lead to improvements in drug design, characterization, and therapeutic effectiveness.

Materials And Methods

Cell Culture

Commercially available MCF-7 cells were obtained from the American Type Culture Collection (Manassas, VA) and were cultured in MEM (Sigma-Aldrich Corp, St. Louis, MO) supplemented with 5% calf serum (HyClone, Logan, UT), 100 µg/ml penicillin/streptomycin (Invitrogen, Carlsbad, CA), and 25 µg/ml gentamicin (Invitrogen). Cells were then seeded in phenol-red free MEM containing 5% charcoal dextran treated calf serum to incubate for 4 days. Two chamber slides (Lab-Tek) with glass bottom coverslips were used to allow for side-by-side imaging of the control and treated samples. The medium was changed on day 2 and 4 prior to treatment with the control vehicle or ligand treatments (Estradiol (E2, 10 nM) and ICI 182,780 (ICI Fulvestrant, 1 µM)). For the colorimetric measurements, a WST1-assay (Roche, Basel, Switzerland) was used and absorbance was measured at 450 nm using a BioRad 680 Microplate Reader.

During imaging the cells were kept at 37°C and in a 5% CO2 atmosphere with an incubator and heated stage insert. Each well was scanned every 30 minutes in a 4×4-tile pattern with a Zeiss EC Plan-Neofluar 10×/0.3 PH 1 objective providing a total field of view of 1.55×1.16 mm^2. A z-stack of 12 slices (48 µm) was recorded at each position. The exposure time was 15 ms for each image at full lamp power (3,200 K, or 10.7 V). For each experiment, one well was left untreated to serve as a control population and the other well was treated with either the E2 or E2+ICI condition. Each condition was measured along with its control two times.

Imaging

Imaging was performed using spatial light interference microscopy (SLIM)[30,41]. SLIM is a white-light optical interferometry modality designed as an add-on module to a commercial phase contrast microscope. In brief, SLIM operates by projecting the back focal of a phase contrast objective onto a liquid crystal phase modulator (LCPM). The LCPM is calibrated to precisely shift the phase of the light scattered by the sample relative to the un-scattered light. Intensity maps are recorded at phase shifts of zero, $\pi/2$, π, and $3\pi/2$.

The SLIM setup used in this study is based on a Zeiss Axio Observer Z1 (Zeiss catalog # 431007901000) motorized inverted research imaging microscope. The microscope base is equipped with a motorized focus drive (minimum step width 10 nm). The objectives used for this study is a Zeiss EC Plan-Neofluar 10×/0.3 PH 1 M27. The intermediate image following the objective and tube lens is directed to left port of the microscope where the SLIM module is attached. The intermediate image is magnified by a 4f system with a focal length 150 mm doublet (Thorlabs, AC508-150-A1-ML) and a focal length 200 mm doublet (Thorlabs, AC508-150-A1-ML). A second 4f system following the magnifying system is comprised of a Fourier lens L1 (doublet with focal length

300 mm, Thorlabs, AC508-300-A1-ML) and Fourier lens L2 (doublet with focal length 500 mm, Thorlabs, AC508-500-A1-ML). The LCPM (array size 7.68 mm×7.68 mm, Boulder Nonlinear, XY Phase series, Model P512-0635) is placed at the back focal plane of L1 and is thus overlaid with the back focal plan of the objective. A polarizer (Edmund Optics, Stock # NT47-316) is placed in front of the LCPM to operate it in phase modulation mode. A Zeiss AxioCam MRm (1388×1040 pixels, pixel size 6.45 µm×6.45 µm, Zeiss catalog #4265099901000) is used for image acquisition. The SLIM module adds 2.22× magnification to the intermediate image. The microscope is also equipped with live cell environmental controls optimized for long time studies, including incubator XL S1 W/CO2 kit (Zeiss catalog #1441993KIT010) and a heating insert P S1/Scan stage (Zeiss catalog #4118609020000). The microscope is automatically controlled by AxioVision (Zeiss catalog #4101300300000) with multi-position, time-lapse, mosaic and Z-stack acquisition capabilities. The LCPM is automatically controlled using Labview. Matlab and ImageJ are used for image processing and visualization. Four intensity maps are recorded in this manner at phase shifts of zero, $\pi/2$, π, and $3\pi/2$. Remarkably, since the initial calibration of the system the accuracy has remained stable and thus no re-calibration or adjustment is required between experiments.

Data Analysis

The quantitative phase image is reconstructed from the four phase shifted intensity images as:

$$\Delta\phi(\mathbf{r}) = \arg\left[\frac{I(\mathbf{r}; -\pi/2) - I(\mathbf{r}; \pi/2)}{I(\mathbf{r}; 0) - I(\mathbf{r}; -\pi)}\right]$$

The dry mass density at each pixel is calculated as $\rho(x,y) = \frac{\lambda}{2\pi\gamma}\phi(x,y)$ where $\gamma = 0.2$ ml/g is the refractive increment of protein, λ is the center wavelength of the illumination and φ is the measured phase difference [31]. The dry mass density map is calculated at each z-location, and the projected maximum of the density is then calculated over the entire stack. The total mass is then calculated by integrating the dry mass density map over a region of interest. It should be noted that the accuracy of the dry mass measurement might be affected by debris present in the culture. Although this was not necessary for any of the experiments in this work, this affect may be mitigated by periodically replacing the culture media. The noise in the dry mass measurements due to such affects is shown in Fig. S2.

For the cluster analysis in this study the images were manually segmented using ImageJ and cells were counted at the beginning and end frames of each time series. In cases where the culture reaches confluence segmentation may become prohibitively difficult, thus it is important to control the initial seeding density to avoid this. The dry mass data was then smoothed using a cubic smoothing spline. For the binned data shown in Fig. 1 and 2, the smoothed data was sorted according to the variable over which the binning is performed. At least five clusters were analyzed per group.

Supporting Information

Figure S1. E2 vs. Veh. (A) Average dry mass (left axis, solid lines) and WST-1 assay data (right axis, dashed lines). (B) Growth rate vs. Time, a significant shift between E2 and Veh can be seen at 10 hours.

Figure S2 Sensitivity of dry mass measurement. Due to debris in the field of view, the noise in the mass measurement is higher (~pgs) than SLIM's capabilities (~fgs).

Movie S1 SLIM images from Veh, E2 and E2+ICI experiments. A clear difference in the growth rates and size of clusters is apparent.

Author Contributions

Conceived and designed the experiments: MM AB BSK GP. Performed the experiments: MM AB. Analyzed the data: MM. Contributed reagents/materials/analysis tools: MM AB. Wrote the paper: MM AB BSK GP.

References

1. Tzur A, Kafri R, LeBleu VS, Lahav G, Kirschner MW (2009) Cell Growth and Size Homeostasis in Proliferating Animal Cells. Science 325: 167–171.
2. Godin M, Delgado FF, Son S, Grover WH, Bryan AK, et al. (2010) Using buoyant mass to measure the growth of single cells. Nat Methods 7: 387–390.
3. Park K, Millet L, Huan J, Kim N, Popescu G, et al. (2010) Measurement of Adherent Cell Mass and Growth. Proc Nat Acad Sci.
4. Son S, Tzur A, Weng Y, Jorgensen P, Kim J, et al. (2012) Direct observation of mammalian cell growth and size regulation. Nat Methods 9: 910–912.
5. Mir M, Wang Z, Shen Z, Bednarz M, Bashir R, et al. (2011) Optical measurement of cycle-dependent cell growth. Proc Nat Acad Sci 108: 13124.
6. Popescu G, Park Y, Lue N, Best-Popescu C, Deflores L, et al. (2008) Optical imaging of cell mass and growth dynamics. Am J Physiol Cell Physiol 295: C538–544.
7. Dunn GA, Zicha D (1998) Using DRIMAPS system of transmission interference microscopy to study cell behavior. In: Celis JE, editor. Cell biology: a laboratory handbook San Diego: Academic press.
8. Barer R (1952) Interference microscopy and mass determination. Nature 169: 366–367.
9. Society AC (2012) Cancer Facts and Figures 2012. Atlanta.
10. Prall OWJ, Rogan EM, Musgrove EA, Watts CKW, Sutherland RL (1998) c-Myc or cyclin D1 mimics estrogen effects on cyclin E-Cdk2 activation and cell cycle reentry. Molecular and Cellular Biology 18: 4499–4508.
11. Prall OWJ, Rogan EM, Sutherland RL (1998) Estrogen regulation of cell cycle progression in breast cancer cells. Journal of Steroid Biochemistry and Molecular Biology 65: 169–174.
12. Dubik D, Shiu RPC (1992) Mechanism of Estrogen Activation of C-Myc Oncogene Expression. Oncogene 7: 1587–1594.
13. Frasor J, Danes JM, Komm B, Chang KCN, Lyttle CR, et al. (2003) Profiling of estrogen up- and down-regulated gene expression in human breast cancer cells: Insights into gene networks and pathways underlying estrogenic control of proliferation and cell phenotype. Endocrinology 144: 4562–4574.
14. Soulez M, Parker MG (2001) Identification of novel oestrogen receptor target genes in human ZR75-1 breast cancer cells by expression profiling. Journal of Molecular Endocrinology 27: 259–274.
15. Dalvai M, Bystricky K (2010) Cell cycle and anti-estrogen effects synergize to regulate cell proliferation and ER target gene expression. PLoS One 5: e11011.
16. Frasor J, Stossi F, Danes JM, Komm B, Lyttle CR, et al. (2004) Selective estrogen receptor modulators: discrimination of agonistic versus antagonistic activities by gene expression profiling in breast cancer cells. Cancer Res 64: 1522–1533.
17. Obiorah I, Jordan VC (2011) Progress in endocrine approaches to the treatment and prevention of breast cancer. Maturitas 70: 315–321.
18. DeVita VT Jr, Chu E (2008) A history of cancer chemotherapy. Cancer Res 68: 8643–8653.
19. Driscoll JS (1984) The Preclinical New Drug Research-Program of the National-Cancer-Institute. Cancer Treatment Reports 68: 63–76.
20. Teicher BA, Selwood DL, Andrews PA (2004) Anticancer drug development: preclinical screening, clinical trials and approval (vol 91, pg 1000, 2004). British Journal of Cancer 91: 1977–1977.
21. Boyd MR, Pauli KD (1995) Some Practical Considerations and Applications of the National-Cancer-Institute in-Vitro Anticancer Drug Discovery Screen. Drug Development Research 34: 91–109.
22. Alley MC, Scudiero DA, Monks A, Hursey ML, Czerwinski MJ, et al. (1988) Feasibility of Drug Screening with Panels of Human-Tumor Cell-Lines Using a Microculture Tetrazolium Assay. Cancer Research 48: 589–601.
23. Paull KD, Shoemaker RH, Boyd MR, Parsons JL, Risbood PA, et al. (1988) The Synthesis of Xtt - a New Tetrazolium Reagent That Is Bioreducible to a Water-Soluble Formazan. Journal of Heterocyclic Chemistry 25: 911–914.
24. Rubinstein LV, Shoemaker RH, Paull KD, Simon RM, Tosini S, et al. (1990) Comparison of in vitro anticancer-drug-screening data generated with a tetrazolium assay versus a protein assay against a diverse panel of human tumor cell lines. J Natl Cancer Inst 82: 1113–1118.
25. Skehan P, Storeng R, Scudiero D, Monks A, McMahon J, et al. (1990) New colorimetric cytotoxicity assay for anticancer-drug screening. J Natl Cancer Inst 82: 1107–1112.
26. Mosmann T (1983) Rapid colorimetric assay for cellular growth and survival: application to proliferation and cytotoxicity assays. J Immunol Methods 65: 55–63.
27. Manual (2013) WST-1 Cell Proliferation Assay Kit. Ann Arbor, MI: Cayman Chemical Company.
28. McGowan EM, Alling N, Jackson EA, Yagoub D, Haass NK, et al. (2011) Evaluation of Cell Cycle Arrest in Estrogen Responsive MCF-7 Breast Cancer Cells: Pitfalls of the MTS Assay. Plos One 6: e20623.
29. Popescu G (2011) Quantitative phase imaging of cells and tissues. New York: McGraw-Hill. 385 p.
30. Wang Z, Millet L, Mir M, Ding H, Unarunotai S, et al. (2011) Spatial light interference microscopy (SLIM). Opt Express 19: 1016–1026.
31. Mir M, Wang Z, Shen Z, Bednarz M, Bashir R, et al. (2011) Optical measurement of cycle-dependent cell growth. Proc Natl Acad Sci U S A 108: 13124–13129.
32. Soule HD, Vazquez J, Long A, Albert S, Brennan M (1973) Human Cell Line from a Pleural Effusion Derived from a Breast Carcinoma. Journal of the National Cancer Institute 51: 1409–1416.
33. Brooks SC, Locke ER, Soule HD (1973) Estrogen Receptor in a Human Cell Line (Mcf-7) from Breast Carcinoma. Journal of Biological Chemistry 248: 6251–6253.
34. Wakeling AE, Dukes M, Bowler J (1991) A Potent Specific Pure Antiestrogen with Clinical Potential. Cancer Research 51: 3867–3873.
35. Lloyd D (2013) The regulation of cell size. Cell 154: 1194–1205.
36. Doisneau-Sixou SF, Sergio CM, Carroll JS, Hui R, Musgrove EA, et al. (2003) Estrogen and antiestrogen regulation of cell cycle progression in breast cancer cells. Endocrine-Related Cancer 10: 179–186.
37. Sutherland RL, Hall RE, Taylor IW (1983) Cell-Proliferation Kinetics of Mcf-7 Human Mammary-Carcinoma Cells in Culture and Effects of Tamoxifen on Exponentially Growing and Plateau-Phase Cells. Cancer Research 43: 3998–4006.
38. Collins P, Webb C (1999) Estrogen hits the surface. Nature Medicine 5: 1130–1131.
39. Hah N, Danko CG, Core L, Waterfall JJ, Siepel A, et al. (2011) A Rapid, Extensive, and Transient Transcriptional Response to Estrogen Signaling in Breast Cancer Cells. Cell 145: 622–634.
40. Sridharan S, Mir M, Popescu G (2011) Simultaneous optical measurement of cell motility and growth. Biomed Opt Exp 2: 2815–2820.
41. Wang Z, Popescu G (2010) Quantitative phase imaging with broadband fields. Applied Physics Letters 96: 051117.

12

Impact of the *Superoxide Dismutase 2* Val16Ala Polymorphism on the Relationship between Valproic Acid Exposure and Elevation of γ-Glutamyltransferase in Patients with Epilepsy: A Population Pharmacokinetic-Pharmacodynamic Analysis

Naoki Ogusu[1], **Junji Saruwatari**[1*], **Hiroo Nakashima**[1], **Madoka Noai**[1], **Miki Nishimura**[1], **Mariko Deguchi**[1], **Kentaro Oniki**[1], **Norio Yasui-Furukori**[2], **Sunao Kaneko**[2], **Takateru Ishitsu**[3,4], **Kazuko Nakagaswa**[1,5]

1 Division of Pharmacology and Therapeutics, Graduate School of Pharmaceutical Sciences, Kumamoto University, Kumamoto, Japan, **2** Department of Neuropsychiatry, Hirosaki University School of Medicine, Hirosaki, Japan, **3** Kumamoto Saishunso National Hospital, Kumamoto, Japan, **4** Kumamoto Ezuko Ryoiku Iryo Center, Kumamoto, Japan, **5** Center for Clinical Pharmaceutical Sciences, Kumamoto University, Kumamoto, Japan

Abstract

Background: There has been accumulating evidence that there are associations among γ-glutamyltransferase (γ-GT) elevation and all-cause mortality, cardiovascular diseases and metabolic diseases, including nonalcoholic fatty liver disease. The primary objective of this study was to evaluate the impact of the most common and potentially functional polymorphisms of antioxidant enzyme genes, i.e. *superoxide dismutase 2 (SOD2)*, *glutathione S-transferase M1* and *glutathione S-transferase T1*, on the γ-GT elevation during valproic acid (VPA) therapy.

Methods and Findings: This retrospective study included 237 and 169 VPA-treated Japanese patients with epilepsy for population pharmacokinetic and pharmacokinetic-pharmacodynamic analyses, respectively. A nonlinear mixed-effect model represented the pharmacokinetics of VPA and the relationships between VPA exposure and γ-GT elevation. A one-compartment model of the pharmacokinetic parameters of VPA adequately described the data; while the model for the probability of the γ-GT elevation was fitted using a logistic regression model, in which the logit function of the probability was a linear function of VPA exposure. The *SOD2* Val16Ala polymorphism and complication with intellectual disability were found to be significant covariates influencing the intercept of the logit function for the probability of an elevated γ-GT level. The predicted mean percentages of the subjects with γ-GT elevation were about 2- to 3-fold, 3- to 4-fold and 4- to 8-fold greater in patients with the *SOD2* Val/Val genotype but without any intellectual disability, those with the *SOD2* Val/Ala or Ala/Ala genotype and intellectual disability and those with the *SOD2* Val/Val genotype and intellectual disability, respectively, compared to those with the *SOD2* Val/Ala or Ala/Ala genotype without intellectual disability.

Conclusion: Our results showed that the *SOD2* Val16Ala polymorphism has an impact on the relationship between VPA exposure and γ-GT elevation in patients with epilepsy. These results suggest that determining the *SOD2* genotype could be helpful for preventing the VPA-induced γ-GT elevation.

Editor: Barbara Bardoni, CNRS UMR7275, France

Funding: This work was supported by grants from the Japan Research Foundation for Clinical Pharmacology and KAKENHI (Nos. 24590652, 25860117, 26360049), and in part by a grant from the Smoking Research Foundation. Norio Yasui-Furukori has received grant/research support or honoraria from and spoken for Asteras, Dainippon, Eli Lilly, GlaxoSmithKline, Janssen-Pharma, Meiji, Mochida, Merck Sharp & Dohme, Otsuka, Pfizer, Takada, and Yoshitomi. The funders had no role in study design, data collection and analysis, decision to publish, or preparation of the manuscript.

Competing Interests: Norio Yasui-Furukori has received grant/research support or honoraria from and spoken for Asteras, Dainippon, Eli Lilly, GlaxoSmithKline, Janssen-Pharma, Meiji, Mochida, Merck Sharp & Dohme, Otsuka, Pfizer, Takada, and Yoshitomi. There are no patents, products in development or marketed products to declare. The remaining authors have declared that no competing interests exist.

* Email: junsaru@gpo.kumamoto-u.ac.jp

Introduction

γ-Glutamyltransferase (γ-GT) is a hepatic and biliary enzyme synthesized by hepatocytes as well as the epithelial cells of the intra-hepatic bile ducts [1]. Measurements of the γ-GT activity in the serum are used clinically as a liver function parameter [1,2]. The serum γ-GT level is also a biomarker of excessive alcohol consumption [1,2]. The available evidence indicates that an elevated γ-GT level is related to nonalcoholic fatty liver disease (NAFLD) [3,4]. The oxidative stress and inflammation caused by NAFLD might contribute to the elevation of γ-GT [5,6]. There is also strong evidence for associations between the γ-GT activity and all-cause mortality, cardiovascular disease, type 2 diabetes, metabolic syndrome, insulin resistance and obesity [2,7,8].

Valproic acid (VPA) is one of the most widely prescribed antiepileptic drugs worldwide [9]. VPA is also used to treat migraines and bipolar, mood, anxiety and psychiatric disorders [9]. Therapeutic drug monitoring is the measurement of the blood level of a drug to ensure that its concentration is within the therapeutic range [10]. Since the dose requirements for VPA are highly variable, therapeutic drug monitoring of VPA is commonly used [10]. Long-term treatment with VPA has been associated with metabolic and endocrine disorders, such as weight gain and hyperinsulinemia, which may contribute to the increased cardiovascular risk observed in patients with epilepsy [9]. Recently, NAFLD has emerged as a common chronic liver condition in VPA-treated patients [9,11,12].

Mitochondrial dysfunction has been implicated in the pathogenesis of VPA-induced hepatotoxicity [9,13]. Superoxide dismutase 2 (SOD2, also known as manganese superoxide dismutase) plays a critical role in the detoxification of mitochondrial reactive oxygen species [13,14]. The T to C nucleotide polymorphism (rs4880, Val16Ala) has been identified in exon 2 of the human *SOD2* gene [15]. The Ala variant is more efficiently imported into the mitochondria than the Val variant, thus resulting in increased mitochondrial SOD2 homotetramer activity derived from the Ala precursor variant [15]. Our previous case-control study demonstrated a possible association between the *SOD2* Val/Val genotype and the VPA-induced elevation of γ-GT [16].

The glutathione *S*-transferase (GST) supergene family consists of phase 2 detoxifying enzymes [17]. GST plays a crucial role in antioxidant defense mechanisms by detoxifying electrophilic xenobiotics and inactivating a variety of endogenous byproducts of oxidative stress [17]. The most extensively studied *GST* polymorphisms occur in two isozymes, i.e. GST mu 1 (GSTM1) and GST theta 1 (GSTT1) [17]. The most common polymorphism in the human *GSTM1* or *GSTT1* gene is a deletion of the whole gene ("null" genotype), which results in a lack of functional activity of the enzyme [17]. The two common deletion polymorphisms of *GSTM1* and *GSTT1* have been reported to be associated with an increased susceptibility to certain oxidative stress-related diseases [18–20]. In a previous case-control study, an association of the *GSTM1* null and *GSTT1* null genotypes with an increased γ-GT levels was reported in VPA-treated Japanese patients with epilepsy [21].

In this study, we applied population pharmacokinetic (PK)-pharmacodynamic (PD) modeling to describe the VPA-induced γ-GT elevation in patients with epilepsy. The primary objective of this retrospective study was to evaluate the impact of the most common and potentially functional polymorphisms in three antioxidant enzyme genes, i.e. *SOD2*, *GSTM1* and *GSTT1*, on the relationship between the VPA exposure and the risk of γ-GT elevation during long-term VPA therapy.

Materials and Methods

Participants and Study Design

This retrospective study was approved by the ethics committees of Kumamoto Saishunso National Hospital and the Faculty of Life Sciences, Kumamoto University (Kumamoto, Japan). This study included patients who were being treated at Kumamoto Saishunso National Hospital (Kumamoto, Japan) between June 1989 and

April 2011. Four hundred and fifty-six Japanese patients with epilepsy and/or their parents gave their written informed consent to participate in this study. For the PK analysis, patients were included if they fulfilled all of the following conditions: had been receiving sustained-release VPA for three weeks or longer and were not taking any drugs that might alter the clearance of VPA, except for antiepileptic drugs; and having detailed medical data available. For the PK-PD analysis, patients were included if they fulfilled all of the criteria for the PK analysis, as well as the following conditions: a history of treatment with VPA for one year or longer; not taking any drugs that may affect the liver function, except for antiepileptic agents; and no history of either viral or alcoholic liver disease.

For all patients, the most appropriate antiepileptic drug was chosen according to the treatment guidelines of the Japan Epilepsy Society. The treatment was changed to another drug if the seizures remained uncontrolled, if drug-precipitated seizures were suspected or if the patient had any intolerable adverse drug reaction(s). At each follow-up visit, the clinical information was recorded. For all patients, VPA was initiated at a dose of 15–40 mg/kg/day for children (400–1,200 mg/day for adults) and was escalated at weekly intervals by 5–10 mg/kg/day (for children) or 200 mg/day (for adults) for each step up to the maximum tolerated dose.

The patients' medical information was retrospectively obtained from their medical records. For every patient, the data included demographics, the VPA dose and schedule, diagnoses, seizure frequency and concomitant medications evaluated at every visit during the VPA therapy. The types of seizures and epileptic syndromes were classified according to the guidelines of the International League Against Epilepsy [22]. We used the International Classification of Diseases, 10th Revision (ICD-10) to identify individuals with moderate or severe intellectual disability (ICD-10 F70–F79, consistent with IQ scores <50), since intellectual disability is known to be common in patients with epilepsy [23]. Clinical laboratory tests, including serum γ-GT measurements, were performed regularly and when necessary. Blood samples were collected for routine therapeutic drug monitoring or to assess the patient for adverse events. Therefore, blood sampling was performed when necessary at the time of the visit for each patient, and thus, there were differences in the timing of blood collection among the patients (e.g., morning and afternoon). The data were retrospectively reviewed independently by a physician and by clinical pharmacists.

Genotyping

Genomic DNA was isolated from EDTA blood samples using a DNA extractor WB kit (Wako Pure Chemical Industries, Ltd. Osaka, Japan). Null genotypes of *GSTM1* and *GSTT1* were determined using polymerase chain reaction (PCR) amplification based on the presence or absence of a PCR amplification product according to the previously described method [20]. The *GST* genotypes were classified as follows: subjects with homozygous deleted alleles (i.e. the "null" genotype) and others (i.e. the "present" genotype). The *SOD2* Val16Ala (c.47T>C; rs4880) polymorphism and the three most common polymorphisms of *cytochrome P450 (CYP) 2C9* and *CYP2C19* enzymes that are involved in VPA metabolism [24], i.e. *CYP2C9*3* (c.1075A>C; rs1057910), *CYP2C19*2* (c.681G>A; rs4244285) and *CYP2C19*3* (c.636G>A; rs4986893), were genotyped using real-time PCR with 5′-nuclease allele discrimination assays (Step One Plus Real-Time PCR system version 2.1; Applied Biosystems, Tokyo, Japan). Genotyping for rs4880, rs1057910, rs4244285 and rs4986893 was performed using commercially available assays (assay IDs: C_8709053_10, C_27104892_10, C25986767_70 and

C_27861809_10, respectively), according to the manufacturer's protocol [25,26]. All reagents were purchased from Applied Biosystems (Tokyo, Japan). Regarding *SOD2* and *CYP2C9*, the genotypes were classified as follows: homozygous for the wild-type allele (i.e. the *SOD2* Val allele or *CYP2C9*1* allele), heterozygous for the wild-type and mutant alleles and homozygous for the mutant allele (i.e. the *SOD2* Ala allele or *CYP2C9*3* allele). Regarding *CYP2C19*, the genotypes were classified into three groups: homozygous extensive metabolizers (EMs) (*1/*1 genotype), heterozygous EMs (*1/*2 or *1/*3 genotype) and poor metabolizers (PMs) (*2/*2, *3/*3 or *2/*3 genotype).

To ensure the quality of the genotyping, we included DNA samples as internal controls, hidden samples of known genotypes and a negative control (water). The genotype distributions of *SOD2* Val16Ala, *CYP2C9*3*, *CYP2C19*2* and *CYP2C19*3* were tested for Hardy-Weinberg equilibrium using the χ^2 test. A *P* value <0.05 was considered to be statistically significant. The statistical analyses were performed using the R software program (version 3.0.0; R Foundation for Statistical Computing, Vienna, Austria).

Assessment of the Serum VPA Concentrations

The serum VPA concentrations were evaluated using the steady-state therapeutic drug monitoring data from clinical practice using a homogenous enzyme immunoassay (Cobas Mira; Roche Diagnostics, Basel, Switzerland). The measurements were obtained in accordance with the manufacturer's protocol. The within- and between-day coefficients of variation for determining VPA were $<10\%$ and the lower limit of quantification was 1 mg/L. Any therapeutic drug monitoring data obtained from patients with suspected temporary noncompliance were excluded from the analysis. The suspected temporary noncompliance was determined by assessing whether the serum concentrations were under the limit of quantification, as well as whether the medications were taken based on the pill counts.

Assessment of the Serum γ-GT Levels

The γ-GT levels were measured using the standard method recommended by the Japan Society of Clinical Chemistry in daily practice at Kumamoto Saishunso National Hospital. Since the γ-GT level shows large inter-individual variability and it is correlated with age and sex [27], we defined an elevated γ-GT level as an increase over the upper limit of the normal range, which was stratified by age and sex [28]. For PK-PD modeling, we included all γ-GT levels measured after the start of VPA therapy in each patient, with the exception of the data collected in the early phase of VPA therapy (i.e. <6 months after the initiation of VPA therapy), in order to exclude any confounding effects due to transient γ-GT elevation after the commencement of VPA therapy [9,29].

Population PK and PK-PD Modeling

All analyses used during the population PK and PK-PD modeling were carried out with a nonlinear mixed-effect model (NONMEM, version 7.2.0; ICON Dev Soln, Ellicott City, MD). First-order conditional estimation with the ADVAN 2 TRANS 2 subroutine was used for PK parameter estimation. The ADVAN 2 subroutine contained the appropriate equations for a one-compartment model with first-order absorption and elimination, while the TRANS 2 subroutine parameterized the models in terms of the clearance and volume. The first-order conditional estimation with the use of laplacian estimation was used for the development of the PK-PD model.

PK Modeling

A one-compartment model with first-order absorption and lag time was used to select the structural model for VPA. During model development, all compartment models were parameterized in terms of values of the absorption rate constant (Ka), apparent oral clearance (CL/F), volume of distribution (Vd/F) and the absorption lag time ($ALAG$). A variance model was established by separately evaluating an additive error model, a proportional error model and an exponential error model for the inter-individual variability of each parameter and the variability of any residual errors. The inter-individual variability was best described using an exponential error model. The residual unexplained variability, which includes other unexplained factors of variability (e.g., model misspecification, assay errors), was best described using a proportional error model.

A regression model was developed using the forward-inclusion and backward-elimination methods. First, each covariate was incorporated nonlinearly into the basic regression model. The influence of covariates on the PK parameters was systematically tested in a forward-building model using different equations for continuous covariates (e.g., age) and categorical covariates (e.g., *CYP2C9* genotype) according to the previously described method [30]. From the basic model, important covariates were identified by plotting the estimates versus the covariates. The influence of these fixed effects was evaluated using the objective function. The full model was created by incorporating all covariates, which thus led to a significant decrease in the objective function. The objective function of the full model was used to test the effects of removing each covariate from the full model. Changes in the objective function of at least 3.84 [χ^2, $P<0.05$; degree of freedom (df) = 1] and 5.99 (χ^2, $P<0.05$; df = 2) were considered to be significant during the forward-inclusion and backward-elimination analyses. The covariates tested were the age, gender, body weight, daily VPA dose, *CYP2C9* genotype, *CYP2C19* genotype and co-administered antiepileptic drugs on the CL/F and body weight and the daily VPA dose on the Vd/F. At this step, typical values of the PK parameters were also considered.

PK-PD Modeling

The final individual PK parameters, determined from the population PK model, were fixed in the PK-PD analysis. A binomial scale was used to represent the serum γ-GT elevation, with 0 indicating data that were within the normal range and 1 indicating an increase over the upper limit of the normal range. A logistic regression model was used to relate the probability of having an elevated γ-GT level. The area under the concentration-time curve (AUC) of VPA was used as the exposure variable. The AUC values were predicted from the population PK model. The probability, *Pr*, of having an elevated γ-GT level was expressed as the inverse logit function:

$$\mathrm{Pr} = \frac{e^{logit(\mathrm{Pr})}}{1 + e^{logit(\mathrm{Pr})}} \quad (1)$$

in which the logit (Pr) is a linear function of the AUC:

$$Logit(\mathrm{Pr}) = Ln\frac{\mathrm{Pr}}{1-\mathrm{Pr}} = BASE + SLOPE \times AUC + \eta \quad (2)$$

where BASE represents the intercept, SLOPE is the slope relating the AUC to the effect and η is the individual random effect.

The logit (Pr) that described a nonlinear E_{max} relationship was also tested, and the equation is described below:

$$Logit(\mathrm{Pr}) = Ln\frac{\mathrm{Pr}}{1-\mathrm{Pr}} = BASE + \frac{E_{max} \times AUC}{EC_{50} + AUC} + \eta \qquad (3)$$

in which E_{max} is the maximum increase in the probability of an elevated γ-GT level and EC_{50} is the exposure at which a half maximal increase in the probability is reached.

The influence of covariates on the logit (Pr) was systematically tested in the same manner as the PK analysis, except for using the equations described below:

$$PD\ parameter = \theta_p + \theta_{cov} \times \text{covariate} \qquad (4)$$

where θ_p is the parameter estimate in an individual patient, while θ_{cov} is a fraction change in the PD parameter, i.e. logit (Pr), for each covariate group. The covariates tested were the age, gender, body weight, daily dose and duration of VPA therapy, CYP2C9 genotype, CYP2C19 genotype, SOD2 genotype, GSTM1 genotype, GSTT1 genotype, complication with intellectual disability and co-administered antiepileptic drugs on the BASE, SLOPE, E_{max} and/or EC_{50}. Typical values of the PD parameters were also considered at this step.

Model Evaluation

A stratified nonparametric bootstrap analysis was performed to investigate the precision of the parameters of the population PK and PK-PD models implemented in the NONMEM and Wings for NONMEM programs (version 720; http://wfn.sourceforge.net/). One thousand replicated datasets were generated by random sampling with replacement, and were stratified according to the study population to ensure a representative study population distribution using the individual as the sampling unit. The population parameters of each dataset were subsequently estimated as described for the original estimation procedure.

For the population PK model, the goodness of fit was assessed by visually inspecting the scattered plots of the population model-predicted versus observed concentrations, the individually model-predicted versus observed concentrations and the conditional weighted residuals versus the population model-predicted concentrations.

A visual predictive check regarding the proportion of there being γ-GT elevation was also performed using 1,000 datasets that were randomly sampled from the original dataset, and was stratified by the statistically significant covariates identified in the final model. The visual predictive check is an internal validation tool that shows how well the model predicts the data on which the model was conditioned, and it compares the dependent variables derived from the original and the simulated datasets. [31]. The R-based software program, Xpose (version 4.4.1), was used for the graphical visualization of the results, and the PsN tool kit (version 3.5.3) was used for the post-processing of the results.

Simulations of the PK-PD Parameters

Based on the final population PK-PD parameter estimates, the probability of there being γ-GT elevation were also simulated at the steady state in 1,000 individuals. The simulation processes were performed using the NONMEM program.

Results

Patient Demographics

237 patients fulfilled all of the inclusion criteria for the PK analysis and 169 fulfilled all of the inclusion criteria for the PK-PD

analysis. The patient characteristics are presented in Table 1. The mean durations of follow-up were 3.2±4.0 and 6.6±5.1 years, respectively. Among the 237 patients included for the PK modeling, the allele frequencies of CYP2C9*3, CYP2C19*2 and CYP2C19*3 were 3.2%, 29.3% and 11.2%, respectively. The frequencies of the CYP2C9*1/*1, *1/*3 and *3/*3 genotypes were 93.7%, 6.3% and 0%, respectively, and those of CYP2C19 homozygous EMs, heterozygous EMs and PMs were 35.9%, 47.2% and 16.9%, respectively. Among the 169 patients included for the PK-PD modeling, the frequency of the SOD2 16Ala allele was 12.7%, and the frequencies of the Val/Val, Val/Ala and Ala/Ala genotypes were 77.6%, 20.7% and 1.7%, respectively. The observed genotype frequency distributions for CYP2C9, CYP2C19 and SOD2 were consistent with the Hardy-Weinberg equilibrium ($P > 0.05$). The number of patients with the SOD2 Ala/Ala genotype (two patients among the 169 PK-PD modeling population) was too small to assess the effect of the genotype on the serum γ-GT elevation; therefore, the Ala/Ala and the Val/Ala genotypes were combined in the subsequent PK-PD analyses. The frequencies of the GSTM1 null and GSTT1 null genotypes were 56.8% and 47.9%, respectively, among the 169 patients included for the PK-PD modeling.

Population PK Model

A total of 827 steady-state VPA concentrations were collected and made available for the PK analysis. The interval between the time of the last dose and the sampling time was distributed over 24 hours. A one-compartment model with exponential inter-individual variability on the Ka, Vd/F, CL/F and ALAG adequately described the data. The best residual error model was an additive model.

The daily VPA dose significantly influenced the Vd/F and CL/F of VPA. The covariates gender, co-administered carbamazepine (CBZ), phenobarbital (PB), phenytoin (PHT) and clobazam (CLB) significantly decreased the objective function values of the CL/F (Table S1). The CYP2C9 and CYP2C19 genotypes did not have any statistically significant influence on the CL/F in the forward-inclusion analysis (Table S1). Compared with the base model, the residual error was reduced by 17.9% in the final model. The final population pharmacokinetic model for VPA was as follows:

$$Ka\ (h^{-1}) = 0.109 \times e^{\eta Ka} \qquad (5)$$

$$Vd/F\ (L) = 21.4 \times \left(\frac{Dose}{1000}\right)^{1.52} \times e^{\eta Vd} \qquad (6)$$

$$CL/F\ (L/h) = 0.559 \times \left(\frac{Dose}{1000}\right)^{0.596} \times 0.917^{female}$$
$$\times 1.19^{CBZ} \times 1.12^{PB} \times 1.43^{PHT} \times 0.906^{CLB} \times e^{\eta CL} \qquad (7)$$

$$ALAG\ (h) = 3.00 \times e^{\eta ALAG} \qquad (8)$$

where Dose is the daily VPA dose (mg/day); female = 1, male = 0; CBZ, PB, PHT or CLB = 1 if CBZ, PB, PHT or CLB was co-administered, and was otherwise 0; and η is the individual random effect.

Among 1,000 bootstrap runs, 965 runs exhibited successful minimization and were included in the bootstrap analysis. Table 2 shows the median parameter estimates obtained using the

Table 1. A summary of the patient characteristics.

Patient Characteristics	PK analysis (N = 237)	PK-PD analysis (N = 169)
	N (%) or mean ± SD (range)	N (%) or mean ± SD (range)
Body weight [kg]	48.8±20.9 (9.6–120.5)	51.0±20.1 (13.0–120.5)
Age [years]	17.2±8.3 (2.2–52.2)	18.0±7.8 (3.0–52.2)
Gender (men/women)	137 (57.8%)/100 (42.2%)	102 (60.4%)/67 (39.6%)
VPA dose [mg/day]	934.3±540.2 (100–2600)	903.8±502.7 (100–2600)
VPA concentration [µg/mL]	68.15±26.54 (7.70–165.0)	67.8±25.7 (7.7–143.0)
Seizure locus		
Generalize	111 (46.8%)	75 (44.4%)
Partial	119 (50.2%)	87 (51.5%)
Unidentified	7 (3.0%)	7 (4.1%)
Seizure type		
Idiopathic	64 (27.0%)	42 (24.8%)
Symptomatic	75 (31.7%)	50 (29.6%)
Cryptogenic	98 (41.3%)	77 (45.6%)
γ-GT [IU/L]	51.3±68.6 (7–515)	48.3±65.1 (2.4–515)
ALT [IU/L]	19.1±15.7(5–134)	18.8±15.1 (4–134)
AST [IU/L]	23.0±10.2 (9–103)	23.4±9.9 (9–103)
Creatinine [mg/dL]	0.5±0.2 (0.1–1.5)	0.6±0.2 (0.1–1.5)
BUN [mg/dL]	12.7±3.7 (3.5–28.3)	13.0±3.7 (3.5–28.3)
Intellectual disability	131 (55.3%)	97 (57.4%)
Monotherapy	378 (45.7%)	226 (47.8%)
Co-administration		
CBZ	190 (23.0%)	94 (19.9%)
CLB	128 (15.5%)	90 (19.0%)
GBP	8 (1.0%)	5 (1.1%)
PB	73 (8.8%)	28 (5.9%)
PHT	88 (10.6%)	45 (9.5%)
TPM	44 (5.3%)	29 (6.1%)
ZNS	59 (7.1%)	27 (5.7%)

PK = pharmacokinetic; PD = pharmacodynamic; N = number; SD = standard deviation; VPA = valproic acid; γ-GT: γ-glutamyltransferase; ALT: alanine aminotransferase; AST: aspartate aminotransferase; BUN = blood urea nitrogen; CBZ = carbamazepine; CLB = clobazam; GBP = gabapentine; PB = phenobarbital; PHT = phenytoin; TPM = topiramate; ZNS = zonisamide.

NONMEM program and the values with 95% confidence intervals (CIs) obtained using the bootstrap approach. The 95% CIs for all parameters obtained using the bootstrap approach was generally comparable to the estimates obtained using the NONMEM program (Table 2).

A scatter plot of the population model-predicted and individually model-predicted concentrations versus the observed concentrations showed no bias, and the conditional weighted residuals were homogeneously distributed over the population model-predicted VPA concentrations (see Figure S1).

PK-PD Model

A total of 472 γ-GT levels were collected and made available for the PK-PD analysis. The best fitted model for the probability of γ-GT elevation was a logistic regression model, in which the logit (Pr) was a linear function of the individual AUC value of VPA. During the forward-inclusion and the backward-elimination analyses, the *SOD2* Val/Val genotype, complication with intellectual disability and co-administered CBZ, PB and PHT

were found to be significant covariates influencing the BASE of the logit (Pr) (Table S2). During the forward-inclusion analysis, the daily VPA dose, age, gender, body weight and duration of VPA therapy significantly influenced the SLOPE. During the backward-elimination analysis, the influence of the gender and duration of VPA therapy on the SLOPE were not statistically significant (Table S2), and therefore, these were removed from the full covariate model. The presence of an intellectual disability was associated with an increased number of co-administered CBZ, PB and PHT drugs ($P<0.0001$), whereas age, body weight and the daily VPA dose significantly correlated with each other ($P<0.05$). Therefore, we excluded the parameters of patient age, body weight and the use of co-administered CBZ, PB and PHT from the final model in order to increase the stability by reducing the degree of multicollinearity.

The final population PK-PD model for the probability of the γ-GT elevation was as follows:

Table 2. The median values of the PK parameter estimates of VPA in the final population PK models obtained using the NONMEM program and the bootstrap analysis.

Parameter	NONMEM	Bootstrap Evaluation	
	Final Estimates	Median	95% CIs
ALAG (h)	3.00 (Fixed)	–	–
Ka (h^{-1})	0.109	0.104	0.0317–0.748
Vd/F (L)	21.4	21.2	8.01–68.1
CL/F (L/h)	0.559	0.558	0.520–0.589
Dose on Vd/F (L)	1.52	1.46	0.457–3.74
Dose on CL/F (L/h)	0.596	0.592	0.525–0.652
Gender on CL/F (L/h)	0.917	0.915	0.847–0.998
CBZ on CL/F (L/h)	1.19	1.20	1.13–1.29
CLB on CL/F (L/h)	0.906	0.907	0.852–0.970
PB on CL/F (L/h)	1.12	1.12	1.03–1.24
PHT on CL/F (L/h)	1.43	1.43	1.31–1.56
ω^2 on ALAG	4.48×10^{-9}	6.69×10^{-5}	6.69×10^{-5}–6.69×10^{-5}
ω^2 on Ka	7.77×10^{-7}	8.82×10^{-4}	8.81×10^{-4}–8.82×10^{-4}
ω^2 on Vd/F	1.83×10^{-7}	4.28×10^{-4}	4.28×10^{-4}–4.28×10^{-4}
ω^2 on CL/F	0.0587	0.241	0.202–0.281
σ^2 (proportional error)	0.0617	0.247	0.224–0.268

VPA = valproic acid; PK = pharmacokinetic; NONMEM = nonlinear mixed-effect model; CIs = confidence intervals; ALAG = absorption lag time; Ka = absorption rate constant; Vd/F = volume of distribution; CL/F = apparent oral clearance; Dose = daily dose of VPA; CBZ = carbamazepine; CLB = clobazam; GBP = gabapentine; PB = phenobarbital; PHT = phenytoin; ω = coefficient of variation of inter-individual variability; σ = coefficient of variation of intra-individual variability; – = data not available.

$$Logit(\Pr) = Ln \frac{\Pr}{1-\Pr} = -6.63 + 3.62^{Intellectual}_{disability}$$
$$+ 1.96^{SOD2Val/Val}_{genotype} + Dose^{1.55} \times AUC + e^{\eta} \quad (9)$$

where AUC is the individual AUC value of VPA that was simulated based on the population PK analysis; intellectual disability = 1 if an intellectual disability was present, and was otherwise 0; SOD2 Val/Val genotype = 1, SOD2 Val/Ala or Ala/Ala genotype = 0; and η is the individual random effect.

Among 1,000 bootstrap runs, 997 runs exhibited successful minimization and were included in the bootstrap analysis. Table 3 shows the median parameter estimates obtained using the NONMEM program and the values with 95% CIs obtained using the bootstrap approach. The 95% CIs for all parameters obtained using the bootstrap approach was generally comparable to the estimates obtained using the NONMEM program (Table 3).

A visual predictive check regarding the proportion of γ-GT elevation using 1,000 datasets according to the SOD2 genotype and complication with intellectual disability is shown in Figure 1. In this study, we included patients 2 to 52 years of age among the original population in the PK-PD analysis (Table 1); however, 93.3% of the patients were 30 years of age or younger (see Figure S2). Therefore, for the visual predictive assessment, we selected patients 30 years of age or younger treated with 100 to 1,300 mg/day of VPA (the usual dose in Japan) in order to predict the data for our PK-PD model appropriately by reducing the variability among the patient ages in the simulated 1,000 datasets. The visual predictive check indicated that the final parameter estimates were reliable (Figure 1).

When 800 mg/day of VPA was administered to patients without any co-treatment, the predicted mean percentages of the subjects with γ-GT elevation were 9.4%, 20.2%, 31.6% and 52.6%, and the mean odds ratios (95% CIs) for the γ-GT elevation during VPA therapy were 1 [reference value], 2.44 (1.88–3.17), 4.47 (3.48–5.74) and 10.74 (8.30–13.75) in patients with the SOD2 Val/Ala or Ala/Ala genotype without intellectual disability, those with the SOD2 Val/Val genotype without intellectual disability, those with the SOD2 Val/Ala or Ala/Ala genotype and intellectual disability and those with the SOD2 Val/Val genotype and intellectual disability, respectively (Table 4). The predicted mean percentages of the subjects with γ-GT elevation were about 2- to 3-fold, 3- to 4-fold and 4- to 8-fold higher in the patients with the SOD2 Val/Val genotype without intellectual disability, those with the SOD2 Val/Ala or Ala/Ala genotype and intellectual disability and those with the SOD2 Val/Val genotype and intellectual disability, respectively, than in those with the SOD2 Val/Ala or Ala/Ala genotype without intellectual disability (Table 4).

Discussion

In this study, we developed an equation to describe the relationship between the serum VPA concentrations and the risk of γ-GT elevation by developing population PK and PK-PD models. During the model developments, we evaluated the associations of the VPA-induced γ-GT elevation with patient-specific covariates, including the SOD2, GSTM1 and GSTT1 genotypes, in Japanese patients with epilepsy (see Figure 2). A one-compartment model with exponential inter-individual variability of the PK parameters adequately described the data; while a logistic model was successfully applied to describe the VPA-

Table 3. The median values of the PD parameter estimates of VPA in the final population PK-PD models obtained using the NONMEM program and the bootstrap analysis.

Parameter	NONMEM	Bootstrap Evaluation	
	Final Estimates (RSE, %)	Median	95% CIs
Base	−6.63 (17.5)	−6.68	−11.6−−4.82
Dose on SLOPE	1.55 (19.4)	1.56	0.83−2.29
Intellectual disability on BASE	3.62 (28.4)	3.62	1.87−8.94
SOD2 genotype on BASE	1.96 (44.1)	2.02	0.33−4.42
ω^2 on logit (Pr)	12.3 (43.4)	3.48	2.29−10.7

VPA = valproic acid; PD = pharmacodynamic; PK = pharmacokinetic; NONMEM = nonlinear mixed-effect model; RES = relative standard error; CIs = confidence intervals; Dose = daily dose of VPA; BASE = intercept; SLOPE = slope relating the AUC of VPA; SOD2 = superoxide dismutase 2; ω = coefficient of variation of inter-individual variability; logit (Pr) = logit function of probability of having an elevated γ-GT level.

induced γ-GT elevation, in which the logit function of probability was a linear function of the VPA exposure (Tables 2 and 3). The results of our PK-PD model indicated that the risk of γ-GT elevation was significantly related to the VPA exposure.

γ-GT is an established liver function test parameter used to determine whether there has been alcohol-associated toxicity [1]. It has also been reported to be a strong independent biomarker for metabolic syndrome, cardiovascular diseases and metabolic diseases, as well as the all-cause mortality [2,7,8]. Recent studies suggested that the γ-GT level is a significant predictor of NAFLD [3,4]. Meanwhile, the potential metabolic abnormalities and hepatotoxicity of VPA are of major concern [9]. Long-term VPA therapy is associated with a high prevalence of NAFLD in adolescents (36.0%) [12] and adults (60.9%) [11] with epilepsy.

Since VPA is a fatty acid that can be metabolized through endogenous pathways in the mitochondria [24], mitochondrial dysfunction has been implicated in the pathogenesis of VPA-induced hepatotoxicity [9,13]. SOD2 represents the first line of cellular defense against mitochondrial reactive oxygen species [14]. In our previous case-control study, we found that the SOD2 Val16Ala polymorphism was associated with the risk of a mild increase in the γ-GT level in VPA-treated patients [16]. The findings of the present study demonstrated that the SOD2 Val/Val genotype could contribute to the relationship between VPA exposure and γ-GT elevation during long-term VPA therapy. Based on the results of this study, the dose adjustment of VPA should be performed to reduce the risk of γ-GT elevation, especially in patients with the SOD2 Val/Val genotype (Figure 1 and Table 4).

The GSTM1 null and GSTT1 null genotypes have been reported to be associated with the risk of cardiovascular or metabolic diseases, including NAFLD, in the general population [18,19]. A previous case-control study reported that the GSTM1 null and GSTT1 null genotypes were associated with elevation of the γ-GT level in VPA-treated patients [21]. However, we did not identify these polymorphisms as statistically significant covariates in our PK-PD model (Table S2). The findings of this study may therefore indicate that the GSTM1 null or GSTT1 null genotype does not play a major independent role in the VPA-induced γ-GT elevation.

The association between epilepsy and intellectual disability has been well described in the literature [23]. A population-based retrospective cohort study showed that the risk of developing intellectual disability was high in patients with epilepsy (hazard ratio: 31.5, 95% CIs: 18.9 to 52.4) [23]. In this study, intellectual disability was also identified as a statistically significant covariate

for γ-GT elevation in the VPA-treated patients (Figure 2 and equation 9). In our study subjects, the complication with intellectual disability was associated with the increased numbers of co-administered CBZ, PB and PHT ($P<0.0001$). These enzyme-inducing antiepileptic drugs are known to increase the γ-GT levels [9,32]. A previous study indicated that VPA-induced γ-GT elevation was found in patients with polytherapy, but not in those with monotherapy [29]. Meanwhile, individuals with intellectual disabilities have also been reported to have higher levels of overweight and obesity than those without [33]. Therefore, we speculated that the patients with intellectual disability may be more likely to be co-administered with enzyme-inducing antiepileptic drugs and/or to have a weight gain, thus resulting in the γ-GT elevation, although the underlying mechanism remains unknown. Nevertheless, the findings of this study may suggest that patients with intellectual disability should be carefully monitored for VPA-induced γ-GT elevation (Figure 1 and Table 4).

VPA is highly protein bound (87–95%), thus resulting in low clearance [24]. There are at least three routes of VPA metabolism in humans: glucuronidation and β-oxidation in the mitochondria (both considered to be major routes accounting for 50% and 40% of the dose, respectively), and CYP-, such as CYP2C9 and CYP2C19, mediated-oxidation in the liver (considered to be a minor route, accounting for ~10% of the dose) [24]. Similar to previous published population PK models for VPA [34–36], in the present study, a one-compartment model adequately described the VPA concentrations (Figure S1).

In this study, we could not find any influence of the CYP2C9 and CYP2C19 polymorphisms on the PK parameters of VPA. These results are in line with a recent Iranian study, showing that no association was observed between the CYP2C9*3 genotype and plasma VPA concentrations [37]. However, two other studies demonstrated an association between the CYP2C9 or CYP2C19 genotype and the PK parameters of VPA. Jiang et al. reported that the CYP2C9 and CYP2C19 genotypes significantly influenced the population PK parameters of VPA in Chinese patients with epilepsy [34]. Tan et al. indicated that subjects who were CYP2C9*3 allele carriers had higher mean plasma VPA concentrations than the non-carriers [38]. The discrepancy between the findings may be attributed to the sample sizes, ages, co-administered antiepileptic drug(s) or races evaluated in the studies. On the other hand, female gender, CBZ, PB, PHT and CLB were identified as statistically significant PK covariates in this study. There is evidence for females having lower UDP-glucuronosyltransferases (UGTs) activity [39]. CBZ, PB and

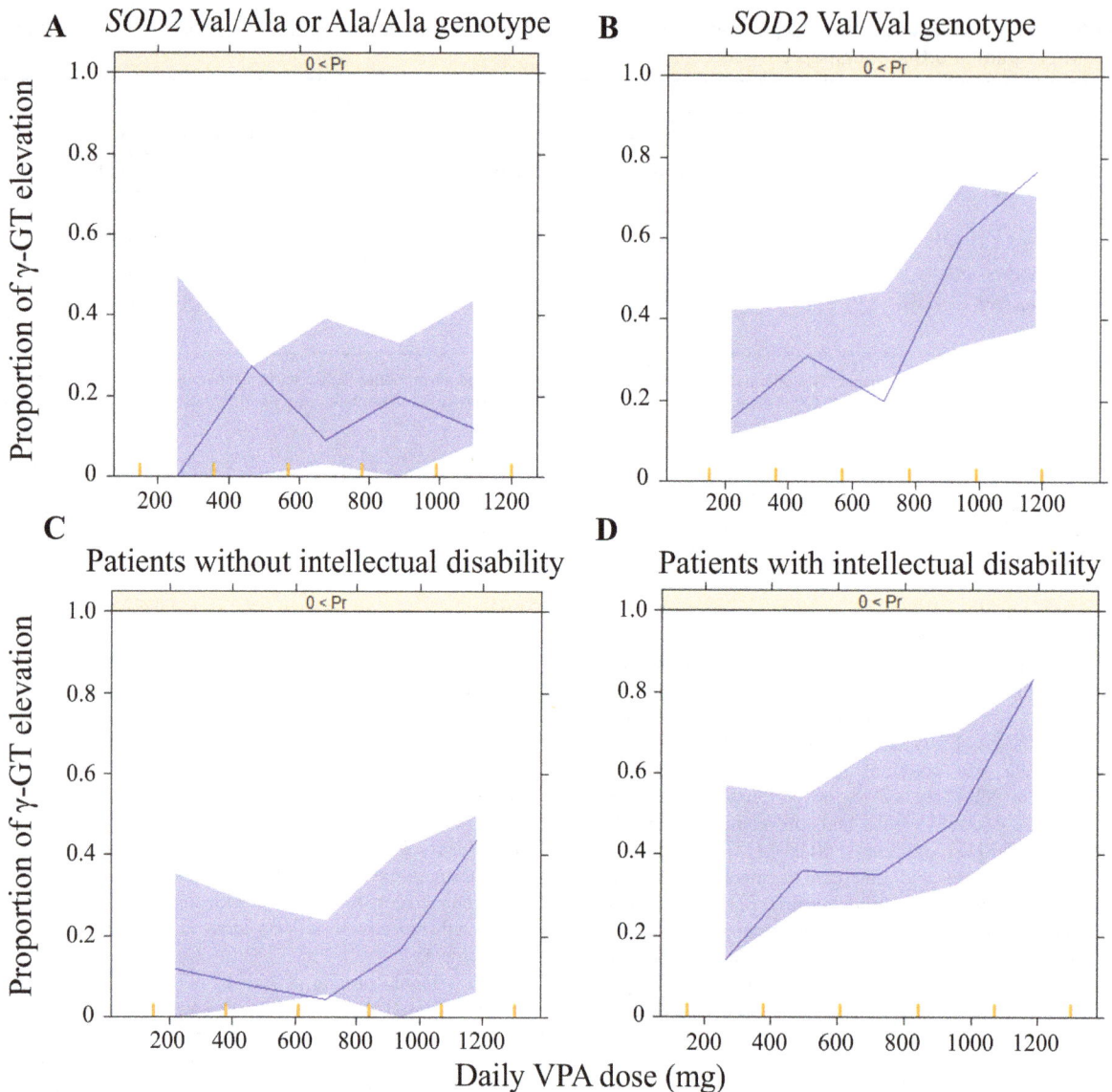

Figure 1. The visual predictive check of the PK-PD model in patients with the *SOD2* Ala/Ala or Val/Ala genotype (A), those with *SOD2* Val/Val genotype (B), those without intellectual disability (C) and those with intellectual disability (D), using the dataset of the study patients aged 30 years old or younger who were treated with 100 to 1,300 mg/day of VPA. The solid line represents the observed proportion of γ-GT elevation and the solid area represents the 90% prediction interval. PK = pharmacokinetic; PD = pharmacodynamics; SOD2 = superoxide dismutase 2; VPA = valproic acid γ-GT: γ-glutamyltransferase.

PHT are all inducers of CYP2C9, CYP2C19 and UGTs [40]. Several population PK studies indicated that female gender decreases the clearance of VPA, whereas co-treatments with enzyme-inducing antiepileptic drugs increase it [35,36]. Additionally, one previous study of pediatric patients reported that CLB reduced the apparent clearance of VPA [41], although the underlying mechanism remains unknown. Therefore, our PK parameter estimates of VPA might support these previous findings.

A major limitation of this study was the retrospective study design that investigated a small number of patients, which may have resulted in a lack of power. First, in this study, we could not determine the standard errors of the PK parameters in the final PK model developed (Table 2). This finding may be due to the complexity of our PK models incorporating many covariates (i.e. age, body weight, genotypes and co-administered drugs) using a

limited number of samples per individual and the routine therapeutic drug monitoring data (i.e. sparse sampling). Second, we could not include the influence of several statistically significant covariates, such as enzyme-inducing antiepileptic drugs (Table S2), on the risk of γ-GT elevation in our final PK-PD model in order to increase the model stability. Third, since we included patients 2 to 52 years of age (Table 1 and Figure S2), further studies with larger numbers of patients are needed to verify the influence of the patient age on the findings of the present study. Fourth, possible effects of other polymorphisms in the genes involved in the disposition of VPA, such as *UGTs* [24] and those involved in the VPA-induced liver dysfunction, such as *PLOG* [9,24], also cannot be ruled out. Lastly, we included only Japanese subjects; therefore, it is unclear whether our results can be generalized to other populations, such as white or black populations. The current

Table 4. The predicted mean percentages of the subjects with γ-GT elevation and the mean odds ratios (95% CIs) for γ-GT elevation during VPA therapy according to the *SOD2* Val16Ala genotype and complication with intellectual disability when different daily doses of VPA were administered to patients without any co-treatment.

Dose (mg)	Intellectual disability	*SOD2* genotype	γ-GT elevation (%)	Odds ratio (95% CIs)
400	–	Val/Ala or Ala/Ala	5.8	1
	–	Val/Val	13.0	2.42 (1.75–3.34)
	+	Val/Ala or Ala/Ala	24.9	5.38 (3.98–7.27)
	+	Val/Val	42.4	11.91 (8.89–15.98)
500	–	Val/Ala or Ala/Ala	6.0	1
	–	Val/Val	14.1	2.56 (1.87–3.51)
	+	Val/Ala or Ala/Ala	25.5	5.32 (3.95–7.16)
	+	Val/Val	43.8	12.12 (9.08–16.17)
600	–	Val/Ala or Ala/Ala	5.2	1
	–	Val/Val	16.9	3.67 (2.66–5.07)
	+	Val/Ala or Ala/Ala	27.8	6.96 (5.10–9.49)
	+	Val/Val	44.8	14.68 (10.82–19.91)
700	–	Val/Ala or Ala/Ala	7.7	1
	–	Val/Val	17.2	2.50 (1.88–3.32)
	+	Val/Ala or Ala/Ala	30.6	5.30 (4.05–6.94)
	+	Val/Val	48.1	11.17 (8.58–14.54)
800	–	Val/Ala or Ala/Ala	9.4	1
	–	Val/Val	20.2	2.44 (1.88–3.17)
	+	Val/Ala or Ala/Ala	31.6	4.47 (3.48–5.74)
	+	Val/Val	52.6	10.74 (8.30–13.75)
900	–	Val/Ala or Ala/Ala	9.6	1
	–	Val/Val	21.1	2.52 (1.94–3.27)
	+	Val/Ala or Ala/Ala	34.9	5.04 (3.94–6.46)
	+	Val/Val	55.6	11.77 (9.22–15.03)
1000	–	Val/Ala or Ala/Ala	10.8	1
	–	Val/Val	24.2	2.65 (2.07–3.39)
	+	Val/Ala or Ala/Ala	35.6	4.57 (3.60–5.80)
	+	Val/Val	56.2	10.63 (8.40–13.46)
1100	–	Val/Ala or Ala/Ala	13.1	1
	–	Val/Val	27.8	2.55 (2.02–3.20)
	+	Val/Ala or Ala/Ala	42.6	4.90 (3.93–6.13)
	+	Val/Val	57.8	9.05 (7.24–11.30)
1200	–	Val/Ala or Ala/Ala	14.8	1
	–	Val/Val	28.1	2.25 (1.80–2.81)
	+	Val/Ala or Ala/Ala	46.6	5.01 (4.04–6.20)
	+	Val/Val	65.3	10.83 (8.71–13.46)

γ-GT: γ-glutamyltransferase; VPA = valproic acid; Dose = daily dose of VPA; SOD2 = superoxide dismutase 2; CIs = confidence intervals; − = absent; + = present.

findings are thus needed to be verified with a larger number of patients, including those from other ethnic groups. Nevertheless, our population PK results of the bootstrap analysis showed that the median parameter estimates obtained from 965 bootstrap data sets were generally comparable with the estimates obtained using the NONMEM program (Table 2), whereas the goodness of fit suggests that our PK model adequately described the original data (Figure S1). Furthermore, the PK-PD results of the bootstrap analysis also showed that the median parameter estimates obtained from 997 bootstrap data sets were generally comparable with the

estimates obtained using the NONMEM program (Table 3), and the visual predictive check among 1,000 datasets indicated that the final parameter estimates were reliable (Figure 1).

In conclusion, this study demonstrated that the *SOD2* Val16Ala polymorphism has an impact on the relationship between VPA exposure and γ-GT elevation in patients with epilepsy, as determined using a population PK-PD modeling approach. Since patients with epilepsy usually receive long-term VPA from childhood, our results suggest that VPA-treated patients should be carefully monitored for γ-GT elevation, especially those with

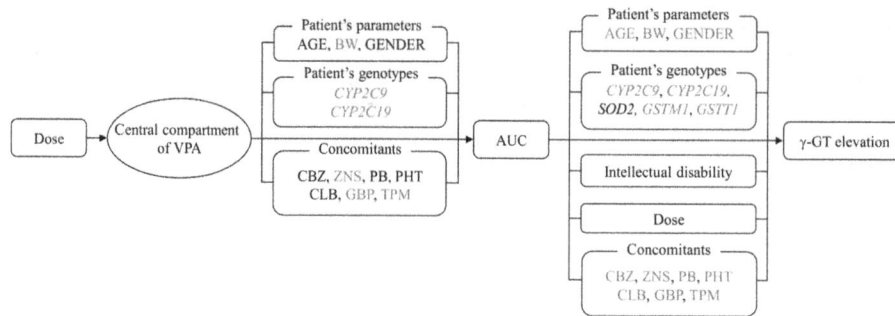

Figure 2. The relationships evaluated in the framework for the γ-GT elevation during VPA therapy. The solid lines indicate the relationships included in the final population PK and PK-PD models. Black letters indicate relationships included in the final models, and grey letters indicate relationships investigated, but not included, in the final models. PK = pharmacokinetic; PD = pharmacodynamics; VPA = valproic acid γ-GT: γ-glutamyltransferase.

the *SOD2* Val/Val genotype. Furthermore, the findings of this study indicate that determining the *SOD2* genotype may be helpful for preventing the VPA-induced γ-GT elevation.

Supporting Information

Figure S1 The goodness of fit of the final population PK model. The population-predicted (A) and individually-predicted (B) versus observed VPA concentrations in Japanese patients with epilepsy. The conditional weighted residuals versus population-predicted VPA concentrations in patients with epilepsy (C).

Table S1 The effects of the tested covariates on the objective function of the PK parameters of VPA.

Table S2 The effects of the tested covariates on the objective function of the PK-PD parameters regarding the probability of a VPA-induced γ-GT elevation.

Acknowledgments

The authors would like to thank all of our co-workers for their skilful contributions to the data collection and management.

Author Contributions

Conceived and designed the experiments: NO JS HN M. Noai M. Nishimura MD SK KO NYF TI KN. Performed the experiments: NO JS HN M. Noai M. Nishimura MD SK KO NYF TI KN. Analyzed the data: NO HN M. Nishimura. Contributed reagents/materials/analysis tools: NO JS HN M. Noai M. Nishimura MD SK KO NYF TI. Contributed to the writing of the manuscript: NO JS HN M. Noai M. Nishimura MD KO NYF TI KN. NO JS HN.

References

1. Whitfield JB (2001) Gamma glutamyl transferase. Crit Rev Clin Lab Sci 38: 263–355.
2. Castellano I, Merlino A (2012) gamma-Glutamyltranspeptidases: sequence, structure, biochemical properties, and biotechnological applications. Cell Mol Life Sci 69: 3381–3394.
3. Verrijken A, Francque S, Mertens I, Talloen M, Peiffer F, et al. (2010) Visceral adipose tissue and inflammation correlate with elevated liver tests in a cohort of overweight and obese patients. Int J Obes (Lond) 34: 899–907.
4. Petta S, Macaluso FS, Barcellona MR, Camma C, Cabibi D, et al. (2012) Serum gamma-glutamyl transferase levels, insulin resistance and liver fibrosis in patients with chronic liver diseases. PLoS One 7: e51165.
5. Lioudaki E, Ganotakis ES, Mikhailidis DP (2011) Liver enzymes: potential cardiovascular risk markers? Curr Pharm Des 17: 3632–3643.
6. Irie M, Sohda T, Iwata K, Kunimoto H, Fukunaga A, et al. (2012) Levels of the oxidative stress marker gamma-glutamyltranspeptidase at different stages of nonalcoholic fatty liver disease. J Int Med Res 40: 924–933.
7. Targher G (2010) Elevated serum gamma-glutamyltransferase activity is associated with increased risk of mortality, incident type 2 diabetes, cardiovascular events, chronic kidney disease and cancer - a narrative review. Clin Chem Lab Med 48: 147–157.
8. Jiang S, Jiang D, Tao Y (2013) Role of gamma-glutamyltransferase in cardiovascular diseases. Exp Clin Cardiol 18: 53–56.
9. Nanau RM, Neuman MG (2013) Adverse drug reactions induced by valproic acid. Clin Biochem 46: 1323–1338.
10. Patsalos PN, Berry DJ, Bourgeois BF, Cloyd JC, Glauser TA, et al. (2008) Antiepileptic drugs–best practice guidelines for therapeutic drug monitoring: a position paper by the subcommission on therapeutic drug monitoring, ILAE Commission on Therapeutic Strategies. Epilepsia 49: 1239–1276.
11. Luef G, Rauchenzauner M, Waldmann M, Sturm W, Sandhofer A, et al. (2009) Non-alcoholic fatty liver disease (NAFLD), insulin resistance and lipid profile in antiepileptic drug treatment. Epilepsy Res 86: 42–47.
12. Verrotti A, Agostinelli S, Parisi P, Chiarelli F, Coppola G (2011) Nonalcoholic fatty liver disease in adolescents receiving valproic acid. Epilepsy Behav 20: 382–385.
13. Begriche K, Massart J, Robin MA, Borgne-Sanchez A, Fromenty B (2011) Drug-induced toxicity on mitochondria and lipid metabolism: Mechanistic diversity and deleterious consequences for the liver. J Hepatol 54: 773–794.
14. Fukai T, Ushio-Fukai M (2011) Superoxide dismutases: role in redox signaling, vascular function, and diseases. Antioxid Redox Signal 15: 1583–1606.
15. Sutton A, Khoury H, Prip-Buus C, Cepanec C, Pessayre D, et al. (2003) The Ala16Val genetic dimorphism modulates the import of human manganese superoxide dismutase into rat liver mitochondria. Pharmacogenetics 13: 145–157.
16. Saruwatari J, Deguchi M, Yoshimori Y, Noai M, Yoshida S, et al. (2012) Superoxide dismutase 2 Val16Ala polymorphism is a risk factor for the valproic acid-related elevation of serum aminotransferases. Epilepsy Res 99: 183–186.
17. Hayes JD, Flanagan JU, Jowsey IR (2005) Glutathione transferases. Annu Rev Pharmacol Toxicol 45: 51–88.
18. Kariz S, Nikolajevic Starcevic J, Petrovic D (2012) Association of manganese superoxide dismutase and glutathione S-transferases genotypes with myocardial infarction in patients with type 2 diabetes mellitus. Diabetes Res Clin Pract 98: 144–150.
19. Oniki K, Hori M, Saruwatari J, Morita K, Kajiwara A, et al. (2013) Interactive effects of smoking and glutathione S-transferase polymorphisms on the development of non-alcoholic fatty liver disease. Toxicol Lett 220: 143–149.
20. Saruwatari J, Yasui-Furukori N, Kamihashi R, Yoshimori Y, Oniki K, et al. (2013) Possible associations between antioxidant enzyme polymorphisms and metabolic abnormalities in patients with schizophrenia. Neuropsychiatr Dis Treat 9: 1683–1698.
21. Fukushima Y, Seo T, Hashimoto N, Higa Y, Ishitsu T, et al. (2008) Glutathione-S-transferase (GST) M1 null genotype and combined GSTM1 and GSTT1 null genotypes are risk factors for increased serum gamma-glutamyltransferase in valproic acid-treated patients. Clin Chim Acta 389: 98–102.

22. Berg AT, Berkovic SF, Brodie MJ, Buchhalter J, Cross JH, et al. (2010) Revised terminology and concepts for organization of seizures and epilepsies: report of the ILAE Commission on Classification and Terminology, 2005–2009. Epilepsia 51: 676–685.

23. Chang HJ, Liao CC, Hu CJ, Shen WW, Chen TL (2013) Psychiatric disorders after epilepsy diagnosis: a population-based retrospective cohort study. PLoS One 8: e59999.

24. Ghodke-Puranik Y, Thorn CF, Lamba JK, Leeder JS, Song W, et al. (2013) Valproic acid pathway: pharmacokinetics and pharmacodynamics. Pharmacogenet Genomics 23: 236–241.

25. Cronin-Fenton DP, Christensen M, Lash TL, Ahern TP, Pedersen L, et al. (2014) Manganese superoxide dismutase and breast cancer recurrence: a Danish clinical registry-based case-control study, and a meta-analysis. PLoS One 9: e87450.

26. Suarez-Kurtz G, Genro JP, de Moraes MO, Ojopi EB, Pena SD, et al. (2012) Global pharmacogenomics: Impact of population diversity on the distribution of polymorphisms in the CYP2C cluster among Brazilians. Pharmacogenomics J 12: 267–276.

27. Jagarinec N, Flegar-Mestric Z, Surina B, Vrhovski-Hebrang D, Preden-Kerekovic V (1998) Pediatric reference intervals for 34 biochemical analytes in urban school children and adolescents. Clin Chem Lab Med 36: 327–337.

28. Wallach J (1996) Interpretation of diagnostic tests. New York: Little, Brown and Company. 1093 p.

29. Jimenez-Rodriguezvila M, Caro-Paton A, Conde M, Duenas-Laita A, Martin-Lorente JL, et al. (1986) Side-effects of sodium valproate, mainly related to its hepatic and pancreatic toxicity. Int J Clin Pharmacol Res 6: 217–224.

30. Saruwatari J, Ogusu N, Shimomasuda M, Nakashima H, Seo T, et al. (2014) Effects of CYP2C19 and P450 Oxidoreductase Polymorphisms on the Population Pharmacokinetics of Clobazam and N-Desmethylclobazam in Japanese Patients With Epilepsy. Ther Drug Monit 36: 302–309.

31. Keizer RJ, Karlsson MO, Hooker A (2013) Modeling and Simulation Workbench for NONMEM: Tutorial on Pirana, PsN, and Xpose. CPT Pharmacometrics Syst Pharmacol 2: e50.

32. Braide SA, Davies TJ (1987) Factors that affect the induction of gamma glutamyltransferase in epileptic patients receiving anti-convulsant drugs. Ann Clin Biochem 24: 391–399.

33. Maiano C (2011) Prevalence and risk factors of overweight and obesity among children and adolescents with intellectual disabilities. Obes Rev 12: 189–197.

34. Jiang D, Bai X, Zhang Q, Lu W, Wang Y, et al. (2009) Effects of CYP2C19 and CYP2C9 genotypes on pharmacokinetic variability of valproic acid in Chinese epileptic patients: nonlinear mixed-effect modeling. Eur J Clin Pharmacol 65: 1187–1193.

35. Birnbaum AK, Ahn JE, Brundage RC, Hardie NA, Conway JM, et al. (2007) Population pharmacokinetics of valproic acid concentrations in elderly nursing home residents. Ther Drug Monit 29: 571–575.

36. Jankovic SM, Milovanovic JR, Jankovic S (2010) Factors influencing valproate pharmacokinetics in children and adults. Int J Clin Pharmacol Ther 48: 767–775.

37. Amini-Shirazi N, Ghahremani MH, Ahmadkhaniha R, Mandegary A, Dadgar A, et al. (2010) Influence of CYP2C9 polymorphism on metabolism of valproate and its hepatotoxin metabolite in Iranian patients. Toxicol Mech Methods 20: 452–457.

38. Tan L, Yu JT, Sun YP, Ou JR, Song JH, et al. (2010) The influence of cytochrome oxidase CYP2A6, CYP2B6, and CYP2C9 polymorphisms on the plasma concentrations of valproic acid in epileptic patients. Clin Neurol Neurosurg 112: 320–323.

39. Franconi F, Brunelleschi S, Steardo L, Cuomo V (2007) Gender differences in drug responses. Pharmacol Res 55: 81–95.

40. Perucca E (2006) Clinically relevant drug interactions with antiepileptic drugs. Br J Clin Pharmacol 61: 246–255.

41. Theis JG, Koren G, Daneman R, Sherwin AL, Menzano E, et al. (1997) Interactions of clobazam with conventional antiepileptics in children. J Child Neurol 12: 208–213.

13

Long Term Effectiveness on Prescribing of Two Multifaceted Educational Interventions: Results of Two Large Scale Randomized Cluster Trials

Nicola Magrini[1]*, Giulio Formoso[1], Oreste Capelli[2], Emilio Maestri[1], Francesco Nonino[1], Barbara Paltrinieri[1], Cinzia Del Giovane[3], Claudio Voci[1], Lucia Magnano[1], Lisa Daya[2], Anna Maria Marata[1], on behalf of the INDRA-NET study group[¶]

1 Drug Evaluation Area, Emilia-Romagna Regional Agency for Health and Social Care, Bologna, Italy, 2 Local Health Authority, Modena, Italy, 3 Department of Clinical and Diagnostic Medicine and Public Health, University of Modena and Reggio Emilia, Modena, Italy

Abstract

Introduction: Information on benefits and risks of drugs is a key element affecting doctors' prescribing decisions. Outreach visits promoting independent information have proved moderately effective in changing prescribing behaviours.

Objectives: Testing the short and long-term effectiveness on general practitioners' prescribing of small groups meetings led by pharmacists.

Methods: Two cluster open randomised controlled trials (RCTs) were carried out in a large scale NHS setting. Ad hoc prepared evidence based material were used considering a therapeutic area approach - TEA, with information materials on osteoporosis or prostatic hyperplasia - and a single drug oriented approach - SIDRO, with information materials on me-too drugs of 2 different classes: barnidipine or prulifloxacin. In each study, all 115 Primary Care Groups in a Northern Italy area (2.2 million inhabitants, 1737 general practitioners) were randomised to educational small groups meetings, in which available evidence was provided together with drug utilization data and clinical scenarios. Main outcomes were changes in the six-months prescription of targeted drugs. Longer term results (24 and 48 months) were also evaluated.

Results: In the TEA trial, one of the four primary outcomes showed a reduction (prescription of alfuzosin compared to tamsulosin and terazosin in benign prostatic hyperplasia: prescribing ratio −8.5%, p = 0.03). Another primary outcome (prescription of risedronate) showed a reduction at 24 and 48 months (−7.6%, p = 0.02; and −9,8%, p = 0.03), but not at six months (−5.1%, p = 0.36). In the SIDRO trial both primary outcomes showed a statistically significant reduction (prescription of barnidipine −9.8%, p = 0.02; prescription of prulifloxacin −11.1%, p = 0.04), which persisted or increased over time.

Interpretation: These two cluster RCTs showed the large scale feasibility of a complex educational program in a NHS setting, and its potentially relevant long-term impact on prescribing habits, in particular when focusing on a single drug. National Health systems should invest in independent drug information programs.

Trial Registration: Controlled-Trials.com ISRCTN05866587

Editor: Barbara Mintzes, University of British Columbia, Canada

Funding: Funding was provided by Agenzia Italiana del Farmaco, 2005 NHS fund for independent research on drugs. The funder had no role in study design, data collection and analysis, decision to publish, or preparation of the manuscript.

Competing Interests: The authors have read the journal's policy and have the following conflicts: Since 2001, the Authors have been involved in the implementation of a pharmacist outreach visit programs in a few Health Districts of Emilia-Romagna, receiving organizational support and NHS funding from the corresponding Local Health Authorities.

* Email: nmagrini@regione.emilia-romagna.it

¶ Membership of the INDRA-NET study group is provided in the Acknowledgments

Introduction

Information on benefits and risks of drug treatments is an important element affecting doctors' prescribing decisions though other factors such as clinical experience and therapeutic traditions, opinion leaders and local context influence, and also information coming from drug industry, play a role. Drug companies invest large sums in informing doctors through a wide range of activities: [1] promotion through drug representatives, sponsored events and symposia, and selective presentation of research findings,[2–5] which seem useful to the purpose of increasing sales, as companies spend on average a quarter of their revenues on marketing activities, almost twice as much as what they invest on research and development.[6–7].

As an international independent expert in drug policy expressed a few years ago *"a major challenge that remains is to reduce the imbalance between promotional and research expenditure, perhaps moving progressively towards a system in which health systems themselves provide the bulk of new drug information rather than indirectly funding, as they presently do, an army of company salesmen"*. [8] Access to the best available information (critically appraised, made easy and brought into small groups) is an important step towards a more balanced view of the actual benefits and risks of drugs allowing a more realistic estimation of the magnitude of the clinically relevant outcomes. Educational outreach visits have been proposed since 1983 as an effective method to promote change in prescribing practices, [9] using either one-to-one meetings with prescribers [10] or group meetings. [11] These methods have been subsequently implemented in various countries, [12] either to provide information from research papers and systematic reviews, free of recommendations, or to favour the use of clinical practice guidelines. Though information is mostly presented in relative terms (RR, OR, HR) there is an increasing tendency of the evidence-based movement towards favouring a presentation of trials results using actual benefits and absolute differences, possibly taking patients baseline risk into account.[13–14] The GRADE approach represents a good example in this regard. [15].

Available evidence on the effectiveness of outreach visits shows variable results, indicating modest to moderate effects (with relatively short-term assessments at 6–12 months), mostly assessing the implementation of clinical practice guidelines. [16–17] There is paucity of evidence formally evaluating the feasibility on a large scale basis of implementing independent information programs, and their long-term prescribing impact – up to several years. Moreover, although specific methods to put these principles into practice have been well conceptualized since about thirty years ago, [10] they have been often applied to academic detailing settings or to single-doctor meetings.

We applied these general principles and methods to a NHS drug information program consisting of twice-a-year small group sessions led by a pharmacist, established in several provinces of the Emilia-Romagna region since 2001. We avoided clinical practice guidelines as supporting material to drive behaviour-change since they were frequently perceived as cost-containment tools. [18].

Two pragmatic cluster randomised trials designed within the same protocol were designed and funded within a public research program.[19–20] Specific aims were to evaluate, in the short and long term, whether an intervention carried out in a natural' NHS setting, consisting of small group meetings of all general practitioners (the clusters), using clear and appealing educational materials, may change doctors' prescribing behaviour. The two trials tested two different approaches: either relatively articulated and rich materials targeting a whole therapeutic area, or more focused materials targeting a newly approved single drug with rapidly increasing prescribing patterns.

Methods

Two consecutive cluster trials, stemming from the same study protocol, were carried out in spring 2007 and autumn-winter 2007–08, respectively, in five Provinces of the Emilia Romagna region (Bologna, Forlì, Modena, Parma and Reggio Emilia, totalling about 2,200,000 inhabitants) involving all practising NHS General Practitioners. [21].

It was initially planned to have also the participation of 40 primary care groups from another region in Northern Italy, Friuli Venezia Giulia (about 400 GPs corresponding to an assisted population of about 440,000 inhabitants), but no agreement was reached between the Regional Health Authority and general practitioners' organisations. For similar reasons, a parallel trial which had been planned in Sardinia was not implemented; such trial aimed to evaluate the effectiveness of different information formats delivered to single general practitioners and discussed by a pharmacist.

In order to evaluate and quantify the impact of such a program, we designed these randomised trials according to the following features:

- improving access to evidence-based clinically relevant information in a NHS setting using available resources;
- helping to assess the relevance and the limits of the available evidence, highlighting the role of systematic reviews and pitfalls due to publication bias, and also critically appraising the most relevant single studies;
- presenting benefit and risks clearly and effectively, [14] to provide better insight on their impact on clinical practice compared to market-driven interpretations from the drug industry; [22]
- integrating information from published studies with assessments from drug regulatory agencies [23] and other relevant contextual information;
- keeping in mind all the organisational factors and settings of what works in changing doctors' behaviour: audit and feedback using prescribing data; [24] strengthening the role of pharmacists as facilitators; [16] favouring active learning in small groups. [12]

We identified doctors' knowledge and attitudes as the main determinants of their prescription; therefore, we used the available resources to address these determinants through a dedicated information program. Specifically, the main principle embraced for our information campaign was the motto "doctor, we give you all the information, you decide".

Primary Care Groups (PCGs) are associations of about 10–15 general practitioners (GPs) constituted to improve the continuity and local provision of primary health care: PCGs were the unit of randomisation in the two cluster trials. All PCGs of the five provinces were asked to participate in two rounds of small group interactive information meetings (one in spring and one in autumn 2007). Within each round of visits, PCGs were randomised in two groups: those receiving information about a topic (A) and those receiving information about a different topic (B), unrelated to (A) (Fig. 1). Groups were compared using for each topic a set of specific prescribing outcomes: group receiving A compared to group "not receiving A" (actually receiving B) and vice versa, so two sets of comparisons were performed in each trial. Each group also received the presentation and discussion of 2 clinical scenarios for each topic and prescribing data concerning the group prescription vs the average prescription in the Local Health Authority (LHA). Feedback on individual prescriptions was avoided to favour a group evaluation rather than flattening the discussion on "who has prescribed what".

The two RCTs had the following distinctive features:

- the 1st RCT (ThErapeutic Area approach or TEA trial), randomised the PCGs in two groups receiving an educational session on a therapeutic topic (treatment of benign prostatic hyperplasia (BPH) or drugs used in the treatment of osteoporosis) using a fairly long information package of 12

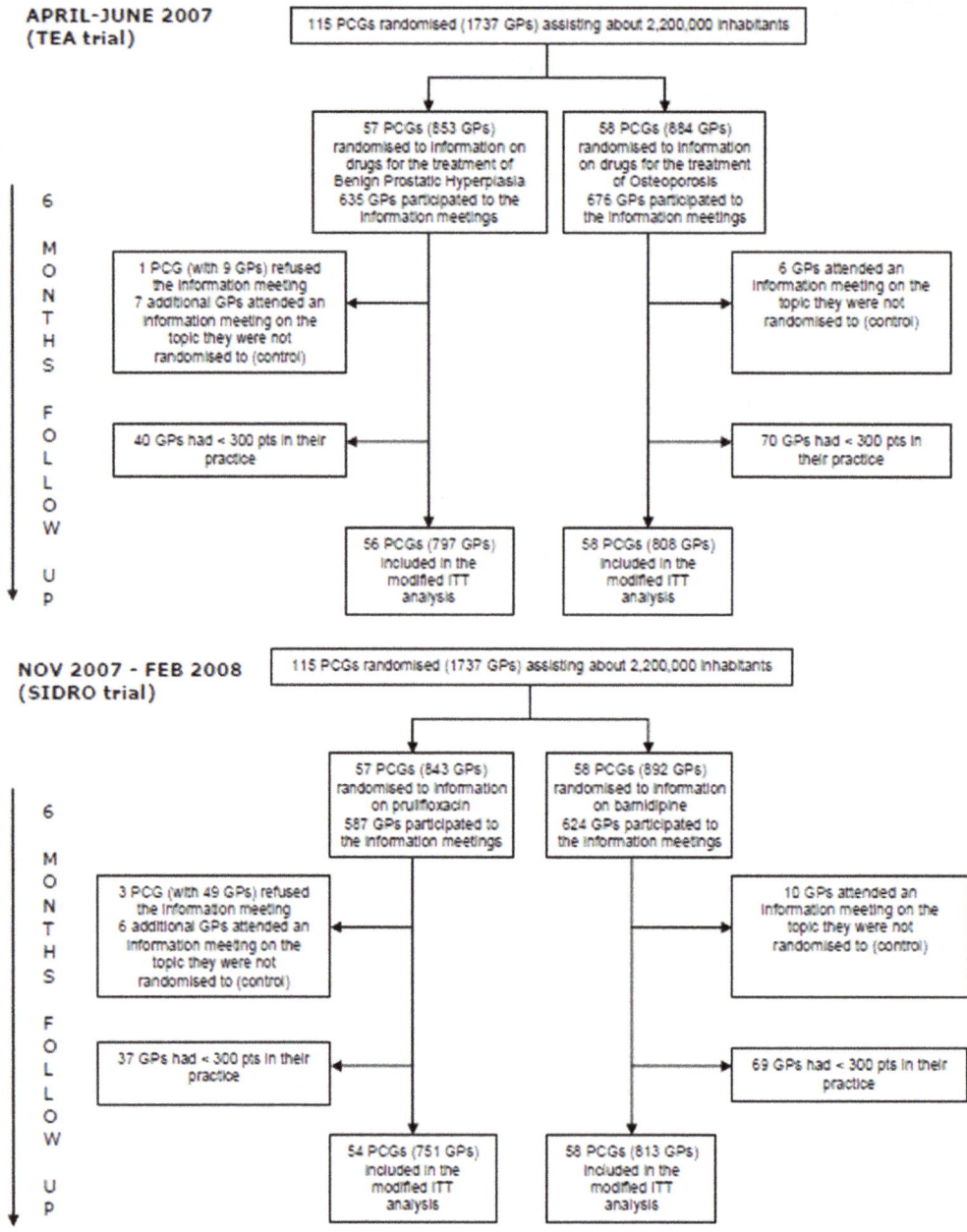

Figure 1. Flow-charts of the two cluster RCTs.

Table 1. The main components of the multifaceted educational intervention.

SETTING	bi-annual small group meetings (each lasting 3–4 hours) with a Primary Care Group (PCG)
TOOLS	ad hoc prepared information packages (pharmacists/referent GPs receive one three-day/half a day courses on the contents of that material); presentation and discussion of real life clinical scenarios; prescribing reports for each PCG comparing with local averages
METHODS	educational outreach visits (small group meetings); audit & feedback; problem-based learning: "we present to you the available evidence and some context, you decide"
ACTORS	a pharmacist acts as facilitator, presenting the evidence-based information packages and commenting on drug utilization data of PCG; a general practitioner acts as referent peer presenting real life clinical scenarios to be discussed in the light of available evidence

Table 2. TEA trial: GPs' mean baseline prescription (in the 3 months preceding the outreach visit) of drugs considered in the primary outcomes, expressed as DDD per 1000 patients.

Drugs considered	Group 1: information on drugs for the treatment of benign prostatic hyperplasia	Group 2: information on drugs for the treatment of osteoporosis
finasteride	5.35	5.46
dutasteride	4.09	4.30
alfuzosin	9.98	9.66
terazosin	4.64	4.73
tamsulosin	11.05	11.11
alendronate	7.35	7.29
risedronate	3.01	2.98

pages on benefits and risks of drugs, highlighting lack of superiority data of newer vs older (originator) drugs, availability of different drug classes and of generic drugs;

• the 2nd RCT (SIngle DRug Oriented – SIDRO trial, meaning cider in Italian), compared the same two groups of PCG, in a meeting occurring 3–4 months later, using more focused information material (4 pages information package) on a single

Table 3. TEA trial: differences in DDD per 1000 patients of prescribed drugs (intervention vs control: 1605 included GPs).

	Absolute mean prescription during follow-up in the 'intervention group' (DDD per 1000 assisted population/day)	Absolute difference at follow-up vs control group (change from baseline expressed as DDD per 1000 assisted population/day)	Relative % variation vs control: m-ITT (95% CI)
Primary outcomes (arm 1: BPH)			
finasteride+dutasteride	6.61	0.24	3.6% (−2.9 to 10.2%)
alfuzosin vs tamsulosin +terazosin †	0.71 (ratio)	−0.06	−8.5% (−16.9 to −0.7%)
Secondary outcomes (arm 1: BPH)			
finasteride	3.60	0.05	1.4% (−6.5 to 9.5%)
dutasteride	3.00	0.18	5.8% (−2.6 to 14.3%)
alfuzosin	6.82	−0.11	−1.7% (−8.9 to 5.6%)
tamsulosin	7.92	0.28	3.7% (−3.1 to 10.4%)
terazosin	3.21	0.17	5.4% (−4.1 to 14.6%)
Primary outcomes (arm 2: osteoporosis)			
alendronate	4.99	<0.01	0.1% (−7.3 to 7.5%)
risedronate	2.03	−0.11	−5.1% (−15.3 to 5.6%)
Secondary outcomes (arm 2: osteoporosis)			
ibandronate	0.48	−0.11	−19.6% (−33.9 to −5.4%)
alendronate vs risedronate + ibandronate §	2.89 (ratio)	0.27	10.4% (−3.5 to 24.6%)
strontium ranelate	0.59	0.03	4.8% (−12.9 to 21.0%)
raloxifene	0.13	<0.01	0.4% (−26.9 to 27.5%)
calcium	1.83	−0.11	−5.4% (−15.6 to 5.4%)
vitamin D	1.72	−0.06	−3.5% (−12.4 to 5.3%)

†56 physicians who had not prescribed tamsulosin or terazosin could not be included in the calculation since this is a ratio.
§300 physicians who had not prescribed risedronate or ibandronate could not be included in the calculation since this is a ratio.

"me too" drug recently approved and with rapidly increasing prescriptions: a calcium antagonist (barnidipine) or a fluoroquinolone (prulifloxacin) were the drugs chosen.

In fact these two RCTs offer two different models of approaching doctors' education: the first approach is disease oriented and closer to thematic courses, requires two ad-hoc trained professionals such as a pharmacist and a physician and tends to provide multiple key messages, often not straightforward for some of the various outcomes considered. The second one is closer to an anti-marketing strategy targeting a single drug, with a pharmacist as the main actor or facilitator of an easy-to-use evidence synthesis, and has more clear-cut outcomes based on prescribing difference of a single drug.

Though the main objective was to estimate the impact of such intervention on the prescribing profile of the various drugs, these two consecutive trials were also designed to allow us to consider differences (in terms of feasibility, acceptability and magnitude of effect) between the two approaches: either a more articulated and "therapeutic area" oriented approach, or a more focused "single drug" approach. They are jointly described in this paper to discuss and contrast these two different approaches, implemented using the same methodology.

The four information packages (the 2007 issues available at http://assr.regione.emilia-romagna.it/it/servizi/pubblicazioni/collane-cessate/archivio-pacchetti/intro) were developed in a clear, simple and appealing format, first reviewing the available evidence, then critically appraising the most relevant or largest among available studies, providing information on absolute benefits and harms of the chosen drugs and some contextual information (e.g. prescribing data and regulatory issues). [22] The idea was to "just present information", without recommending which of the addressed drugs should be prescribed. In particular, during the outreach visits, available evidence on targeted drugs was presented, highlighting the difference between a statistically significant effect on outcomes of questionable clinical relevance, and their meaning expressed in absolute terms (NNT/NNH, absolute reduction in risks, etc).

The small group meetings were organised by the Departments of Primary Care within each LHA and were part of a continuing medical education program (providing CME credits). They were led by a trained pharmacist, supported by a "referent" GP delegate by his/her PCG who had the main role to stimulate the "inter pares" discussion using ad-hoc clinical scenarios and a problem-based approach. Table 1 synthesizes the main components of the multifaceted intervention.

Approximately one pharmacist per 5–10 PCGs (80–150 GPs) was trained through one four-day intensive course (36 hours) on EBM methodology, a three-day course (about 20–22 hours) for each topic in TEA trial (osteoporosis and BPH) and 1 day course for each single drug in SIDRO trial. One GP for each PCG (referent) received a half-day training module on each topic their practice group had been randomised to. Pharmacists were assigned to each PCGs before randomization.

Stratified randomisation was carried out within each Local Health Authority (LHA), using the number of assisted population per PCG (under or over the mean for that LHA) as stratifying factor. Computer generated random numbers were used to assign PCGs to either group, in order to get the minimum possible difference between groups in terms of number of assisted population per PCG.

Outcomes

Main outcomes were referred to differences in NHS prescription of drugs under scrutiny (expressed as DDD per thousand patients) during the six months after the educational intervention, with a parallel comparison of individual doctors who had received the specific information topic versus those who received the other one, adjusted for the cluster effect. Baseline imbalances were taken into account calculating the change from baseline in the prescribing rate. Secondary analyses with 12, 24 and 48 months of follow-up were also performed, to assess the persistence of effects in absence of reminders.

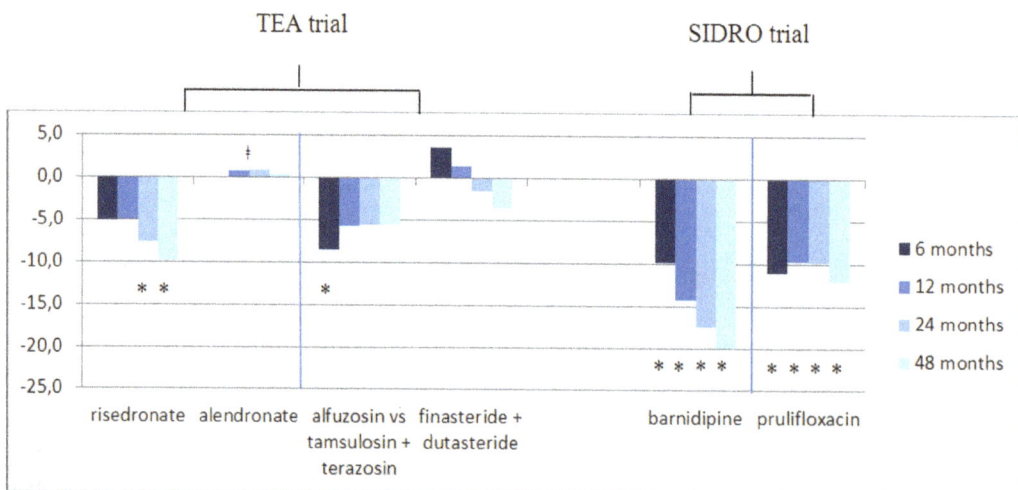

* statistically significant

‡ alendronate was the only bisphosphonate available as generic drug

Figure 2. % differences in primary outcomes at 6 months (main analysis), 12, 24 and 48 months.

Table 4. SIDRO trial: GPs' mean baseline prescription (in the 3 months preceding the outreach visit) of considered drugs, expressed as DDD per 1000 patients.

Drugs considered:	Group 1: information on prulifloxacin	Group 2: information on barnidipine
prulifloxacin	0.19	0.18
barnidipine	1.07	1.06

Specifically, the TEA trial had four primary outcomes and 11 secondary outcomes (see results section). Some outcomes were designed to evaluate a shift toward off-patent drugs (such as tamsulosin and terazosin for BPH or alendronate for osteoporosis) which were also those with more robust evidence. In general, a prescribing reduction was expected since evidence-based data show that prescription of drugs in those therapeutic areas may be excessive.

In the SIDRO trial a reduction was expected for both the 2 two main outcomes (one for each arm), representing the prescription of me-too drugs.

All data were collected through a regional routine data collection system, containing information (including date of prescription) about all prescriptions written by each doctor to residents of Emilia-Romagna.

In addition to prescribing outcomes, a questionnaire exploring doctors' knowledge on the addressed topics and attitudes on the information materials was distributed before and after the information meetings. Questionnaires assessing knowledge were specifically designed for each topic and were nominal' (for receiving CME credits), whereas those assessing attitudes were anonymous for a more unbiased evaluation of opinions on completeness, balance and usefulness of the information.

Statistical considerations

From a sample of 40 clusters (about 600 general practitioners) and using a dedicated software (Cluster Randomisation Sample Size Calculator version 1.0.2, Health Services Research Unit, Aberdeen University) we estimated the intracluster correlation coefficients (ICC) and the sample size that would have been required to see a difference of 10–15% in the prescription of the specific drugs, assuming an average cluster (PCG) size of 15. [25].

With the recruitment of 115 PCGs, and using correction for multiplicity considering primary outcomes of both trials, we had 80% power to detect a 9–15% difference for the various drugs considered.

Doctors' prescriptions were analysed according to the randomisation scheme, independently of their participation in the outreach visits. A few exceptions leading to a modified intention-to-treat analysis (m-ITT) are described below. In particular, the following were excluded from the main analyses:

- general practitioners with fewer than 300 patients; these could have abnormal rates in the prescription of specific drugs if people using these drugs were over-represented among their patients, distorting the trial results; moreover, their practice populations may rapidly grow over time, since they are usually young doctors beginning their activity (in fact no prescribing reports are produced for these GPs since they would not be reliable);

- general practitioners who participated in a different information meeting (different topic) from the assigned one because they had moved to a different PCG after randomization. Since these cases occurred mostly for administrative reasons (re-arranging of PCGs at LHA level) rather than through doctors' choice, we judged that this specific modification to the ITT would not limit generalizability, whereas keeping those doctors in the original randomization scheme even if receiving a different topic could have led to biased results;

- one PCG refused its consent to participate.

Generalised linear models (random effects models) were used to correct primary outcomes for baseline imbalances in the prescription of targeted drugs.

STATA version 11 was used for data analysis.

Ethics approval

The two RCTs have been approved by each of the Ethics Committees of the Local Health Authorities (Parma, Reggio Emilia, Modena, Bologna, Forlì) involved in the research. Randomized doctors were not asked to sign an informed consent form: their participation to the information meetings was part of a compulsory program set by the Local Health Authorities. Prescribing data are routinely collected and informed consent is not needed for their collection and analysis. Ethics Committees were of course aware of the recruitment procedure: one of the Committees (Modena) declared that a formal approval was not even necessary for the reasons described above.

Table 5. SIDRO trial: differences in DDD per 1000 patients of prescribed drugs (intervention vs control).

prescribing outcomes (primary)	Absolute mean prescription during follow-up in the 'intervention group' (DDD per 1000 patients)	Absolute difference at follow-up vs control group (change from baseline expressed as DDD per 1000 patients)	m-ITT (95% CI) (1564 included GPs)
prulifloxacin	0.17	−0.02	−11.1% (−0.5 to −22,2%)
barnidipine *	1.94	−0.21*	−9.8% (−1.9 to −18.2%)

*a lower increase was observed in the intervention group.

Table 6. Participants' opinions about usefulness of information received (question: Do you think the information you have received will be useful?).

Information package	Very much	Quite	Little	Not at all	No answer
Osteoporosis	42.5%	53.5%	1.8%	0.1%	2.1%
BPH	29.7%	62.3%	4.5%	0.9%	2.6%
Prulifloxacin	31.0%	43.6%	19.1%	3.1%	3.2%
Barnidipine	37.3%	35.8%	18.2%	6.3%	2.3%

Even if not strictly necessary (having randomized general practitioners and not patients) we registered the trials on the ISRCTN register (trial registration n.: ISRCTN05866587).

Results

First RCT: ThErapeutic Area approach (TEA) trial: Information on drugs for the treatment of benign prostatic hyperplasia (arm 1) and drugs for the treatment of osteoporosis (arm 2)

The flow charts of cluster participants is shown in Figure 1. All 115 PCGs, corresponding to 1737 GPs assisting about two millions inhabitants, were randomised. A total of 1605 GPs (92.4%) were included in the m-ITT analysis, excluding 110 GPs (6.3%) who had less than 300 subjects in their assisted population, one PCG (with 9 GPs –0,5%) refusing to participate to the study, and 13 single GPs (0,7%) who had moved to a different PCG after randomisation. A total of 1311 of the included GPs (81.7%) participated in the information meetings (per protocol population).

Table 2 shows GPs' mean baseline prescription of drugs considered in the primary outcomes. Limited imbalances between the two groups (less than 5%) had to be considered. Table S1 shows number and characteristics of PCGs and GPs in the ITT analysis.

Table 3 synthesizes differences in change from baseline between intervention and control groups in prescribing outcomes. In the ITT analysis, one BPH-related primary outcome showed a statistically significant reduction: specifically, the ratio between alpha blocker drugs alfuzosin (still under patent) and tamsulosin+terazosin (off patent) decreased by 8.5% (p = 0.03; intracluster correlation coefficient or ICC of almost 0), suggesting a shift towards off patent drugs, as expected. The other BPH-related primary outcome, prescription of finasteride+dutasteride did not reach statistically significant differences (ICC = 0.06).

As for osteoporosis related outcomes, no primary outcome showed a statistically significant reduction in the ITT analysis (ICC for alendronic acid and risedronic acid were 0.04 and 0.31, respectively);

One secondary outcome, prescription of ibandronic acid, showed a statistically significant reduction (−19.6%; p = 0.01; ICC = 0.002), although its prescription was very limited in absolute terms. This drug was shown to lack evidence on primary prevention of osteoporotic fractures.

Fig. 2 provides a clear representation of results also related to longer term follow-ups (after 12, 24 and 48 months), allowing for an evaluation of persistence of effects: similar direction to 6-month results are showed, except for combined prescription of finasteride and dutasteride in BPH. Ratio between alpha blocker drugs alfuzosin and tamsulosin+terazosin lost statistical significance after 12 months. Surprisingly, prescription of risedronate in osteoporo-

sis was further reduced and was statistically significant after 24 and 48 months (−7.6%, p = 0.02; and −9,8%, p = 0.03).

Second RCT: SIngle DRug Oriented (SIDRO) trial: A new antibiotic and a new antihypertensive (a calcium-channel blocker): prulifloxacin (arm 1) and barnidipine (arm 2)

In this subsequent trial, all 115 PCGs, corresponding to 1735 GPs, were randomised (two general practitioners retired in the period between the first and the second trial – Fig. 1).

A total of 1564 GPs (90.1%) were included in the ITT analysis, excluding 106 GPs (6.1%) who had fewer than 300 subjects in their assisted population, three PCGs (with 49 GPs –2,8%) refusing the small group meeting, and 16 single GPs (0,9%) who had moved to a different PCG after randomization receiving the "control" information (Fig. 1); 1211 of the included GPs (77,4%) participated in the information meetings (per protocol population).

Table 4 shows GPs' mean baseline prescription for the drugs of interest. Limited imbalances between the two groups (about 6%) had to be considered. Table S2 shows number and characteristics of PCGs and GPs in the ITT analysis.

Table 5 synthesizes differences in change from baseline between intervention and control groups in prescribing outcomes related to the prulifloxacin and barnidipine information meeting. In the modified ITT analysis, both the primary outcomes showed a statistically significant reduction of about 10%: prulifloxacin −11.1% (p = 0.04; ICC = 0.05); barnidipine −9.8% (p = 0.02; ICC = 0.08). This suggests that information focused on a single drug rather than on more complex therapeutic strategies can be successful in changing doctors' behaviours and this result is stable or even increasing over time (up to 4 years); however, caution is needed in interpreting these data, considering the limited prescription of these drugs in absolute terms (in particular of prulifloxacin).

Results after 12, 24 and 48 months showed, surprisingly, a progressively larger reduction in the prescription of barnidipine, doubled after 48 months, and similar reductions in the prescription of prulifloxacin, suggesting that the effect of the intervention might have persisted over time (Fig. 2).

Assessment of doctors' knowledge and attitudes

The majority of doctors could identify the correct answers to several questions and to improve their baseline knowledge after the intervention, although answers were given collectively in most of the information meetings, limiting the usefulness of such analysis. For this reason, those results are not shown.

As for doctors' opinions on completeness and usefulness of the information received, the vast majority of general practitioners evaluated it as "very much" or "quite", as shown in Table 6. Even if the more articulated information presented in the first RCT was associated with less evident changes in the prescribing outcomes, compared with the more focused information of the second RCT (as described above), such information was more appreciated by doctors: more than 90% considered information packages in the first RCT either "very" or "quite" useful compared to 72–75% in the second RCT.

Discussion

These two cluster RCTs confirm that pharmacists' outreach visits can be an effective way of promoting evidence-based prescribing in a large NHS setting and show that effects can persist in the long-term (up to 4 years). They are also the largest studies done in terms of number of doctors involved. A cluster design was used since group meetings are held regularly (at least twice a year) with Primary Care Groups in the intervention areas and because they represent a natural setting where to deliver information, stimulate analysis and discussion through a problem-based approach. [26–27].

In the first RCT (TEA trial) in which information materials addressed a therapeutic area and had broader clinical scope and extent (drugs in the treatment of benign prostatic hyperplasia/osteoporosis), only one of the four predefined primary outcome showed a statistically significant reduction (prescription of alfuzosin compared to tamsulosin and terazosin in benign prostatic hyperplasia). The fairly ambitious quantitative hypothesis to be tested (10–15% difference in doctors' prescriptions) was thus substantially not demonstrated, in spite of the involvement of about 1800 general practitioners. Among the other three primary outcomes in the first RCT, one (prescription of risedronate) has become statistically significant after two years of follow-up, further reducing its prescription in the intervention group, and this finding is not easy to interpret; another primary outcome (prescription of alendronate) was affected by its availability as generic drug just before the start of the trial, as well as by its better assessed benefit-risk profile compared to the other bisphosphonates; this may have reduced the potential to show a difference between the two groups. As for bisphosphonates, the prescription of ibandronate (a secondary outcome) showed a reduction in the intervention group, but this drug was little prescribed.

Conversely, in the second RCT (SIDRO trial) which concerned information on a single drug, both primary outcomes showed clear and statistically significant prescribing reductions (10% or more) lasting a long time. Although doctors generally appreciated the therapeutic area approach used in the first RCT - addressing both diagnostic and therapeutic questions in a broad range of clinical scenarios - more than the more focused single drug approach, the latter seems to have affected doctors' prescribing behaviour more clearly.

These studies confirm findings from previous RCTs conducted mostly in Northern Europe and North America, showing that pharmacists delivering evidence-based information and prescribing data through outreach visits may influence doctors' prescribing behaviour in the short term. Our findings add that positive results are mostly obtained with an intervention focused on a single drug, suggesting that the more complex the information, the more complex and the less likely the related behaviour/prescribing change. Contrary to the findings of previous educational intervention trials, we found high persistence of the effects (measured initially as stated in the study protocol at 6 and 12 months, and in subsequent periods up to 48 months) even in absence of reminders. This result was particularly sharp for barnidipine, a calcium antagonist possibly suffering from the competition of many drugs in the same class.

The evaluation of educational interventions is fairly complex given the many different variables in play. [28] Among these, we did not consider patient demand as a main driver of drug prescription, giving priority to feasibility and replicability of the intervention. However, the pragmatic nature of these RCTs and their large-scale implementation in a natural setting strengthen the external validity of the results.

The context may determine the success of these educational programs, by hindering or facilitating the implementation of small group meetings. In this regard, general practitioners from Friuli Venezia-Giulia (another region in Northern Italy), initially supposed to take part in the RCTs, did not in the end do so because their representatives and the Regional Health Authority disagreed. Moreover, one more RCT was originally planned in Sardinia (a large island in Southern Italy), to compare three different strategies of information delivery to solo general practitioners: [21] this trial did not take place for similar reasons as in Friuli Venezia-Giulia. Involvement of doctors' organizations and strong endorsement of Health Authorities are crucial in implementing such an anti-promotional intervention; doctors may see these interventions as top-down, cost-saving approaches.

In conclusion, the confirmation of a positive impact of independent information programs in a large-scale natural setting, in particular when information on single drugs is provided, can be considered as a fairly relevant finding and the persistence of the observed differences for up to 4 years is quite a new one. If the organizational environment is "good enough" and a strong endorsement from Health Authorities (with the sole aim to promote public health optimizing treatments) is assured, information programs led by National Health Systems Agencies may provide a critical alternative to industry-led information to physicians. Future studies should focus on assessing whether positive findings are driven by how information is delivered (small groups versus one-to-one meetings) and presented, evaluating different formats and ways of presenting the actual magnitude of benefits and risks of drugs and other health interventions.

Acknowledgments

We want to thank Prof. David Sackett (McMaster University, Canada) for useful suggestions and great encouragement in developing the research project.

Contributors

Members of the INDRA-NET (INformation on DRugs And NEw Therapies) study group are:
- Local Health Authority of Bologna: C. Castelvetri, P. Falcone, M. Magnani, M. Manzoli, P. Pagano, E. Pasi, G. Santilli, S. Scaramagli, P. Tomasi, L. Toni, P. Zuccheri.
- Local Health Authority of Forlì: F. Carnaccini, R. Consiglio.
- Local Health Authority of Modena: M. Ghelfi, C. Orsi, M. Pagani.
- Local Health Authority of Parma: M. Boffetti, G. Negri, F. Pinelli.
- Local Health Authority of Reggio Emilia: R. Ballestri, R. Montanari.

Steering Committee: M. Bobbio (Chairman); P. Malavasi, G. Negri, M. Salera, E. Sapigni (Emilia-Romagna); P. Carossino, G. Carta, M. Cicalò, D. Garau, G. Sanna (Sardinia); L. Crapesi, L. Marcuzzo, R. Paduano, G. Tosolini (Friuli Venezia Giulia); G. Formoso, N. Magrini, A. M. Marata (coordinating group).

Author Contributions

Conceived and designed the experiments: NM GF AMM. Analyzed the data: CDG CV. Wrote the paper: GF NM. Development of information tools: OC EM AMM GF BP LM LD FN. Coordination of educational meetings: AMM OC EM GF FN LM LD.

References

1. Collier J, Iheanacho I (2002) The pharmaceutical industry as an informant. Lancet 360: 1405–1409.
2. Melander H, Ahlqvist-Rastad J, Meijer G, Beermann B (2003) Evidence b(i)ased medicine – selective reporting from studies sponsored by pharmaceutical industry: review of studies in new drug applications. BMJ 326: 1171–1173.
3. Ridker PM, Torres J (2006) Reported outcomes in major cardiovascular clinical trials funded by for-profit and not-for-profit organizations: 2000–2005. JAMA 295: 2270–2276.
4. Dickersin K (2005) Publication bias: Recognizing the problem, understanding its origins and scope, and preventing harm. In: Rothstein H, Sutton A, Borenstein M (eds). Publication bias in meta-analysis: prevention, assessment, and adjustments. London: Wiley, p 11–33.
5. Chan AW (2008) Bias, spin, and misreporting: time for full access to trial protocols and results. PLoS Medicine 5(11): e230. DOI:10.1371/journal.pmed.0050230.
6. Light DW, Lexchin JR (2012) Pharmaceutical research and development: what do we get for all that money? BMJ 345: e4348.
7. The Congress of the United States – Congressional Budget Office (2006) Research and Development in the Pharmaceutical Industry.
8. Graham Dukes MN (2002) Accountability of the pharmaceutical industry. Lancet 360: 1682–1684.
9. Avorn J, Soumerai SB (1983) Improving drug-therapy decisions through educational outreach - a randomized controlled trial of academically based detailing. New Engl J Med 308: 1457–1463.
10. Soumerai SB, Avorn J (1990) Principles of educational outreach (academic detailing) to improve clinical decision making. JAMA 263: 549–556.
11. Simon SR, Majumdar SR, Prosser LA, Salem-Schatz S, Warner C, et al. (2005) Group versus individual academic detailing to improve the use of antihypertensive medications in primary care: a cluster-randomized controlled trial. Am J Med 118: 521–528.
12. O'Brien MA, Rogers S, Jamtvedt G, Oxman AD, Odgaard-Jensen J, et al. (2007) Educational outreach visits: effects on professional practice and health care outcomes. *Cochrane Database of Systematic Reviews*, Issue 4. Art. No.: CD000409. DOI: 10.1002/14651858.CD000409.pub2.
13. Woloshin S, Schwartz LM (2011) Communicating data about the benefits and harms of treatment: a randomized trial. Ann Intern Med 155: 87–96.
14. Woloshin S, Schwartz LM, Welch HG (2008) Know Your Chances. Understanding Health Statistics. Berkeley (CA): University of California Press 2008.
15. Guyatt GH, Oxman AD, Vist GE, Kunz R, Falck-Ytter Y, et al. (2008) GRADE: an emerging consensus on rating quality of evidence and strength of recommendations. BMJ 336: 924–926.
16. Nkansah N, Mostovetsky O, Yu C, Chheng T, Beney J, et al. (2010) Effect of outpatient pharmacists' non-dispensing roles on patient outcomes and prescribing patterns. Cochrane Database of Systematic Reviews Issue 7. Art. No.: CD000336. DOI: 10.1002/14651858.CD000336.pub2.
17. Grimshaw JM, Thomas RE, MacLennan G, Fraser C, Ramsay CR, et al. (2004) Effectiveness and efficiency of guideline dissemination and implementation strategies. Health Technol Assess 8: 1–352.
18. Formoso G, Liberati A, Magrini N (2001) Practice Guidelines: Useful and "Participative" Method? Survey of Italian Physicians by Professional Setting. Arch Intern Med 161: 2037–2042.
19. Italian Medicines Agency (AIFA) Research & Development Working Group (2010) Feasibility and challenges of independent research on drugs: the Italian Medicines Agency (AIFA) experience. Eur J Clin Invest 40: 69–86.
20. Garattini S, Chalmers I (2009) Patients and the public deserve big changes in evaluation of drugs. BMJ 338: b1025.
21. Magrini N, Formoso G, Marata AM, Capelli O, Maestri E, et al. (2007) Randomised controlled trials for evaluating the prescribing impact of information meetings led by pharmacists and of new information formats, in General Practice in Italy. BMC Health Services Research 7: 158.
22. Formoso G, Marata AM, Magrini N (2007) Social marketing: should it be used to promote evidence-based information? Soc Sci Med 64: 949–953.
23. Schwartz LM (2009) Lost in Transmission – FDA Drug Information That Never Reaches Clinicians. New Engl J Med 361: 1717–1720.
24. Ivers N, Jamtvedt G, Flottorp S, Young JM, Odgaard-Jensen J, et al. (2012) Audit and feedback: effects on professional practice and healthcare outcomes. Cochrane Database of Systematic Reviews Issue 6. Art. No.: CD000259. DOI: 10.1002/14651858.CD000259.pub3.
25. Donner A, Klar N (1996) Statistical considerations in the design and analysis of community intervention trials. J Clin Epidemiol 49: 435–439.
26. Norman G (2002) Research in medical education: three decades of progress. BMJ 324: 1560–1562.
27. Godwin M, Ruhland L, Casson I, MacDonald S, Delva D, et al. (2003) Pragmatic controlled clinical trials in primary care: the struggle between external and internal validity. BMC Medical Research Methodology 3: 28.
28. Craig P, Dieppe P, Macintyre S, Michie S, Nazareth I, et al. (2008) Developing and evaluating complex interventions: the new Medical Research Council guidance. BMJ 337: a1655 doi:10.1136/bmj.a1655.

14

A Polymeric Prodrug of 5-Fluorouracil-1-Acetic Acid Using a Multi-Hydroxyl Polyethylene Glycol Derivative as the Drug Carrier

Man Li[Ə], Zhen Liang[Ə], Xun Sun, Tao Gong*, Zhirong Zhang*

Key Laboratory of Drug Targeting and Drug Delivery Systems, Ministry of Education, West China School of Pharmacy, Sichuan University, Chengdu, Sichuan, PR China

Abstract

Purpose: Macromolecular prodrugs obtained by covalently conjugating small molecular drugs with polymeric carriers were proven to accomplish controlled and sustained release of the therapeutic agents *in vitro* and *in vivo*. Polyethylene glycol (PEG) has been extensively used due to its low toxicity, low immunogenicity and high biocompatibility. However, for linear PEG macromolecules, the number of available hydroxyl groups for drug coupling does not change with the length of polymeric chain, which limits the application of PEG for drug conjugation purposes. To increase the drug loading and prolong the retention time of 5-fluorouracil (5-Fu), a macromolecular prodrug of 5-Fu, 5-fluorouracil-1 acid-PAE derivative (5-FA-PAE) was synthesized and tested for the antitumor activity *in vivo*.

Methods: PEG with a molecular weight of 38 kDa was selected to synthesize the *multi-hydroxyl polyethylene glycol* derivative (PAE) through an addition reaction. 5-fluorouracil-1 acetic acid (5-FA), a 5-Fu derivative was coupled with PEG derivatives via ester bond to form a macromolecular prodrug, 5-FA-PAE. The *in vitro* drug release, pharmacokinetics, *in vivo* distribution and antitumor effect of the prodrug were investigated, respectively.

Results: The PEG-based prodrug obtained in this study possessed an exceedingly high 5-FA loading efficiency of 10.58%, much higher than the maximum drug loading efficiency of unmodified PEG with the same molecular weight, which was 0.98% theoretically. Furthermore, 5-FA-PAE exhibited suitable sustained release in tumors.

Conclusion: This study provides a new approach for the development of the delivery to tumors of anticancer agents with PEG derivatives.

Editor: Ronald Hancock, Laval University Cancer Research Centre, Canada

Funding: The authors acknowledge the financial support from the National Natural Science Foundation of China (no. 30873167) and the National Basic Research Program of China (973 program, No: 2013CB932504). The funders had no role in study design, data collection and analysis, decision to publish, or preparation of the manuscript.

Competing Interests: The authors have declared that no competing interests exist.

* Email: gongtaoy@126.com (TG); zrzzl@vip.sina.com (ZZ)

Ə These authors contributed equally to this work.

Introduction

Cancer is one of the most life-threatening diseases worldwide, which seriously endangers human health and survival [1,2]. Surgery, radiotherapy, chemical medication, biological immunization therapies are the major treatment strategies, among which chemotherapy plays an important role in the treatment of cancer [3–9]. Regarding chemotherapies, 5-fluorouracil (5-Fu) is one of the most widely used antimetabolites in clinic [10], which shows significant inhibitory effect against a broad spectrum of solid tumors [11–13]. Traditional chemotherapies such as 5-Fu are cytotoxic agents that inhibit rapidly proliferating cancer cells. Due to its low specificity, side effects such as myelosuppression, mucositis, dermatitis and diarrhea are commonly observed during the clinical application of 5-Fu [14–16]. Additionally, 5-Fu has a very short half life of about 20 minutes and is rapidly eliminated

after administration. The irregular oral absorption and the low bioavailability often results in poor clinical therapeutic outcome [17–19].

To address the aforementioned problems, researchers have tried various methods to improve the efficacy and to reduce the toxicity of 5-Fu, including modification of the chemical structure, formulation strategies and novel delivery systems. Several small molecular prodrugs of 5-Fu were developed, such as 5-fluoro-2'-deoxyuridine, 1-(2-tetrahydrofuryl)-5-fluorouracil and 3, 5-dioctanoyl 5-fluoro-2-deoxyuridine [20–22]. Various delivery systems have been developed for the targeted delivery of 5-Fu [23]. Menei *et al* developed biodegradable microspheres to obtain sustained delivery of 5-Fu for the treatment of glioblastoma [24]. Liposomes have been used as a sustained delivery system for 5-Fu [25]. In recent years, macromolecular carrier/delivery systems have been studied extensively. Macromolecular prodrugs obtained by combining small molecular drugs with polymeric carriers could slowly release the therapeutic agents *in vivo* with an improved half-life [26–31]. Moreover, the enhanced permeability and retention (EPR) effect may contribute to the accumulation of macromolecular prodrugs within the solid tumor, which would lead to a tumor-targeted drug delivery and reduced toxicity to normal tissues [32–34]. Moreover, the EPR effect has been regarded as the "golden rule" in the design of antitumor drugs. Based on the EPR effect, numerous tumor-targeted drug delivery systems were developed using macromolecules such as albumin (65 kDa), transferrin (90 kDa), IgG (immunoglobulin, 150 kDa), α2-macroglobulin (240 kDa) and ovomucoid of chicken eggwhite (29 kDa, highly glycosylated protein), and some have entered clinical trials [35].

In addition to the aforementioned macromolecular materials, polyethylene glycol (PEG) has become a material of great interests due to its low toxicity, low immunogenicity and high biocompatibility [36–38]. The molecular weight of PEG used in forming macromolecular prodrugs would impact the *in vivo* behaviors of the conjugates because the retention time of the prodrugs increased with the molecular weight of the carriers [30]. Prolonged retention of the prodrug is critical to the tumor accumulation of the therapeutic agents loaded. However, for linear PEG macromolecules, the number of available hydroxyl groups for drug coupling does not change with the length of the polymeric chain, which limits the application of PEG for drug conjugation purposes. Therefore, the development of new PEG derivatives to improve its drug loading efficiency has become a hot topic in material science and is of great significance to the tumor-targeted delivery of small molecular agents and 4-arm PEG derivatives were thus developed [39], and the 4-arm PEG based prodrugs have entered clinical trials with promising results [40–44]. For small molecular drugs such as 5-Fu, treatment requires a high therapeutic concentration, while the macromolecular based prodrugs have a relatively low drug loading efficiency. Thus, the modification of linear PEG creates derivatives with high drug loading efficiency which will have great significance for anticancer drug development [45].

In this study, a macromolecular prodrug, 5-fluorouracil-1 acid-PAE derivative (5-FA-PAE), was designed and synthesized to increase the drug loading efficiency, achieve delivery to the tumor and prolong the retention time. PEG with a molecular weight of 38 kDa was selected as the starting material to obtain the multi-hydroxyl PEG derivative, which was then coupled with 5-fluorouracil-1 acetic acid (5-FA), to afford the prodrug. The *in vitro* drug release, pharmacokinetics, *in vivo* distribution and antitumor effect of the prodrug were investigated, respectively.

Materials and Methods

Materials

Polyethylene glycol (PEG, average molecular weight ~38 kDa), allyl glycidyl ether (AGE), mercaptoethanol, 1-(3-dimethylaminopropyl)-3-ethylcarbodiimide hydrochloride (EDC·HCl) and N-hydroxysuccinimide (NHS) were purchased from Sigma-Aldrich (USA). Sodium hydride (NaH) was supplied by Damao Chemical Reagent Factory (Tianjin, China). 5-Fluorouracil (USP29) was purchased from Nantong Jinghua Pharmaceuticals Co., Ltd (Jiangsu, China). All other chemicals used were of reagent grade.

Synthesis of multi-hydroxyl polyethylene glycol derivative (polyethylene glycol-allyl glycidyl ether-mercaptoethanol, PAE)

Polyethylene glycol-allyl glycidyl ether (PA) was synthesized as described before [46,47] with some modifications. Briefly, 10.0 g of PEG was melted in an oil bath at 120°C with stirring under vacuum for about 3 h to remove the adsorbed moisture before adding 120 mg of NaH. The mixture was stirred for 4 h at 120°C, and 2.0 ml of AGE was added. The product was recrystallized with isopropanol to remove the micromolecular materials.

Synthesis of 5-FA-PAE prodrug

5-FA was synthesized as previously described [48,49] with some modification. Briefly, 6.5 g of 5-Fu was dissolved in 25 ml of aqueous solution of potassium hydroxide (4 M), then 15 ml of aqueous solution of chloroacetic acid (5 M) was added dropwise with stirring. The pH value of the reaction mixture was monitored and kept at 10 by adding an aqueous solution of potassium hydroxide (10 M) during the addition of chloroacetic acid and throughout the whole course of the reaction. The mixture was heated to 50°C in an oil bath with stirring for 8 h, and then acidified by HCl to obtain 5-FA.

A solution of 5-FA (0.496 g) in 1 ml of dimethylformamide was added dropwise to a solution of 0.5 g of PAE in 20 ml of dimethylformamide, then 0.196 g (1.7 mmol) of NHS and 0.4 g (2.09 mmol) of EDC·HCl were added sequentially. After a further 16 h of incubation at room temperature away from light, the mixture was precipitated with 150 ml of isopropanol. The obtained residue was recrystallized by isopropanol several times until the reagents and uncoupled 5-FA were totally removed (monitored by TLC and HPLC), then dried in vacuum at 40°C overnight.

HPLC analysis

HPLC assay was established for the determination of 5-FA in PBS, plasma or tissues homogenates, which was performed using Shimadzu instruments (Chiyoda-Ku, Japan) consisting of a CTO-10A column thermostat, two LC-10AT pumps and a SPD-10A UV detector. A Scienhome ODS column (5 μm, 150×4.6 mm, Tianjin, China) was used to separate samples. Phosphate buffer (0.05 M, pH 2.5) was used as the mobile phase at a flow rate of 1 ml/min. The temperature of the column was kept at 35°C and the effluent was detected at 270 nm. Studies showed that the precision, accuracy, and recovery of this HPLC method all met the measurement requirements.

Safety evaluation

All animal experiments were approved by the Institutional Animal Care and Ethic Committee of Sichuan University (Approved No. SYXK2013-185). All animals were fed on a light and dark cycle and allowed free access to standard chow and water. Temperature and relative humidity were kept at 25°C and 50%, respectively. After experiment, mice were sacrificed by neck dislocation, and all efforts were made to minimize suffering. Myelosuppression is one of the major side effects of 5-Fu [14]. To assess the suppression level, 60 male Kunming mice (20–25 g, purchased from Laboratory Animal Center of Sichuan University) were randomly divided into 5 groups (n = 12) and were intravenously administered with 5-Fu (27.66 mg/kg), 5-FA (40 mg/kg), PAE (338 mg/kg) or 5-FA-PAE (378 mg/kg) (equivalent to 0.213 mmol/kg 5-FA). The control group was given physiological saline (0.009 g/ml). Zero point one mL blood samples were collected at prearranged time intervals (one day before injection and 1, 4, 7, and 10 days post injection). The white blood cells (WBC) and the blood platelets number were counted by MEK-6318K Automated Hematology Analyzer (Nihonkohden, Shinjuku-ku, Japan) as an index of myelosuppression.

In vitro drug release

The *in vitro* drug release of 5-FA-PAE was investigated in physiological saline (0.009 g/ml), PBS with various pH values, 50% mouse plasma (diluted with PBS, pH 7.4, v/v) and 50% mouse tumor homogenate which was obtained from the H22 tumor loaded mice (homogenized and diluted with physiological saline). An aqueous solution of 5-FA-PAE (100 µl) was added to 4 ml of preheated release medium (physiological saline or PBS with pH = 3.04, 4.51, 6.02, 7.41, 8.99). The mixture was maintained in a water bath at 37°C under continuously stirring, and 100 µl of each sample was collected at fixed time intervals (i.e. 0.25, 1, 3, 6, 10, 24, 48, 72, 96 h). The samples from physiological saline and PBS was acidified by 100 µl hydrochloric acid (1 M), diluted with 300 µl mobile phase and analyzed by HPLC. The samples from mouse plasma and tumor homogenate were obtained in duplicate at each time point (100 µl each). For hydrolysis, samples were mixed with 50 µl of aqueous solution of 5-bromouracil (96 µg/ml, 50 µl) as the internal standard, and then supplemented with 100 µl sodium hydroxide (1 M) and acidified by 100 µl hydrochloric acid (1 M), and extracted by 3.3 ml of ethyl ester for 15 min. After centrifugation at 10,000 rpm for 5 min, 2.7 ml of the ethyl ester portion was collected, concentrated in a nitrogen gas flow, redissolved in 100 µl of the mobile phase and centrifuged at 10,000 rpm for 10 min before HPLC analysis. The other group was not subjected to hydrolysis by substituting sodium hydroxide solution with saline and acidifying with 50 µl hydrochloric acid. The differences of 5-FA in the two groups at the same time point was the unreleased 5-FA in each sample. The decrement method was used to calculate the release rate. All experiments were conducted in triplicate.

Pharmacokinetics study

Male Wistar rats were purchased from The laboratory Animal Center of Sichuan University. 12 Wistar rats (body weight: 200 g±20 g) were divided into two groups randomly (n = 6). The control group and the test group were administered intravenously with 20 mg/kg of 5-FA and 189 mg/kg 5-FA-PAE (equivalent to 20 mg/kg of 5-FA) dissolved in physiological saline, respectively. The blood samples were collected into heparinized centrifuge tubes at predetermined intervals (see Table S2 in file SI) by retro-orbital puncture, and the plasma was separated by centrifugation. Each plasma sample of the test groups was divided into two portions. They were treated as hydrolyzed and unhydrolyzed as described in the "In vitro drug release" section. The two portions of the samples were analyzed by HPLC to determine the plasma concentrations of released 5-FA and total 5-FA of the conjugate whereas the plasma samples of the control group were treated as unhydrolyzed samples.

In vivo distribution

Murine H22 hepatocarcinoma cells (purchased from Type Culture Collection of Chinese Academy of Sciences) were maintained in RPMI 1640 medium supplemented with 2 mM L-glutamine and 10% fetal bovine serum (FBS) at 37°C with 5% CO_2, and were passaged every 2 or 3 days. The tumor-bearing animal model was established by subcutaneous injection of H22 cells (1×10^7 cells/ml, in 0.2 ml saline) into the right axillary region of Kunming mice. The sizes of tumors were monitored 7 days after inoculation and the tumor volumes were calculated as described in the "*Antitumor activity in tumor-bearing mice*" section. The mice with tumor volumes between 0.35 cm^3 and 0.65 cm^3 were randomized into two groups (n = 30). The control group and the test groups were administered intravenously with 20 mg/kg of 5-FA or 189 mg/kg 5-FA-PAE (equivalent to 20 mg/kg of 5-FA) dissolved in physiological saline (0.009 g/ml), respectively. The mice were exsanguinated and sacrificed by neck dislocation at predetermined time points. Tissues including heart, liver, spleen, lung, kidney, brain and tumor were collected, washed with physiological saline, weighed and homogenized with two fold concentrated physiological saline. The samples of the test group were treated as hydrolyzed samples as described in the section "*In vitro drug release*", whereas those of the control group were treated as unhydrolyzed samples. All data are presented as the concentration of 5-FA.

Antitumor activity in tumor-bearing mice

The tumor-bearing mice model was established as previously described in the "*In vivo distribution*" section. 72 h after inoculation, mice with no signs of tumor growth were exclude from this experiment. 48 tumor-bearing mice were randomly divided into 4 groups (n = 12). The control group was administered intravenously with 20 ml/kg of physiological saline. The other groups were administered intravenously with 30 mg/kg (0.160 mmol/kg) of 5-FA or 284 mg/kg 5-FA-PAE (equivalent to 0.160 mmol/kg 5-FA) dissolved in physiological saline. 5-Fu (20.47 mg/kg, 0.160 mmol/kg) was administered as a control. All animals were administered once on day 3, 5, 7, 9, 11, 13, 15 after the inoculation of H22 cells and sacrificed on day 20. Tumors and organs (heart, liver, spleen, lung, kidney, brain and thymus) were removed and weighed. The tumor volume and tumor control rate were evaluated. The tumor volume, organ/body weight index and tumor control rate were calculated as follows:

$$\text{Tumor volume (mm}^3) = 0.5 \times \text{Width}^2 \times \text{Length}$$

$$Organ/body\ weight\ index = weight\ of\ each\ organ\ (tumor)/$$
$$weight\ of\ mouse \times 100$$

$$Tumor\ control\ rate\ (\%) =$$
$$\left(\begin{array}{c} average\ tumor\ weight\ of\ control\ group- \\ average\ tumor\ weight\ of\ test\ group \end{array} \right) \bigg/ \begin{array}{c} average\ tumor\ weight \\ of\ control\ group \end{array}$$

Data analysis

The data of pharmacokinetics and *in vivo* distribution study were processed using the Drug and Statistics Software 2.0 (DAS 2.0, Shanghai, China). The statistical analysis of the samples was performed by using one-way ANOVA and Student's *t*-test. *p*-values <0.05 were considered as statistically different.

Results and Discussion

Synthesis and characterization of 5-FA-PAE prodrug

As a polyether macromolecule, PEG is widely used for its suitable solubility and bioavailability in developing drug delivery systems [50–53]. However, as a drug carrier, the loading efficiency of prodrugs based on PEG is significantly constrained due to the limited positions for drug conjugation, *i.e.*, two hydroxy groups in the linear PEG molecule [45]. Thus, the modification of PEG to create derivatives with higher drug loading efficiency is greatly needed. PEG with a molecular weight of 38 kDa was selected as the starting material to synthesize the derivative (Fig. 1A). Allyl glycidyl ether was coupled to both ends of PEG under the catalysis of sodium hydride to form an intermediate, namely PA, with multi-double bonds on the side chains. PA was further reacted with small molecules through the addition reaction of the double bonds and the thiol group to afford various PEG derivatives with multi-hydroxyl groups. ^{1}H-NMR showed that the double bonds disappeared completely in PAE (Figure S1 in file SI). The GPC analysis demonstrated that PA and PAE had similar molecular weight distribution as the starting material PEG (Table 1). As a common drug carrier, the molecular weight of PEG greatly influenced the *in vivo* behaviors of prodrugs [54]. As the molecular weight increases, the *in vivo* clearance rate decreases. Thus, PEG with a higher Mw is likely to prolong the retention time of prodrugs and increase the drug accumulation in a tumor. It is suggested that the Mw of PEG should be no less than 30 kD to

prevent the prodrug from quick elimination from kidney [55]. Accordingly, PEG of 38 kD was used as the starting material.

However, 5-Fu could not be directly coupled with the carriers due to the lack of available hydroxyl groups in the structure. The derivative of 5-Fu, 5-fluorouracil-1-acetic acid (5-FA), was synthesized first. The macromolecular prodrug multi-hydroxyl polyethylene glycol-5-fluorouracil-1-acetic acid (5-FA-PAE) was obtained by covalently conjugating 5-FA with the PEG derivative under the catalysis of carbodiimide condensing agents (Figure 1B). The successful synthesis of the 5-fluorouracil derivative and the prodrug was confirmed by ^{1}H-NMR (Figure S1 in file SI). A higher molecular weight (Mw) and polydispersity (PDI) of 5-FA-PAE were observed compared with those of PAE (Table 1). HPLC analysis indicated that after the double bond-thiol addition reaction, multiple hydroxyl groups were introduced on the PEG backbone thus making it capable of loading more drugs. The drug loading efficiency of 5-FA-PAE was determined as 10.58%, much higher than the maximum drug loading efficiency of PEG with the same molecular weight, which was calculated as 0.98% theoretically. The drug loading efficiency of 5-FA-PAE was improved by

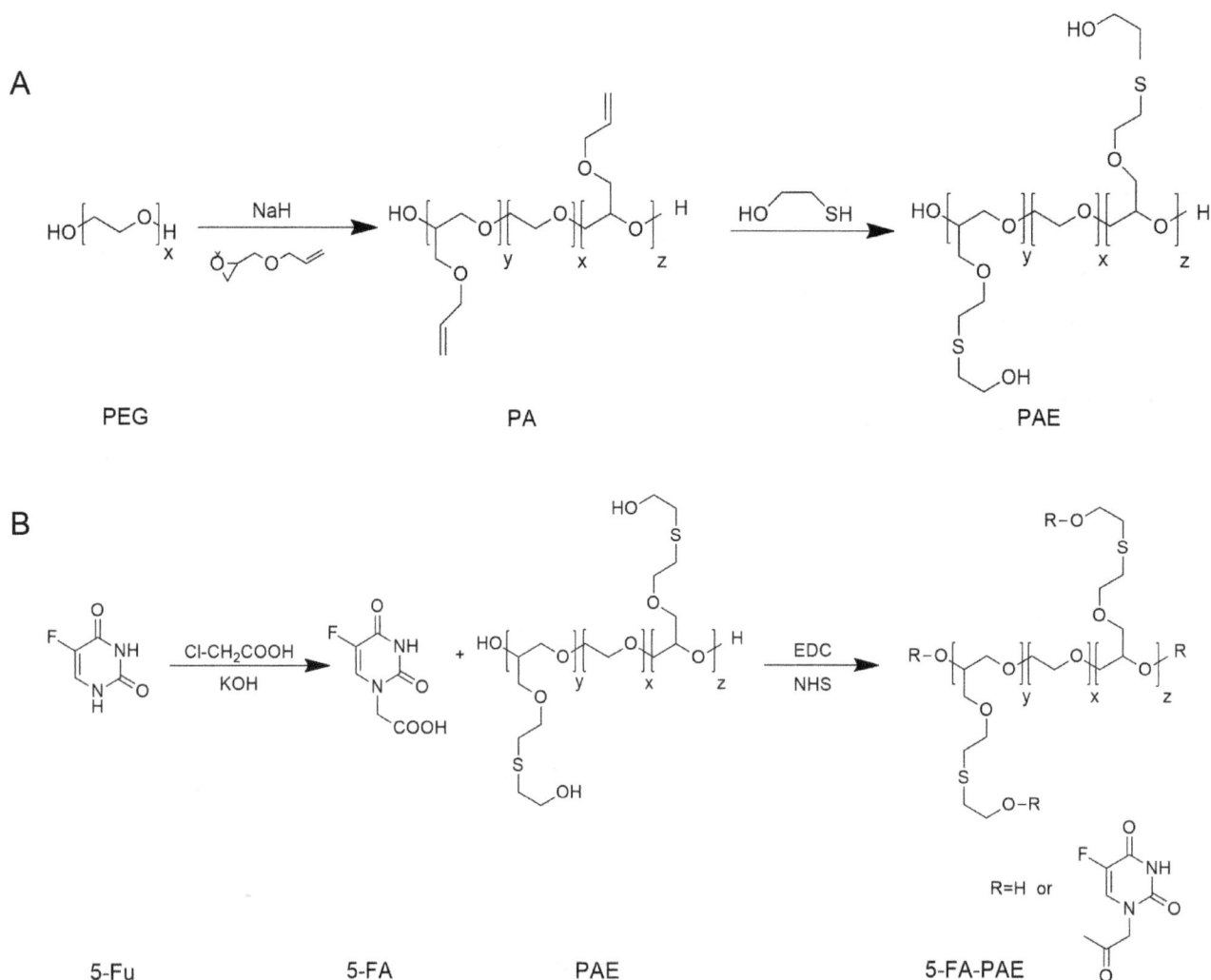

Figure 1. Synthesis routes of PAE (A) and 5-FA-PAE conjugates (B). (A) PA was synthesized by adding NaH to PEG and the mixture was stirred for 4 h at 120°C. Then PAE was obtained by adding AGE to the mixture. (B) 5-FA was added dropwise to PAE in dimethylformamide, then NHS and EDC·HCl were added. After incubation, the mixture was precipitated with isopropanol. The obtained residue was recrystallized by isopropanol several times and dried in vacuum at 40°C overnight to produce 5-FA-PAE.

Table 1. The molecular weight of the polymeric carrier (PEG, PA, PAE) and the prodrug (5-FA-PAE).

Compound	MP (Da)	Mw (Da)	Mn (Da)	PDI
PEG	38914	38045	27596	1.38
PA	33984	36039	21322	1.69
PAE	34282	36628	20842	1.76
5-FA-PAE	35413	44629	19998	2.23

PDI: polydispersity.

10.8-fold compared to that of 5-FA. The significant enhancement in drug loading efficiency would greatly increase the drug concentration within a tumor via the EPR effect.

Safety evaluation

To investigate the myelosuppression levels after 5-FA or 5-FA-PAE treatment, hematological parameters (i.e. the number of white blood cells and blood platelets) were measured at different time points after drug administration. Changes in these parameters presumably reflect the occurrence of myelosuppression and abnormality in the immune system. As shown in Table 2, the WBC count decreased after intravenous injection of 5-Fu, 5-FA and 5-FA-PAE. Only the group of 5-Fu exhibited significant reduction of WBC ($5.39 \pm 2.17 \times 10^9$/L one day after injection, $p < 0.05$). Then the WBC level increased gradually. Notably, the increase of WBC in the 5-Fu group was slower, leading to a lower WBC level at day 10 ($8.59 \pm 2.39 \times 10^9$/L) compared with the level before administration ($9.55 \pm 1.28 \times 10^9$/L), while the WBC level of other groups recovered within 4 days. Another major indicator of myelosuppression is the change in blood platelets number. Table S1 in file SI shows that though the platelets number of 5-Fu decreased 1 day after injection, the blood platelets of all groups didn't exhibit any significant changes, indicating that both 5-FA and 5-FA-PAE hardly affect the platelets level at such doses. Taken together, these results indicated that the prodrug of 5-Fu, 5-FA-PAE, showed a lower toxicity than 5-Fu.

In vitro drug release

The *in vitro* drug release behavior of 5-FA-PAE was investigated using phosphate buffered saline (PBS) of various pH values, physiological saline, mouse plasma and tumor homogenate as the release media. The release rate of 5-FA-PAE was pH-dependent. As the pH increased, the release rate increased significantly, reaching $94.1\% \pm 5.88\%$ at 96 h when the pH was 8.99 (Figure 2A). This is mostly likely due to the hydrolysis of ester bonds under basic conditions. However, if the conjugation with

the PEG derivative increased the retention time in plasma, this would possibly enhance the drug accumulation in a tumor (Figure 2B). The release rate of prodrug 5-FA-PAE in plasma was $89.46\% \pm 6.36\%$ at 10 h, and reached $98.15\% \pm 1.96\%$ at 24 h, while the rate was $55.9\% \pm 0.61\%$ in tumor homogenate at 24 h, suggesting that the ester bond can be easily degraded by easterases in plasma.

Pharmacokinetics study

A major drawback of 5-Fu is the relatively short half-life, which results in poor patient compliance and side effects. 5-FA, the derivative of 5-Fu, shows the same metabolism and clearance rate as 5-Fu. Moreover, after conjugation with PEG, the retention time in plasma was greatly prolonged, which might enhance tumor accumulation. After administration intravenously, 5-FA was rapidly eliminated from the blood circulation, which led to a complete removal at 6~8 h after administration, whereas the elimination rate of 5-FA-PAE was much lower than that of 5-FA, and the blood retention time of this macromolecular prodrug reached more than 96 h (Figure 3). The detailed plasma concentration of 5-FA and 5-FA-PAE at different time points are shown in Table S2 in file SI. Some pharmacokinetic parameters, such as the area under the curve (AUC), the mean retention time (MRT) and the elimination half-life ($t_{1/2}$) of 5-FA-PAE were much higher than those of 5-FA, *i.e.*, 25.6 times for AUC (546.6 ± 36.7 μg/ml ·h vs 21.37 ± 4.36 μg/ml ·h), 11.7 times for MRT (7.962 ± 0.400 h vs 0.679 ± 0.142 h) and 14.4 times for $t_{1/2}$ (22.10 ± 5.92 h vs 1.538 ± 0.419 h), indicating a much longer blood circulation times and a remarkably enhanced bioavailability of the macromolecular prodrug (Table 3). Meanwhile, the amount of 5-FA released from 5-FA-PAE in rat plasma was determined. Although the total amount of 5-FA-PAE in rat plasma was significantly higher than that of 5-FA, the concentration of released 5-FA from 5-FA-PAE was not as much as 5-FA. It was lower than the 5-FA group within 30 min after administration and then increased slightly afterwards (Table S2 in file SI). This may

Table 2. The number of white blood cells in mice administered with saline, 5-Fu, 5-FA, PAE or 5-FA-PAE ($\times 10^9$/L).

	1 day before injection	1 day after injection	4 days after injection	7 days after injection	10 days after injection
saline	9.77±1.99	8.86±2.79	11.19±6.78	12.24±4.37	12.06±7.58
5-FA-PAE	9.35±1.39	8.73±1.90	11.73±5.44	12.00±2.02	12.52±3.78
5-FA	9.13±2.23	8.99±1.86	10.32±5.71	10.24±4.50	11.55±3.62
PAE	9.54±1.64	8.46±1.85	9.85±3.09	10.74±5.13	11.93±3.40
5-Fu	9.55±1.28	5.39±2.17*	6.84±5.76	7.34±2.82	8.59±2.39

Each value represents the mean ± SD (n = 12).
*$p < 0.05$ vs. 5-Fu, 1 day before injection.

A

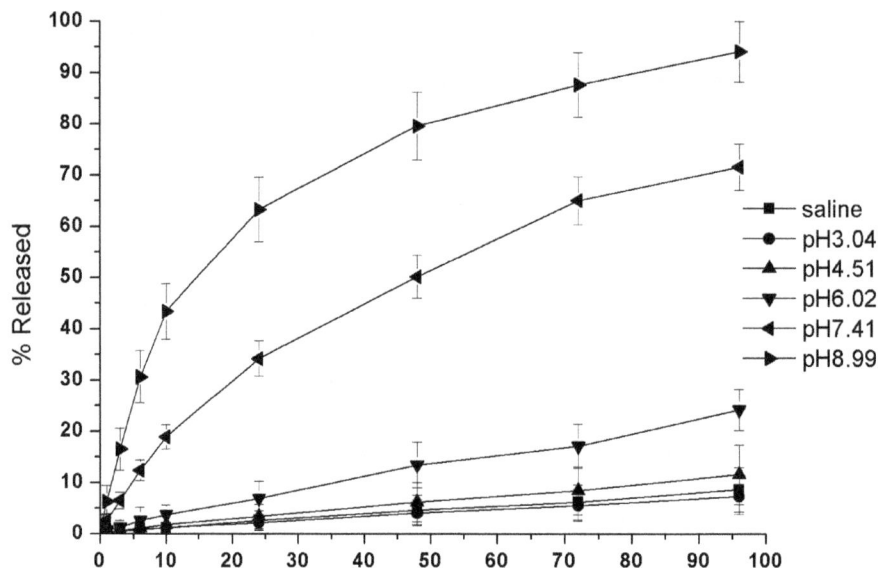

B

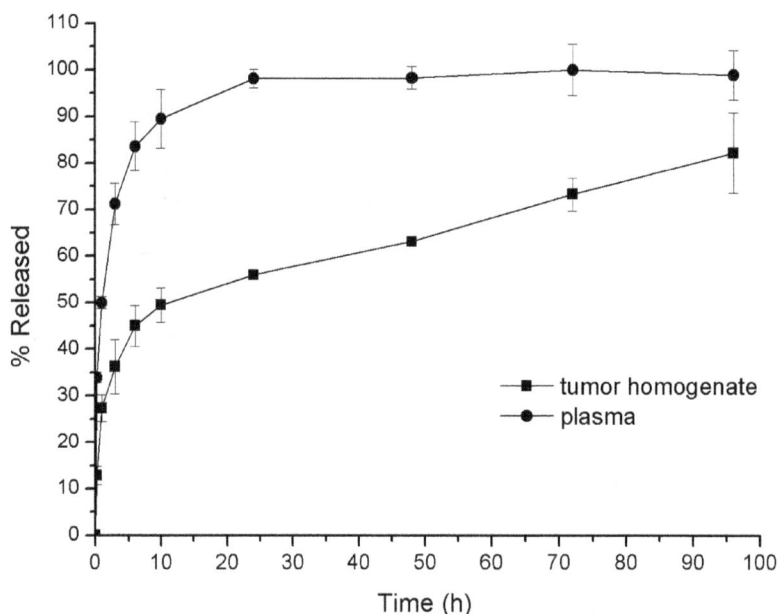

Figure 2. *In vitro* **drug release of 5-FA-PAE.** (A) Drug release profiles of 5-FA-PAE in PBS and saline. 100 µl 5-PA-PAE was added to preheated release media (PBS of different pH values or saline) and incubated at 37°C with stirring. Samples were collected at fixed time intervals, acidified by hydrochloric acid (1 M) and analyzed by HPLC. (B) Drug release profiles of 5-FA-PAE in murine tumor homogenate and plasma. The samples from mouse plasma and tumor homogenate were obtained in duplicate at each time point (100 µl each). For hydrolysis, 100 µl sodium hydroxide (1 M) were added to samples followed by 100 µl hydrochloric acid (1 M). The other group was not subjected to hydrolysis by substituting sodium hydroxide solution with saline and acidifying with 50 µl hydrochloric acid. The differences of 5-FA in the two groups at the same time point was the unreleased 5-FA in each sample. Each value represents the mean $\pm$ SD (n = 3).

have an impact on the antitumor efficacy of 5-FA-PAE, but could avoid certain possible side effects.

Due to the obvious discrepancy of retention time between 5-FA and 5-FA-PAE, two sets of different time points were adopted to fully describe the *in vivo* fate of 5-FA and 5-FA-PAE. The first time point for 5-FA and 5-FA-PAE was 1 min and 5 min after administration, respectively.

In the *in vitro* release study, about 98% of 5-FA was released from 5-FA-PAE in plasma at 24 h, in other words, 2% 5-FA-PAE remained intact, while in the pharmacokinetics study, the concentration of unreleased 5-FA-PAE was 228.276 ± 5.441 µg/ml 5 min after administration (the difference between total concentration of 5-FA-PAE and free 5-FA released from 5-FA-PAE), and decreased to 2.439 ± 0.258 at 24 h (about 1.1% of the

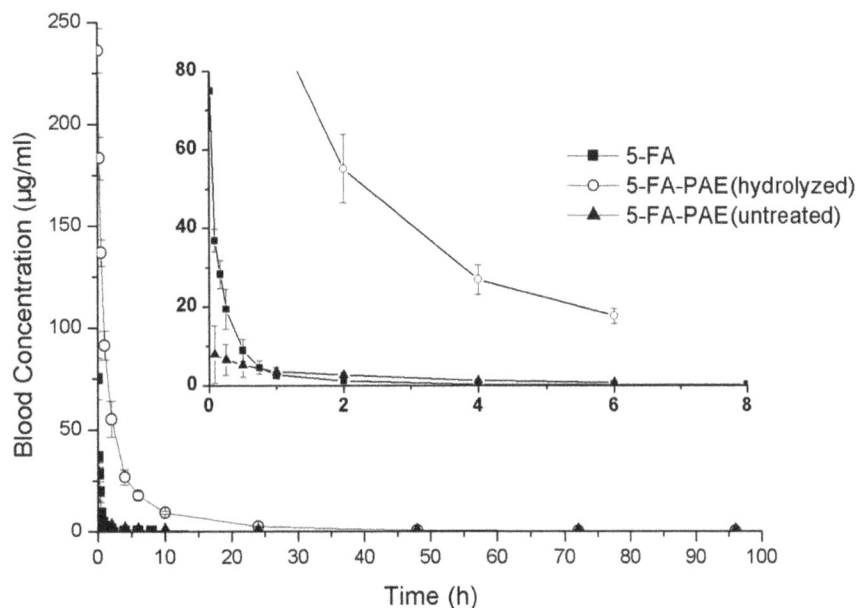

Figure 3. Pharmacokinetics of 5-FA and 5-FA-PAE after _i.v._ injection. The control group and the test groups were administered intravenously with 20 mg/kg of 5-FA or 189 mg/kg of 5-FA-PAE (equivalent to 20 mg/kg of 5-FA) dissolved in physiological saline, respectively. Each plasma sample of the 5-FA-PAE group was divided into two portions (treated as hydrolyzed and unhydrolyzed), which were analyzed by HPLC to determine the plasma concentrations of released 5-FA and total 5-FA of the conjugate whereas the plasma samples of the control group were treated as unhydrolyzed samples. Each value represents the mean $\pm$ standard deviation (n = 6).

concentration at 5 min), which is consistent with the previous _in vitro_ release study. Comparing the concentration of the free 5-FA of unhydrolyzed and hydrolyzed 5-FA-PAE group, it can be concluded that the unreleased 5-FA-PAE was intact in the blood circulation, which could accumulate in tumor tissue in the form of prodrug and then slowly release 5-FA at the tumor site to achieve antitumor effect. 5-FA was shown to be rapidly eliminated from blood, while after conjugation with PAE, the retention time was significantly prolonged, which may be attributed to a protective role of PEG. Thus, the prolonged retention time of 5-FA not only extended the duration time and enhanced the bioavailability, but also improved the delivery of macromolecular drugs to a tumor.

In vivo distribution

Small molecular drugs eliminate quickly after intravenous administration, which could distribute them to normal tissues through capillaries nonspecifically. To analyze the _in vivo_ biodistribution of 5-FA-PAE, the murine hepatic cancer cell line (H22) was used to establish the tumor-bearing animal model. The hepatoma H22 model has been widely use as a tumor model in the study of antitumor drugs and its mechanism. Generally, it is believed that the orthotopic tumor can better simulate the pathologic process of tumor development. However, due to the high mortality rate of animals and the complexity of operation, we

Table 3. Pharmacokinetic parameters of 5-FA and 5-FA-PAE after i.v. injection in rats.

Parameters	Unit	5-FA	5-FA-PAE
AUC $_{0-t}$	µg/ml·h	21.37±4.36	546.6±36.7
AUC $_{0-\infty}$	µg/ml·h	21.63±4.47	551.5±35.0
MRT $_{0-t}$	h	0.679±0.142	7.962±0.400
MRT $_{0-\infty}$	h	0.795±0.240	9.072±0.513
VRT $_{0-t}$	h^2	1.519±0.326	190.2±19.7
VRT $_{0-\infty}$	h^2	2.703±1.558	335.8±79.4
t$_{1/2}$	h	1.538±0.419	22.10±5.92
T$_{max}$	h	0.0167±0	0.097±0.034
V	ml/g	2.107±0.620	1.172±0.358
Cl	ml/g/h	0.967±0.259	0.036±0.002
C$_{max}$	µg/ml	74.92±10.16	232.4±13.5

AUC, area under the plasma concentration−time curve; MRT, mean residence time; VRT, variance of mean residence time; t$_{1/2}$: elimination half life; T$_{max}$, time of maximum concentration; V, apparent volume of distribution; CL, clearance; Cmax, the maximum of 5-FA concentration in plasma.
Each value represents the mean $\pm$ SD (n = 5).

A

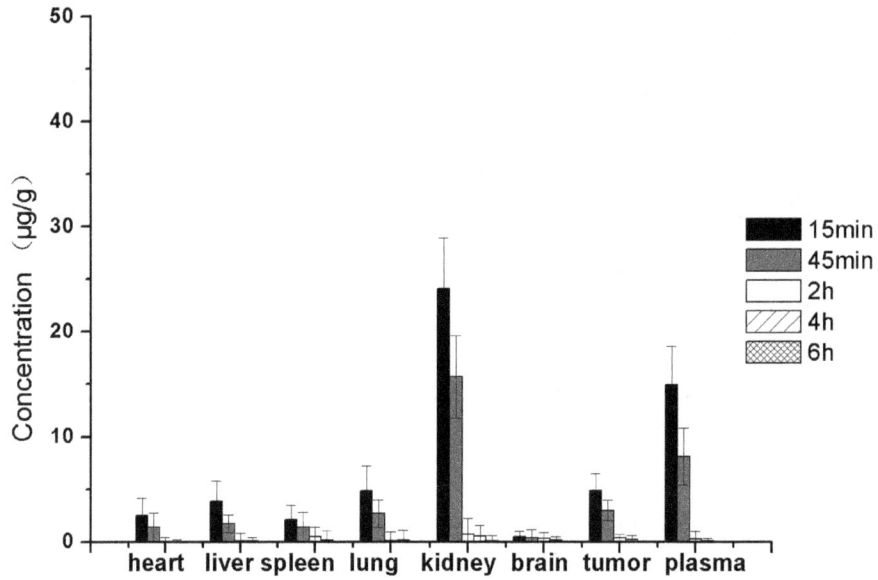

B

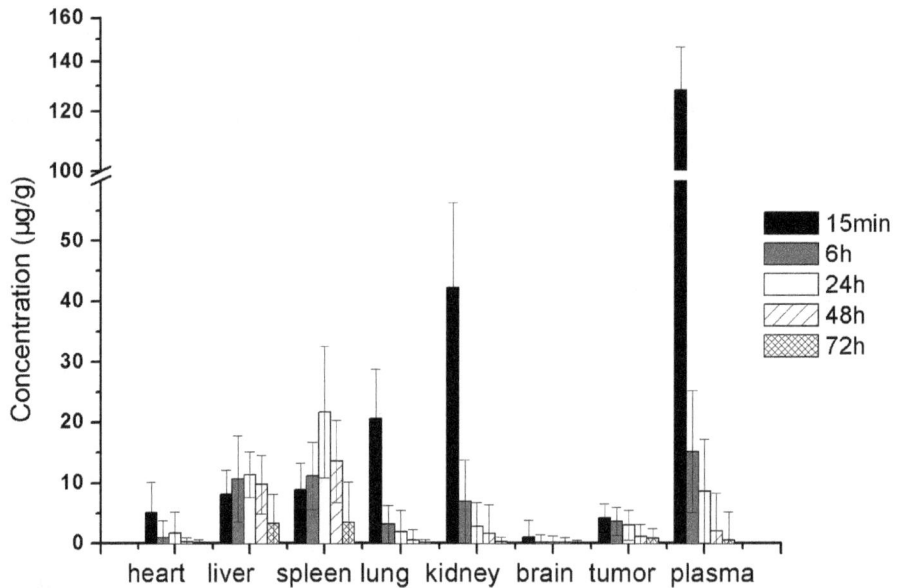

Figure 4. Biodistribution of 5-FA (A) and 5-FA-PAE (B) after *i.v.* injection. The tumor-bearing animal model was established by subcutaneous injection of H22 cells into Kunming mice. The control group and the test groups were administered intravenously with 20 mg/kg of 5-FA or 5-FA-PAE (equivalent to 20 mg/kg of 5-FA), respectively. The mice were exsanguinated and sacrificed at predetermined time points. Tissues (heart, liver, spleen, lung, kidney, brain and tumor) were collected, weighed and homogenized with two fold concentrated physiological saline. The samples of the test group were treated as hydrolyzed samples, whereas those of the control group were treated as unhydrolyzed samples. All data are presented as the concentration of 5-FA. Each value represents the mean ± standard deviation (n = 6).

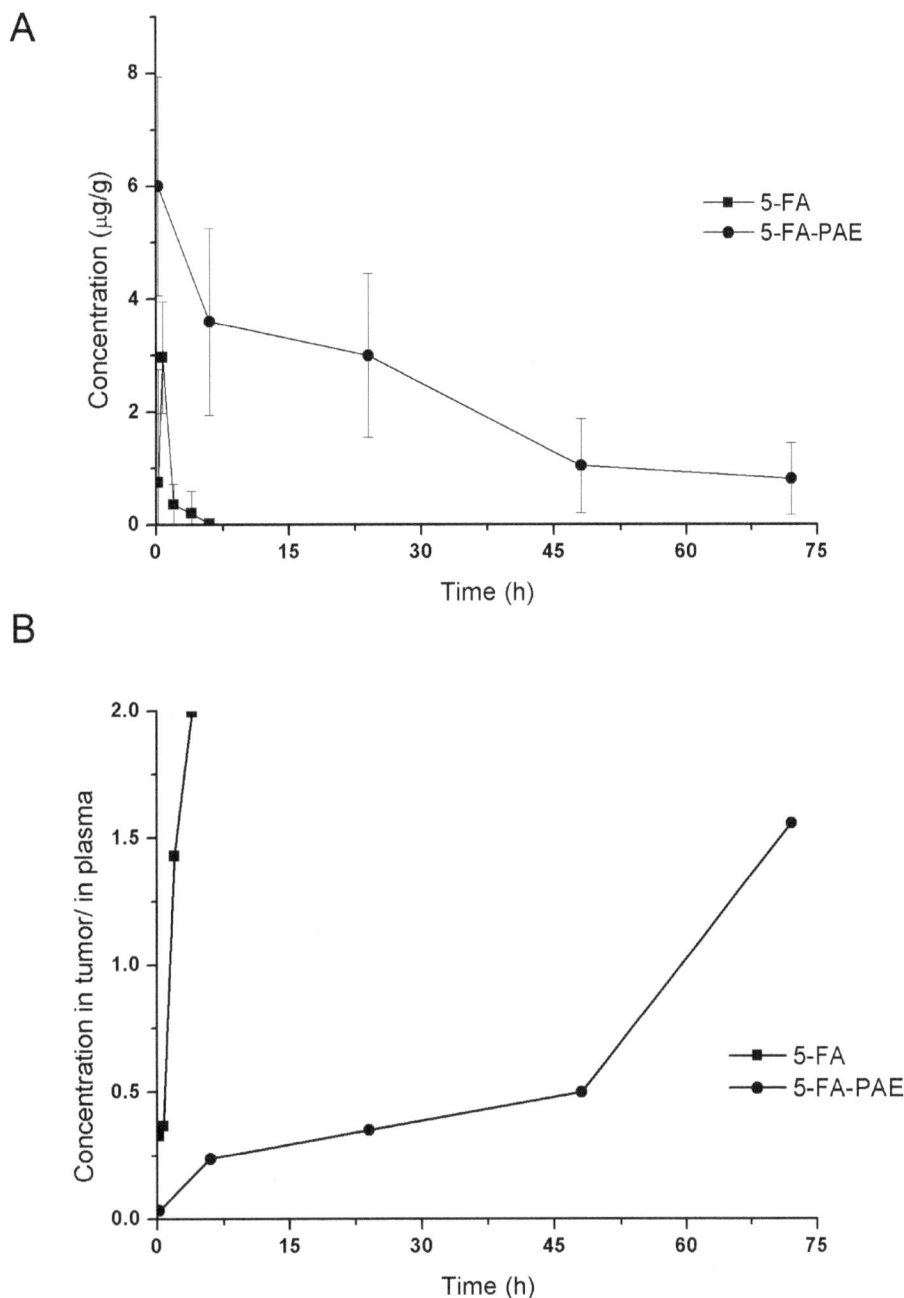

Figure 5. Drug concentration in tumor and plasma. The tumor-bearing mice model was described in the "*In vivo* biodistribution" section. The control group and the test groups were administered intravenously with 20 mg/kg of 5-FA and 5-FA-PAE (equivalent to 20 mg/kg of 5-FA), respectively. (A) Drug concentration of 5-FA and conjugated 5-FA-PAE in tumor at different time points. (B) Ratio of drug concentration in tumor vs. that in plasma of 5-FA and conjugated 5-FA-PAE.

adopted the ectopic model. After intravenous injection, at all time points, the concentration of 5-FA in kidney was significantly higher than other organs and in the tumor, suggesting that renal excretion was the major pathway of 5-FA elimination from the body. Other than kidney, 5-FA did not show any specificity in distribution with similar drug concentrations in heart, liver, spleen, lung and tumor. 15 min after the intravenous injection of 5-FA-PAE, the plasma concentration was the highest of all samples (128.1±18.3 μg/g). However, as the time increased, the plasma concentration of 5-FA-PAE decreased rapidly, dropping to

8,57±3.33 μg/g at 24 h, while the concentration in liver and spleen increased gradually and peaked at 24 h (11.35±3.78 μg/g in liver and 21.68±10.83 μg/g in spleen). 5-FA-PAE was detectable in all organs and tumor at 72 h after injection (consistent with the pharmacokinetics study), indicating that the retention time of 5-FA-PAE was longer than 5-FA (Fig. 4A and 4B).

The concentration of 5-FA and 5-FA-PAE in tumor is shown in Fig 5A. The concentration of 5-FA decreased rapidly after administration and was undetectable after 6 h. Though the

A

B

saline   5-FA-PAE   5-FA   5-FU

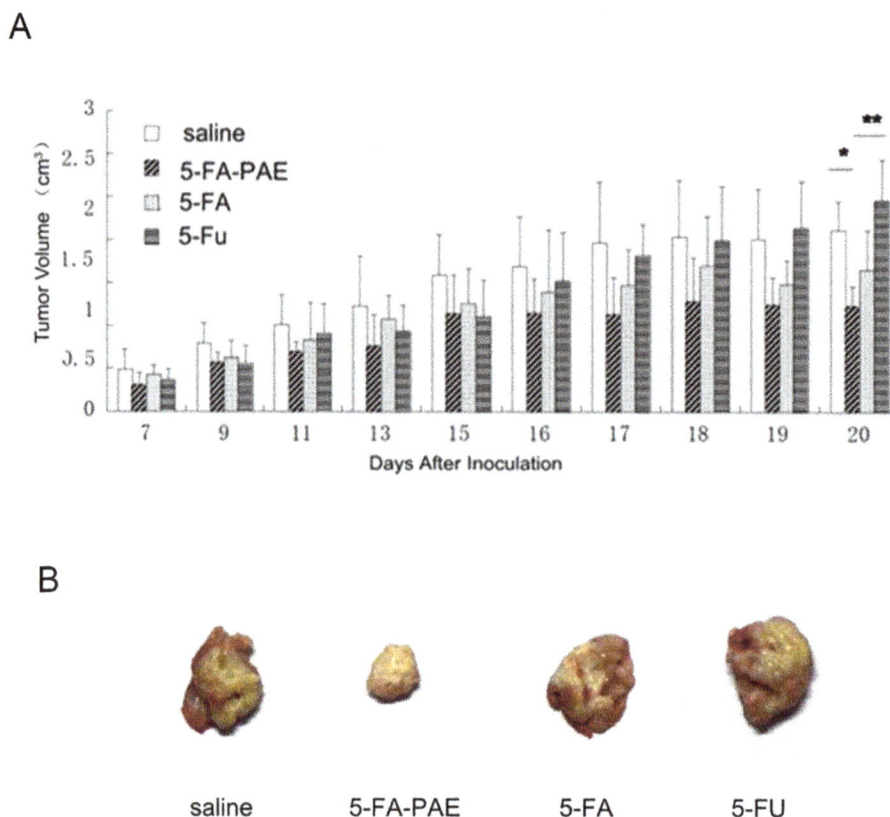

Figure 6. The antitumor effects on tumor-bearing mice. Mice were i.v injected with saline (20 mg/kg, 0.160 mmol/kg), 5-FA-PAE (284 mg/kg, 0.160 mmol/kg), 5-FA (30 mg/kg, 0.160 mmol/kg) or 5-Fu (20.47 mg/kg, 0.160 mmol/kg) on day 3, 5, 7, 9, 11, 13 and 15 after inoculation of H22 cells. On day 20, mice were sacrificed. Tumors and organs were removed and weighed. (A) The tumor volumes after inoculation (n = 6–12). * $p < 0.05$, ** $p < 0.01$. (B) Images of tumors in tumor-bearing mice on day 20 after inoculation of tumor cells (n = 6).

maximum concentration of 5-FA-PAE was slightly lower than 5-FA at 15 min after injection (4.22 ± 2.3 µg/g for 5-FA-PAE and 4.86 ± 1.62 µg/g for 5-FA), the concentration of 5-FA-PAE remained at a relatively high level and lasted for 72 h, indicating that 5-FA-PAE could slowly release 5-FA in the tumor and exert an antitumor effect. The concentration in the tumor vs. those in plasma of 5-FA-PAE and 5-FA is displayed in Fig. 5B. 45 min after administration, the concentration of 5-FA in tumor was lower than that in plasma, and then increased rapidly afterwards. 4 h after injection, the ratio of tumor/plasma concentration reached 1.99, suggesting that 5-FA could distribute from plasma to tumor

within a short time, and that the clearance rate of 5-FA in plasma was higher than that in the tumor. 6 h after administration, the 5-FA concentration was almost undetectable in both plasma and tumor. The ratio of tumor/plasma concentration of 5-FA-PAE increased steadily within 48 h after injection and was lower than 0.5. Between 48 h to 72 h, the ratio increased quickly and reached 1.56 at 72 h, indicating that the clearance of 5-FA-PAE from tumor was much lower than that from the plasma. These results indicated that the amount of 5-FA-PAE in tumor lasted longer compared with that of 5-FA, exhibiting a sustained-release profile.

Table 4. Tumor weight and tumor control rate of mice administrated with saline, 5-Fu, 5-FA or 5-FA-PAE.

Treatment	Tumor weight (g)	Tumor control rate (%)
saline	2.229 ± 0.521	-
5-FA-PAE	1.072 ± 0.249 **	$51.9 \pm 11.2^{\Delta}$
5-FA	1.449 ± 0.392 *	$35.0 \pm 17.6^{\Delta}$
5-Fu	2.383 ± 0.841	-6.9 ± 37.7

*$p < 0.05$ vs. saline group.
**$p < 0.01$ vs. saline group.
$^{\Delta}p < 0.05$ vs. 5-Fu group.
Each value represents the mean ± SD (n = 6).

Table 5. The organ/body weight index of mice administrated with saline, 5-Fu, 5-FA or 5-FA-PAE.

Tissue	saline	5-FA-PAE	5-FA	5-Fu
Heart	0.440±0.047	0.431±0.042	0.443±0.031	0.424±0.038
Liver	5.643±0.291	6.255±1.023	5.737±1.068	5.601±0.897
Spleen	1.226±0.390	1.360±0.543	1.398±0.478	1.264±0.694
Lung	0.978±0.236	0.955±0.141	1.068±0.407	0.900±0.109
Kidney	1.368±0.131	1.377±0.083	1.426±0.113	1.298±0.089
Brain	1.355±0.110	1.317±0.203	1.421±0.302	1.452±0.308
Thymus	0.192±0.097	0.261±0.070	0.221±0.155	0.167±0.086
Tumor	7.088±1.961	3.381±1.224*$^\Delta$	4.957±2.336	8.816±3.578

*$p<0.05$ vs. saline group.
$^\Delta p<0.05$ vs. 5-Fu group.
Each value represents the mean ± SD (n = 6).

Though the initial concentration and tumor/blood concentration ratio of 5-FA were higher than 5-FA-PAE, a high elimination rate of 5-FA severely limited its therapeutic effect in clinic. In comparison, the concentration of 5-FA-PAE in the tumor could be maintained at a relatively high level, which lasted for more than 70 h, despite the large variation (probably due to inter-individual difference). Similarly, the tumor/blood concentration ratio of 5-FA-PAE showed a gradually increasing trend.

Antitumor effect in tumor-bearing mice

5-Fu is the first-choice antimetabolite in the treatment of colon cancer and colorectal cancer. 5-FA, a derivative of 5-Fu, has been reported to be effective and safe [56–59]. To address the antitumor activity of the prodrug, 5-FA and 5-Fu were both used as controls. In the pharmacokinetics studies of anticancer drugs, two dosing regimens are commonly used. One is the preventive administration strategy in which drugs are administered at the beginning of the tumor growth. The other one is the therapeutic administration with drugs administered when the tumor growth reached a certain size. Since the relatively high mortality rate of the H22 tumor model in the later period of this experiment, we adopted a prophylactic administration scheme, i.e. 72 h after inoculation, mice with no signs of tumor growth were excluded from this experiment. Based on the pharmacokinetics and biodistribution results, we administered the drugs every other day (from day 3 to day 15 after inoculation). The antitumor effect of 5-FA-PAE was assessed by analyzing tumor volume, tumor control rate and the organ/body weight index of tumor-bearing mice. From the beginning of administration, the tumor volume of 5-FA-PAE group was smaller than that of the saline group, showing the highest antitumor activity (Figure 6A and 6B). The 5-FA and 5-Fu groups also displayed some antitumor effect. However, after the last administration on day 15, the tumor volume of these two groups increased obviously, while the tumor size of the 5-FA-PAE group did not, which suggested that the antitumor activity of 5-FA-PAE could last for a longer time. This is compatible with the pharmacokinetics results in which 5-FA-PAE showed a much longer retention time than that of 5-FA. 20 days after inoculation, the average tumor volume of 5-FA-PAE group was significantly smaller than that of the 5-Fu and saline groups ($p<0.01$). However, no significant differences were observed between the 5-FA and 5-FA-PAE groups. This may be due to the large variation of the 5-FA group.

Though the tumor control rates of the 5-FA-PAE and 5-FA groups were not significantly different ($p>0.05$), the tumor control rates of the 5-FA-PAE group (51.9±11.2%) and the 5-FA group (35.0±17.6%) were significantly higher than that of the 5-Fu and saline groups (Table 4). Since the tumor growth can affect the weight of normal organs, the organ/body weight index was used to assess the impact. The tumor/body index of the 5-FA-PAE (3.381±1.224) group was much lower than those of the 5-Fu (8.816±3.578) and saline groups (7.088±1.961, $p<0.05$, Table 5). No significant differences were observed in other organ/body indices.

Owing to the conjugation with PEG, 5-FA-PAE exhibited a longer retention time, which led to a long-lasting antitumor effect. Notably, during the administration period, the death rate in the tumor-bearing mice of the 5-FA-PAE group is relatively high. This is probably due to the tumor growth and the toxicity of 5-FA-PAE, which is also a drawback of our present regimen and needs further refinement. However, after administration of all doses, no more deaths were observed in the 5-FA-PAE group, indicating that the toxicity caused by repeated administration of 5-FA-PAE was reversible. While in the 5-FA and 5-Fu groups, large number of animal deaths were observed after all administrations, suggesting a shorter duration of their antitumor effect.

Conclusion

To solve the paradox of drug loading and the molecular weight of PEG, we synthesized a PEG multi-hydroxyl derivative (PAE). PAE was coupled with 5-FA via ester bonds to afford 5-FA-PAE, and the drug loading efficiency was shown to be 10.8-fold higher than using unmodified PEG. Besides, the retention time and bioavailability of 5-FA-PAE were greatly improved compared to 5-FA, showing a prolonged half-life and improved antitumor efficacy *in vivo*. Owing to the improved drug loading efficiency and prolonged half-life, the multi-hydroxyl PEG derivative PAE proves to be an efficient carrier for 5-Fu. Future study should focus on further improving the tumor-targeting efficiency and the antitumor effect of 5-FA-PAE while reducing its toxicity. This paper provides some insights for the future development of antitumor drugs using PEG as a drug carrier.

Supporting Information

File S1 Supporting files. Figure S1, Identification of different polymers. The ^{1}H-NMR spectra of 5-Fu (A), 5-FA (B), PEG (C), the polymeric carrier PAE (D) and the prodrug 5-FA-PAE (E). **Table S1**, The number of blood platelets in mice administered with saline, 5-Fu, 5-FA, PAE or 5-FA-PAE. ($\times 10^9$/

L). **Table S2**, Plasma concentration of 5-FA and 5-FA-PAE at different time points.

Author Contributions

Conceived and designed the experiments: ZL XS TG ZZ. Performed the experiments: ZL. Analyzed the data: ML. Wrote the paper: ML.

References

1. Sarkar FH (2010) Recent trends in anti-cancer drug discovery. Mini Rev Med Chem 10: 357–358.
2. Na Y (2009) Recent cancer drug development with xanthone structures. J Pharm Pharmacol 61: 707–712.
3. Meada H (2001) SMANCS and polymer-conjugates macromolecular drug: advantages in cancer chemotherapy. Adv Drug Deliv Rev 46: 169–185.
4. Dang CT (2006) Drug treatments for adjuvant chemotherapy in breast cancer: recent trials and future directions. Expert Rev Anticancer Ther 6: 427–436.
5. Thompson N, Lyons J (2005) Recent progress in targeting the Raf/MEK/ERK pathway with inhibitors in cancer drug discovery. Curr Opin Pharmacol 5: 350–356.
6. Kelloff GJ, Boone CW, Malone W, Steele V (1993) Recent results in preclinical and clinical drug development of chemopreventive agents at the National Cancer Institute. Basic Life Sci 61: 373–386.
7. Sartor O, Halstead M, Katz L (2010) Improving outcomes with recent advances in chemotherapy for castrate-resistant prostate cancer. Clin Genitourin Cancer 8: 23–28.
8. Deeken JF, Figg WD, Bates SE, Sparreboom A (2007) Toward individualized treatment: prediction of anticancer drug disposition and toxicity with pharmacogenetics. Anti-cancer Drugs 18: 111–126.
9. Kintzel PE, Dorr RT (1995) Anticancer drug renal toxicity and elimination: dosing guidelines for altered renal function. Cancer Treat Rev 21: 33–64.
10. Duschinsky R, Pleven E, Heidelberger C (1957) The synthesis of 5-fluoropyrimidines. J Chem Soc 79: 4559–4560.
11. Ogiso T, Noda N, Asai N, Kato Y (1976) Antitumor agents. I. Effect of 5-fluorouracil and cyclophosphamide on liver microsomes and thymus of rat. Jpn J Pharmacol 26: 445–453.
12. Ogiso T, Noda N, Masuda H, Kato Y (1978) Antitumor agents. II. Effect of 5-fluorouracil and cyclophosphamide on immunological parameters and liver microsomes of tumor-bearing rats. Jpn J Pharmacol 28: 175–183.
13. Parker WB, Cheng YC (1990) Metabolism and mechanism of action of 5-fluorouracil. Pharmacol Ther 48: 381–395.
14. Macdonald JS (1999) Toxicity of 5-fluorouracil. Oncology 13: 33–34.
15. Shuey DL, Setzer RW, Lau C, Zucker RM, Elstein KH, et al. (1995) Biological modeling of 5-fluorouracil developmental toxicity. Toxicology 102: 207–213.
16. Van Kuilenburg AB, Meinsma R, Van Gennip AH (2004) Pyrimidine degradation defects and severe 5-fluorouracil toxicity. Nucleosides, Nucleotides and Nucleic Acids 23: 1371–1375.
17. Iyer L, Ratain MJ (1999) 5-fluorouracil pharmacokinetics: causes for variability and strategies for modulation in cancer chemotherapy. Cancer Invest 17: 494–506.
18. Milano G, Chamorey AL (2002) Clinical pharmacokinetics of 5-fluorouracil with consideration of chronopharmacokinetics. Chronobiol Int 19: 177–189.
19. Schalhorn A, Kühl M (1992) Clinical pharmacokinetics of fluorouracil and folinic acid. Semin Oncol 19: 82–92.
20. Pazdur R, Hoff PM, Medgyesy D, Royce M, Brito R (1998) The oral fluorouracil prodrugs. Oncology 12: 48–51.
21. Malet-Martino M, Martino R (2002) Clinical studies of three oral prodrugs of 5-fluorouracil (capecitabine, UFT, S-1): a review. Oncologist 7: 288–323.
22. Wang JX, Sun X, Zhang ZR (2002) Enhanced brain targeting by synthesis of 3′,5′-dioctanoyl-5-fluoro-2′-deoxyuridine and incorporation into solid lipid nanoparticles. Eur J Pharm Biopharm 54: 285–290.
23. Arias JL (2008) Novel strategies to improve the anticancer action of 5-fluorouracil by using drug delivery systems. Molecules 13: 2340–2369.
24. Menei P (1999) Local and sustained delivery of 5-Fluorouracil from biodegradable microspheres for the radiosensitization of glioblastoma. Cancer 86: 325–330.
25. Gupta Y, Jain A, Jain P, Jain SK (2007) Design and development of folate appended liposomes for enhanced delivery of 5-FU to tumor cells. J.Drug Targeting 15: 231–240.
26. Azori M (1987) Polymeric prodrugs. Crit Rev Ther Drug Carrier Syst 4: 39–65.
27. Hoste K, De Winne K, Schacht E (2004) Polymeric prodrugs. Int J Pharm 277: 119–131.
28. D'Souza AJM, Topp EM (2004) Release from polymeric prodrugs: linkages and their degradation. J Pharm Sci 93: 1962–1979.
29. Takakura Y, Hashida M (1995) Macromolecular drug carrier systems in cancer chemotherapy: macromolecular prodrugs. Crit Rev Oncol Hematol 18: 207–231.
30. Onishi H, Machida Y (2008) In vitro and in vivo evaluation of microparticulate drug delivery systems composed of macromolecular prodrugs. Molecules 13: 2136–2155.
31. Huang Y, Park YS, Wang J, Moon C, Kwon YM, et al (2010) ATTEMPTS system: a macromolecular prodrug strategy for cancer drug delivery. Curr Pharm Des 16: 2369–2376.
32. Goh PP, Sze DM, Roufogalis BD (2007) Molecular and cellular regulators of cancer angiogenesis. Curr Cancer Drug Targets 7: 743–758.
33. Maeda H, Fang J, Inutsuka T, Kitamono Y (2003) Vascular permeability enhancement in solid tumor: various factors, mechanisms involved and its implications. Int Immunopharmacol 3: 319–328.
34. Maeda H, Wu J, Sawa T, Matsumura Y, Hori K (2000) Tumor vascular permeability and the EPR effect in macromolecular therapeutics: a review. J Control Release 65: 271–284.
35. Maeda H, Bharate GY, Daruwalla J (2009) Polymeric drugs for efficient tumor-targeted drug delivery based on EPR-effect. Eur J Pharm Biopharm 71: 409–419.
36. Sawa T, Wu J, Akaike T, Maeda H (2000) Tumor-targeting chemotherapy by a xanthine oxidase-polymer conjugate that generates oxygen-free radicals in tumor tissue. Cancer Res 60: 666–671.
37. Pasut G, Veronese FM (2007) Polymer-drug conjugation, recent achievements and general strategies. Prog Polym Sci 32: 933–961.
38. Veronese FM, Harris JM (2002) Theme issue on "Peptide and Protein Pegylation I". Adv Drug Deliv Rev 54: 453–606.
39. Zhao H, Rubio B, Sapra P, Wu D, Reddy P, et al (2008) Novel prodrugs of SN38 using multiarm poly(ethylene glycol) linkers. Bioconjug Chem 19: 849–859.
40. Rowinsky EK, Rizzo J, Ochoa L, Takimoto CH, Forouzesh B, et al. (2003) A phase I and pharmacokinetic study of pegylated camptothecin as a 1-hour infusion every 3 weeks in pantients with advanced solid malignancies. J Clin Oncol 21: 148–157.
41. Guo Z, Wheler JJ, Naing A, Mani S, Goel S, et al. (2008) Clinical pharmacokinetics (PK) of EZN-2208, a novel anticancer agent, in patients (pts) with advanced malignancies: a phase I, first-in-human, dose-escalation study. J Clin Oncol 26: 2556.
42. Ton NC, Parker GJ, Jackson A, Mullamitha S, Buonaccorsi GA, et al. (2007) Phase I evaluation of CDP791, a PEGylated di-Fab' conjugate that binds vascular endothelial growth factor receptor 2. Clin Cancer Res 13: 7113–7118.
43. Michallet M, Maloisel F, Delain M, Hellmann A, Rosas A, et al. (2004) Pegylated recombinant interferon-a lpha-2b vs recombinant interferon-alpha-2b for the initial treatment of chronic-phase chronic myelogenous leukemia: a phase III study. Leukemia 18: 309–315.
44. Hwu WJ, Panageas KS, Menell JH, Lamb LA, Aird S, et al. (2006) Phase II study of temozolomide plus pegylated interferon-alpha-2b for metastatic melanoma. Cancer 106: 2445–2451.
45. Pasut G, Veronese FM (2009) PEG conjugates in clinical development or use as anticancer agents: an overview. Adv Drug Deliv Rev 61: 1177–1188.
46. Koyama Y, Umehara M, Mizuno A, Itaba M, Yasukouchi T, et al. (1996) Synthesis of novel poly(ethylene glycol) derivatives having pendant amino groups and aggregating behavior of its mixture with fatty acid in water. Bioconjug Chem 7: 298–301.
47. Burton SC, Harding DRK (1998) Preparation of chromatographic matrices by free radical addition ligand attachment to allyl groups. J Chromatogr A 796: 273–282.
48. Hao AJ, Deng YJ, Li TF, Suo XB, Cao YH, et al. (2006) Degradation kinetics of fluorouracil-acetic-acid-dextran conjugate in aqueous solution. Drug Dev Ind Pharm 32: 757–763.
49. Udo K, Hokonohara K, Motoyama K, Arima H, Hirayama F, et al. (2010) 5-Fluorouracil acetic acid/beta-cyclodextrin conjugates: drug release behavior in enzymatic and rat cecal media. Int J Pharm 388: 95–100.
50. Smyth HF Jr Carpenter CP, Weil CS (1950) The toxicology of the polyethylene glycols. J Am Pharm Assoc 39: 349–354.
51. Richter AW, Akerblom E (1983) Antibodies against polyethylene glycol produced in animals by immunization with monomethoxy polyethylene glycol modified proteins. Int Arch Allergy Appl Immunol 70: 124–131.
52. Zalipsky S, Gilon C, Zilkha A (1983) Attachment of drugs to polyethylene glycols. Eur Polym J 19: 1177–1183.
53. Sheridan W, Menchaca D (1998) Overview of the safety and biologic effects of PEG-rHuMGDF in clinical trials. Stem Cells 16: 193–198.
54. Riebeseel K, Biedermann E, Löser R, Breiter N, Hanselmann R, et al. (2002) Polyethylene glycol conjugates of methotrexate varying in their molecular weight from MW 750 to MW 40000: synthesis, characterization, and structure-activity relationships in vitro and in vivo. Bioconjug Chem 13: 773–785.

55. Greenwald RB, Gilbert CW, Pendri A, Conover CD, Xia J, et al. (1996) Drug delivery systems: water soluble taxol 2'-poly(ethylene glycol) ester prodrugs-design and in vivo effectiveness. Med Chem 39: 424–431.

56. Chung SM, Yoon EJ, Kim SH, Lee MG, Heejoo L, et al. (1991) Pharmacokinetics of 5-fluorouracil after intravenous infusion of 5-fluorouracil-acetic acid-human serum albumin conjugates to rabbits. Int J Pharm 68: 61–68.

57. Zuo D, Jiang T, Guan H, Wang KQ, Qi X, et al. (2001) Synthesis, Structure and Antitumor Activity of Dibutyltin Oxide Complexes with 5-Fluorouracil Derivatives. Crystal Structure of $[(5\text{-Fluorouracil})\text{-}1\text{-CH}_2\text{CH}_2\text{COOSn(n-Bu)}_2]_4O_2$. Molecules 6: 647–654.

58. Kang NI, Lee SM, Maeda M, Ha CS, Cho WJ (2002) Synthesis, antitumour and DNA replication activities of polymers containing vinyl-(5-fluorouracil)-ethanoate. Polym Int 51: 443–449.

59. Yang ZY, Wang LF, Yang XP, Wang DW, Li YM (2000) Pharmacological study on antitumor activity of 5-fluorouracil-1-acetic acid and its rare earth complexes. J Rare Earth 18: 140–143.

15

Alginate Hydrogel Protects Encapsulated Hepatic HuH-7 Cells against Hepatitis C Virus and Other Viral Infections

Nhu-Mai Tran[1], Murielle Dufresne[1]*, François Helle[2], Thomas Walter Hoffmann[2], Catherine François[2], Etienne Brochot[2], Patrick Paullier[1], Cécile Legallais[1], Gilles Duverlie[2], Sandrine Castelain[2]

1 UMR CNRS 7338 Biomechanics and Bioengineering, University of Technology, Compiègne, France, 2 EA4294 Department of Fundamental and Clinical Virology, University of Picardie Jules Verne, Amiens, France

Abstract

Cell microencapsulation in alginate hydrogel has shown interesting applications in regenerative medicine and the biomedical field through implantation of encapsulated tissue or for bioartificial organ development. Although alginate solution is known to have low antiviral activity, the same property regarding alginate gel has not yet been studied. The aim of this work is to investigate the potential protective effect of alginate encapsulation against hepatitis C virus (HCV) infection for a hepatic cell line (HuH-7) normally permissive to the virus. Our results showed that alginate hydrogel protects HuH-7 cells against HCV when the supernatant was loaded with HCV. In addition, alginate hydrogel blocked HCV particle release out of the beads when the HuH-7 cells were previously infected and encapsulated. There was evidence of interaction between the molecules of alginate hydrogel and HCV, which was dose- and incubation time-dependent. The protective efficiency of alginate hydrogel towards HCV infection was confirmed against a variety of viruses, whether or not they were enveloped. This promising interaction between an alginate matrix and viruses, whose chemical mechanisms are discussed, is of great interest for further medical therapeutic applications based on tissue engineering.

Editor: Eve-Isabelle PECHEUR, UMR Inserm U1052/CNRS 5286, France

Funding: The authors would like to thank the FEDER Program and the Picardy Region, France for providing financial support for this project. The funders had no role in study design, data collection and analysis, decision to publish, or preparation of the manuscript.

Competing Interests: The authors have declared that no competing interests exist.

* Email: murielle.dufresne@utc.fr

Introduction

Among marine algae polysaccharide-based biomaterials, alginate is currently used in biomedical and pharmaceutical areas for wound dressing, as an ointment for burns, or as a formulation aid in controlled drug delivery systems [1–3]. Thanks to its biosafety and biocompatibility, alginate is also commonly used for tissue and cell immobilization by means of a bioencapsulation process [4]. Cells are entrapped within spherical alginate beads whose hydrogel structure protects them from mechanical stress while ensuring exchanges of nutrients or waste molecules within the surrounding medium. The immuno-isolation provided by alginate encapsulation is undoubtedly the major advantage of this technology when intended for transplantation or tissue regeneration. In the case of type I diabetes, twenty-five years of preclinical studies have recently made possible significant progress in the implantation of encapsulated Langerhans islets in patients [5]. Compared to other biopolymers, the considerable success of alginate used for microencapsulation relies upon the middle conditions required for the gelation process. Alginate salts, such as sodium-alginate (Na-alg), are composed of residues of *D*-mannuronic acid (M) and *L*-guluronic acid (G) covalently (1–4)-linked in homo- or hetero-blocks, and which have a high affinity for divalent or trivalent ions. Calcium ions interact through ionic crosslinking with the carboxylate groups of monosaccharide residues allowing the formation of a three dimensional (3D) network between polymeric chains, with limited effects on cell viability.

Numerous works described the antiviral activity of algal carbohydrate polymers [6–7] leading to promising therapeutic applications when used either alone or associated with existing antiviral drugs. These polysaccharides are extracted from the cell walls of red, brown or green algae from which they account for more than 50% of the dry weight. Besides their considerable structural diversity, all of these polymers are negatively charged and, in most cases, present a high sulfation level. Their antiviral activities target a broad spectrum of human pathogens including enveloped viruses such as human immunodeficiency virus (HIV) [8–9], herpes simplex virus (HSV) [10], human cytomegalovirus (HCMV), dengue virus [11], and non-enveloped viruses, such as hepatitis A virus (HAV) and human papillomavirus (HPV) [12–13]. Based on their safety and low toxicity, marine polysaccharides are interesting solutions for limiting viral infections in clinical contexts. Although experiences using marine polymers as an orally-delivered agent have been described [14], only a few clinical studies have been conducted so far [15]. The well-known anticoagulant activity of most sulfated polysaccharides, associated with their high molecular weight which is incompatible with free diffusion towards tissues, explains the obstacles to their use as natural compounds in *in vivo* conditions [14,16–17]. Structural modifications by means of chemical or enzymatic processes can be requested to meet clinical constraints [18].

Although alginate antiviral activity is described as low compared to many other marine polysaccharide compounds, we hypothesized that this property could benefit cells entrapped in calcium-alginate (Ca-alg) beads for further use as implanted tissue or organ supply. For this purpose, using a simple extrusion process, we encapsulated human hepatoma-derived cells (HuH-7), a specific cell line which is up to now the most employed cellular model recognized for both its high permissiveness with regard to hepatitis C virus (HCV) infection and its ability to produce and secrete HCV particles [19]. The aim of this study was thus to investigate the potential protective effect of Ca-alg hydrogel encapsulating hepatic cells against HCV infection.

Materials and Methods

Alginate solution

Na-alg from *Macrocystis pyrifera* (brown algae), medium viscosity (Sigma-Aldrich) was used at 1.5% (w/v). Its molecular weight ranged from 80,000 to 120,000 Da, G/M = 33/67, viscosity at 2% = 2000 cP. To prepare the Na-alg solution, the alginate powder was dissolved within a sterile saline solution (154 mM NaCl solution buffered with 10 mM Hepes, pH 7.4). The mixture was subsequently filtered using a 0.2 μm membrane leading to a sterile Na-alg sol.

2D cell cultures

Hepatoma HuH-7 and transduced HuH-7-RFP-NLS-IPS cell lines were used. HuH-7 (RCB1366) cells were kindly provided by Jean Dubuisson (Institut de Biologie de Lille, France) and were plated in 25 cm^2 flasks, cultured in Glutamax-supplemented DMEM with 10% fetal bovine serum. HuH-7-RFP-NLS-IPS cells were obtained by transduction of HuH-7 cells with lentiviral pseudo-particles expressing the RFP-NLS-IPS reporter. Briefly, lentivirus pseudo-particles were generated by co-transfection of 293T cells with TRIP-RFP-NLS-IPS (kindly provided by C.M. Rice, Rockefeller University, New York, USA), HIV gag-pol, and vesicular stomatitis virus envelope protein G (VSV-G) encoding plasmids as described previously [20]. HuH-7 cells were transduced by overnight incubation with lentivirus pseudo-particles at 37°C to obtain cell lines stably expressing the red fluorescent protein (RFP) on the outer membrane of the mitochondria. The translocation of the cleavage product RFP-NLS from the cytoplasm to the nucleus characterized the HCV infected cells. All cells were grown to 80-90% confluence in the same culture conditions before experiments to avoid any discrepancy in cell passage, cell density or medium quality.

Encapsulated cell cultures

Encapsulated cell cultures were established using HuH-7 or HuH-7-RFP-NLS-IPS cells according to previously described techniques [21]. Cell density in the Na-alg sol was 500 000 cells/mL. Droplets of this mixture were obtained by a classical extrusion process with co-axial air flow. The parameters for the encapsulation process, including air and alginate flows, distance between the needle and the gelation bath surface, were experimentally determined to produce spherical droplets. The droplets formed were gelified in a CaCl$_2$ bath (115 mM CaCl$_2$, 154 mM NaCl buffered with 10 mM HEPES) for 15 min at room temperature, leading to ionically crosslinked alginate beads (Ca-alg beads) with an expected diameter of about 600 μm. Following the cell encapsulation stage, various volumes of beads were transferred to tissue culture 6-well plates with 1 mL or 2 mL of complete DMEM medium added on a 3D moving plate. The encapsulated cell cultures were maintained in a 5% CO$_2$ incubator at 37°C.

Under certain conditions, the encapsulated HuH-7 cells were extracted from the beads after degelification based on alginate lyase treatment. Briefly, Ca-alg beads were washed twice with sterile PBS solution and incubated with alginate lyase solution (Sigma, 1 mg/mL) at v/v for 15 min at 37°C. The solution was then neutralized by addition of PBS and centrifuged. The cell sediment was recovered and plated in tissue culture 6-well plates with 2 mL of complete DMEM medium added.

High-resolution cryo-Scanning Electron Microscopy (cryo-SEM)

High-resolution cryo-SEM (Hitachi S4500 field emission gun SEM equipped with a dedicated Polaron LT 7480 cryopreparation device, Orleans University) was used to investigate the 3D structure of the Ca-alg bead network in the absence of cells, as previously described [21]. Briefly, beads from the samples were cryofixed by plunge-freezing them in nitrogen slush at -210°C then fractured with a cold metal rod. The samples were transferred into the SEM chamber, where sublimation of the surface ice formed from the interstitial water of the sample was obtained by progressively increasing the temperature up to about −70°C. The temperature of the sample was then lowered back to about −110°C, making possible complete stabilization of the sample. The observations were performed at 1 kV without any sample coating.

Epifluorescence microscopy

Cell viability within the beads was assessed qualitatively using fluorescence staining with propidium iodide and acridine orange (Sigma Aldrich, France) under a confocal microscope (DMI 6000B, Leica, France). A fluorescence microscope (Nikon Eclipse TE2000U) was used to characterize the infected HuH-7-RFP-NLS-IPS cells, by translocation of the RFP-NLS product from the cytoplasm to the nucleus. Nuclei were counterstained with DAPI.

HCV infection

HuH-7 and HuH-7-RFP-NLS-IPS cells encapsulated in beads or in 2D cultures used as controls were in contact with one of the two following HCV particle types: (i) JFH1-CS-A4 (i24) virus (JFH1 virus), an adapted version of the full-length JFH1 virus (genotype 2a; GenBank access number AB237837; kindly provided by T. Wakita) which contains mutations leading to amino acid changes F172C and P173S at the C-terminus of the core protein [22]. Both mutations have been shown to increase the viral titers [23]; (ii) JFH1-CS-A4-RLuc-TM virus (JFH1-RLuc virus) which contains a *Renilla* luciferase reporter gene as described previously [22].

Encapsulated and 2D cell cultures were incubated with the viral particles for 4h on 3D moving plates, the medium was then discarded and replaced with fresh medium. All experiments to assay HCV particles in the supernatant were performed 72h post-infection.

HCV particle quantification

The HCV particles were detected using different methods to assess viral RNA replication (RNA quantification) or the particle infectivity of JFH1 and JFH1-RLuc by FFU titration and luciferase activity respectively.

- HCV RNA quantification: in this case, the quantification was performed directly in the supernatant of the encapsulated or 2D (control) cell cultures. Briefly, HCV RNA was extracted using the QiaAmp viral RNA mini kit (Qiagen). cDNAs were synthesized using a High Capacity cDNA

Reverse Transcription kit and random hexamers as described by the manufacturer (Applied Biosystems). Amplifications were carried out with the TaqMan Universal PCR master Mix on an ABI 7900HT Sequence Detection System (Applied Biosystems) using primer and probe sets for HCV RNA [24].

- FFU titration: HCV infectious particle detection in the supernatants could be assessed by secondary infection of naive HuH-7-RFP-NLS-IPS cells, cultivated under 2D conditions. Briefly, 2D cell cultures were incubated for 4h with the bead culture supernatant, the medium was then discarded and replaced with fresh medium. Seventy-two hours post-infection, particle infectivity was determined by Focus Forming Unit (FFU) titration. The infected cells were fixed with paraformaldehyde (4%) and checked for fluorescence translocation in the nucleus using a confocal microscope.

- Luciferase activity: in this case, JFH1-CS-A4-RLuc-TM virus particles had to be used for the infection stage. HCV infectious particle detection could then be performed by quantifying luciferase activity in 2D naive HuH-7 cell cultures incubated with the bead culture supernatant. Two dimension cell cultures were incubated for 4h with the bead culture supernatant, the medium was then discarded and replaced with fresh medium. Seventy-two hours post-infection, the cells were lysed by addition of 100 µl of *Renilla* luciferase Assay Lysis Buffer (Promega). Luminescence was measured according to the manufacturer's instructions on a Centro XS3 LB960 luminometer (Berthold Technologies). Fifty microliters of cell lysate were used to determine luciferase activity. Results are expressed as relative light units (RLU) and are reported as the means ± S.D.

Other virus infection

The infectivity of different viruses from the enveloped virus family such as Sindbis virus (50 nm in diameter), and herpes simplex virus type 1 (HSV-1) (140 nm) or the non-enveloped family such as Poliovirus type 1 (30 nm) was assessed on encapsulated HuH-7 cells in alginate beads. The cytopathic effect of these viruses on HuH-7 cells was observed after 48 h post-infection and the virus titration (Tissue culture infectious dose 50% or $TCID_{50}$) was determined using microscopy imaging analysis as previously described [25].

Data analysis

Data are expressed as mean ± standard error of mean value. All results are representative of 3 independent experiments. Statistical analysis was performed using the non-parametric Kruskal-Wallis test in order to compare the differences between the groups.

Results

HuH-7 cell encapsulation into Ca-alg beads

The 3D cell culture was established by encapsulating HuH-7 cells at 500 000 cells/mL of Na-alg as described in the materials and methods section. The isolated cells were found to be homogeneously distributed into beads and maintained high viability post-encapsulation (Fig. 1A). The beads' mean diameter was about 600 µm. The beads showed a porous inner structure with a pore size estimated at 9.5+/−0.34 µm using cryo-SEM (Fig. 1B).

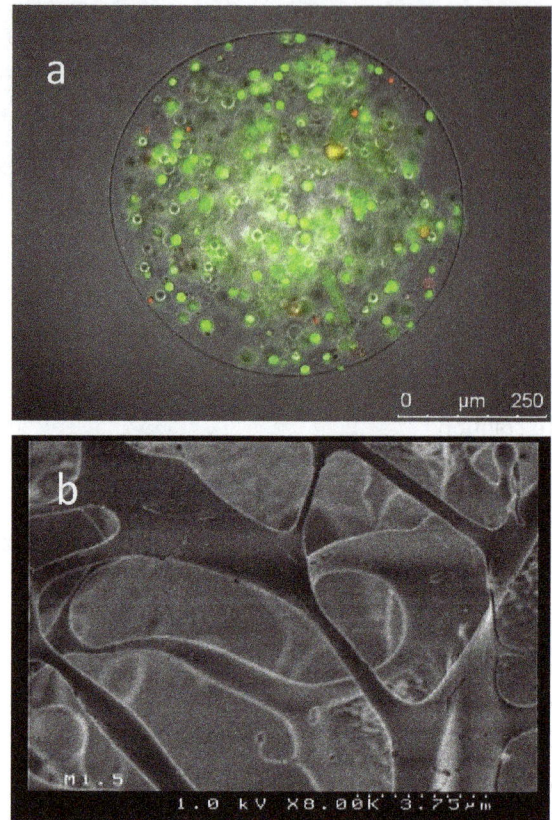

Figure 1. Characterization of HuH-7 cells encapsulated in Ca-alg beads at day 3 in culture. (A) Cell distribution in the Ca-alg beads. Cell viability was assessed using propidium iodide and acridine orange which stained dead and live cells, respectively. Scale bar 250 µm (B) The matrix porosity of Ca-alg beads was visualized by cryoscanning electron microscopy. Scale bar 3.75 µm.

Absence of infection by HCV when HuH-7-RFP-NLS-IPS cells were encapsulated in Ca-alg beads

In these experiments, HuH-7-RFP-NLS-IPS cells were used to characterize the infected cells (Fig. 2A). 48 h after a 4 h incubation period between HCV and Ca-alg bead hosting cells, microscopic visualization of the infected cell foci was performed. Translocation of a cleavage product from the cytoplasm to the nucleus was observed in the control 2D cell cultures, characterized by an overlay of DAPI and RFP fluorescent dyes. Interestingly, an absence of foci in the HuH-7-RFP-NLS-IPS cells was observed in the encapsulated cell system incubated with HCV, the red fluorescence remaining in the cytoplasm (Fig. 2B). To confirm the absence of new HCV cell culture (HCVcc) production in the supernatant of encapsulated HuH-7 cells, after 4 h of JFH1 virus incubation in contact with Ca-alg beads immobilizing HuH-7-RFP-NLS-IPS cells, the medium was removed and replaced by fresh complete DMEM medium. The production of new particles was assessed 72 h post-infection by measuring in the supernatant the amount of HCV RNA expressed as HCV RNA IU/mL (Fig. 2C). The HCV RNA was quantified at very low levels in the supernatant of the Ca-alg encapsulated cells, with no significant difference between the empty Ca-alg beads condition, i.e. beads devoid of cell, unlike the 2D cell cultures used as positive controls, which showed significant differences up to a 6 log fold change between both system cultures ($P<0.0001$). In the same way, no

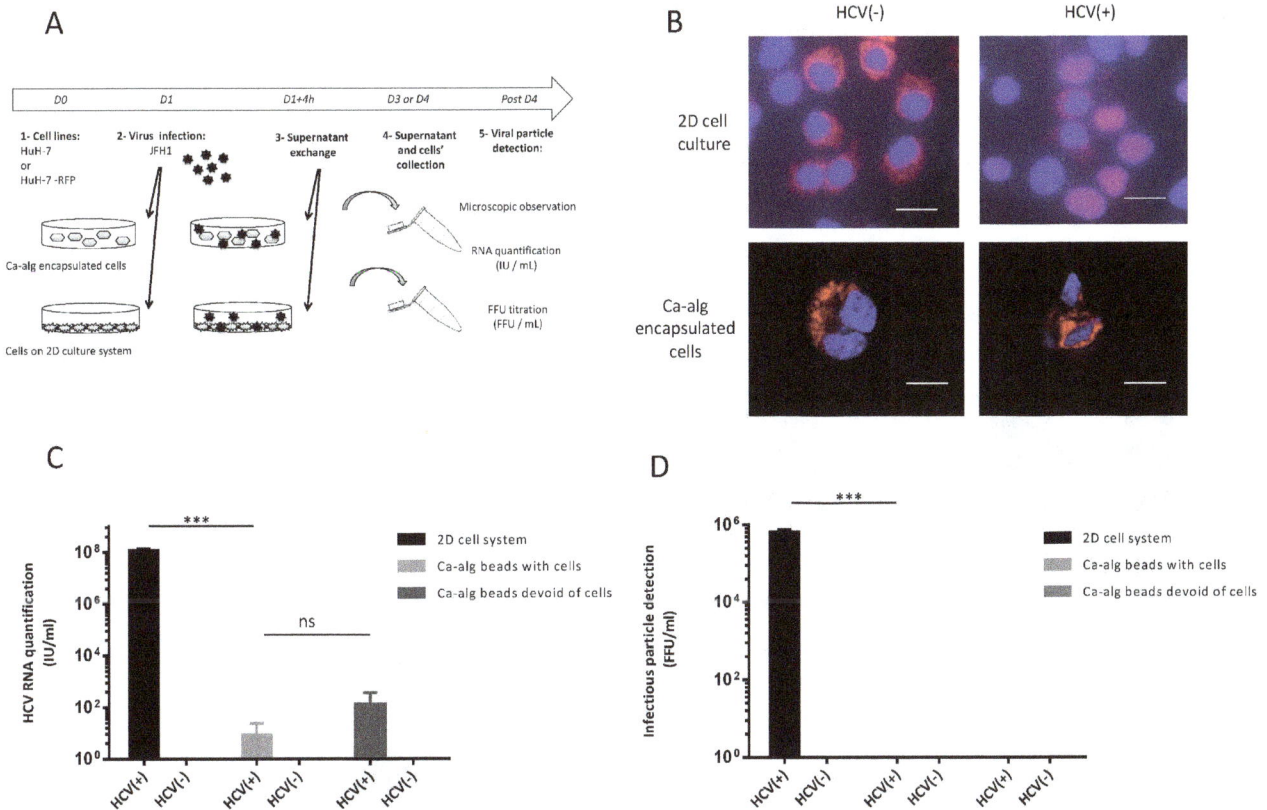

Figure 2. Absence of HCV infection by Ca-alg encapsulated cells. (A) Encapsulated cell cultures were established by encapsulating HuH-7-RFP-NLS-IPS cells within Ca-alg beads (500 000 cells/mL). Following the cell encapsulation stage, 400 μL of beads were transferred to tissue culture 6-well plates with 1 mL of DMEM medium added on 3D moving plates. After 4 h of contact with the JFH1 virus (HCV+) or without (HCV), the medium was removed and replaced with 2 mL of fresh complete DMEM medium. Ca-alg beads devoid of HuH-7 cells were used as controls. (B) Foci of infected cells (in 2D or in beads), identified by translocation of the cleavage product RFP-NLS from cytoplasm to nucleus, were visualized at 48 h by fluorescence microscope. Images are representative of three independent experiments. Nuclei were stained by DAPI. (C) The amount of HCV RNA was quantified in the bead supernatants by RT-qPCR. Results are expressed as HCV RNA IU/mL and are reported as the mean ± S.D. of triplicate measurements. (D) Viral titers were determined in the bead supernatants by FFU assay. Results are expressed as FFU/mL and are reported as the mean ± S.D. of three independent experiments. ***$P < 0.0001$, ns: no significant difference.

production of new HCVcc particles by FFU titration was measured compared to the 2D control cultures (Fig. 2D). This means that HuH-7 cells encapsulated in Ca-alg beads were not infected by the HCV added to the supernatant.

Absence of HCVcc new particle production of previously infected and Ca-alg encapsulated HuH-7 cells

To explore this phenomenon, cells were chronically infected with the JFH1-RLuc virus before their encapsulation in Ca-alg beads (Fig. 3A). After 6 days' culture on 3D moving plates, HuH7-RFP-NLS-IPS encapsulated cells were observed with fluorescence microscopy. The translocation of the RFP product from cytoplasm to nucleus showed that previously infected cells were able to achieve HCV replication when encapsulated in Ca-alg beads (Fig. 3B).

The quantification of HCV RNA was assessed by RT-qPCR (Fig. 3C) and by new HCVcc production in the culture supernatant by measuring luciferase activity 72 h post-infection (Fig. 3D). As expected, in the 2D system used as the control with an equivalent number of cells and encapsulated cells, the HCV RNA in the supernatant was quantified. Conversely, HCV RNA detected in the supernatant of infected and encapsulated cells was a 4 log fold change lower than in the 2D system supernatant ($P <$

0.0001) but superior to the supernatant of the beads hosting non-infected cells. To determine the origin of the RNA detected in the culture medium of the encapsulated infected cells, the production of new HCVcc particles was quantified. In previously infected and encapsulated cell cultures, luciferase activity levels were under the threshold corresponding to non-infected and encapsulated cells. This suggested that no new HCVcc particles were released in the supernatant of the Ca-alg encapsulated infected cells. The viral RNA detected may then correlate with defective or degraded RNA from lysed infected cells in the beads.

In spite of their ability to achieve HCV replication, the stress inherent to the encapsulation process may affect the previously infected cells, as the infected cells are more sensitive than the non-infected ones, and influence viral production. To alleviate this hypothesis, Ca-alg beads were degelified by alginate lyase treatment and the cells recovered were plated on the 2D system. HCVcc particle production in the culture supernatant was assessed by measuring luciferase activity 72 h post-infection. As shown in Figure 3E, the capacity for HCVcc particle production in the chronically infected cells was not altered by the encapsulation and degelification processes. The restoration of HCVcc production in infected HuH-7 cells after bead degelification indicated that the absence of detection of HCVcc particles in the

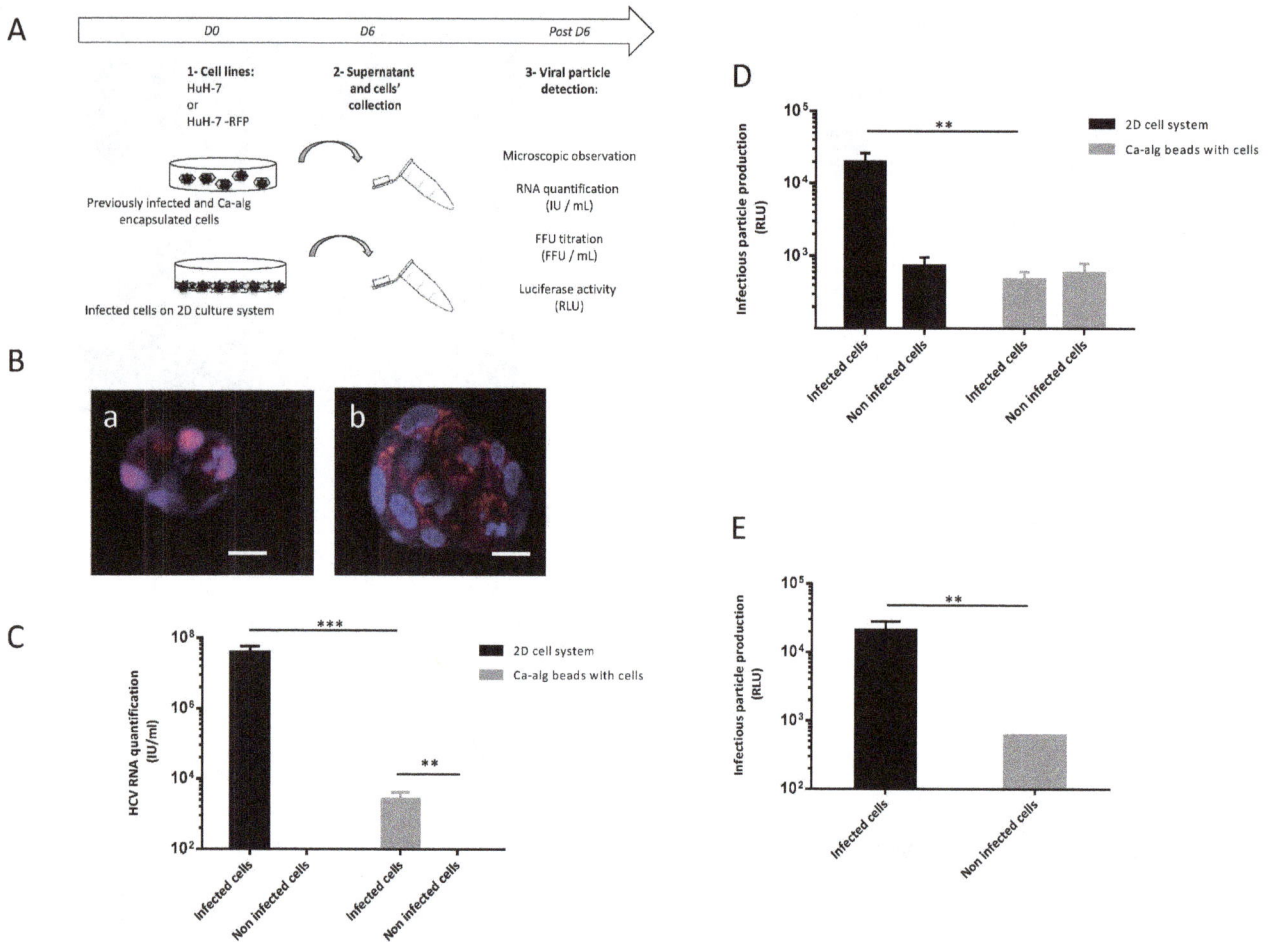

Figure 3. Absence of production of new HCVcc particles by previously infected and encapsulated cells. (A) Encapsulated cell cultures were established using JFH1-RLuc virus-infected HuH-7 cells or non-infected cells within Ca-alg beads. Following the cell encapsulation stage, 400 μL of beads were transferred in tissue culture 6-well plates with 1 mL of complete DMEM medium added on 3D moving plates. (B) Foci of infected (a) or non-infected (b) HuH-7-RFP-NLS-IPS cells identified by translocation of the cleavage product RFP-NLS from cytoplasm to nucleus, were visualized at 6 days post-encapsulation by fluorescence microscope. Images are representative of three independent experiments. Nuclei were stained by DAPI. Scale bar 20 μm. The supernatants of the bead culture cells were collected at day 6 and incubated for 4 h with HuH-7 cell 2D cultures. (C) The amount of HCV RNA was quantified in the bead culture supernatants by RT-qPCR. Results are expressed as HCV RNA IU/mL and are reported as the mean ± S.D. of triplicate measurements. (D) Infectious particle production was assessed luciferase assay on infected cells at 72 h post-infection. Results are expressed as RLU and are reported as the means ± S.D. of three independent experiments. (E) Infectious particle production was also assessed by measuring *Renilla* luciferase activities after bead degelification to free previously infected cells and plating them. Results are expressed as relative light units (RLU) and are reported as the means ± S.D. of three independent experiments. **$P<0.001$, ***$P<0.0001$.

supernatant of Ca-alg encapsulated cells cannot be attributed to cell dysfunctions.

Protective property of Ca-alg beads against HCV infection depends on the Ca-alg bead/virus volume ratio and time of incubation between HCV and Ca-alg beads

Taken together, the previous results suggested that the Ca-alg matrix may interact with HCV particles during the exchanges between the inner and outer parts of the beads. To challenge this assumption, various incubation conditions for Ca-alg beads devoid of cells with the JFH1-RLuc virus were analyzed on a 3D moving support. Firstly, after three incubation times (0.5, 2 and 20 h), the supernatant was collected and submitted to HCV particle detection by measuring luciferase activity. As shown in Fig. 4A, the number of HCV particles decreased in the supernatant after

contact with the Ca-alg beads, and this decrease was directly linked to the time of contact between the virus and beads. The longer the contact time, the lower the number of infectious HCV particles in the supernatant, reaching the level of the condition of the Ca-alg beads without HCV. Secondly, different Ca-alg bead/virus volume ratios were tested (0/1 to 8/1). As could be expected, the interaction between the Ca-alg beads and virus was significantly linked to the bead/virus volume ratio. The absence of detection of HCV particles in the supernatant was observed when a bead/virus volume ratio of 8/1 (Fig. 4B) was attained. All these results suggest that the protective property of the Ca-alg beads against HCV was associated with trapping the viral particles by the Ca-alg hydrogel, which depended on the available and/or accessible surface of the materials in contact with them. Thus, the beads could retain HCV by a confinement of the particles in

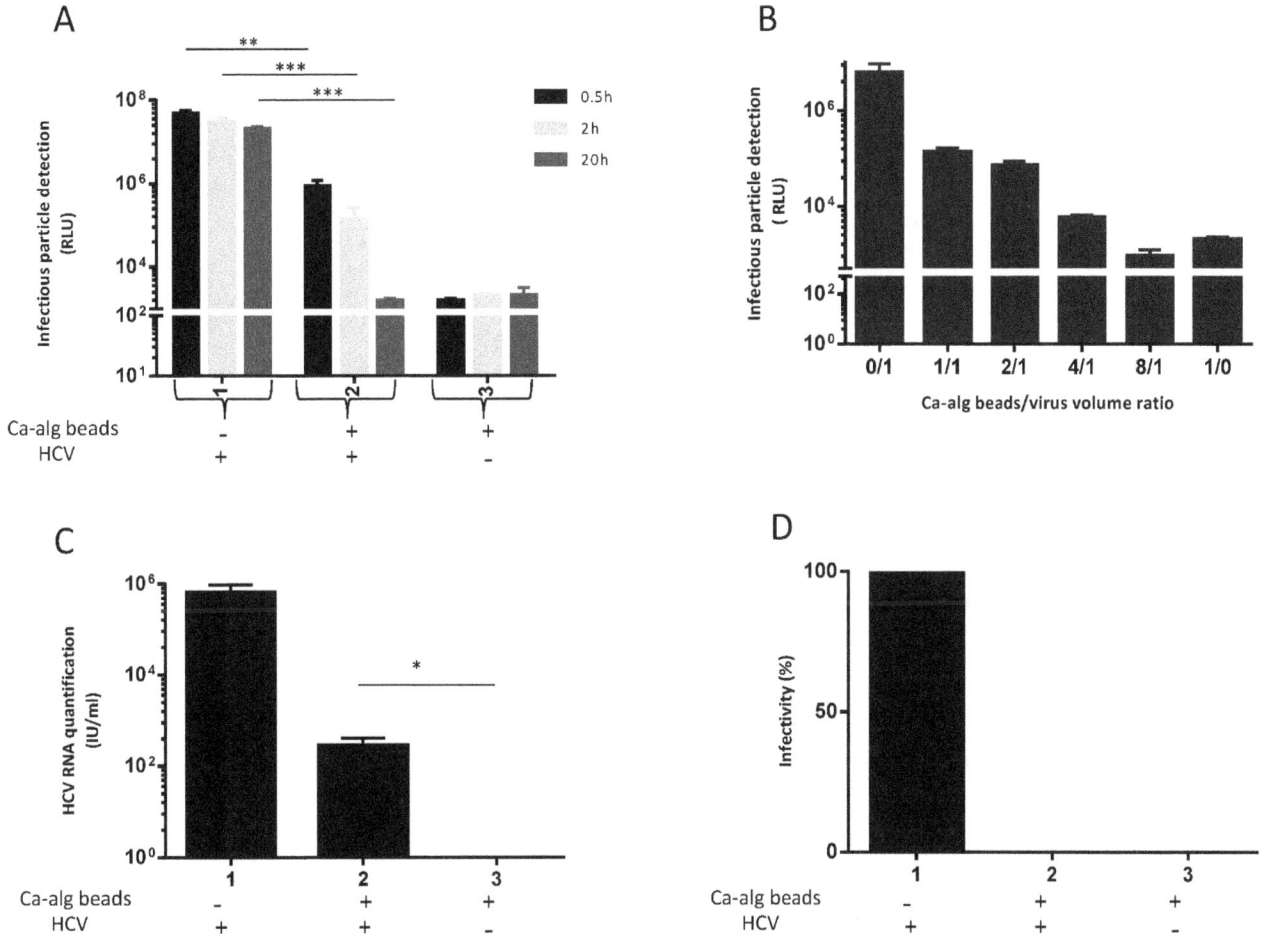

Figure 4. Protective property of Ca-alg beads against HCV infection is dependent on bead/virus volume ratio concentration and time of incubation. Ca-alg beads devoid of cells were produced. (A) 1200 µL of Ca-alg beads were transferred in tissue culture 6-well plates with 1 mL of complete DMEM medium added on 3D moving plates. After three incubation times (0.5, 2 and 20 h) at room temperature of JHF1-RLuc virus with a Ca-alg bead/virus volume ratio of 4/1, the supernatant was recovered and incubated for 4 h with HuH-7 cell 2D cultures. The detection of infectious particles was assessed by luciferase assay on infected cells at 72 h post-infection. Results are expressed as RLU and are reported as the means ± S.D. of three independent experiments. (B) The same experiment was performed with different Ca-alg bead/virus volume ratios (0/1 to 8/1) for 20 h. As previously described, the supernatant was recovered and incubated for 4 h with HuH-7 cell 2D cultures. Luciferase assays were performed on the infected cells at 72 h post-infection. The Ca-alg beads without the JFH1-RLuc virus were used as controls (Ctrl). Results are expressed as RLU and are reported as the means ± S.D. of three independent experiments. (C) After 20 h post-incubation of JFH1 virus in a Ca-alg bead/virus volume ratio of 4/1, the Ca-alg beads were washed, degelified by lyase treatment. Viral titers of the supernatants were determined by FFU assay. Results are converted into a percentage of infectivity. (D) Under the same incubation conditions as C), the amount of HCV RNA was also quantified in the supernatants (condition without beads) and from the Ca-alg bead products after lyase treatment (condition with beads) by RT-qPCR. Results are expressed as HCV RNA IU/mL and are reported as the mean ± S.D. of triplicate measurements. *$P<0.05$, **$P<0.001$, ***$P<0.0001$.

hydrogel porosity or by chemical interactions between the alginate molecules and viral particles.

Protective property of Ca-alg beads against HCV depends on viral particle binding to Ca-alg beads

To determine whether the viral entrapment depended on physical or chemical interactions with the Ca-alg hydrogel, beads devoid of cells were incubated for 20 h with HCV, washed, and enzymatically digested by means of alginate lyase treatment. The alginate lyase is known to cleave the glycosidic bonds, freeing the monomers or oligomers from the alginate molecules [26]. The presence of HCV RNA detected in bead digestion products after alginate lyase treatment (Fig. 4C) associated with the absence of infectious particles (Fig. 4D) suggested that stable interactions link HCV envelope components to the Ca-alg matrix.

Protective activity of Ca-alg beads against other enveloped and non-enveloped viruses

To further characterize whether this Ca-alg gel property is specific to HCVcc particles or not, three other viruses were studied in similar Ca-alg encapsulation culture conditions. One non-enveloped virus (Poliovirus type 1) and two enveloped viruses (HSV-1 and Sindbis virus) were incubated for 4 h with 600 µL of beads encapsulating HuH-7 cells. Then, the supernatant was removed and replaced with fresh complete medium. After 48 h of incubation, the supernatants were used to infect HuH-7 cell 2D cultures at different dilutions. After 24 h, particle infectivity was determined by $TCID_{50}$ titration. As shown in Fig. 5, a drastic decrease in the infectious titer (more than 2 fold for HSV-1 and 3 fold for poliovirus and Sindbis virus) was observed between supernatants harvested in 2D and encapsulated culture systems,

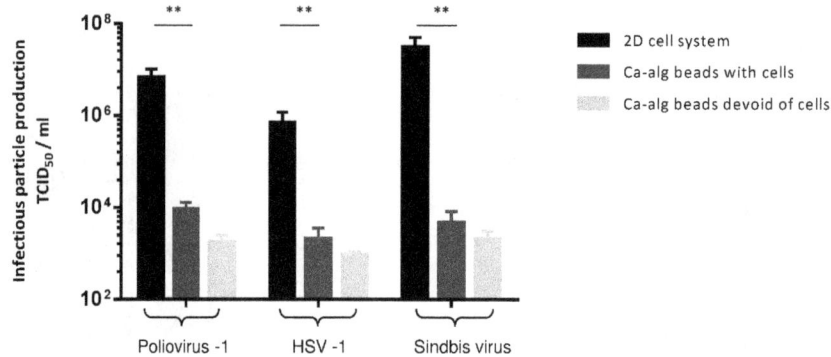

Figure 5. Protective property of Ca-alg beads against various enveloped and non-enveloped viruses. Following the HuH-7 encapsulation stage, 600 μL of beads were transferred to tissue culture 6-well plates with 1 mL of complete DMEM medium added on 3D moving plates. After 4 h of Sindbis virus, HSV-1 and Poliovirus type 1 infection, the medium was removed and replaced with fresh complete DMEM medium. The Ca-alg beads devoid of cells were used as controls. The supernatants of the cultured cells were recovered at 48 h and incubated for 4 h with HuH-7 cell 2D cultures. Infectious particle production was assessed by $TCID_{50}$ titration using microscopy imaging analysis. **$P<0.001$.

respectively. These results were similar to those observed for the HCV infectivity tests. Altogether, these data suggest that the Ca-alg matrix activity was not specific to one virus but that this gelified polymer may interact indifferently with enveloped and non-enveloped viruses.

Discussion

The present study showed for the first time a protective effect of alginate gel used as a matrix for HuH-7 cell microencapsulation against various pathogen viruses. To test the protective effect of Ca-alg beads against HCV infection, we encapsulated either HuH-7-RFP-NLS-IPS cells before submitting this cell system to HCV or previously infected cells. In all cases, no infectious HCVcc particle was produced in the culture medium. More precisely, the non-translocation of the cleavage products RFP-NLS from cytoplasm to the nucleus showed the inability of the HCV to access the entrapped cells or to activate the HCV receptors to enter into cells. However, our previous data suggested HuH-7 cell cultures in Ca-alg beads were a relevant model for HCV infection for two reasons: i) after their encapsulation in Ca-alg beads with optimized alginate composition, isolated HuH-7 cells proliferated and reorganized into multicellular aggregates [27]. The recovery of a differentiated state was confirmed by the polarized structure of the cellular aggregates, characterized by specific localization of tight junctions and polarity markers, providing evidence of the beneficial effect of the 3D environment culture in the Ca-alg matrix to reproduce a hepatic-like tissue. HuH-7 cells expressed specific receptors to HCV, such as receptors SR-BI and CD81, and co-receptors, claudin-1 and occludin, mimicking the *in vivo* configuration. HuH-7 cells embedded in Ca-alg beads were thus expected to recognize and interact with HCV on their plasma membrane, as was confirmed by recent studies when aggregated HuH-7 cells were cultivated without any matrix or embedded in Matrigel or in galactosylated cellulosic sponge [28–30]. ii) The second reason dealt with the structure of the Ca-alg matrix. In a previous work, various concentrations and viscosities of Na-alg solution were tested to produce beads with a porosity allowing the diffusion of VHC size particles. According to the high-resolution cryo-SEM analysis of the Ca-alg matrix and to dynamic diffusion test results, the Na-alg solution at 1.5% with medium viscosity was retained. In particular, the beads produced by this way were permeable to polystyrene nanoparticles up to 100 nm in diameter [27], which is compatible with the diameter of HCV (50 to 80 nm)

[31]. Therefore, neither the biological properties of the HuH-7 cells nor Ca-alg bead porosity could explain the absence of viral production in the supernatant, when naïve or previously infected HuH-7 cells were encapsulated.

The barrier exerted by the Ca-alg network is composed of homo- and hetero-polymers of M and G residues whose negative charges of carboxylate groups interact with calcium to crosslink the polymer chains. The Ca-alg hydrogel maintains high negative charges, as it was analyzed by the potential zeta of beads [32–33]. The viral inhibitory effects due to ionic interactions are well documented, particularly among the sulfated polysaccharides derived from natural sources [16]. Studies on the structure-activity relationships of seaweed polysaccharides have underlined distinct molecular mechanisms for antiviral actions which inhibit different stages in the virion life cycle or prior to cell infection, *i.e.* by inactivating viruses before host cell contact [7]. Our results suggest that the high negative charges of Ca-alg hydrogel may interact with envelope components of HCV, blocking the viral particles in the gel environment or hindering specific interactions between viral compounds and specific membrane receptors. Similar results were obtained with low and medium viscosity alginate (data not shown) supporting the idea that polysaccharide chain length was not involved in the antiviral activity. These data were confirmed using pure alginate of medical grade quality (data not shown), meaning that no overshadowing responses associated to contaminations such as endotoxins were implicated in the viro-protective effect of Ca-alg gel. In addition, the results of the incubation time and dose-effect experiments, using different ratios of empty bead volume-to-viral charge, were in favor of an adsorption mechanism of the viral particles on the Ca-alg matrix.

Nevertheless, alginate molecules in suspension revealed low antiviral activity compared to other marine polysaccharides [16]. The chemical composition of M and G residues, which are naturally devoid of sulfated groups, explains the weak antiviral potency of alginate [34]. As an example, anti-HSV-1 activity of Na-alg was lower than that of sulfated polysaccharides, characterized by 50% inhibitory concentration values (IC_{50}) in a range of 10 to 15 μg/mL, *i.e.* ten times higher than the IC_{50} of fucoidans, sulfated molecules [10,34]. Cermelli *et al.* demonstrated antiviral activity of hyaluronic acid, a non-sulfated negatively-charged glycosaminoglycan, characterized by variable efficiency depending on the type of virus, at effective concentrations ranging from 1 to 4 mg/mL [35]. In the present work, beads were extruded from an Na-alg solution at 15 mg/mL, which is 1000 times greater than that of the alginate solution concentrations classically used for antiviral activity experiments [10,33]. This high alginate concentration in hydrogel, generally varying from 0.5 to 2%, was reinforced by shrinkage of the beads during their immersion in the calcium solution used for the gelification stage [36,37]. The negative charges concentrated in a limited volume and the spatial conformation of the polymers in Ca-alg gels might also support efficient antiviral activity [10]. Finally, our results support a non-specific Ca-alg-virus interaction regarding the efficiency of the Ca-alg viro-protective effect on a variety of viruses, whether enveloped or not. Cermelli *et al.* speculated on a structure-activity relationship of negatively-charged glycosaminoglycan involving general/non specific host cell-virus interactions [35]. Structure and sequence-based statistical analyses have demonstrated that positively-charged basic amino acids on viral proteins participate in binding to glycosaminoglycan receptors [38]. Ca-alg hydrogel may inhibit different viruses by interfering with the viral adsorption process via receptor entry blocking [7].

The recent progress made in bioengineered products provides a hopeful strategy for liver supply, offering a promising alternative to whole liver transplantation which suffers from an allogenic organ shortage crisis [39]. The allo- or xenotransplantation of hepatocytes encapsulated in alginate beads is an attractive approach to support host liver recovery and whose feasibility has been demonstrated in various animal models [40–41]. Mei *et al.* documented the beneficial influence of implantation of porcine encapsulated cells on survival rate and metabolic performances compared to free hepatocyte transplantation in a mouse model of liver failure [41], which was confirmed by the co-encapsulation of stem cells and hepatocytes [42–44]. Nevertheless, the use of allogenic or xenogenic cell microencapsulation for regenerative medicine is associated with certain risks in terms of virus-mediated infectious diseases provided from either the grafts or the recipients [45], which may ultimately have an impact on human health recovery. Given the numerous applications for microencapsulation in Ca-alg beads using a natural biomaterial approved by the U.S. Food and Drug Administration, the promising *in vitro* protective effect against viruses reported here is an innovative and attractive

property of alginate gel with two new interesting advantages: first, viral infection by a retrovirus, an endogenous virus or a potentially unknown virus from the encapsulated cells cannot be transmitted to the patient, and, conversely, encapsulated cell functions cannot be hampered by a viral infection in the host. Numerous applications in the field of regenerative medicine may be concerned, such as cartilage repair, bone regeneration [46] or diabetes treatment by means of a bioartificial pancreas [47]. More generally speaking, the protective property of alginate gel against viruses may have applications extending far beyond biomedicine [48].

Conclusion

Alginate hydrogel used as a matrix for HuH-7 cell microencapsulation has a protective effect against JFH1 HCV, Sindbis virus, HSV-1, and Poliovirus type 1 infection when these viruses were added to the supernatant. In addition, Ca-alg hydrogel blocked the release of HCV particles out of the beads when HuH-7 cells were previously infected and encapsulated. The use of Ca-alg beads devoid of cells in inhibitory experiments showed that the protective activity was dose- and incubation time-dependent, and depended on chemical interactions between the Ca-alg gel and HCV particles. Broadening this protective effect may have appealing applications in regenerative medicine.

Acknowledgments

The authors are grateful to Christian Défarges from Orléans University, for sharing his expertise in cryoSEM microscopy procedures and data analysis and to Véronique Descamps and Virginie Morel, EA4294 - University of Picardie, for their expert technical assistance.

Author Contributions

Conceived and designed the experiments: GD CL SC MD. Performed the experiments: TH NMT SC MD. Analyzed the data: NMT SC MD. Contributed reagents/materials/analysis tools: FH CF EB PP. Wrote the paper: MD SC CL GD.

References

1. de Vos P, Faas MM, Strand B, Calafiore R (2006) Alginate-based microcapsules for immunoisolation of pancreatic islets. Biomaterials 27(32):5603–5617.
2. Orive G, Tam SK, Pedraz JL, Hallé JP (2006) Biocompatibility of alginate-poly-L-lysine microcapsules for cell therapy. Biomaterials 27(20):3691–3700.
3. Tonnesen HH, Karlsen J (2002) Alginate in drug delivery systems. Drug Dev Ind Pharm 28(6):621–630.
4. Steele JA, Hallé JP, Poncelet D, Neufeld RJ (2014) Therapeutic cell encapsulation techniques and applications in diabetes. Adv Drug Deliv Rev 67–68:74–83.
5. Calafiore R, Basta G (2014) Clinical application of microencapsulated islets: Actual prospectives on progress and challenges. Adv Drug Deliv Rev 67–68:84–92.
6. Vo TS, Kim SK (2010) Potential anti-HIV agents from marine resources: an overview. Mar Drugs 8(12):2871–2892.
7. Wang W, Wang SX, Guan HS (2012) The antiviral activities and mechanisms of marine polysaccharides: an overview. Mar Drugs 10(12):2795–2816.
8. Miao B, Geng M, Li J, Li F, Chen H, et al. (2004) Sulfated polymannuroguluronate, a novel anti-acquired immune deficiency syndrome (AIDS) drug candidate, targeting CD4 in lymphocytes. Biochem Pharmacol 68(4):641–649.
9. Queiroz KC, Medeiros VP, Queiroz LS, Abreu LR, Rocha HA, et al. (2008) Inhibition of reverse transcriptase activity of HIV by polysaccharides of brown algae. Biomed Pharmacother 62(5):303–307.
10. Sinha S, Astani A, Ghosh T, Schnitzler P, Ray B (2010) Polysaccharides from Sargassum tenerrimum: structural features, chemical modification and anti-viral activity. Phytochemistry 71:235–242.
11. Talarico LB, Damonte EB (2007) Interference in dengue virus adsorption and uncoating by carrageenans. Virology 363(2):473–485.
12. Girond S, Crance JM, Van Cuyck-Gandre H, Renaudet J, Deloince R (1991) Antiviral activity of carrageenan on hepatitis A virus replication in cell culture. Res Virol 142(4):261–270.
13. Buck CB, Thompson CD, Roberts JN, Müller M, Lowy DR, et al. (2006) Carrageenan is a potent inhibitor of Papillomavirus infection. PLoS Pathog 2(7):e69.
14. Fitton JH (2011) Therapies from fucoidan; multifunctional marine polymers. Mar Drugs 9(10):1731–1760.
15. Araya N, Takahashi K, Sato T, Nakamura T, Sawa C, et al. (2011) Fucoidan therapy decreases the proviral load in patients with human T-lymphotropic virus type-1-associated neurological disease. Antivir Ther 16(1):89–98.
16. Ghosh T, Chattopadhyay K, Marschall M, Karmakar P, Mandal P, et al. (2009) Focus on antivirally active sulfated polysaccharides: from structure-activity analysis to clinical evaluation. Glycobiology 19(1):2–15.
17. Ngo DH, Kim SK (2013) Sulfated polysaccharides as bioactive agents from marine algae. Int J Biol Macromol 62:70–75.
18. Tengdelius ME, Lee CJ, Grenegård M, Griffith M, Påhlsson P, et al. (2014) Synthesis and biological evaluation of fucoidan-mimetic glycopolymers through cyanoxyl-mediated free-radical polymerization. Biomacromolecules 15(7):2359–2368.
19. Wilson GK, Stamataki Z (2012) *In vitro* systems for the study of hepatitis C virus infection. Int J Hepatol 2012:292591.
20. Jones CT, Catanese MT, Law LM, Khetani SR, Syder AJ, et al. (2010) Real-time imaging of hepatitis C virus infection using a fluorescent cell-based reporter system. Nat Biotechnol 28(2):167–171.
21. David B, Dufresne M, Nagel MD, Legallais C (2004) *In vitro* assessment of encapsulated C3A hepatocytes functions in a fluidized bed bioreactor. Biotechnol Prog 20(4):1204–1212.
22. Helle F, Brochot E, Fournier C, Descamps V, Izquierdo L, et al. (2013) Permissivity of primary human hepatocytes and different hepatoma cell lines to cell culture adapted hepatitis C virus. PLoS One 8(8):e70809.
23. Delgrange D, Pillez A, Castelain S, Cocquerel L, Rouillé Y, et al. (2007) Robust production of infectious viral particles in Huh-7 cells by introducing mutations in hepatitis C virus structural proteins. J Gen Virol 88(9):2495–2503.

24. LaBarre DD, Lowy RJ (2001) Improvements in methods for calculating virus titer estimates from TCID50 and plaque assays. J Virol Methods 96:107–126.

25. Castelain S, Descamps V, Thibault V, François C, Bonte D, et al. (2004) TaqMan amplification system with an internal positive control for HCV RNA quantitation. J Clin Virol 31(3):227–234.

26. Kam N, Park YJ, Lee EY, Kim HS (2011) Molecular identification of a polyM-specific alginate lyase from Pseudomonas sp. strain KS-408 for degradation of glycosidic linkages between two mannuronates or mannuronate and guluronate in alginate. Can J Microbiol 57(12):1032–1041.

27. Tran NM, Dufresne M, Duverlie G, Castelain S, Défarge C, et al. (2013) An appropriate selection of a 3D alginate culture model for hepatic Huh-7 cell line encapsulation intended for viral studies. Tissue Eng Part A 19(1-2):103–113.

28. Molina-Jimenez F, Benedicto I, Dao Thi VL, Gondar V, Lavillette D, et al. (2012) Matrigel-embedded 3D culture of Huh-7 cells as a hepatocyte-like polarized system to study hepatitis C virus cycle. Virology 425(1):31–39.

29. Sainz B Jr, TenCate V, Uprichard SL (2009) Three-dimensional HuH-7 cell culture system for the study of Hepatitis C virus infection. Virol J 6:103–111.

30. Ananthanarayanan A, Nugraha B, Triyatni M, Hart S, Sankuratri S, et al. (2014) Scalable spheroid model of human hepatocytes for hepatitis C infection and replication. Mol Pharm 11(7):2106–2114.

31. Revie D, Salahuddin SZ (2011) Human cell types important for hepatitis C virus replication in vivo and in vitro: old assertions and current evidence. Virol J 8:346–371.

32. Kurosaki T, Kitahara T, Kawakami S, Nishida K, Nakamura J, et al. (2009) The development of a gene vector electrostatically assembled with a polysaccharide capsule. Biomaterials 30(26):4427–4434.

33. Nimtrakul P, Atthi R, Limpeanchob N, Tiyaboonchai W (2013) Development of Pasteurella multocida-loaded microparticles for hemorrhagic septicemia vaccine. Drug Dev Ind Pharm available from URL: http://informahealthcare.com/doi/abs/10.3109/03639045.2013.873448 (doi: 10.3109/03639045.2013.873448).

34. Bandyopadhyay SS, Navid MH, Ghosh T, Schnitzler P, Ray B (2011) Structural features and in vitro antiviral activities of sulfated polysaccharides from Sphacelaria indica. Phytochemistry 72(2-3):276–283.

35. Cermelli C, Cuoghi A, Scuri M, Bettua C, Neglia RG, et al. (2011) In vitro evaluation of antiviral and virucidal activity of a high molecular weight hyaluronic acid. Virol J 8:141–149.

36. Saitoh S, Araki Y, Kon R, Katsura H, Taira M (2000) Swelling/deswelling mechanism of calcium alginate gel in aqueous solutions. Dent Mater J 19(4):396–404.

37. Blandino A, Macias M, Cantero D (1999) Formation of calcium alginate gel capsules: influence of sodium alginate and CaCl$_2$ concentration on gelation kinetics. J Bios Bioeng 88(6):686–689.

38. Gandhi NS, Mancera RL (2008) The structure of glycosaminoglycans and their interactions with proteins. Chem Biol Drug Des 72(6):455–482.

39. Abouna GM (2008) Organ shortage crisis: problems and possible solutions. Transplant Proc 40(1):34–38.

40. Aoki T, Jin Z, Nishino N, Kato H, Shimizu Y, et al. (2005) Intrasplenic transplantation of encapsulated hepatocytes decreases mortality and improves liver functions in fulminant hepatic failure from 90% partial hepatectomy in rats. Transplantation 79(7):783–790.

41. Capone SH, Dufresne M, Rechel M, Fleury MJ, Salsac AV, et al. (2013) Impact of alginate composition: from bead mechanical properties to encapsulated HepG2/C3A cell activities for in vivo implantation. PLoS One 8(4):e62032.

42. Mei J, Sgroi A, Mai G, Baertschiger R, Gonelle-Gispert C, et al. (2009) Improved survival of fulminant liver failure by transplantation of microencapsulated cryopreserved porcine hepatocytes in mice. Cell Transplant 18(1):101–110.

43. Shi XL, Zhang Y, Gu JY, Ding YT (2009) Coencapsulation of hepatocytes with bone marrow mesenchymal stem cells improves hepatocyte-specific functions. Transplantation 88(10):1178–1185.

44. Zhang Y, Chen XM, Sun DL (2014) Effects of coencapsulation of hepatocytes with adipose-derived stem cells in the treatment of rats with acute-on-chronic liver failure. Int J Artif Organs 2(37):133–141.

45. Kim J, Choi E, Kwon Y, Lee D, Hwang D, et al. (2009) Characterization of clones of human cell line infected with porcine endogenous retrovirus (PERV) from porcine cell line, PK-15. Infect. Chemother 41:1–8.

46. Sun J, Tan H (2013) Alginate-based biomaterials for regenerative medicine applications. Materials 6:1285–1309.

47. Opara EC, McQuilling JP, Farney AC (2013) Microencapsulation of pancreatic islets for use in a bioartificial pancreas. Methods Mol Biol 1001:261–266.

48. Steenson LR, Klaenhammer TR, Swaisgood HE (1987) Calcium alginate-immobilized cultures of lactic Streptococci are protected from bacteriophages. J Dairy Sci 70(6):1121–1127.

16

Guidelines for Therapeutic Drug Monitoring of Vancomycin

Zhi-Kang Ye[1,2]**, Can Li**[1,2]**, Suo-Di Zhai**[1]*****

1 Department of Pharmacy, Peking University Third Hospital, Beijing, China, **2** Department of Pharmacy Administration and Clinical Pharmacy, School of Pharmaceutical Sciences, Peking University Health Science Center, Beijing, China

Abstract

Background and Objective: Despite the availability of clinical practice guidelines (CPGs) for therapeutic drug monitoring (TDM) of vancomycin, vancomycin serum concentrations still do not reach therapeutic concentrations in many patients. Thus, we sought to systematically review the quality and consistency of recommendations for an international cohort of CPGs regarding vancomycin TDM.

Methods: PubMed, Embase, guidelines' websites and Google were searched for CPGs for vancomycin TDM. Two independent assessors rated the quality of each CPG using the Appraisal of Guidelines for Research & Evaluation II (AGREEII) instrument and data were independently extracted.

Results: Twelve guidelines were evaluated and the overall quality of guidelines for vancomycin TDM was moderate. The highest score was recorded in the domain of clarity of presentation, and the lowest score was recorded in the domain of rigor of development and stakeholder involvement. The specific recommendations for vancomycin TDM were moderately consistent and guidelines varied in trough concentration monitoring, frequency of TDM, and serum concentration targets.

Conclusion: The overall guideline quality for vancomycin TDM was not optimal and effort is needed to improve guideline quality, especially in the domain of rigor of development and stakeholder involvement.

Editor: John Conly, University of Calgary, Canada

Funding: These authors have no support or funding to report.

Competing Interests: The authors have declared that no competing interests exist.

* E-mail: zhaisuodi@163.com

Introduction

Vancomycin is a first-line therapy for methicillin-resistant *Staphylococcus aureus* (MRSA) [1] and this drug is recommended for therapeutic drug monitoring (TDM) to minimize the risk of nephrotoxicity and to ensure successful therapeutic outcomes [2]. To improve the quality of vancomycin TDM, several organizations have developed clinical practice guidelines (CPGs) for appropriate vancomycin TDM. More patients have appropriate trough concentration measurement and sample timing when the guideline is followed [3]. However, many studies suggest that significant numbers of patients do not achieve therapeutic vancomycin serum concentrations [4–13].

CPGs are "statements that include recommendations intended to optimize patient care. They are informed by a systematic review of evidence and an assessment of the benefits and harms of alternative care option" [14]. Properly developed, high quality CPGs should offer better patient outcomes, reduce risk, and allow cost-effective clinical care [15,16]. However, many CPGs offer poor quality, highly variable recommendations [17–21]. To our knowledge, a systematic evaluation of the quality and the consistency of vancomycin TDM guidelines have not been reported. Thus, the objective of this review was to systematically evaluate the quality and consistency of recommendations for an international cohort of CPGs regarding vancomycin TDM, and in

an effort to help develop or update vancomycin TDM guidelines to achieve higher quality recommendations.

Methods

Identification of Guidelines

Guidelines for vancomycin TDM were identified (until June 25, 2013) in PubMed and Embase. Search terms included text words and Medical Subject Headings (MeSH) terms as follows: ("guideline" or "practice guideline" or "guidelines" or "practice guidelines" or "recommendation" or "consensus review" or "guideline" as TopicMeSH) and ("vancomycin" MeSH) and ("therapeutic drug monitoring" or "TDM" or "drug monitoring" or "therapeutic monitoring" or "serum concentration monitoring" or "therapeutic drug" or "drug monitoring" MeSH). Guideline websites and Google were searched to include more relevant CPGs: these included the National Guideline Clearinghouse (www.guideline.gov), Guidelines International Network (www.g-i-n.net/), National Institute for Health and Clinical Excellence (www.nice.org.uk), Scottish Intercollegiate Guidelines Network (www.sign.ac.uk) and China Guideline Clearinghouse (cgc.bjmu.edu.cn:820/). The search term was "vancomycin" and all results were reviewed. Google was searched using the words "vancomycin" and "guideline" and the first 100 items were reviewed. To ensure that all potentially relevant guidelines were retrieved, we conducted a search by country in Google and no language restriction was applied.

Selection of Guidelines

CPGs for vancomycin TDM included those that both provided practical clinical recommendations and were endorsed by medical specialty associations, relevant professional societies or governmental agencies. Documents lacking such recommendations and secondary publications were excluded.

Evaluation of Guidelines

Two assessors (Z.K.Y and C.L) used online training tools recommended by the AGREE collaboration before conducting appraisals. Two assessors independently scored each guidelines using AGREE II [22]. AGREE II consists of 23 items organized into six domains: "scope and purpose" (3 items), "stakeholder involvement" (3 items), "rigor of development" (8 items), "clarity of presentation" (3 items), "applicability" (4 items), and "editorial independence" (2 items). Each item is scored from 1 (strongly disagree) to 7 (strongly agree). We referred to methods of a previous study to resolve discrepancies between the two assessors: Briefly, if scores by both assessors differed by two points, they were averaged but if they differed by one point, the lower score was kept. Next, if scores between assessors varied by three points or more, a consensus was reached after a discussion. If consensus was not reached, a third person (S.D.Z) participated in the discussion and resolved the discrepancy [20]. The standard score of each domain was calculated as a percentage of the maximum possible score:

The scaled domain scores =

(obtained score − minimum possible score) divided by

(maximum possible score − minimum possible score).

A score of 50% was chosen to establish the proportion of guidelines which scored greater than or equal to the level in six domains. The overall assessment of included CPGs was based on the overall quality of each guideline.

Synthesis of results

The included CPGs were summarized according to specific recommendations, including indications for TDM, pharmacokinetics-pharmacodynamics, methods of TDM, target of serum concentrations and initial administration plan.

Results

Study selection

Figure 1 shows the study selection process for inclusion in this review. A total of 635 records were retrieved and after application of the inclusion and exclusion criteria, 12 CPGs (AME [23], LOS [24], JAP [25], VAN [26], ALB [27], NHS [28], CAL [29], DEV [30], COR [31], BAT [32], SAP [33], WOR [34]) were included in the review. Table 1 depicts the demographic characteristics for included guidelines. Among the twelve CPGs, three (AME, JAP, NHS) were national CPGs [23,25,28], and the remaining CPGs were regional guidelines. The AME and JAP CPGs were found in medical literature databases [23,25], and the others were found by Google searches. The AME and JAP CPGs rated the quality of evidence and graded the strength of recommendations using the classification schemata of the Canadian Medical Association.

Scope and Purpose

Table 2 shows the standardized scores of each domain and overall recommendation. The mean score for the domain of scope and purpose was 63% (range 28–100%). Nine guidelines scored greater than or equal to 50% [23,25–27,29–31,33,34], two of them scored greater than or equal to 94% [23,25]. Most guidelines clearly specifically described their scope, related clinical questions and target populations.

Stakeholder Involvement

The mean score for the domain of stakeholder involvement was 27% (range 6–50%). Only three guidelines scored 50% [23,25,31]. No guidelines appeared to include or consider the views or preferences of the target population. Also, members of the guideline development group were not well identified for many guidelines.

Rigor of development

The mean score for the domain of rigor of development was 20% (4–73%). Two guidelines scored above 70% [23,25], the remaining guidelines scored below 20%. Only the AME CPG clearly described the systematic methods for searching evidence [23] and the JAP CPG clearly described the procedure of updating the guideline [25]. No guideline reported their recommendations on an underlying systematic review.

Clarity of presentation

The mean score for the domain of clarity of presentation was 77%. All CPGs scored above 50%. Three CPGs scored greater than 90% [23,25,27]. Most guidelines presented specific, easily identified recommendations for the management of vancomycin TDM.

Applicability

The mean score for the domain of applicability was 47% (range 38–54%). Only four CPGs scored greater than 50% [23,25–27]. No guideline considered the cost of vancomycin TDM, and little information was offered to describe TDM barriers or facilitators.

Editorial independence

The mean score for the editorial independence was 45% (25–67%). Four CPGs scored greater than or equal to 50% [23,25,31,34]. Only the AME and JAP CPGs reported the information about competing interests of guideline development group members [23,25].

Clinical practice guideline recommendations

Indication of TDM. In Table 3, TDM indication reporting is described for the CPGs. Four CPGs (JAP, AME, ALB and VAN) recommended that TDM should be performed in patients receiving aggressive dosing, patients with high risk of nephrotoxicity, unstable renal function, and in those receiving prolonged therapy (more than three or five days). Three CPGs (JAP, VAN and ALB) specifically recommended that TDM should be performed in patients undergoing hemodialysis, those who were obese or had low body weight, those with special conditions that cause fluctuating volumes of distribution, and in pregnant and pediatric patients. The ALB CPG recommended vancomycin TDM should be performed in patients with anticipated therapy of more than two weeks, and the LOS CPG recommended that vancomycin TDM should be performed in patients receiving more than 48 h of vancomycin therapy (Table 3).

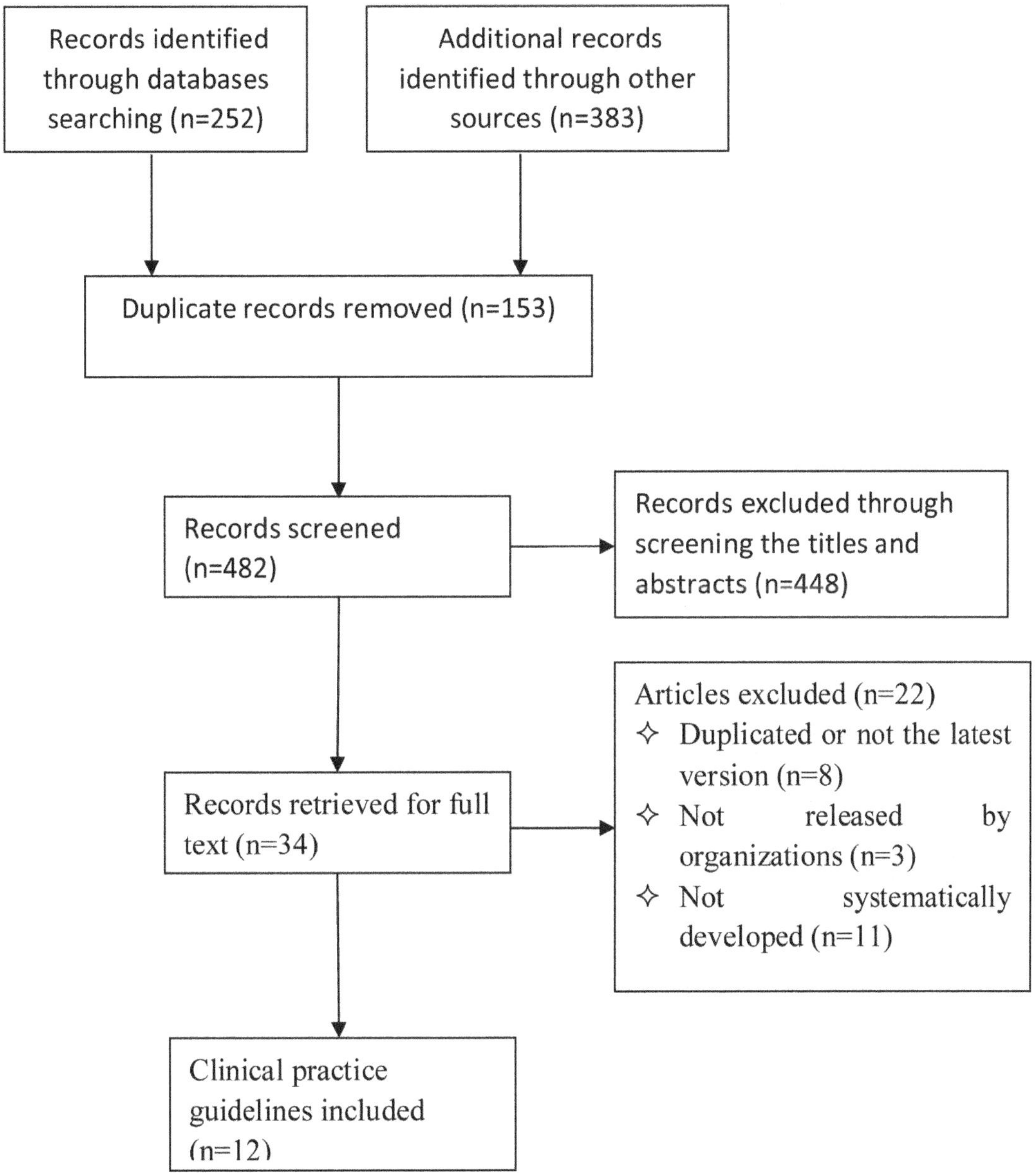

Figure 1. Flow chart for the systematic review.

Pharmacokinetic and pharmacodynamics monitoring (PK-PD) parameters. Three CPGs (JAP, AME and VAN) recommended that an area under the curve (AUC)/minimum inhibitory concentration (MIC) ratio of more than 400 was associated with clinical efficacy of vancomycin therapy. Trough concentrations were the best surrogates for AUC. Other CPGs did not consider a monitoring parameter associated with clinical efficacy (Table 3).

Peak or trough concentrations. Ten CPGs (JAP, AME, LOS, ALB, NHS, CAL, DEV, BAT, SAP and WOR) recommended monitoring trough concentrations or pre-dose levels rather than peak serum concentrations. The VAN CPG recommended monitoring pre- and post-dose concentrations to obtain precise pharmacokinetics for some special patients. The COR CPG recommended monitoring peak and trough serum concentrations (Table 3).

Time to first sample. Most CPGs recommended obtaining the first trough sample at steady state (before the 3rd, 4th, or 5th dose in patients with normal renal function). The SAP CPG recommended monitoring troughs within the 48 h of starting therapy. The DEV CPG did not report a time for obtaining the first trough (Table 3).

Frequency of TDM. Five CPGs (AME, JAP, ALB, VAN and DEV) recommended weekly monitoring after initial TDM in patients with normal renal function, and more frequent follow-up trough concentration monitoring was required in patients with hemodynamic instability, high-dose vancomycin administration, unstable renal function, and those at high risk for nephrotoxicity. The LOS CPG recommended more frequent monitoring in patients with complicated infections (goal trough was 15–20 µg/mL) or those with longer courses of therapy. Other CPGs recommended additional drug concentration measurements 4 days or less for patients with normal renal function, and

Table 1. Characteristics of clinical practice guideline.

Title	Year of publication	Country/Region	Level of development	Organization behind the guideline	Number of authors	Number of references
Therapeutic monitoring of vancomycin in adult patients: A consensus review of the American Society of Health-System Pharmacists, the Infectious Diseases Society of America, and the Society of Infectious Diseases Pharmacists (AME) [23]	2009	America	National	ASHP/IDSA/SIDP	15	129
Vancomycin dosing and monitoring of serum vancomycin levels Infectious diseases section guidelines (LOS) [24]	2013	Los Angeles	Regional	VAGLAHS	NR	20
Practice guidelines for therapeutic drug monitoring of vancomycin: a consensus review of the Japanese Society of Chemotherapy and the Japanese Society of Therapeutic Drug Monitoring (JAP) [25]	2013	Japan	National	JSC/JSTDM	18	116
Vancomycin Therapeutic Drug Monitoring Vancouver Coastal Health & Providence Health Care Regional Guideline (VAN) [26]	2011	Canada, Vancouver	Regional	VCH/PHC	9	7
Vancomycin Monitoring and Dosing Guideline (ALB) [27]	2011	Canada, Edmonton	Regional	AHS	NR	11
Vancomycin Guideline for Adults (NHS) [28]	NR	United Kingdom	National	File NHS ADTC	NR	NR
Prescribing Guidelines for Intravenous Vancomycin in Adults (CAL) [29]	2009	United Kingdom, Calderdale and Huddersfield	Regional	CHNHS	NR	7
Guidelines on Intravenous (IV) Vancomycin Dosing in Adults (DEV) [30]	2010	United Kingdom, Devon and Exeter	Regional	RDENHS	NR	NR
Vancomycin prescription and therapeutic drug monitoring guideline (COR) [31]	2010	United Kingdom, Cornwall	Regional	RCHNHS	7	3
Guidelines for the Dosing and Monitoring of Gentamicin, Vancomycin and Teicoplanin (BAT) [32]	2009	United Kingdom, Bath	Regional	RUHBNHS	NR	6
Intravenous Vancomycin Use in Adults Intermittent (Pulsed) Infusion (SAP) [33]	2013	United Kingdom, Scottish	Regional	SAPG	NR	NR
Guidelines for Vancomycin Dosing and Monitoring in Adult Patients (WOR) [34]	2008	United Kingdom, Worcestershire	Regional	WAHNHS	10	5

AME: American; ASHP: American Society of Health-System Pharmacists; IDSA: Infectious Diseases Society of America; SIDP: Society of Infectious Diseases Pharmacists; LOS: Los Angeles; VAGLAHS: VA Greater Los Angeles Healthcare System; JAP: Japanese; JSC: Japanese Society of Chemotherapy; JSTDM: Japanese Society of Therapeutic Drug Monitoring; VAN: Vancouver; VCH: Vancouver Costal Health; PHC: Providence Health Care; AHS: Alberta; ALB: Alberta Health Services; NHS: National Health Services; File NHS ADTC: File National Health Services Board Area Drugs and Therapeutics Committee; CAL: Calderdale; CHNHS: Calderdale and Huddersfield NHS; DEV: Devon; RDENHS: Royal Devon and Exeter NHS; COR: Cornwall; RCHNHS: Royal Cornwall Hospitals NHS; BAT: Bath; RUHBNHS: Royal United Hospitals Bath NHS; SAP: Scottish Antimicrobial Prescribing; SAPG: Scottish Antimicrobial Prescribing Group; WOR: Worcestershire; WAHNHS: Worcestershire Acute Hosptials NHS; NR: not reported.

Table 2. AGREE II domain-standardized scores for CPGs on vancomycin TDM.

Guideline	Scope and Purpose (%)	Stakeholder Involvement (%)	Rigor of development (%)	Clarity and presentation (%)	Applicability (%)	Editorial independence (%)	Overall assessment
AME	100	50	71	100	54	67	Recommend
LOS	39	6	4	78	38	25	Not recommend
JAP	94	50	73	100	58	67	Recommend
VAN	89	33	13	78	54	42	Recommend with modification
ALB	50	17	13	94	54	42	Recommend with modification
NHS	28	11	4	61	42	33	Not recommend
CAL	50	11	4	78	42	42	Not recommend
DEV	50	22	8	56	46	42	Not recommend
COR	83	50	13	72	46	50	Recommend with modification
BAT	33	17	8	73	46	42	Not recommend
WOR	78	44	19	67	42	50	Recommend with modification
SAP	56	17	6	72	46	42	Not recommend
Mean (Range)	63 (28–100)	27 (6–50)	20 (4–73)	77 (56–100)	47 (38–58)	45(25–67)	

recommended more frequent monitoring for patients with unstable renal function, hemodynamic instability, or in patients who experienced changes in renal function (Table 3).

Sample time. Three CPGs (JAP, AME and ALB) recommended a trough sample should be obtained within 30 min prior to next dose. The DEV CPG recommended a trough measurement within 60 min prior to the next dose. Other CPGs did not recommend trough sample timing (Table 3).

The VAN CPG defined a 3 or 24 h post-dose serum concentration as a "post levels". The COR CPG recommended measuring peak concentrations 1 h after the end of infusion. In addition, the JAP CPG did not recommend routine monitoring peak concentrations, but if peak concentrations are needed in some special circumstances, peak concentrations should be measured 1–2 h after the end of infusion.

Target of serum concentrations in TDM. Only three CPGs (ALB, BAT and WOR) recommended that vancomycin trough concentrations should be more than 5 µg/mL, and most CPGs recommended that vancomycin trough concentrations should be maintained above 10 µg/mL to avoid development of drug resistance. Most CPGs recommended higher trough concentrations in patients with bacterial infections, infective endocarditis, osteomyelitis, meningitis and hospital-acquired pneumonia, but no CPG recommend trough concentrations greater than 20 µg/mL. The VAN CPG recommended 15–20 µg/mL for patients with complicated infections and suggested less than 10 µg/mL for patients with urinary tract infections or skin and soft tissue infections not due to MRSA. The ALB CPG recommended trough concentrations at 5–20 µg/mL. If therapy was combined with aminoglycosides, recommended trough concentrations were lower than those for patients without aminoglycoside combination therapy. The COR CPG recommended trough concentrations of 10–15 µg/mL, and peak concentrations of 18–26 µg/mL. The VAN CPG recommended 3 h post vancomycin concentrations of 20–40 µg/ml (Table 3).

Initial administration plan. All guidelines recommended calculating the vancomycin dose according to renal function.

Three CPGs (JAP, LOS and AME) recommended giving a loading dose of 25–30 mg/kg to facilitate rapid attainment of target trough concentrations for serious or complicated infections. Four CPGs (VAN, NHS, DEV and SAP) recommended prescribing a loading dose according to the patients' actual body weight. Five CPGs (ALB, CAL, COR, BAT and WOR) did not recommend a loading dose (Table 3).

Overall assessment

Two CPGs (AME, JAP) were recommended [23,25], and four CPGs (VAN, ALB, COR and WOR) were recommended with modification [26,27,31,34]. Six CPGs (LOS, NHS, CAL, DEV, BAT and SAP) were not recommended. The two CPGs that were recommended have a higher score in domain of rigor of development and a standard search strategy, and they classified the quality of evidence and graded the strength of recommendations. The six CPGs that were not recommended scored below 10% in the domain of rigor of development and the other domains' scores was not high.

Discussion

To our knowledge, this is the first study to evaluate the quality and consistency of vancomycin TDM guidelines; although, CPG quality has been investigated in a variety of clinical areas [17–21]. We made three important findings: first, the overall guideline quality was moderate, and more efforts are needed to improve these guidelines, especially with respect to the domain of rigor of development and stakeholder involvement. Second, vancomycin TDM guideline recommendations were moderately consistent. Third, regional guidelines were of lower quality than national guidelines. In the United Kingdom and Canada, national guidelines may be of sufficient quality to replace regional guidelines of those areas.

Guidelines consistently scored well with respect to clarity and presentation, suggesting that this domain may be easier to achieve or may be more highly emphasized by guideline developers. The

Table 3. Recommendations from CPGs.

Item	AME	LOS	JAP	VAN	ALB	NHS	CAL	DEV	COR	BAT	SAP	WOR
Indication of TDM	✓	✓	✓	✓	✓	NR	NR	NR	NR	NR	NR	NR
PK-PD parameter	✓	NR	✓	✓	NR	NR	NR	NR	NR	NR	NR	NR
Method of TDM												
Peak or trough concentration	trough	trough	trough	Pre-levels and post-levels	trough	trough	Pre-dose levels	Pre-dose levels	Peak and trough	Pre-dose levels trough	Pre-dose levels trough	trough
Time for trough sample	Within 30 min	NR	Within 30 min	NR	Within 30 min	NR	NR	Within 60 min	NR	NR	NR	NR
Time to first level (patients with normal renal function)	Before 4th dose	Before 5th dose	Before 4th or 5th dose	not earlier than 3rd dose and within 48 h	After at least two dose	before 2nd maintenance dose	Before 3rd, 4th or 5th dose	NA	before 3rd or 4th dose	Before 3rd or 4th dose	within 48 h of starting therapy	Before 3rd, 4th dose
Frequency of TDM (patients with normal renal function)	weekly	Depend on clinical condition	weekly	weekly	weekly	Twice weekly	Twice weekly	weekly	After 4 days	Twice weekly	Every 2-3 days	Every 3-4 days
Target of trough concentration (µg/mL)	10-20	10-20	10-20	Lower than 20	5-20	10-20	10-20	10-20	10-15	5-15	10-20	5-15
Target trough concentration in complicated infections	15-20	15-20	15-20	15-20	10-20	15-20	15-20	NR	NR	10-15	15-20	Higher levels[a]
Loading dose	25-30 mg/kg	25-30 mg/kg	25-30 mg/kg	(ma×2,500 mg/dose)	NR	Loading dose	NR	Loading dose	NR	NR	Loading dose	NR

NR: not reported.
[a]Higher levels may be required in specific situations as directed by the microbiologist.

lowest score was recorded in rigor of development, perhaps due to the fact that most guidelines did not report the systematic methods for evidence searching, and many had poorly described information about selection criteria, evidential strengths and limitations, and procedures for updating guidelines. The AME and JAP CPG had the highest scores in this domain and all rated the quality of evidence and graded the recommendation strength, indicating that using a formal system might improve scores for developmental rigor. Developmental rigor is closely related to guideline quality and guideline developers should pay more attention to this domain. The mean score for stakeholder involvement was 27%. No guidelines have considered the views and preferences of patients or of the public, but patient involvement in decision making about care management may improve physician and patient guideline adherence and improve clinical outcomes [35].

The mean score for applicability was 47%, and only four guidelines scored greater than 50% in this area. No guideline considered the cost of vancomycin TDM and no guideline provided enough evidence to support the necessity of vancomycin TDM. Guideline developers did not address potential barriers of guideline implementation and this may have contributed to many hospitals not monitoring vancomycin serum concentrations and many patients not achieving target therapeutic concentrations. The mean score for the scope and purpose was 63%, and most guidelines described their scope, related clinical questions and target populations well. The mean score for editorial independence was 45%. No guidelines described funding sources, although they were developed by medical societies. Most guidelines did not offer data regarding competing interests among guideline development group members. Guideline developers should emphasize these points in future studies.

Specific recommendations of vancomycin TDM guidelines were moderately consistent and varied with respect to trough concentration monitoring, TDM frequency and target serum concentrations across guidelines, which was possibly attributed to unique references for each guideline and only two guidelines (AME, JAP) describing their systematic search strategy. Also, few prospective or randomized trials for vancomycin TDM were available and most of the published literature regarding vancomycin monitoring are observational studies.

The AME and JAP CPG rated the quality of evidence and graded recommendations using the same classification schemata recommended by the Canadian Medical Association. However,

evidence and strength of recommendations were inconsistent, and this may be attributed to the search strategy, criteria for selecting evidence, methods for formulating recommendations, and experts' consensus [36]. The Grading of Recommendations Assessment, Development and Evaluation (GRADE) approach for rating the quality of evidence and grading the strength of recommendations is increasingly being adopted by organizations because this rating system is explicit, comprehensive, transparent and pragmatic [37].We advise guideline developers to adopt GRADE for this reason.

Our search identified all potentially relevant studies but limitations of our approach included the fact that included CPGs were written in English or Chinese. So other CPGs written in other languages were likely missed, even though no restriction on language was applied. Second, AGREE II did not provide criteria about the overall assessment to guide assessors in determining scores, so two assessors may fail to properly weigh domain scores.

In conclusion, the overall quality of vancomycin TDM guidelines was moderate and warrant improvement. Specifically, rigor of development and stakeholder involvement would benefit from increased scrutiny. Guideline recommendations were moderately consistent, especially with respect to regional guidelines. Local adaptation of existing high-quality CPGs to national use is worth considering and a national, high quality guideline to replace various regional guidelines would avoid duplicate efforts. The developers of guidelines should adhere more closely to the AGREE instrument when developing or updating vancomycin TDM guidelines.

Acknowledgments

We thank the study team for their cooperation and the original authors of the included studies for their thoughtful work.

Author Contributions

Conceived and designed the experiments: ZKY SDZ. Performed the experiments: ZKY CL. Analyzed the data: ZKY CL. Contributed reagents/materials/analysis tools: ZKY CL. Wrote the manuscript: ZKY. Revised the manuscript: ZKY CL SDZ. Approved the final version of the manuscript: ZKY CL SDZ.

References

1. Cataldo MA, Tacconelli E, Grilli E, Pea F, Petrosillo N (2012) Continuous versus intermittent infusion of vancomycin for the treatment of Gram-positive infections: systematic review and meta-analysis. J Antimicrob Chemother 67: 17–24.

2. Ye ZK, Tang HL, Zhai SD (2013) Benefits of Therapeutic Drug Monitoring of Vancomycin: A Systematic Review and Meta-Analysis. PLoS ONE 8.

3. Swartling M, Gupta R, Dudas V, Guglielmo BJ (2012) Short term impact of guidelines on vancomycin dosing and therapeutic drug monitoring. Int J Clin Pharm 34: 282–285.

4. Eiland LS, English TM, Eiland EH (2011) Assessment of Vancomycin Dosing and Subsequent Serum Concentrations in Pediatric Patients. Annals of Pharmacotherapy 45: 582–589.

5. De Cock P, Haegeman E, Goerlandt N, Vanhaesebrouck P, Stove V, et al. (2010) Focused Conference Group: P13 - Maximising benefits and minimizing harms from drugs vancomycin dosing and monitoring in children: Compliance with guidelines in a belgian teaching hospital. Basic and Clinical Pharmacology and Toxicology 107: 250–251.

6. Li J, Udy AA, Kirkpatrick CM, Lipman J, Roberts JA (2012) Improving vancomycin prescription in critical illness through a drug use evaluation process: a weight-based dosing intervention study. Int J Antimicrob Agents 39: 69–72.

7. Khotaei GT, Jam S, SeyedAlinaghi S, Motamed F, Nejat F, et al. (2010) Monitoring of serum vancomycin concentrations in pediatric patients with normal renal function. Acta Medica Iranica 48: 91–94.

8. Delicourt A, Touzin K, Lavoie A, Therrien R, Lebel D (2012) [Monitoring of vancomycin in pediatrics]. Med Mal Infect 42: 167–170.

9. Mariani-Kurkdjian P, Nebbad H, Aujard Y, Bingen E (2008) [Monitoring serum vancomycin concentrations in the treatment of Staphylococcus infections in children]. Arch Pediatr 15: 1625–1629.

10. Commandeur D, Giacardi C, Danguy Des Deserts M, Huynh S, Buguet-Brown ML, et al. (2011) [Monitoring vancomycin in an intensive care unit: A retrospective survey on 66 patients]. Med Mal Infect 41: 410–414.

11. Wilson FP, Berns JS (2012) Vancomycin levels are frequently subtherapeutic during continuous venovenous hemodialysis (CVVHD). Clin Nephrol 77: 329–331.

12. Hochart C, Berthon C, Corm S, Gay J, Cliquennois M, et al. (2011) Vancomycin serum concentration during febrile neutropenia in patients with acute myeloid leukemia. Med Mal Infect 41: 652–656.

13. Marengo LL, Del Fiol Fde S, Oliveira Sde J, Nakagawa C, Croco EL, et al. (2010) Vancomycin: the need to suit serum concentrations in hemodialysis patients. Braz J Infect Dis 14: 203–208.

14. Institute of Medicine (2011) Clinical Practice Guidelines We Can Trust. Washington, DC: The National Academies Press.

15. Grimshaw J, Freemantle N, Wallace S, Russell I, Hurwitz B, et al. (1995) Developing and implementing clinical practice guidelines. Qual Health Care 4: 55–64.

16. Cluzeau F, Littlejohns P, Grimshaw JM (1994) Appraising clinical guidelines: towards a "which" guide for purchasers. Qual Health Care 3: 121–122.

17. Acuna-Izcaray A, Sanchez-Angarita E, Plaza V, Rodrigo G, Montes de Oca M, et al. (2013) Quality assessment of asthma clinical practice guidelines: a systematic appraisal. Chest.

18. Zhang ZW, Liu XW, Xu BC, Wang SY, Li L, et al. (2013) Analysis of quality of clinical practice guidelines for otorhinolaryngology in China. PLoS One 8: e53566.

19. Grilli R, Magrini N, Penna A, Mura G, Liberati A (2000) Practice guidelines developed by specialty societies: the need for a critical appraisal. Lancet 355: 103–106.

20. Holmer HK, Ogden LA, Burda BU, Norris SL (2013) Quality of clinical practice guidelines for glycemic control in type 2 diabetes mellitus. PLoS One 8: e58625.

21. de Haas ER, de Vijlder HC, van Reesema WS, van Everdingen JJ, Neumann HA (2007) Quality of clinical practice guidelines in dermatological oncology. J Eur Acad Dermatol Venereol 21: 1193–1198.

22. The AGREE Next Steps Consortium (2009) Appraisal of Guidelines for Research and Evaluation. Available: http://www.agreetrust.org/. Accessed 2 June 2013.

23. Rybak M, Lomaestro B, Rotschafer JC, Moellering R Jr, Craig W, et al. (2009) Therapeutic monitoring of vancomycin in adult patients: a consensus review of the American Society of Health-System Pharmacists, the Infectious Diseases Society of America, and the Society of Infectious Diseases Pharmacists. Am J Health Syst Pharm 66: 82–98.

24. VA Greater Los Angeles Healthcare System (2013) Vancomycin Dosing and Monitoring of Serum Vancomycin Levels Infectious Diseases Section Guidelines.

25. Matsumoto K, Takesue Y, Ohmagari N, Mochizuki T, Mikamo H, et al. (2013) Practice guidelines for therapeutic drug monitoring of vancomycin: a consensus review of the Japanese Society of Chemotherapy and the Japanese Society of Therapeutic Drug Monitoring. J Infect Chemother 19: 365–380.

26. de Lemos J, Lau T, Legal M, Betts T, Collins M, et al. (2011) Vancomycin Therapeutic Drug Monitoring Vancouver Coastal Health & Providence Health Care Regional Guideline. http://www.vhpharmsci.com/Resources/Vancomycin%20Regional%20Guidelines%20_27SEP11_%20FINAL.pdf. Accessed 24 June 2013.

27. Alberta Health Services (2011) Vancomycin Monitoring and Dosing Guideline. http://www.albertahealthservices.ca/LabServices/wf-lab-vancomycin-monitoring-and-dosingguideline.pdf. Accessed 24 June 2013.

28. National Health Services Board Area Drugs and Therapeutics Committee Vancomyin Guideline for Adults. http://www.fifeadtc.scot.nhs.uk/support/antibiotics/Vancomycin%20Guideline.pdf. Accessed 24 June 2013.

29. Calderdale and Huddersfield NHS Foundation Trust (2009) Prescribing Guidelines for Intravenous Vancomycin in Adults. http://www.formulary.cht.nhs.uk/pdf,_doc_files_etc/MMC/094_Antibiotic_Guidelines_December_2009/88-90_Vancomycin.pdf. Accessed 25 June 2013.

30. Royal Devon and Exeter NHS (2010) Guidelines on Intravenous (IV) Vancomycin Dosing in Adults. http://www.rdehospital.nhs.uk/docs/prof/antimicrobial/Vancomycin_EXETER__FINAL_2010_(3)1.pdf. Accessed 25 June 2013.

31. Kendall J, Adie K, Parry R, Powell N, Bendall R, et al. (2010) Vancomycin prescription and therapeutic drug monitoring guideline. http://www.rcht.nhs.uk/DocumentsLibrary/RoyalCornwallHospitalsTrust/Clinical/Pharmacy/Vancomyc inPrescriptionAndTherapeuticDrugMonitoringGuideline.pdf. Accessed 25 June 2013.

32. Royal United Hospitals Bath NHS (2009) Guidelines for the Dosing and Monitoring of Gentamicin, Vancomycin and Teicoplanin. http://www.ruh.nhs.uk/For_Clinicians/departments_ruh/Pathology/documents/haematology/Dosing_of_Gentamicin_Vancomycin_and_Teicoplanin.pdf. Accessed 25 June 2013.

33. Scottish Antimicrobial Prescribing Group (2013) Intravenous Vancomycin Use in Adults Intermittent (Pulsed) Infusion. http://www.scottishmedicines.org.uk/files/sapg/SAPG_Intravenous_vancomycin_adults_Pulsed_infusion_.pdf. Accessed 25 June 2013.

34. Worcestershire Acute Hosptials NHS (2008) Guidelines for Vancomycin Dosing and Monitoring in Adult Patients.

35. Hahn DL (2009) Importance of evidence grading for guideline implementation: the example of asthma. Ann Fam Med 7: 364–369.

36. Campbell F, Dickinson HO, Cook JV, Beyer FR, Eccles M, et al. (2006) Methods underpinning national clinical guidelines for hypertension: describing the evidence shortfall. BMC Health Serv Res 6: 47.

37. Guyatt GH, Oxman AD, Vist GE, Kunz R, Falck-Ytter Y, et al. (2008) GRADE: an emerging consensus on rating quality of evidence and strength of recommendations. BMJ 336: 924–926.

17

Hidden Drug Resistant HIV to Emerge in the Era of Universal Treatment Access in Southeast Asia

Alexander Hoare[1], Stephen J. Kerr[1,2], Kiat Ruxrungtham[2,3], Jintanat Ananworanich[1,2,3], Matthew G. Law[1], David A. Cooper[1], Praphan Phanuphak[2,3], David P. Wilson[1]*

1 National Centre in HIV Epidemiology and Clinical Research, The University of New South Wales, Sydney, Australia, 2 The HIV Netherlands Australia Thailand Research Collaboration, The Thai Red Cross AIDS Research Centre, Bangkok, Thailand, 3 Faculty of Medicine, Chulalongkorn University, Bangkok, Thailand

Abstract

Background: Universal access to first-line antiretroviral therapy (ART) for HIV infection is becoming more of a reality in most low and middle income countries in Asia. However, second-line therapies are relatively scarce.

Methods and Findings: We developed a mathematical model of an HIV epidemic in a Southeast Asian setting and used it to forecast the impact of treatment plans, without second-line options, on the potential degree of acquisition and transmission of drug resistant HIV strains. We show that after 10 years of universal treatment access, up to 20% of treatment-naïve individuals with HIV may have drug-resistant strains but it depends on the relative fitness of viral strains.

Conclusions: If viral load testing of people on ART is carried out on a yearly basis and virological failure leads to effective second-line therapy, then transmitted drug resistance could be reduced by 80%. Greater efforts are required for minimizing first-line failure, to detect virological failure earlier, and to procure access to second-line therapies.

Editor: Mark Wainberg, McGill University AIDS Centre, Canada

Funding: The authors acknowledge funding from the Australian Research Council (DP0771620, FT0991990), National Health and Medical Research Council (CDA568705), and National Institutes of Health (U01-AI069907). The National Centre in HIV Epidemiology and Clinical Research is funded by the Australian Government Department of Health and Ageing, and is affiliated with the Faculty of Medicine, University of New South Wales. The funders had no role in the study design, data collection, analysis, decision to publish or preparation of the manuscript.

Competing Interests: The authors have declared that no competing interests exist.

* E-mail: Dwilson@nchecr.unsw.edu.au

Introduction

HIV/AIDS arose in Asia in the early-to-mid 1980s. By the 1990s HIV epidemics had established in numerous countries; among the worst affected were Thailand and Cambodia with HIV prevalence levels of 1–2%. Currently Thailand, Cambodia, and Myanmar have been experiencing declines in HIV prevalence [1,2], however, countries such as Vietnam, Indonesia, Pakistan and China have observed growth in their epidemics [3].

Effective antiretroviral therapy (ART) is currently being scaled up in most countries in the region. In principle, anyone who is treatment eligible, according to country-specific guidelines but generally similar to the WHO treatment guidelines for resource limited settings [4], can receive ART to slow disease progression [5]. But with greater treatment coverage there is concern about the development of drug resistance, especially in countries where second-line therapy is not widely available. The transmission of drug-resistant strains can potentially lead to ineffective treatment for individuals [6] and reduce their treatment options.

Transmitted drug resistance is a problem around the world, including the Southeast Asia region. Documented rates of transmitted drug resistance include 4% in 2003–2004 in Japan [7] and increases in Taiwan from 6.6% in 1999–2003 to 12.7% in 2003–2006 [8] and Thailand from <1% in 2003 to 5.2% in 2006 [9]. The vast majority of patients (~80%) in Asia start treatment

on AZT/d4T plus 3TC plus EFZ/NVP [10]. This regimen is likely to be the standard for the foreseeable future (perhaps with tenofovir replacing AZT/d4T). If mutations that confer resistance to this standard regimen become widespread, ART rollout strategies could be compromised in a way that is not seen in developed countries with more treatment options.

The primary means to detect transmitted drug resistance is to perform blood tests on newly infected treatment-naïve individuals. Resistance strains can be divided up into two broad categories, namely, majority-resistant and minority-resistant variants. Majority resistant strains are detected through conventional nucleotide sequencing methods after polymerase chain reaction (PCR) amplification, however, these methods are not sensitive enough to detect minority-resistant strains that comprise less than ~25% of the viral population [11]. These minority-resistant variants can be detected using advanced real time PCR assays [12,13]. There is potential for these minority strains to go undetected in the population, leading to under-estimates of transmitted resistance levels.

We sought to estimate the potential levels of acquired and transmitted (majority and minority) drug resistant strains of HIV that could emerge in a typical Southeast Asian population. We do this through the development of a biologically realistic mathematical transmission model. We use the situation in Thailand as a representation for a general Asian epidemic and thus calibrated the model to reflect the epidemic in Thailand. Thailand is a leading example of treatment scale-up with the introduction of ART through the National Access to Antiretroviral Program for People who have AIDS by the Ministry of Public Health Access to Care program [14,15] and extended to the government's National AIDS Program by the National Health Security Office in 2004 [16]. Our mathematical model is parameterized using specific clinical, demographic, biological, and behavioral data in and around Bangkok, Thailand, before second-line therapy became available. Although second-line therapy is rolling out in Thailand, it is not available for many HIV-infected people in other countries. Our model extends previous mathematical models of HIV drug resistance applied to other settings (e.g. [17,18,19,20]) and models that incorporate at-risk groups for the Southeast Asian setting [21].

Methods

Our model describes the unique nature of Asian HIV epidemics whereby epidemics typically emerge and are initially driven by injecting drug use and sex work. Waves of infection occurred in these population groups, followed by infection among clients of sex workers and their regular sexual partners which led to generalized epidemics. In recent years HIV epidemics have emerged among

men who have sex with men. This epidemic pattern has been observed in numerous Southeast Asian countries [22,23] and is captured by our model (see Figure S1). To reflect disease progression, we assumed that all HIV-infected people progress from primary/acute HIV infection, to chronic/asymptomatic infection, to a treatment-eligible stage, and then may receive treatment (Fig. 1). Each disease stage is associated with a different viral load and hence a different level of infectiousness [24,25]. Disease progression rates are assumed to be different in the presence of a majority-resistant strain due to lower viral fitness, but we assume minority-resistant strains have the same fitness as wild-type virus. We assume that reduced viral fitness of majority-resistant strains diminishes their replicative capacity and thus their ability to be transmitted. A multiplying factor was used to model a decrease in viral fitness between 5% and 50% [18,19]. Mathematical Details S1 contains more details about the implementation of this viral fitness factor. Once on treatment, we assume that patients will continue using their ART regimen, even if treatment failure occurs, as limited second or third line treatment options are available in many settings.

The level of adherence to ART is associated with clinical success [26,27] as systemic drug concentrations determine the degree of pressure to select for drug resistant strains [28,29,30,31,32].

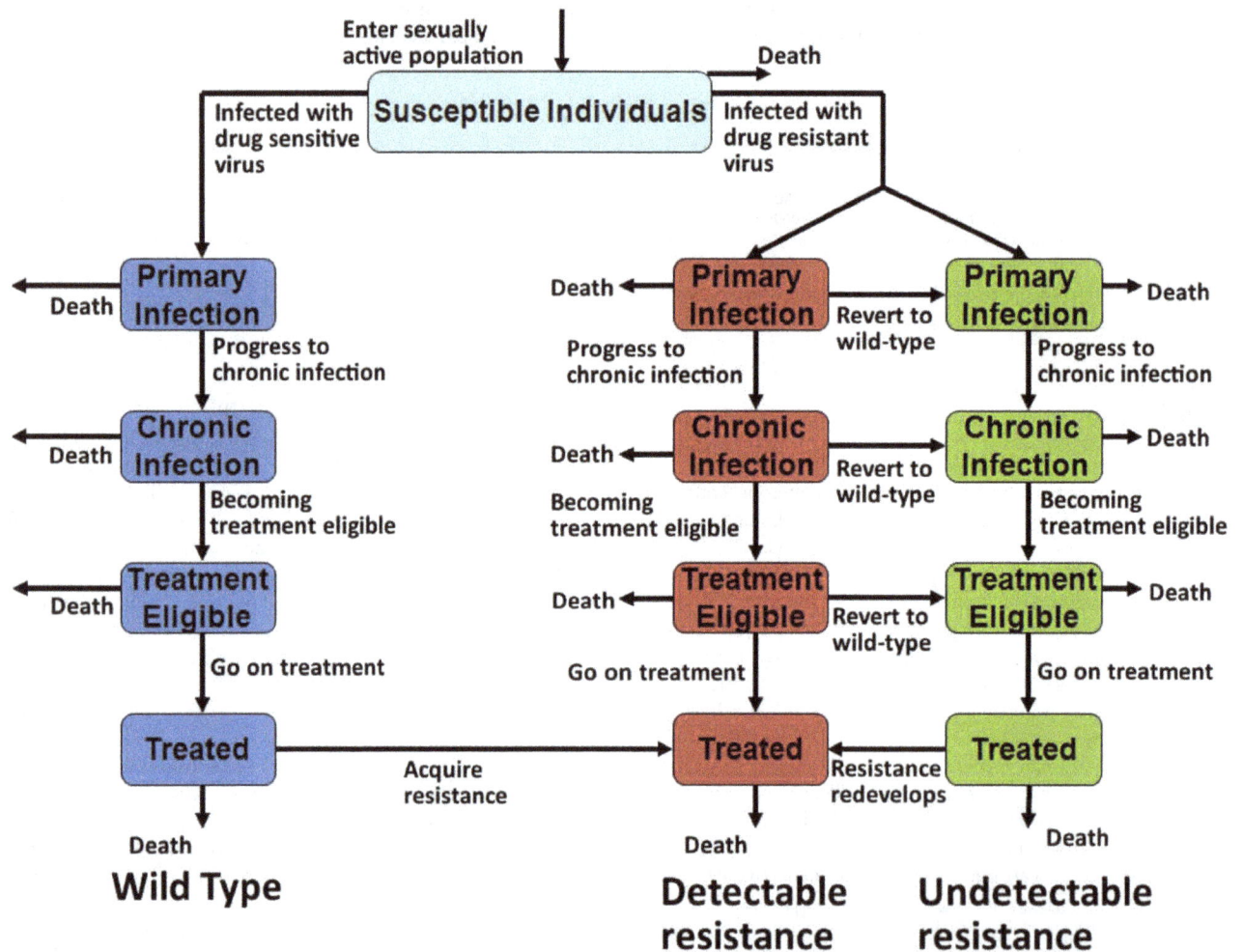

Figure 1. Schematic diagram of our mathematical model. The natural progression of HIV infection captured by our model, with disease progression illustrated vertically; the model is also divided into three arms: each arm governs a different type of virus (wild-type, majority-resistant variants, minority-resistant variants).

Although there is variability in adherence between people, in our model we do not explicitly model adherence to ART but based on international clinical data [33,34,35] we assume that 3–5% of people on first-line ART select for drug resistant mutations each year and acquire drug-resistant strains. We track populations of people infected with either wild-type HIV or strains of drug-resistant HIV that are detectable or appear to have reverted to wild-type. Those people who have strains that appear to revert to wild-type have minority-resistant variants and it is assumed that majority-resistant variants will quickly emerge under pressure of ART. We use our model (and uncertainty and sensitivity analyses [36,37]) to estimate the future trajectories of wild-type and drug-resistant HIV epidemics, determine the biological, clinical, and behavioral factors that are most important in giving rise to these evolving epidemics and how they might change with time in order to plan public health prevention and clinical practice strategies most appropriately. Some mathematical modeling has been carried out to forecast HIV epidemics in Southeast Asia [21], but no previous model has investigated the impact of drug resistance in this region.

The model was then used to assess the impact of regular viral load testing in a setting where second line treatment is available and commenced once virological failure is detected. We assumed that viral load tests could be performed at regular intervals on all those who are receiving treatment. We simulated different scenarios of frequency of viral load testing: once every 2 years, every year, twice yearly, or quarterly. We also assumed that a period of one week was required between the time of the test and receiving the test results and starting the patient on effective second-line treatment. Full technical detail of the model structure, assumptions and parameter values can be found in the supporting information.

Results

Emergence of Drug Resistance

After 10 years of universal ART without access to any second line therapies, moderately high levels of drug resistance can be expected in the HIV-infected population. People on ART will start to acquire drug resistant strains of virus. If second and subsequent lines of therapy are not widely available and failed regimens continue to be used then the emergent drug-resistant strains can be transmitted to susceptible individuals. Subsequently, the proportion of newly-infected treatment-naïve HIV cases that have drug-resistant strains could be substantial. Our model estimates that after 10 years of universal ART without monitoring of treatment failure and optimizing therapy ~24% of new infections could include drug-resistant mutations (Fig. 2a). Approximately one-

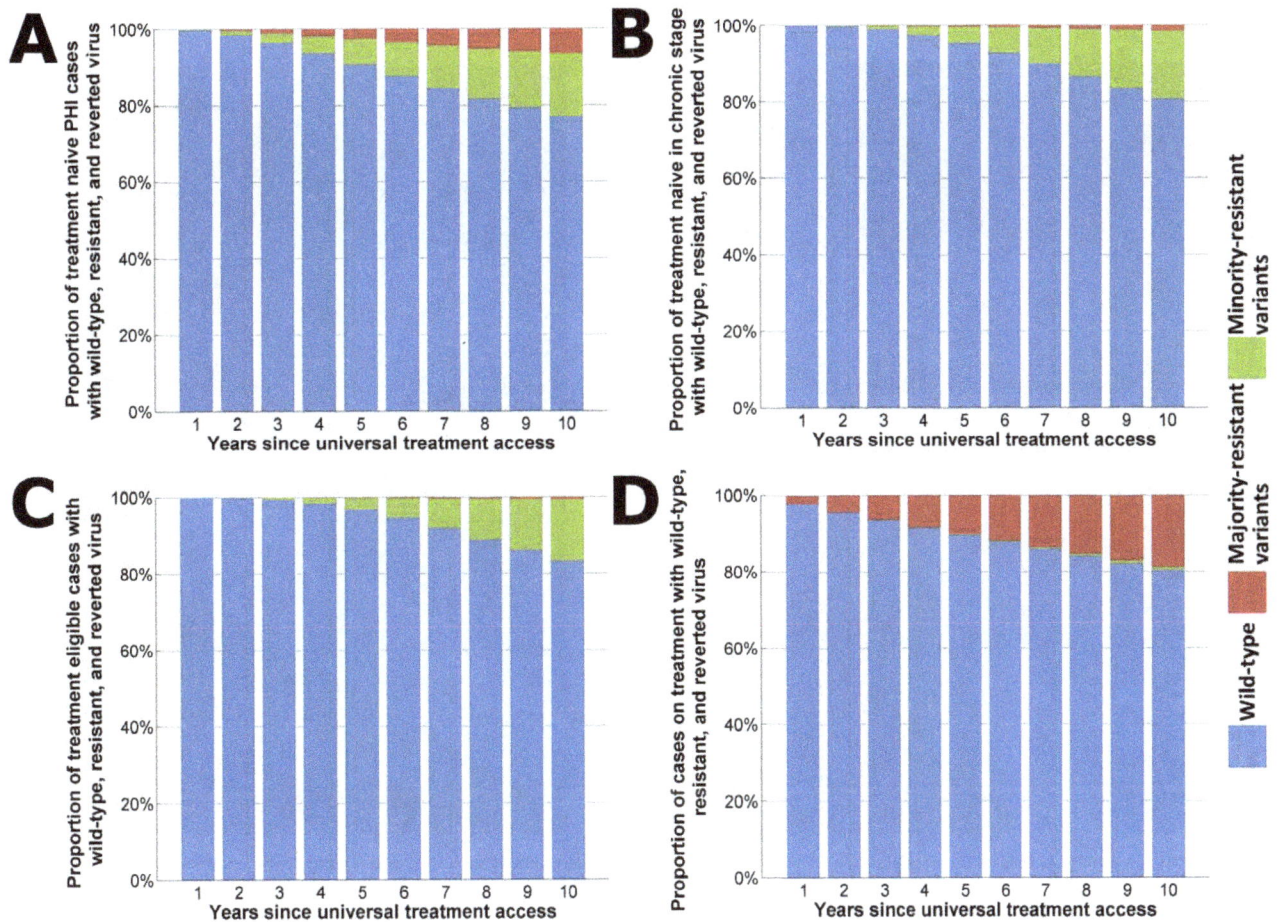

Figure 2. Stacked column charts indicating proportions of HIV viral types. Proportions of all HIV infections that are predominantly wild-type virus (blue), drug-resistant strains that are undetectable/minority-resistant variants (green), or drug-resistant strains that can be detected/majority-resistant variants (red) for HIV-infected cases in (**a**) primary infection, (**b**) chronic infection, (**c**) treatment-eligible stage, and (**d**) on treatment. Plots are over the time period since the introduction of universal access, and without any options for second-line therapy.

third of cases in the primary/acute stage of infection with drug-resistant mutations could have majority-resistant variants of HIV that are detectable and the remainder would have minority-resistant variants (Fig. 2a).

Most subjects infected with transmitted resistant virus appear to revert to wild type

In the absence of the pressure of ART, majority-resistant strains of HIV tend to revert to become minority-resistant variants that appear to be exclusively wild-type and not detected by standard sequencing methods. According to our model, after 10 years of universal access to ART without second-line options ~20% of treatment-naïve cases in asymptomatic stage would have some drug-resistant strains and ~17% of cases at treatment-eligible stage of infection would have some drug-resistant strains (Fig. 2b, c). However, it is likely that the vast majority of these cases would have minority-resistant variants: only ~1% and <1% of the respective HIV cases would have detectable majority-resistant variants after 10 years (Fig. 2b,c). Thus, drug-resistant HIV could remain hidden and will only re-emerge when selective pressure of ART is applied. Of course, the rate of reversion could differ between different antiretroviral drug-based mutations. The re-emergence of drug-resistant strains could be quick once treatment is commenced by individuals. The vast majority (~95%) of individuals on ART who have drug-resistant strains would have

majority-resistant variants (Fig. 2d). Based on our model we estimate that after 10 years of universal treatment access ~20% of all people that are on ART would have drug-resistant strains of HIV (Fig. 2d).

Factors determining the prevalence of drug resistance

Key factors giving rise to the prevalence of drug resistance differ between populations of treatment-naïve and treatment-experienced individuals. Multivariate sensitivity analyses revealed that the average time for resistant strains to appear to revert to wild-type virus and the relative fitness of drug-resistant strains were the most important parameters for determining the prevalence of majority-resistant variants in treatment-naïve cases (Fig. 3a). The relative fitness of viral strains with resistant mutations is a key determinant in the prevalence of transmitted drug resistance. The greater the fitness of these strains the larger the prevalence of 'hidden' resistance in the treatment-naïve population. Transmitted drug resistance increases with fitter drug-resistant strains and slower majority-to-minority variant reversion times. In contrast, the average time for drug-resistant strains to re-emerge upon pressure of ART (in individuals with minority-resistant variants; that is, to become majority-resistant variants upon applying pressure of ART) and the percentage of patients that acquire drug resistance per year (in individuals with wild-type) were found to be the most important factors in determining the proportion of

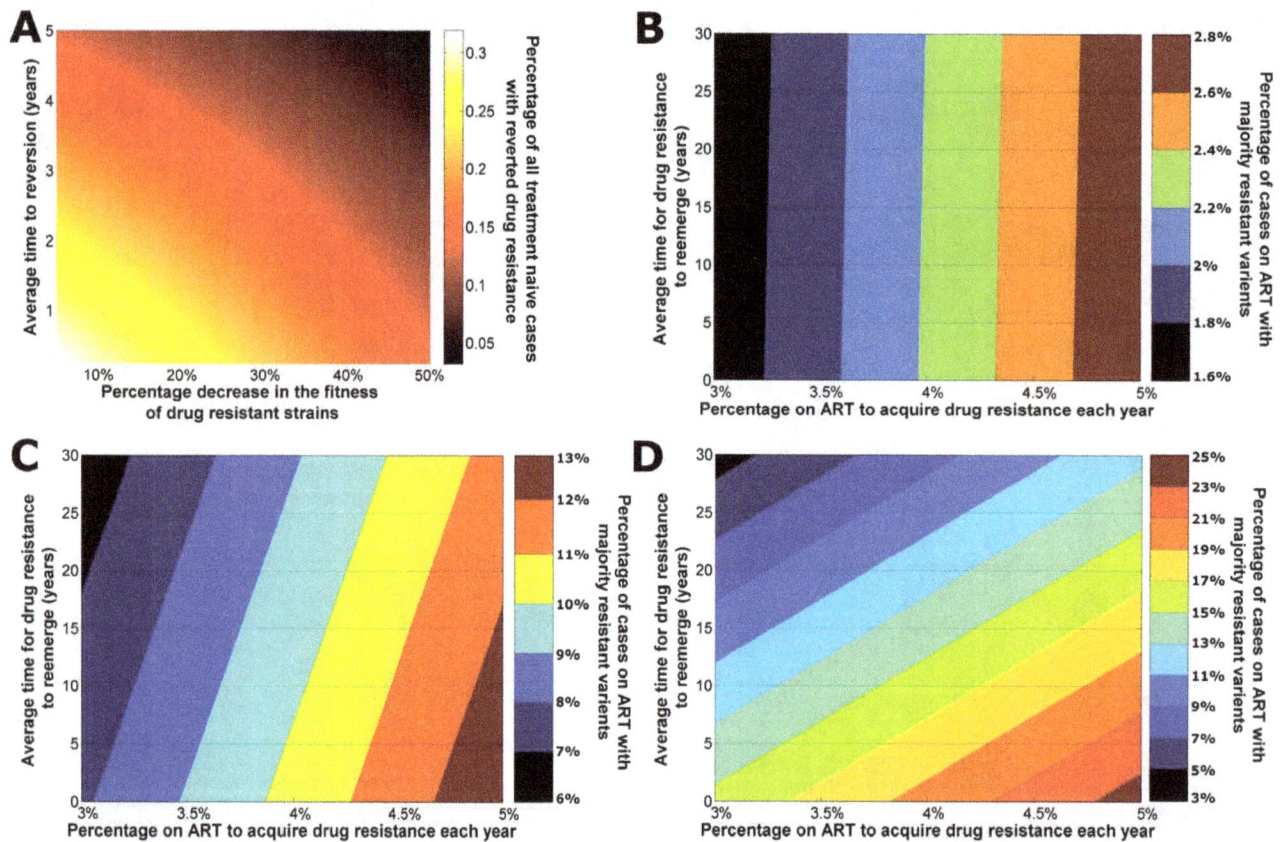

Figure 3. Series of response surfaces from sensitivity analyses. (a) A response surface plot of the proportion of treatment-naïve HIV-infected cases with minority-resistant variants versus viral fitness of drug-resistant strains and the average time for majority-resistant variants to revert to minority-resistant variants in the absence of ART. **(b)–(d)** Contour plots of the proportion of cases on ART that have majority-resistant variants (colored contours) versus the rate at which people infected with wild-type acquire drug resistant virus (x-axis) and the average time for majority-resistant variants to emerge for people infected with minority-resistant variants (y-axis) after **(b)** 1 year, **(c)** 5 years, and **(d)** 10 years of universal treatment access.

treated individuals with majority-resistant variants (Fig. 3b–d). Interestingly, the relative importance of these two factors changes over time. To illustrate this, in Figure 3b–d we present a series of contour plots of the prevalence of majority-resistant variants among the treated population after 1 year (Fig. 3b), 5 years (Fig. 3c), and 10 years (Fig. 3d) after commencing universal treatment access. We found that the number of people receiving treatment that have detectable drug resistance after one year of universal access to treatment is almost completely dependent on the percentage that acquire resistance per year, as indicated by the close to vertical lines in Figure 3b. After five years, the dependence has begun to shift such that the average time for resistance to reemerge begins to have an impact on the prevalence of drug-resistant HIV (Fig. 3c). After 10 years, the prevalence of detectable drug resistance is now more dependent on the average time for drug resistance to reemerge for transmitted drug-resistant strains than on the rate of acquired resistance (Fig. 3d). When projected even further, after 20 years the vast majority of drug-resistant cases are due to transmitted resistance (see Figure S2). This suggests that the nature of the drug-resistant HIV epidemic could change considerably, initially being driven by acquired resistance and then evolve to be dominated by cases who have transmitted (but hidden) drug resistance.

Reducing transmitted drug resistance through viral load testing

In many Southeast Asian countries, treatment failure is often realized due to clinical symptoms rather than the presence of mutations or virological or immunological failure. Frequent viral load testing is generally infeasible due to financial constraints. However, viral load testing for monitoring patients' responses to ART is available in some settings and it could be expected that it will become more common across the region in the future. Therefore, we used our model to estimate the expected proportion of newly acquired HIV infections to have drug-resistant strains versus the frequency of viral load testing of individuals on ART (assuming that treated cases that experience virological failure commence and are maintained on second and subsequent lines of therapy that successfully suppresses

viral load). In Figure 4 we present the expected levels of transmitted drug resistance versus the frequency of viral load testing. As the testing frequency is increased, a substantial reduction in the prevalence of transmitted drug resistance is observed. Providing a test every two years will reduce the prevalence by more than 50% compared to no viral load testing. With yearly testing, the proportion of all new infections with transmitted resistance drops below 5% (that is, an 80% relative reduction). According to our model, if viral load testing is further increased to every three months, transmitted drug resistance will make up only ~2.5% of all infections (reducing transmitted resistance by 90% compared to the situation where no testing is carried out). When compared to yearly testing, our model found that six and three monthly testing offered a relative reduction of 28% and 44% in transmitted drug resistance levels, respectively.

Discussion

Effective treatment with antiretroviral drugs reduces viral load which improves the health of treated individuals and also decreases infectiousness and the potential to transmit the virus to others [24,25,38]. However, persons infected with drug-resistant HIV have reduced therapeutic options for their survival [39,40]. Antiretroviral resistance was detected against the first drug used against HIV, AZT, shortly after it was introduced [41]. Subsequently, resistance to every currently licensed antiretroviral drug has been observed. Drug-resistant strains of HIV that are acquired through use of ART can then be transmitted to susceptible people. The first report of observed transmission of drug-resistant HIV was in 1993 [42]. The transmission of drug resistance is becoming an increasing problem among many nations with long histories of ART. Data on rates of transmitted and acquired resistance in Southeast Asian countries is limited. In the few areas in which HIV transmitted resistance have been measured in Asia, already moderate levels (~4–5%) have been observed in some countries [43,44,45]. In other regions of the world, prevalence of drug resistant HIV among treatment-naïve persons has been estimated to be up to 25% [46]. It is important to implement strategies in Southeast Asian countries to avoid the

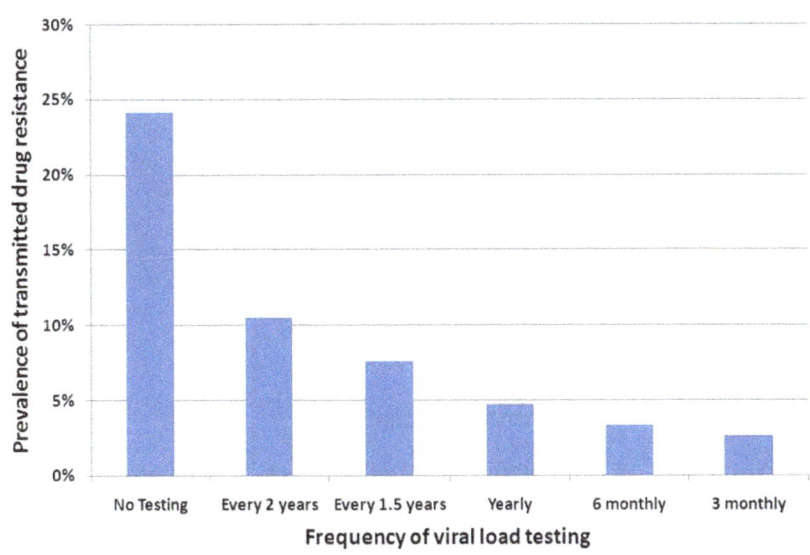

Figure 4. Prevalence of transmitted drug resistance after 10 years with various viral load testing frequencies. Testing scenarios include: no testing, once every two years, once every 1.5 years, yearly, twice yearly, and quarterly. Once tested, it is assumed that anyone failing treatment is taken off the failed regimen and given access to new treatment.

high prevalence of transmitted drug resistance that has occurred elsewhere.

We demonstrated that if treatment options are limited for those who fail first-line therapy then the prevalence of acquired and transmitted drug resistant strains of HIV could be relatively large. The prevalence of transmitted drug resistance could be ~24% after ten years of universal treatment access if there is no viral load monitoring and access to second-line therapy. However, most (99%) of the drug resistance could remain 'hidden' as minority-resistant variants that are not detectable by standard sequencing methods. Majority-resistant variants are likely to emerge at significantly faster rates than expected once treatment is initiated [47]. While there is some uncertainty about whether minority-resistant strains have a substantial [12,48] or limited [13] impact on the success of antiretroviral therapy, the impact of majority-resistant strains on treatment is known to be significant. Majority-resistant strains may be more likely to survive in the presence of antiretroviral therapy than wild-type strains, however, they are likely to have reduced replicative capacity leading to lower viral loads in plasma and genital fluids and thus lower potential to be transmitted to other people. Our model demonstrated the importance of viral fitness whereby strains with higher fitness are more likely to lead to higher population levels of transmitted drug resistance (Figure 3a).

To reduce the prevalence of drug resistance among treatment-naïve individuals it is recommended that treated cases are regularly monitored and that second-line and subsequent lines of therapy are made available for those who have failed first-line regimens. We investigated the expected impact on transmitted drug resistance of different frequencies of viral load monitoring and access to second-line therapy when required. Even with a modest testing frequency of once every two years for patients on ART, the model demonstrates a large reduction in the amount of transmitted drug resistance would be achieved. Testing as frequently as quarterly could reduce the prevalence of transmitted drug resistance by ~90%. In Thailand, since 2008 second-line therapy with TDF/3TC/LPV/r has been widely available as well as once yearly viral load monitoring and genotyping (for those with viral load of more than 2000 copies per ml). However, there are limited treatment options in Thailand and patients with TDF resistance will have difficulties in finding effective second line treatment options. Wide availability of third line treatments for patients in this region will be unlikely in the near future. Therefore, it is highly important to minimise drug resistance. Based on our model, yearly testing can reduce transmitted drug resistance to below 5%. It is important for countries in Southeast Asia to procure access to second-line therapies and determine ways of implementing regular viral load monitoring. It will then be important to procure third-line and salvage therapies for patients in this region, however, this is unlikely to be feasible in the near future. Viral load testing is not widely available in many Asian countries and the emergence of drug resistant HIV is not typically assessed during patient consultation [49,50]. Without viral load or genotypic monitoring, late detection of treatment failure may facilitate the acquisition of numerous additional resistance mutations [51]. Monitoring of patients' CD4 counts and viral load levels is being carried out in the Treat Asia HIV Observational Database (TAHOD) study [52]. TAHOD and other surveillance activities such as the Treat Asia Studies to Evaluate Resistance (TASER) study are important foundations for monitoring treatment success and detecting the development of resistance to antiretrovirals. In some countries governments pay for the first triple combination, but patients pay for other drugs if the first regimen fails. This barrier to accessing second-line therapy

needs to be overcome else persistent use of sub-optimal or failed regimens will occur. Continued use of a failed regimen may select for increases in drug-resistant HIV strains that may then be transmitted to others.

Limited combinations of antiretrovirals are available for first-line treatment in most Southeast Asian countries. In Thailand, first-line therapy is based on NNRTIs and usually consists of a fixed dose combination of d4T/3TC/NVP, with a newer regimen of ZDV/3TC/NVP recently rolled out [53]. The prevalence of resistance in Thailand to NNRTI and NRTI based drug combinations can restrict second-line options in close to half of patients [54]. The World Health Organization has recently made recommendations against use of Triomune (d4T/3TC/NVP) in initiation of first line therapy [55,56]. New treatment guidelines for Thailand will also be released shortly [57]. These guidelines recommend AZT- and TDF- with EFV or NVP and 3TC as preferred first-line. There is a planned 2-year phase out of d4T for patients already receiving d4T. Similar clinical approaches may not be achievable in all resource-limited settings and the use of Triomune is likely to continue. Obtaining access to more first-line antiretroviral combinations will also assist with treatment options and could prolong the time until second-line therapies are required and reduce the risk of resistant strains being transmitted.

While first-line therapy continues to scale-up around Southeast Asia it is important to plan for, and control, the emergence of drug-resistant HIV, particularly as most drug-resistant cases in the future could be 'hidden' as minority-resistant variants. Current surveillance programs, which are based around testing newly diagnosed subjects aged less than 25 years rather than genuinely acute infections, will not detect the scale of the problem. Hidden transmitted drug resistance has the potential to drive relatively high levels of drug resistance over the next 5–10 years unless treated cases are monitored regularly and initiate second-line therapies soon after the failure of first-line options. Data from TAHOD suggest that around half of patients beginning ART will require second-line therapies 3 years after beginning treatment [10]. Diagnosing newly acquired infections is important for understanding the true degree of transmitted drug resistance [9,58] and should be prioritized as we approach the next phase of HIV epidemics in an era of universal treatment access.

While our model is specifically constructed and calibrated to reflect the unique epidemiology of HIV transmission in Southeast Asia, the conclusions drawn from our study can also be applied to other settings. Most countries in Southeast Asia still use d4T-based first-line therapy, which is similar to Sub-Saharan Africa. Access to antiretrovirals is similarly limited in both regions. Our results are generally applicable to non resource-rich settings in which suboptimal regimens are used and there are limited therapeutic options. Our conclusions concerning the dangers of continued use of failed treatment regimens and important value of regular viral load monitoring coupled with access to second-line therapies may assist countries in their scale-up of antiretroviral treatment.

Supporting Information

Mathematical Details S1 Detailed description of mathematical model.

Figure S1 The seven population subgroups contained within the model. Lines between groups indicate interactions for sexual mixing.

Figure S2 Response surface plot from sensitivity analysis. This plot shows the proportion of cases on ART that have majority-resistant variants (colored contours) versus the rate at which people infected with wild-type acquire drug resistant virus (x-axis) and the average time for majority-resistant variants to emerge for people infected with minority-resistant variants (y-axis) after 20 years of universal treatment access.

Author Contributions

Conceived and designed the experiments: DPW. Performed the experiments: AH. Analyzed the data: AH. Wrote the paper: AH SK KR JA ML DAC PP DPW. Supervised the project: DPW. Provided data to inform the mathematical model: SK. Provided advice and assisted in the interpretation and presentation of results: KR JA ML DAC PP.

References

1. Rojanapithayakorn W (2006) The 100% Condom Use Programme in Asia. Reproductive Health Matters 14: 41–52.
2. (2009) Annual Repot 2008. NCHADS.
3. UNAIDS (2008) 2008 Report on the global AIDS epidemic. Geneva: UNAIDS.
4. WHO (2003) Scaling up antiretroviral therapy in resource-limited settings: treatment guidelines for a public health approach; Geneva World Health Organization; Available at http://www.who.int.
5. Chasombat S, McConnell MS, Siangphoe U, Yuktanont P, Jirawattanapisal T, et al. (2009) National Expansion of Antiretroviral Treatment in Thailand, 2000–2007: Program Scale-Up and Patient Outcomes. J Acquir Immune Defic Syndr 50: 506–512.
6. Yam WC, Chen JH, Wong KH, Chan K, Cheng VC, et al. (2006) Clinical utility of genotyping resistance test on determining the mutation patterns in HIV-1 CRF01_AE and subtype B patients receiving antiretroviral therapy in Hong Kong. J Clin Virol 35: 454–457.
7. Gatanaga H, Ibe S, Matsuda M, Yoshida S, Asagi T, et al. (2007) Drug-resistant HIV-1 prevalence in patients newly diagnosed with HIV/AIDS in Japan. Antiviral Res 75: 75–82.
8. Chang SY, Chen MY, Lee CN, Sun HY, Ko W, et al. (2008) Trends of antiretroviral drug resistance in treatment-naive patients with human immuno-deficiency virus type 1 infection in Taiwan. J Antimicrob Chemother 61: 689–693.
9. Apisarnthanarak A, Jirayasethpong T, Sa-nguansilp C, Thongprapai H, Kittihanukul C, et al. (2008) Antiretroviral drug resistance among antiretrovi-ral-naive persons with recent HIV infection in Thailand. HIV Med 9: 322–325.
10. Srasuebkul P, Calmy A, Zhou J, Kumarasamy N, Law M, et al. (2007) Impact of drug classes and treatment availability on the rate of antiretroviral treatment change in the TREAT Asia HIV Observational Database (TAHOD). AIDS Res Ther 4: 18.
11. Schuurman R, Demeter L, Reichelderfer P, Tijnagel J, de Groot T, et al. (1999) Worldwide evaluation of DNA sequencing approaches for identification of drug resistance mutations in the human immunodeficiency virus type 1 reverse transcriptase. J Clin Microbiol 37: 2291–2296.
12. Johnson JA, Li JF, Wei X, Lipscomb J, Irlbeck D, et al. (2008) Minority HIV-1 drug resistance mutations are present in antiretroviral treatment-naive populations and associate with reduced treatment efficacy. PLoS Med 5: e158.
13. Peuchant O, Thiebaut R, Capdepont S, Lavignolle-Aurillac V, Neau D, et al. (2008) Transmission of HIV-1 minority-resistant variants and response to first-line antiretroviral therapy. AIDS 22: 1417–1423.
14. Chasombat S, Lertpiriyasuwat C, Thanprasertsuk S, Suebsaeng L, Lo YR (2006) The National Access to Antiretroviral Program for PHA (NAPHA) in Thailand. Southeast Asian J Trop Med Public Health 37: 704–715.
15. Bunjumnong O. Thailand: access to antiretroviral treatment under Universal Health Care Scheme; 2002; Barcelona.
16. Maneesriwongul WL, Tulathong S, Fennie KP, Williams AB (2006) Adherence to antiretroviral medication among HIV-positive patients in Thailand. J Acquir Immune Defic Syndr 43 Suppl 1: S119–122.
17. Wilson DP, Kahn J, Blower SM (2006) Predicting the epidemiological impact of antiretroviral allocation strategies in KwaZulu-Natal: the effect of the urban-rural divide. Proc Natl Acad Sci U S A 103: 14228–14233.
18. Blower S, Bodine E, Kahn J, McFarland W (2005) The antiretroviral rollout and drug-resistant HIV in Africa: insights from empirical data and theoretical models. AIDS 19: 1–14.
19. Blower S, Ma L, Farmer P, Koenig S (2003) Predicting the impact of antiretrovirals in resource-poor settings: preventing HIV infections whilst controlling drug resistance. Curr Drug Targets Infect Disord 3: 345–353.
20. Sanchez MS, Grant RM, Porco TC, Gross KL, Getz WM (2005) A decrease in drug resistance levels of the HIV epidemic can be bad news. Bull Math Biol 67: 761–782.
21. Brown T, Peerapatanapokin W (2004) The Asian Epidemic Model: a process model for exploring HIV policy and programme alternatives in Asia. Sex Transm Infect 80 Suppl 1: i19–24.
22. Ruxrungtham K, Brown T, Phanuphak P (2004) HIV/AIDS in Asia. Lancet 364: 69–82.
23. Weniger BG, Limpakarnjanarat K, Ungchusak K, Thanprasertsuk S, Choopanya K, et al. (1991) The epidemiology of HIV infection and AIDS in Thailand. AIDS 5 Suppl 2: S71–85.
24. Quinn TC, Wawer MJ, Sewankambo N, Serwadda D, Li C, et al. (2000) Viral load and heterosexual transmission of human immunodeficiency virus type 1. Rakai Project Study Group. N Engl J Med 342: 921–929.
25. Wilson DP, Law MG, Grulich AE, Cooper DA, Kaldor JM (2008) Relation between HIV viral load and infectiousness: a model-based analysis. Lancet 372: 314–320.
26. King MS, Brun SC, Kempf DJ (2005) Relationship between adherence and the development of resistance in antiretroviral-naive, HIV-1-infected patients receiving lopinavir/ritonavir or nelfinavir. J Infect Dis 191: 2046–2052.
27. Wood E, Hogg RS, Yip B, Harrigan PR, O'Shaughnessy MV, et al. (2003) Effect of medication adherence on survival of HIV-infected adults who start highly active antiretroviral therapy when the CD4+ cell count is 0.200 to $0.350 \times 10(9)$ cells/L. Ann Intern Med 139: 810–816.
28. Tam LW, Chui CK, Brumme CJ, Bangsberg DR, Montaner JS, et al. (2008) The relationship between resistance and adherence in drug-naive individuals initiating HAART is specific to individual drug classes. J Acquir Immune Defic Syndr 49: 266–271.
29. Bangsberg DR, Acosta EP, Gupta R, Guzman D, Riley ED, et al. (2006) Adherence-resistance relationships for protease and non-nucleoside reverse transcriptase inhibitors explained by virological fitness. AIDS 20: 223–231.
30. Bangsberg DR, Porco TC, Kagay C, Charlebois ED, Deeks SG, et al. (2004) Modeling the HIV protease inhibitor adherence-resistance curve by use of empirically derived estimates. J Infect Dis 190: 162–165.
31. Bangsberg DR, Charlebois ED, Grant RM, Holodniy M, Deeks SG, et al. (2003) High levels of adherence do not prevent accumulation of HIV drug resistance mutations. AIDS 17: 1925–1932.
32. Harrigan PR, Hogg RS, Dong WW, Yip B, Wynhoven B, et al. (2005) Predictors of HIV drug-resistance mutations in a large antiretroviral-naive cohort initiating triple antiretroviral therapy. J Infect Dis 191: 339–347.
33. Maggiolo F, Airoldi M, Kleinloog HD, Callegaro A, Ravasio V, et al. (2007) Effect of adherence to HAART on virologic outcome and on the selection of resistance-conferring mutations in NNRTI- or PI-treated patients. HIV Clin Trials 8: 282–292.
34. Phillips AN, Dunn D, Sabin C, Pozniak A, Matthias R, et al. (2005) Long term probability of detection of HIV-1 drug resistance after starting antiretroviral therapy in routine clinical practice. AIDS 19: 487–494.
35. Phillips AN, Leen C, Wilson A, Anderson J, Dunn D, et al. (2007) Risk of extensive virological failure to the three original antiretroviral drug classes over long-term follow-up from the start of therapy in patients with HIV infection: an observational cohort study. Lancet 370: 1923–1928.
36. Blower SM, Dowlatabadi H (1994) Sensitivity and Uncertainty Analysis of Complex-Models of Disease Transmission: an HIV Model, as an Example. International Statistical Review 62: 229–243.
37. Hoare A, Regan DG, Wilson DP (2008) Sampling and sensitivity analyses tools (SaSAT) for computational modelling. Theoretical Biology and Medical Modelling 5: 4.
38. Attia S, Egger M, Muller M, Zwahlen M, Low N (2009) Sexual transmission of HIV according to viral load and antiretroviral therapy: systematic review and meta-analysis. AIDS 23: 1397–1404.
39. Ruxrungtham K, Pedro RJ, Latiff GH, Conradie F, Domingo P, et al. (2008) Impact of reverse transcriptase resistance on the efficacy of TMC125 (etravirine) with two nucleoside reverse transcriptase inhibitors in protease inhibitor-naive, nonnucleoside reverse transcriptase inhibitor-experienced patients: study TMC125-C227. HIV Med 9: 883–896.
40. Hogg RS, Bangsberg DR, Lima VD, Alexander C, Bonner S, et al. (2006) Emergence of drug resistance is associated with an increased risk of death among patients first starting HAART. PLoS Med 3: e356.
41. Larder BA, Darby G, Richman DD (1989) HIV with reduced sensitivity to zidovudine (AZT) isolated during prolonged therapy. Science 243: 1731–1734.
42. Ho DD, Moudgil T, Alam M (1989) Quantitation of human immunodeficiency virus type 1 in the blood of infected persons. N Engl J Med 321: 1621–1625.
43. Choi JY, Kim EJ, Park YK, Lee JS, Kim SS (2008) National survey for drug-resistant variants in newly diagnosed antiretroviral drug-naive patients with HIV/AIDS in South Korea: 1999–2005. J Acquir Immune Defic Syndr 49: 237–242.
44. Jittamala P, Puthanakit T, Chaiinseeard S, Sirisanthana V (2009) Predictors of virologic failure and genotypic resistance mutation patterns in thai children receiving non-nucleoside reverse transcriptase inhibitor-based antiretroviral therapy. Pediatr Infect Dis J 28: 826–830.
45. Chetchotisakd P, Anunnatsiri S, Kiertiburanakul S, Sutthent R, Anekthananon T, et al. (2006) High rate multiple drug resistances in HIV-infected patients failing nonnucleoside reverse transcriptase inhibitor regimens

in Thailand, where subtype A/E is predominant. J Int Assoc Physicians AIDS Care (Chic Ill) 5: 152–156.

46. Booth CL, Geretti AM (2007) Prevalence and determinants of transmitted antiretroviral drug resistance in HIV-1 infection. J Antimicrob Chemother 59: 1047–1056.

47. Tang JW, Pillay D (2004) Transmission of HIV-1 drug resistance. J Clin Virol 30: 1–10.

48. Van Laethem K, De Munter P, Schrooten Y, Verbesselt R, Van Ranst M, et al. (2007) No response to first-line tenofovir+lamivudine+efavirenz despite optimization according to baseline resistance testing: impact of resistant minority variants on efficacy of low genetic barrier drugs. J Clin Virol 39: 43–47.

49. Cohen GM (2007) Access to diagnostics in support of HIV/AIDS and tuberculosis treatment in developing countries. Aids 21 Suppl 4: S81–87.

50. WHO (2008) Towards Universal Access: Scaling up priority HIV/AIDS interventions in the health sector.

51. Kumarasamy N, Madhavan V, Venkatesh KK, Saravanan S, Kantor R, et al. (2009) High frequency of clinically significant mutations after first-line generic highly active antiretroviral therapy failure: implications for second-line options in resource-limited settings. Clin Infect Dis 49: 306–309.

52. Zhou J, Kumarasamy N, Ditangco R, Kamarulzaman A, Lee CK, et al. (2005) The TREAT Asia HIV Observational Database: baseline and retrospective data. J Acquir Immune Defic Syndr 38: 174–179.

53. Sirivichayakul S, Phanuphak P, Pankam T, R OC, Sutherland D, et al. (2008) HIV drug resistance transmission threshold survey in Bangkok, Thailand. Antivir Ther 13 Suppl 2: 109–113.

54. Sungkanuparph S, Manosuthi W, Kiertiburanakul S, Piyavong B, Chumpathat N, et al. (2007) Options for a second-line antiretroviral regimen for HIV type 1-infected patients whose initial regimen of a fixed-dose combination of stavudine, lamivudine, and nevirapine fails. Clin Infect Dis 44: 447–452.

55. (2009) Rapid advice Antiretroviral therapy for HIV infection in adults and adolescents. Geneva: The World Health Organisation.

56. (2009) Meeting report: revision of WHO ART guidelines for adults and adolescents. Geneva: The World Heath Organisation.

57. Sungkanuparph S, Techasathi W, Teeraratkul A, Chasombat S, Bhakeecheepe S, et al. (2010) Thai National Guidelines for Antiretroviral Therapy in HIV-1 Infected Adults and Adolescents 2010. Asian Biomedicine (in press).

58. Apisarnthanarak A, Mundy LM (2008) Antiretroviral drug resistance among antiretroviral-naive individuals with HIV infection of unknown duration in Thailand. Clin Infect Dis 46: 1630–1631.

18

Therapeutic Drug Monitoring and Pharmacogenetic Study of HIV-Infected Ethnic Chinese Receiving Efavirenz-Containing Antiretroviral Therapy with or without Rifampicin-Based Anti-Tuberculous Therapy

Kuan-Yeh Lee[1], Shu-Wen Lin[2,3], Hsin-Yun Sun[4], Ching-Hua Kuo[3,5], Mao-Song Tsai[6], Bing-Ru Wu[7], Sue-Yo Tang[2], Wen-Chun Liu[4], Sui-Yuan Chang[7,8]*, Chien-Ching Hung[4,9,10]*

1 Department of Internal Medicine, National Taiwan University Hospital Hsin-Chu Branch, Hsin-Chu, Taiwan, 2 Graduate Institute of Clinical Pharmacy, National Taiwan University, Taipei, Taiwan, 3 Department of Pharmacy, National Taiwan University Hospital and National Taiwan University College of Medicine, Taipei, Taiwan, 4 Department of Internal Medicine, National Taiwan University Hospital and National Taiwan University College of Medicine, Taipei, Taiwan, 5 School of Pharmacy, National Taiwan University, Taipei, Taiwan, 6 Department of Internal Medicine, Far Eastern Memorial Hospital, New Taipei City, Taiwan, 7 Department of Clinical Laboratory Sciences and Medical Biotechnology, National Taiwan University College of Medicine, Taipei, Taiwan, 8 Department of Laboratory Medicine, National Taiwan University Hospital and National Taiwan University College of Medicine, Taipei, Taiwan, 9 Department of Medical Research, China Medical University Hospital, Taichung, Taiwan, 10 China Medical University, Taichung, Taiwan

Abstract

Objectives: Plasma efavirenz concentrations in HIV-infected patients with tuberculosis (TB) may be affected by cytochrome P450 (CYP) 2B6 single-nucleotide polymorphisms and concurrent rifampicin use. We aimed to investigate the effects of *CYP2B6* G516T polymorphisms and concomitant rifampicin use on the plasma efavirenz concentrations in HIV-infected Taiwanese.

Methods: HIV-infected patients with or without TB who had received combination antiretroviral therapy containing efavirenz (600 mg daily) for two weeks or greater were enrolled for determinations of *CYP2B6* G516T polymorphism and plasma efavirenz concentrations with the use of polymerase-chain-reaction restriction fragment-length polymorphism and high-performance liquid chromatography, respectively.

Results: From October 2009 to August 2012, 171 HIV-infected patients, including 18 with TB, were enrolled 113 (66.1%) with *CYP2B6* G516G, 55 (32.2%) GT, and 3 (1.8%) TT genotype. Patients receiving rifampicin had a significantly lower median plasma efavirenz concentration than the control group (2.16 vs 2.92 mg/L, $P = 0.003$); however, all patients achieved target plasma concentration (>1 mg/L). Patients with GT or TT genotype had a significantly higher plasma concentration than those with GG genotype (2.50 vs 3.47 mg/L for GT genotype and 8.78 mg/L for TT genotype, $P<0.001$). Plasma efavirenz concentration >4 mg/L was noted in 38 (22.2%) patients, which was associated with a lower weight (per 10-kg increase, odds ratio, 0.52; 95% confidence interval, 0.33–0.83) and GT or TT genotype (odds ratio, 4.35; 95% confidence interval, 1.97–9.59) in multivariate analysis.

Conclusions: Despite combination with rifampicin, sufficient plasma efavirenz concentrations can be achieved in HIV-infected Taiwanese with TB who receive efavirenz 600 mg daily. Carriage of *CYP2B6* 516 GT and TT genotypes and a lower weight are associated with higher plasma efavirenz concentrations.

Editor: Pierre Roques, CEA, France

Funding: This study was supported by grants from the Centers for Disease Control, Taiwan and Institute for Biotechnology and Medicine Industry, Taiwan. The funding sources played no role in study design and conduct, data collection, analysis or interpretation, writing of the manuscript, or the decision to submit it for publication.

Competing Interests: The authors have declared that no competing interests exist.

* E-mail: hcc0401@ntu.edu.tw (CCH); sychang@ntu.edu.tw (SYC)

Introduction

Efavirenz is a potent non-nucleoside reverse-transcriptase inhibitor (NNRTI) and its combination with tenofovir and emtricitabine remains one of the preferred antiretroviral regimens for antiretroviral-naive patients without resistance-associated mutations to NNRTIs [1]. The recommended therapeutic levels of efavirenz at 12 hours are 1 to 4 mg/L [2]. Sub-therapeutic drug concentrations may increase the risk of drug resistance and treatment failure; on the other hand, concentrations above the therapeutic range may increase the risk of drug-related toxicities, such as neuropsychiatric side effects, which may lead to emergence of resistance resulting from treatment interruptions [2].

Efavirenz is metabolized primarily through hepatic cytochrome P450 (CYP) 2B6. The wide inter-patient variability of efavirenz concentrations has been reported, which may be related to sex, weight, ethnicity, drug-drug interactions, and single-nucleotide polymorphism (SNP) of *CYP2B6* [3–8]. However, conflicting data regarding the aforementioned factors makes dose adjustment while co-administration with other drugs or weight-based adjustment problematic [9,10].

Efavirenz-containing antiretroviral therapy has been recommended for HIV-infected patients with tuberculosis (TB) when rifampicin-containing anti-tuberculous therapy is co-administered. Rifampicin may induce activity of CYP enzymes, which may lower the plasma concentrations of efavirenz. The early pharmacokinetic studies reported a reduction by 26% in the efavirenz concentration when co-administered with rifampicin [11], and the package insert of efavirenz recommends a compensatory increase of efavirenz from a standard dose of 600 mg to 800 mg per day for patients who are taking concomitant rifampicin and have a weight greater than 50 kg [9,12]. However, a recently published clinical trial demonstrated the opposite findings and did not support weight-based dosing of efavirenz in combination with rifampicin [10]. In addition, prior studies have shown that *CYP2B6* polymorphism, particularly G516T, is associated with high plasma concentrations of efavirenz and its drug-related toxicity [7,13,14]. The frequency of *CYP2B6* G516T polymorphisms may vary with different racial populations [15], and the pharmacogenetic data of efavirenz concentrations in Taiwanese patients are lacking. In this study, we aimed to investigate the effect of concurrent use of rifampicin and *CYP2B6* G516T polymorphisms on the plasma efavirenz concentrations in HIV-infected Taiwanese patients.

Materials and Methods

Study Population

From October 2009 to August 2012, HIV-infected patients who were aged 18 years or greater and had been receiving an efavirenz-containing combination antiretroviral therapy at a daily dose of 600 mg for more than 14 days were enrolled when they sought routine HIV care at the National Taiwan University Hospital, the largest referral hospital for inpatient and outpatient HIV care in Taiwan. For patients who received a clinical or microbiologically confirmed diagnosis of TB, the daily dose of rifampicin was 450 mg for those with a weight less than 50 kg and 600 mg for those with a weight of 50 kg or greater. Patients were excluded from the study if they were pregnant; infected with HIV that was shown to harbor resistance-associated mutations to efavirenz or other NNRTIs; receiving anti-tuberculous regimens that did not contain rifampicin; infected with rifampicin-resistant *Mycobacterium tuberculosis*; or had hepatic transaminases greater than five times the upper limit of normal. The protocol was approved by the Research Ethics Committee of the National Taiwan University Hospital (registration number, 200908014M) and all patients provided written informed consent prior to enrollment.

Data Collection and Sample Preparation

We used a computerized case record form to collect data on the demographics, weight and height, and clinical characteristics including CD4 lymphocyte counts and plasma HIV RNA loads at baseline and during the follow-up, serostatus of hepatitis B virus and hepatitis C virus, concomitant medications (including antiretroviral therapy and rifampicin), and the date and time of the last efavirenz dose that was usually taken at bedtime. Blood samples were collected 12 ± 1 hours after the last dose of efavirenz into tubes containing EDTA as anticoagulant for *CYP2B6* G516T genotyping and determination of efavirenz concentration. Plasma samples were stored at $-20°C$ until analysis.

Laboratory Investigations

Determination of plasma HIV RNA load and CD4 lymphocyte count. Plasma HIV RNA load was quantified using the Cobas Amplicor HIV-1 Monitor test (Cobas Amplicor version 1.5, Roche Diagnostics Corporation, IN) with a lower detection limit of 40 copies/mL, and CD4 lymphocyte count was determined using FACFlow (BD FACS Calibur, Becton Dickinson, CA). The CD4 counts and plasma HIV RNA loads were monitored one month after initiation of combination antiretroviral therapy in antiretroviral-naive patients, or change of regimens in the presence of virological failure; and every three to six months thereafter according to the national HIV treatment guidelines.

***CYP2B6* G516T genotyping.** High molecular weight genomic DNA was extracted from PBMC using the Wizard® Genomic DNA purification kit (Promega, WI, USA). The concentration of extracted DNA was determined by spectrophotometry and stored at $-20°C$ before further analysis. Polymerase-chain-reaction restriction fragment-length polymorphism (PCR-RFLP) was performed to determine the SNPs of *CYP2B6* G516T.

Determination of efavirenz concentrations. The plasma concentration of efavirenz was analyzed using high-performance liquid chromatography (HPLC) based on a validated method reported by Ramachandran et al. [16] with minor modifications. In brief, 300 µL of plasma was added to 300 µL of acetonitrile for deproteinization, and the organic layer was dried under nitrogen. The extract was then dissolved with 150 µL of methanol and 200 µL of 10 mM phosphate buffer (pH 4.0) and acetonitrile in a 57:43 (volume/volume) ratio. The HPLC system consisted of a L-2130 HTA solvent delivery pump, a L-2200 autosampler, a UV1000 wavelength detector programmable UV detector wavelength 245 nm and the computing integrator for HPLC D-2000 Elite on Windows (version 1.2, Hitachi High Technologies Corporation, Tokyo, Japan). Chromatography was performed on a C18 column (Mightsil RP-18 GP, 250×4.6 nm with 5 µm beads, particle size 3.5 mm; Kanto Corporation, Portland, OR, USA) protected by a guard column (1033 mm I.D.; Phenomenex, Torrance, CA, USA), and a flow rate of 1 mL/min. The mobile phase was composed of the same phosphate buffer mixed with acetonitrile (57:43). The retention time of efavirenz was 13.43 min. The calibration curve was linear within the range 0.5 to 10.0 mg/L, and data more than 10.0 mg/L was designated as 10.0 mg/L. The lower limit of quantification was 0.5 mg/L. Recovery after extraction from plasma was 101%. Accuracy ranged from 97.7 to 101.6%. Intra-assay and inter-assay coefficients of variation at 5 µg/mL ranged from 0.2 to 0.97% and 1.15 to 1.93%, respectively.

Statistical Analysis

Statistical analysis was performed using SPSS software (version 17.0; SPSS Inc., Chicago, IL, USA). Continuous variables were reported as medians and ranges, and were compared using the Mann-Whitney test. Categorical variables were expressed as numbers and percentages, and were compared using the Pearson $\chi2$ test or Fisher's exact test, as appropriate. Multivariate logistic regression analysis was used to evaluate the association between each independent variable and risk of high plasma efavirenz concentration (>4 mg/L). Variables with P values <0.10 in the univariate analyses were entered into a multivariate logistic regression model with the backward elimination method. Pear-

Table 1. Clinical characteristics of 171 HIV-infected patients who received efavirenz-containing combination antiretroviral therapy with or without receiving concurrent rifampicin-containing anti-tuberculous therapy.

	All patients (n=171)	Concurrent Rifampicin Use			CYP2B6 G516T Polymorphisms			
		Rifampicin (n=18)	Control (n=153)	P value	GG (n=113)	GT (n=55)	TT (n=3)	P value
Age, median (range), years	38 (19–87)	44 (24–69)	37 (19–87)	0.08	38 (19–87)	38 (21–72)	37 (31–38)	0.74
Male sex, n (%)	160 (93.6)	18 (100)	142 (92.8)	0.61	105 (92.9)	52 (94.5)	3 (100)	>0.99
Homosexual male, n (%)	136 (79.5)	16 (88.9)	120 (78.4)	0.48	86 (76.1)	47 (85.5)	3 (100)	0.31
Body weight, kg, median (range) [patients with available data]	62 (40.5–95) [170]	59 (41–73) [18]	62 (40.5–95) [152]	0.040	62 (40.5–95) [113]	62 (47–81) [54]	61 (61–65) [3]	0.97
Body-mass index, median (range), kg/m^2 [patients with available data]	21.5 (14.5–29.8) [167]	20.7 (14.5–25.0) [18]	21.5 (15.4–29.8) [149]	0.26	21.9 (14.5–21.8) [110]	21.3 (17.5–29.7) [54]	21.0 (20.1–21.2) [3]	0.69
CART-naive, n (%)	45 (26.3)	9 (50.0)	36 (23.5)	0.041	26 (23.0)	18 (32.7)	1 (33.3)	0.39
Plasma HIV viral load at baseline, median (range), log$_{10}$ copies/mL	1.6 (1.6–6.3)	4.2 (1.6–5.8)	1.6 (1.6–6.3)	<0.001	1.6 (1.6–6.1)	1.6 (1.6–6.3)	1.6 (1.6–4.8)	0.57
Plasma HIV viral load <200 copies/mL at baseline, n (%)	121 (70.8)	6 (33.3)	115 (75.2)	<0.001	83 (73.5)	36 (65.5)	2 (66.7)	0.56
CD4 at baseline, median (range), cells/μL	401 (3–1377)	119 (3–1100)	413 (11–1377)	0.001	430 (3–1377)	358 (14–1037)	300 (232–586)	0.33
Chronic HBV infection, n (%)	37 (21.6)	3 (16.7)	34 (22.2)	0.77	20 (17.7)	17 (30.9)	0 (0)	0.12
Chronic HCV infection, n (%)	14 (8.2)	3 (16.7)	11 (7.2)	0.17	8 (7.1)	6 (10.9)	0 (0)	0.53
Total bilirubin, median (range), mg/dL [patients with available data]	0.51 (0.13–5.64) [161]	0.94 (0.2–3.93) [16]	0.49 (0.13–5.64) [145]	0.001	0.53 (0.13–3.17) [108]	0.48 (0.21–5.64) [50]	0.41 (0.34–0.57) [3]	0.64
AST, median (range), U/L [patients with available data]	25 (12–241) [163]	37 (15–76) [18]	24 (12–241) [145]	0.07	24 (12–241) [109]	25 (12–135) [51]	32 (24–42) [3]	0.57
CYP2B6 G516T polymorphisms, n (%)								
GG	113 (66.0)	12 (66.7)	101 (66.0)	0.84				
GT	55 (32.2)	6 (33.3)	49 (32.0)	0.88				
TT	3 (1.8)	0 (0)	3 (2.0)	>0.99				
Concurrent rifampicin use, n (%)					12 (10.6)	6 (10.9)	0 (0)	>0.99

* Abbreviations: AST, aspartate aminotransferase; cART, combination antiretroviral therapy; HBV, hepatitis B virus; HCV, hepatitis C viru.

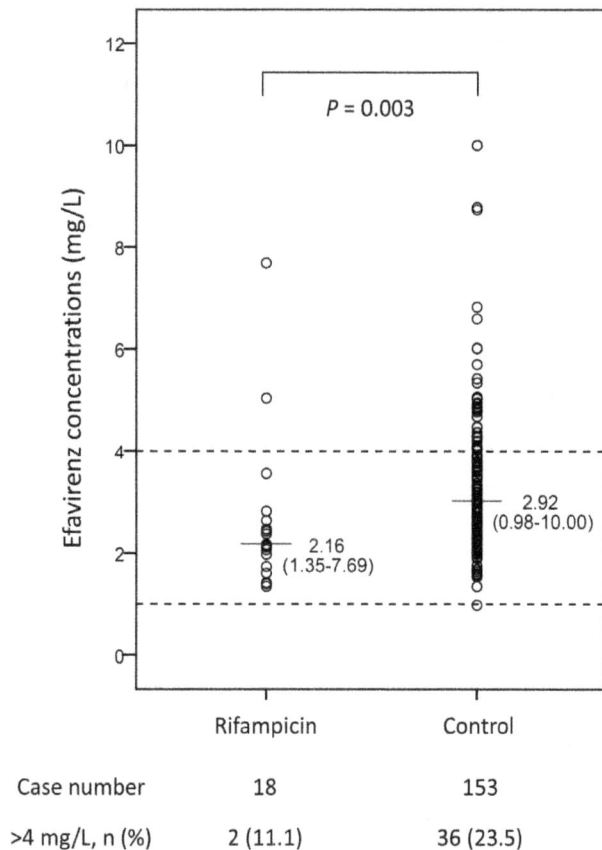

Figure 1. Plasma efavirenz concentrations of HIV-infected patients with (n = 18) and without taking rifampicin (n = 153). Dash lines indicate the target plasma concentrations of efavirenz for wild-type HIV-1 isolate.

son's correlations were used to evaluate the relationships between body weight and plasma efavirenz concentration. P values <0.05 were considered statistically significant.

Results

During the study period, 171 HIV-infected patients, all of whom were ethnic Chinese, were enrolled. The baseline characteristics of the patients are shown in Table 1. Most of the patients were male (93.6%) with a median age of 38 years (range, 19–87 years). The median weight was 62 kg (range, 40.5–95 kg). About three quarters of the patients (126, 73.7%) had been receiving combination antiretroviral therapy for 24 weeks or more with a plasma HIV RNA load <200 copies/mL in 121 (96.0%). The median CD4 count was 401 cells/μL (range, 3–1377 cells/μL). Eighteen patients (10.5%) were also taking rifampicin-containing anti-tuberculous therapy, including 15 with microbiologically-confirmed TB, two with subsequently microbiologically-confirmed non-tuberculous mycobacteriosis, and one with TB diagnosed based on clinical presentation. Seventy-seven (45.0%) patients received concomitant medications other than antiretroviral and anti-tuberculous therapy, and none of these drugs had been reported to cause significant drug-drug interaction with efavirenz.

All 171 patients had determinations of *CYP2B6* G516T polymorphism: 113 patients (66.1%) had carriage of GG genotype (wild-type), 55 (32.2%) GT genotype (heterozygous mutant), and 3 (1.8%) TT genotype (homozygous mutant). Compared with those

who did not have TB, patients with TB and receiving rifampicin had a lower weight (median, 59 vs 62 kg, $P = 0.040$), though the body-mass index (BMI) between the two groups was similar (Table 1); were less likely to have had combination antiretroviral therapy before enrollment into this study (50.0% vs 76.5%, $P = 0.041$); and were more likely to have higher levels of total bilirubin levels in the serum (median, 0.94 vs 0.49 mg/dL, $P = 0.001$). The demographics, HIV-related variables, and laboratory data were all similar among the patients with different genotypes of *CYP2B6* G516T (Table 1).

The median plasma concentration of efavirenz at 12 hours for all patients was 2.82 mg/L (range, 0.98–10.00 mg/L), and almost all of the patients achieved plasma efavirenz concentration of more than 1 mg/L except one with a level of 0.98 mg/L. Figure 1 shows the comparison of plasma efavirenz concentrations between the patients with and those without receiving rifampicin. Compared with the patients not receiving rifampicin, patients receiving rifampicin had a significantly lower median plasma concentration by 26% (median [range], 2.16 [1.35–7.69] vs 2.92 [0.98–10.00] mg/L, $P = 0.003$). Nevertheless, all patients receiving rifampicin achieved plasma efavirenz concentrations above the recommended target concentration (>1 mg/L), even in the eight patients who weighted 60 kg or more (the plasma concentrations ranging from 1.35 to 2.82 mg/L). Figure 2 shows the plasma efavirenz concentrations in patients with different *CYP2B6* G516T genotypes. Patients with heterozygous or homozygous mutants had significantly higher plasma efavirenz concentrations compared to those with wild type (median [range], 2.50 mg/L [0.98–10.00] for GG genotype vs 3.47 mg/L [1.35–8.73] for GT genotype and 8.78 mg/L [4.77–10.00] for TT genotype; $P < 0.001$).

More than one fifth of the patients (38, 22.2%) had plasma efavirenz concentrations greater than 4 mg/L, a concentration that was reported to be associated with a higher risk for neuropsychiatric adverse effects [2]. Univariate and multivariate analyses revealed that a lower weight and heterozygous or homozygous mutant of *CYP2B6* G516T genotypes were statistically significantly associated with elevated plasma efavirenz concentrations above 4 mg/L (Table 2). Figure 3 shows that plasma efavirenz concentrations were inversely correlated with weight, and leaner patients (especially those <50 kg) had plasma efavirenz concentrations greater than 4 mg/L.

Fourteen of 18 patients (77.8%) receiving rifampicin and 143 of 153 patients (93.5%) not receiving rifampicin continued efavirenz-containing combination antiretroviral therapy for at least 24 weeks. Among the patients receiving rifampicin, three died of bacterial pneumonia complicated with respiratory failure and one was transferred to another hospital. On the other hand, among the patients not receiving rifampicin, one patient died of bacterial pneumonia complicated with respiratory failure; two discontinued efavirenz due to intolerable neuropsychiatric side effects with plasma efavirenz concentrations of 4.08 and >10.0 mg/L, respectively; three changed antiretroviral regimen because of genotypic resistance to efavirenz; and the other four were lost to follow-up. The proportion of patients with successful virological suppression (plasma HIV RNA load <200 copies/mL) at week 24 was similar between the patients receiving rifampicin and those not receiving rifampicin (92.9% vs 99.3%, $P = 0.34$). As for the 45 antiretroviral-naïve patients, 8 and 32 patients in each group continued efavirenz-containing combination antiretroviral therapy for at least 24 weeks, and the proportions of patients who achieved virological suppression was also similar (87.5% vs 96.9%, $P = 0.73$).

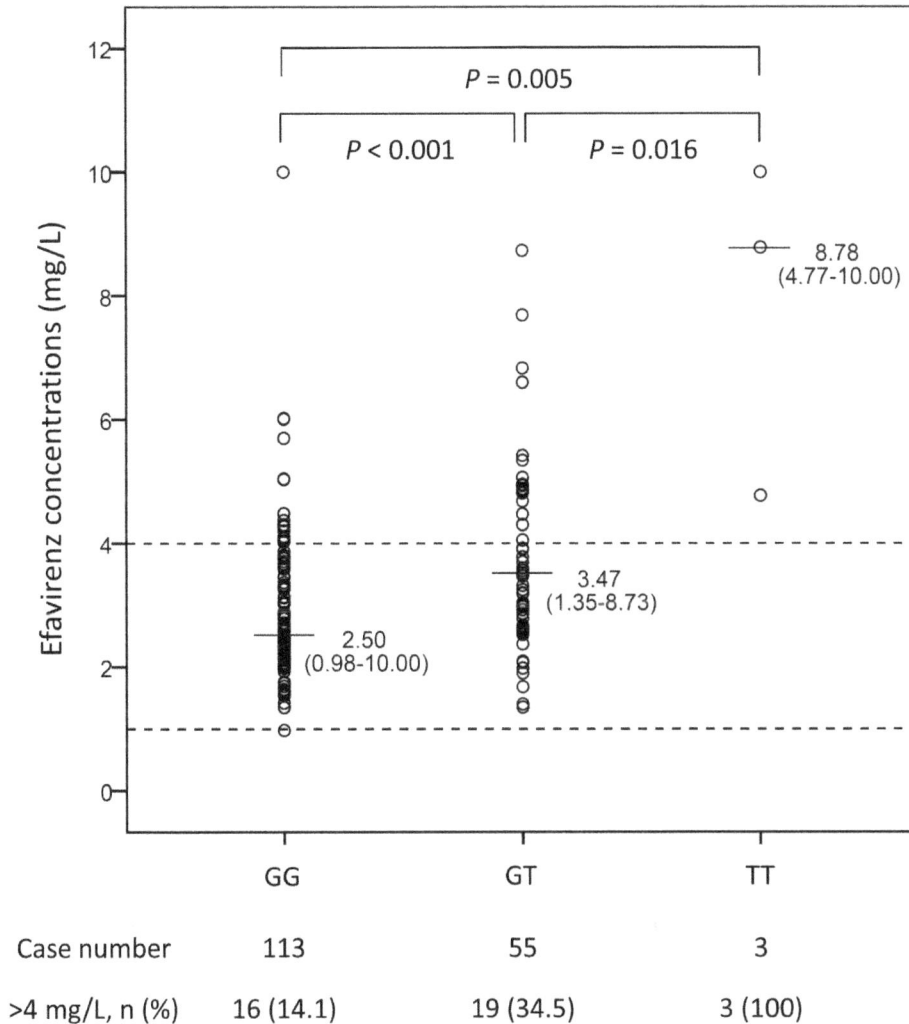

Figure 2. Plasma efavirenz concentrations of 171 HIV-infected patients with different genotypes of *CYP2B6* G516T polymorphisms.
Dash lines indicate the target plasma concentrations of efavirenz for wild-type HIV-1 isolate.

Discussion

This therapeutic drug monitoring and pharmacogenetic study that was performed in HIV-infected Taiwanese individuals showed that almost all patients could achieve therapeutic efavirenz concentrations (>1 mg/L) regardless of *CYP2B6* G516T polymorphism, rifampicin use, or body weight. In contrast, a significant proportion of the patients had toxic levels (>4 mg/L), which was statistically significantly associated with a lower weight and GT or TT genotypes of *CYP2B6* G516T.

Efavirenz-containing combination antiretroviral therapy is the preferred antiretroviral therapy for HIV-related TB for which rifampicin-based anti-tuberculous therapy is co-administered [1]. However, data are conflicting on the appropriate efavirenz dose when co-administered with rifampicin among the published studies [7,10–12,17,18]. The discrepancy may be related to the study populations with different body habitus and pharmacogenetics. Early studies reported a 26% reduction in the plasma efavirenz concentration when co-administered with rifampicin [11,12], and the possible mechanism is that rifampicin induces the activity of the main metabolic enzyme, CYP2B6, which results in enhanced efavirenz clearance and reduced plasma levels. As a

result, the US Food and Drug Administration approved a revised efavirenz package insert recommending efavirenz be increased from a standard daily dose of 600 mg to 800 mg for patients taking concomitant rifampicin who weigh greater than 50 kg [9], based on empirical data from the two drug-drug interaction trials [11,12] and semi-mechanistic population pharmacokinetic modeling.

In contrast, more recent and larger studies in HIV-infected patients with TB indicated either that there was no significant impact of rifampicin on efavirenz concentrations [7,17]; or that rifampicin co-administration increased efavirenz concentrations [10,18]. The study by Ramachandran et al. conducted in South India [7] and another study by Cohen et al. in South Africa (with a mean weight of 66 kg among participants) [17] both demonstrated that *CYP2B6* G516T polymorphism but not rifampicin co-administration significantly influenced the pharmacokinetics of efavirenz. The study by Kwara et al. found that patients receiving rifampicin had significantly higher mean efavirenz concentrations in those with the *CYP2B6* 516TT genotype [18]. The authors hypothesized that the paradoxical effect may be due to increased susceptibility of the CYP2B6 (172-histidine) variant allozyme (resulting from the 516G→T polymorphism) to inhibition by one

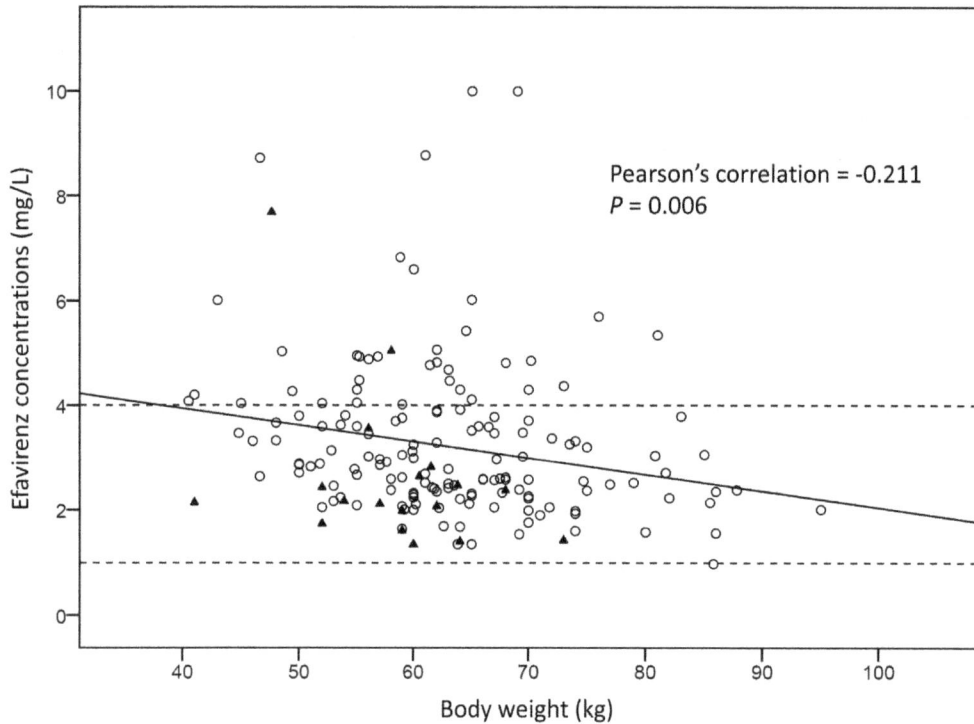

Body weight, kg	40-49	50-59	60-69	70-79	>80
Case number	14	51	67	25	13
>4 mg/L, n (%)	8 (57.1)	11 (21.6)	14 (20.9)	4 (16.0)	1 (7.7)

Figure 3. Relationship between efavirenz plasma concentrations (mg/L) and body weight (kg). Triangles indicate cases with concurrent rifampicin use, and circles indicate cases without taking rifampicin.

(or more) of the anti-tuberculous drugs as compared with the reference CYP2B6 (172-glutamine) enzyme, and metabolic inhibition on the non-CYP2B6 accessory pathways, including CYP2A6 by isoniazid. More studies are warranted to determine the underlying mechanism. The large multinational and multi-center STRIDE Study that enrolled 543 participants showed that efavirenz and rifampicin co-administration was associated with a trend toward higher, not lower, efavirenz trough concentrations compared to efavirenz alone in all patients (median, 1.96 vs

1.80 mg/L, $P = 0.067$), and the concentrations were significantly higher in blacks (median, 2.08 vs 1.75 mg/L, $P = 0.005$) [10]. CYP2B6 genotyping for the participants of the STRIDE pharmacokinetic study is planned for further analysis to determine whether the CYP2B6 genetic polymorphisms play an important role in the paradoxical increases in efavirenz concentrations with rifampicin co-administration.

In our study, patients taking rifampicin had significantly lower plasma efavirenz concentrations compared to the patients not

Table 2. Univariate and multivariate logistic regression analyses of variables associated with toxic plasma efavirenz concentrations (>4 mg/L).

	Univariate analysis		Multivariate analysis	
	OR (95% CI)	P value	OR (95% CI)	P value
Age, years	0.98 (0.95, 1.02)	0.36		
Body weight, per 10-kg increase	0.59 (0.39, 0.89)	**0.011**	0.52 (0.33, 0.83)	**0.006**
Chronic HBV infection	0.96 (0.40, 2.31)	0.92		
Chronic HCV infection	0.56 (0.12, 2.62)	0.46		
Rifampicin use	0.41 (0.09, 1.85)	0.24		
CYP2B6 516 GT or TT genotypes	3.71 (1.75, 7.84)	**0.001**	4.35 (1.97, 9.59)	**<0.001**

Abbreviations: 95% CI, 95% confidence interval; OR, odds ratio.

receiving rifampicin, but all of them could achieve plasma efavirenz concentrations above the therapeutic target. Besides, most of the patients (88.9%) weighed greater than 50 kg. As a result, our findings suggest that the standard daily 600 mg efavirenz dose is adequate for patients on efavirenz-containing combination antiretroviral therapy who receive concurrent rifampicin for the treatment of TB. Of note, there were only three patients with the *CYP2B6* 516TT genotype, and none of them were taking rifampicin concomitantly in our study. Therefore, more studies are needed to determine if the same phenomenon of paradoxically elevated efavirenz concentrations in patients with *CYP2B6* 516TT genotype receiving rifampicin will be seen in Chinese population.

Efavirenz is mainly metabolized by CYP2B6, and the *CYP2B6* gene is highly polymorphic. Many previous studies have shown *CYP2B6* SNP, particularly G516T, to be associated with higher plasma efavirenz concentrations and its drug-related toxicity, which could result in early discontinuation of antiretroviral therapy [19,20]. The allele frequency of *CYP2B6* G516T varies among the different ethnicities, ranging from 14% to 21% in Asian populations [15,21,22], 22% to 30% in Caucasians [8,20,23], and up to near 50% in Africans [13,24]. In our study, the frequency of *CYP2B6* G516T was 17.8% (32.2% of GT genotype and 1.8% of TT genotype), which was similar to those in prior Asian studies [15,21,22]. To avoid high plasma efavirenz concentrations and related drug toxicities, therapeutic drug monitoring and pharma-cogenetic-guided dosing strategy that have been described by Gatanaga et al. [25] would be helpful and should be introduced into clinical practice.

Several studies have demonstrated that a higher weight were associated with lower efavirenz levels [5,6], but how to adjust doses according to the weight remains a debatable issue. Some studies suggested an increase of efavirenz dose for heavy patients taking rifampicin [26], while other studies showed data arguing against this suggestion [10,27]. In our study, nearly all patients could achieve therapeutic concentrations, and a significant proportion of the patients who had a lower weight achieved plasma efavirenz concentrations of greater than 4 mg/L (figure 3). As a result, a reduced dose of efavirenz with the information of therapeutic drug monitoring will be beneficial to Taiwanese patients with a lower weight to minimize the risk of adverse events and save treatment costs.

Our study has several limitations. First, it was performed at a single hospital in Taiwan, with most patients being male. Information on the efavirenz concentrations among HIV-infected female patients remains limited. Second, only patients who could tolerate efavirenz for two weeks or more were included in this study, and three quarters of the patients had been receiving efavirenz for more than 24 weeks. Therefore, the proportion of patients with toxic drug levels may be underestimated since patients with significantly higher drug concentrations may have interrupted or changed regimen earlier than two weeks because of severe psychiatric side effects and skin rashes. Third, this was a cross-sectional study, and we did not collect serial blood samples when the patients received and after they discontinued rifampicin-containing anti-tuberculous therapy, to avoid inter-patient variations. Last, we did not collect information on neuropsychiatric adverse effects to correlate with plasma efavirenz concentrations.

In conclusion, with information obtained from therapeutic drug monitoring and pharmacogenetic study in HIV-infected Taiwanese, we have shown that most patients could achieve therapeutic efavirenz concentrations, with or without combination with rifampicin, when receiving a standard 600 mg of efavirenz daily; and lower weights and *CYP2B6* 516 GT and TT genotypes were associated with higher plasma efavirenz concentrations that might be associated with an increased risk of neuropsychiatric adverse effects.

Acknowledgments

Footnote: Preliminary analyses of these data were presented as a poster abstract no.983 at the *50th Annual Interscience Conference on Antimicrobial Agents and Chemotherapy* held in Boston, 12–15 September, 2010.

Author Contributions

Conceived and designed the experiments: K-YL S-WL S-YC C-CH. Performed the experiments: K-YL S-WL H-YS C-HK M-ST B-RW S-YT W-CL S-YC C-CH. Analyzed the data: K-YL S-WL S-YC C-CH. Contributed reagents/materials/analysis tools: S-WL S-YC C-CH. Wrote the paper: K-YL C-CH.

References

1. Panel on Antiretroviral Guidelines for Adults and Adolescents (2013) Guidelines for the use of antiretroviral agents in HIV-1-infected adults and adolescents. Department of Health and Human Services. Available at: http://aidsinfo.nih.gov/contentfiles/lvguidelines/AdultandAdolescentGL.pdf. Accessed: 16 June 2013.

2. Marzolini C, Telenti A, Decosterd LA, Greub G, Biollaz J, et al. (2001) Efavirenz plasma levels can predict treatment failure and central nervous system side effects in HIV-1-infected patients. AIDS 15: 71–75.

3. Burger D, van der Heiden I, la Porte C, van der Ende M, Groeneveld P, et al. (2006) Interpatient variability in the pharmacokinetics of the HIV non-nucleoside reverse transcriptase inhibitor efavirenz: the effect of gender, race, and CYP2B6 polymorphism. Br J Clin Pharmacol 61: 148–154.

4. Pfister M, Labbe L, Hammer SM, Mellors J, Bennett KK, et al. (2003) Population pharmacokinetics and pharmacodynamics of efavirenz, nelfinavir, and indinavir: Adult AIDS Clinical Trial Group Study 398. Antimicrob Agents Chemother 47: 130–137.

5. Stohr W, Back D, Dunn D, Sabin C, Winston A, et al. (2008) Factors influencing efavirenz and nevirapine plasma concentration: effect of ethnicity, weight and co-medication. Antivir Ther 13: 675–685.

6. Poeta J, Linden R, Antunes MV, Real L, Menezes AM, et al. (2011) Plasma concentrations of efavirenz are associated with body weight in HIV-positive individuals. J Antimicrob Chemother 66: 2601–2604.

7. Ramachandran G, Hemanth Kumar AK, Rajasekaran S, Kumar P, Ramesh K, et al. (2009) CYP2B6 G516T polymorphism but not rifampin coadministration influences steady-state pharmacokinetics of efavirenz in human immunodeficiency virus-infected patients in South India. Antimicrob Agents Chemother 53: 863–868.

8. Haas DW, Ribaudo HJ, Kim RB, Tierney C, Wilkinson GR, et al. (2004) Pharmacogenetics of efavirenz and central nervous system side effects: an Adult AIDS Clinical Trials Group study. AIDS 18: 2391–2400.

9. Food and Drug Administration. Sustiva labeling update/dosing adjustment with rifampin. Available: http://www.fda.gov/ForConsumers/ByAudience/ForPatientAdvocates/HIVandAIDSActivities/ucm294476.htm. Accessed: 16 June 2013.

10. Luetkemeyer AF, Rosenkranz SL, Lu D, Marzan F, Ive P, et al. (2013) Relationship Between Weight, Efavirenz Exposure, and Virologic Suppression in HIV-Infected Patients on Rifampin-Based Tuberculosis Treatment in the AIDS Clinical Trials Group A5221 STRIDE Study. Clin Infect Dis 57: 586–593.

11. Benedek IH, Joshi A, Fiske WD, et al. Pharmacokinetic interaction between efavirenz and rifampin in healthy volunteers [abstract 42280]; 1998 June 28-July 3; Geneva, Switzerland.

12. Lopez-Cortes LF, Ruiz-Valderas R, Viciana P, Alarcon-Gonzalez A, Gomez-Mateos J, et al. (2002) Pharmacokinetic interactions between efavirenz and rifampicin in HIV-infected patients with tuberculosis. Clin Pharmacokinet 41: 681–690.

13. Nyakutira C, Roshammar D, Chigutsa E, Chonzi P, Ashton M, et al. (2008) High prevalence of the CYP2B6 516G−>T(*6) variant and effect on the population pharmacokinetics of efavirenz in HIV/AIDS outpatients in Zimbabwe. Eur J Clin Pharmacol 64: 357–365.

14. Uttayamakul S, Likanonsakul S, Manosuthi W, Wichukchinda N, Kalambaheti T, et al. (2010) Effects of CYP2B6 G516T polymorphisms on plasma efavirenz and nevirapine levels when co-administered with rifampicin in HIV/TB co-infected Thai adults. AIDS Res Ther 7: 8.

15. Guan S, Huang M, Chan E, Chen X, Duan W, et al. (2006) Genetic polymorphisms of cytochrome P450 2B6 gene in Han Chinese. Eur J Pharm Sci 29: 14–21.

16. Ramachandran G, Kumar AK, Swaminathan S, Venkatesan P, Kumaraswami V, et al. (2006) Simple and rapid liquid chromatography method for determination of efavirenz in plasma. J Chromatogr B Analyt Technol Biomed Life Sci 835: 131–135.

17. Cohen K, Grant A, Dandara C, McIlleron H, Pemba L, et al. (2009) Effect of rifampicin-based antitubercular therapy and the cytochrome P450 2B6 516G> T polymorphism on efavirenz concentrations in adults in South Africa. Antivir Ther 14: 687–695.

18. Kwara A, Lartey M, Sagoe KW, Court MH (2011) Paradoxically elevated efavirenz concentrations in HIV/tuberculosis-coinfected patients with CYP2B6 516TT genotype on rifampin-containing antituberculous therapy. AIDS 25: 388–390.

19. Ingelman-Sundberg M, Sim SC, Gomez A, Rodriguez-Antona C (2007) Influence of cytochrome P450 polymorphisms on drug therapies: pharmacogenetic, pharmacoepigenetic and clinical aspects. Pharmacol Ther 116: 496–526.

20. Wyen C, Hendra H, Siccardi M, Platten M, Jaeger H, et al. (2011) Cytochrome P450 2B6 (CYP2B6) and constitutive androstane receptor (CAR) polymorphisms are associated with early discontinuation of efavirenz-containing regimens. J Antimicrob Chemother 66: 2092–2098.

21. Cho JY, Lim HS, Chung JY, Yu KS, Kim JR, et al. (2004) Haplotype structure and allele frequencies of CYP2B6 in a Korean population. Drug Metab Dispos 32: 1341–1344.

22. Hiratsuka M, Takekuma Y, Endo N, Narahara K, Hamdy SI, et al. (2002) Allele and genotype frequencies of CYP2B6 and CYP3A5 in the Japanese population. Eur J Clin Pharmacol 58: 417–421.

23. Haas DW, Smeaton LM, Shafer RW, Robbins GK, Morse GD, et al. (2005) Pharmacogenetics of long-term responses to antiretroviral regimens containing Efavirenz and/or Nelfinavir: an Adult Aids Clinical Trials Group Study. J Infect Dis 192: 1931–1942.

24. Kwara A, Lartey M, Sagoe KW, Xexemeku F, Kenu E, et al. (2008) Pharmacokinetics of efavirenz when co-administered with rifampin in TB/HIV co-infected patients: pharmacogenetic effect of CYP2B6 variation. J Clin Pharmacol 48: 1032–1040.

25. Gatanaga H, Hayashida T, Tsuchiya K, Yoshino M, Kuwahara T, et al. (2007) Successful efavirenz dose reduction in HIV type 1-infected individuals with cytochrome P450 2B6 *6 and *26. Clin Infect Dis 45: 1230–1237.

26. Manosuthi W, Sungkanuparph S, Tantanathip P, Mankatitham W, Lueang-niyomkul A, et al. (2009) Body weight cutoff for daily dosage of efavirenz and 60-week efficacy of efavirenz-based regimen in human immunodeficiency virus and tuberculosis coinfected patients receiving rifampin. Antimicrob Agents Chemother 53: 4545–4548.

27. Borand L, Laureillard D, Madec Y, Chou M, Pheng P, et al. (2013) Plasma concentrations of efavirenz with a 600 mg standard dose in Cambodian HIV-infected adults treated for tuberculosis with a body weight above 50 kg. Antivir Ther 18: 419–423.

19

The Oral Commensal *Streptococcus mitis* Shows a Mixed Memory The Cell Signature That Is Similar to and Cross-Reactive with *Streptococcus pneumoniae*

Stian André Engen[1]*, Håkon Valen Rukke[1], Simone Becattini[2], David Jarrossay[2], Inger Johanne Blix[1,3], Fernanda Cristina Petersen[1◊], Federica Sallusto[2◊], Karl Schenck[1◊]

1 Department of Oral Biology, University of Oslo, Oslo, Norway, 2 Institute for Research in Biomedicine, Università della Svizzera Italiana, Bellinzona, Switzerland, 3 Department of Periodontology, University of Oslo, Oslo, Norway

Abstract

Background: Carriage of and infection with *Streptococcus pneumoniae* is known to predominantly induce T helper 17 (Th17) responses in humans, but the types of Th cells showing reactivity towards commensal streptococci with low pathogenic potential, such as the oral commensals *S. mitis* and *S. salivarius*, remain uncharacterized.

Methods: Memory CD4+ T helper (Th) cell subsets were isolated from healthy human blood donors according to differential expression of chemokine receptors, expanded *in vitro* using polyclonal stimuli and characterized for reactivity against different streptococcal strains.

Results: Th cells responding to *S. mitis*, *S. salivarius* and *S. pneumoniae* were predominantly in a CCR6+CXCR3+ subset and produced IFN-γ, and in a CCR6+CCR4+ subset and produced IL-17 and IL-22. Frequencies of *S. pneumoniae*-reactive Th cells were higher than frequencies of *S. mitis*- and *S. salivarius*-specific Th cells. *S. mitis* and *S. pneumoniae* isogenic capsule knock-out mutants and a *S. mitis* mutant expressing the serotype 4 capsule of *S. pneumoniae* showed no different Th cell responses as compared to wild type strains. *S. mitis*-specific Th17 cells showed cross-reactivity with *S. pneumoniae*.

Conclusions: As Th17 cells partly control clearance of *S. pneumoniae*, cross-reactive Th17 cells that may be induced by commensal bacterial species may influence the immune response, independent of capsule expression.

Editor: Bernard Beall, Centers for Disease Control & Prevention, United States of America

Funding: This work was supported by the European Research Council grant number 323183 PREDICT (to FS). The Institute for Research in Biomedicine, Bellinzona, is supported by the Helmut Horten Foundation (http://www.helmut-horten stiftung.org/en/homepage.html). The funders had no role in study design, data collection and analysis, decision to publish, or preparation of the manuscript.

Competing Interests: The authors have declared that no competing interests exist.

* Email: s.a.engen@odont.uio.no

◊ These authors contributed equally to this work.

Introduction

A reciprocal beneficial relationship has developed between hosts and their symbionts throughout evolution. In the human oral cavity, more than 700 bacterial species can be found [1,2] of which a healthy person can host more than 200 [3]. In order for the commensals to persist in their niches, it is important that adequate host-microbe interplay is established. This comprises immune exclusion by keeping microbes from interacting with host cell by mucus, SIgA and/or antimicrobial peptides, and immune elimination by innate and adaptive responses without the induction of inflammation [4].

S. mitis is a pioneer bacterial species that colonizes the nasopharynx and all sites of the oral cavity from early infancy. Its predominance persists during life and in adults *S. mitis* is found in the oral cavity of nearly all persons. *S. mitis* is closely related to *S. pneumoniae* which also resides in the oronasopharynx: the species may share as much as 39% of their genes, including many of the virulence genes [5]. Despite their genetic similarity, *S. pneumoniae* causes serious infections in about 14.5 million children every year, whereas *S. mitis* rarely causes disease [6].

After the second year of life, a drastic reduction in carriage and disease rate caused by *S. pneumoniae* occurs, independent of capsular serotype [7]. This reduction is attributed to the development of serum IgG and secretory antibodies [8], and to antigen-specific T cell responses [9,10]. Oral carriage state of *S. mitis* is probably partly regulated by secretion of salivary SIgA [11,12], but the role of Th cells has not been explored.

Naïve T helper (Th) cells develop into different polarized effector Th subsets that are tailored to effectively cope with the type of infection, including Th1 and Th2 that produce IFN-γ or IL-4, respectively [13]. More recently, Th17 [14], Th22 [15,16], and Th9 [17] have been described, which produce IL-17, IL-22 or IL-9, respectively. Th cell subsets with a mixed phenotype have been also identified, including T cells producing IL-17 and IFN-γ, or IL-17 and IL-4 [18–20]. In this study, we set out to examine the phenotype and functional property of *in vivo*-primed memory CD4$^+$ Th cells reactive with antigens from the oral commensal species *S. mitis* and *Streptococcus salivarius*, and compare it to that of *S. pneumoniae*.

Utilizing a T cell screening method, we found that memory Th cells reactive against *S. mitis* and *S. salivarius* are predominantly found in the CCR6$^+$ Th1 and Th17 subsets, a distribution similar to that obtained for *S. pneumoniae*. In addition, we observed interspecies cross-reactivity among *S. mitis*–reactive and *S. pneumoniae*-reactive T cell clones.

Material and methods

Bacterial strains

Bacterial strains included *S. mitis* (CCUG 31611T, 62644, 62641), *S. pneumoniae* (TIGR4, Sero 1, D39) and *S. salivarius* (JIM8777) (Table 1). Isogenic capsule deletion mutants of *S. mitis* 31611T (*S. mitis* Δ*cps*) and *S. pneumoniae* TIGR4 (*S. pneumoniae* Δ*cps*) and a capsule switch mutant of *S. mitis* 31611T expressing the serotype 4 capsule of *S. pneumoniae* TIGR4 (*S. mitis* 31611T TIGR4) were constructed as described before [21]. All strains were grown in Todd Hewitt Broth (THB) (BD Biosciences, Franklin Lakes, NJ). Over night cultures were diluted in THB and grown to OD = 1 at 600 nm. Cells were harvested by centrifugation at 5000 g for 10 min at 4°C, washed in endotoxin free Dulbecco's-PBS (Sigma-Aldrich, St. Louis, MO) and UV-inactivated for 30 min using UVC 500 Crosslinker (GE Healthcare, Fairfield, CT). The UV-treated bacterial suspensions were aliquoted and frozen at −80°C.

Blood samples and cell sorting

Blood from anonymized healthy donors was obtained from the Swiss Blood Donation Centers of Basel and Lugano, and used in compliance with the Swiss Federal Office of Public Health (authorization n. A000197/2 to F.S). No submission to a local ethics committee was needed because volunteer donors from the national registry sign an informed consent form (Swiss Red Cross, Medical Questionnaire and Informed Consent Form, version 09), stating that their blood could be used for medical research after definitive anonymization. PBMCs were obtained using Ficoll-Paque PLUS (GE Healthcare) gradient centrifugation. CD14$^+$ monocytes and CD4$^+$ T cells were isolated by positive selection using magnetic beads (Miltenyi Biotec, Bergisch Gladbach, Germany). CD14$^+$ cells were collected and frozen at −80°C for later use. In order to sort distinct Th subsets, CD14$^-$CD4$^+$ cells were incubated with the following antibodies: anti-CD45RA (Qdot655, Invitrogen, Carlsbad, CA); anti-CXCR3 (APC, BD Biosciences); anti-CCR4 (PE-Cy7, BD Biosciences); anti-CCR6 (Brilliant Violet 605, BioLegend, San Diego, CA); anti-CCR10 (PE, R&D systems, Minneapolis, MN); anti-CD8 (PECy5, Beckman Coulter, Brea, CA); anti-CD19 (PECy5, Beckman Coulter); anti-CD25 (PECy5, Beckman Coulter); anti-CD56 (PECy5, Beckman Coulter). CD45RA$^-$CD8$^-$CD19$^-$CD25$^-$CD56$^-$ cells were sorted on a FACSAria (BD Biosciences) into the following subsets: i. CXCR3$^+$CCR4$^-$CCR6$^-$CCR10$^-$, ii. CCR6$^+$CXCR3$^+$CCR4$^-$CCR10$^-$ (both enriched in Th1 and defined thereafter as Th1 and CCR6$^+$ Th1, respectively), iii. CCR4$^+$CXCR3$^-$CCR6$^-$CCR10$^-$ (enriched in Th2); iv. CCR6$^+$CCR4$^+$CXCR3$^-$CCR10$^-$ (Th17), and v. CCR6$^+$CCR4$^+$CCR10$^+$CXCR3$^-$ (enriched in Th22). The sorting strategy is summarized in Table S1. Cytokine production by the sorted cell subsets was measured in the 24-hour culture supernatants after activation with immobilized anti-CD3 (clone TR66, 5µg/ml) and anti-CD28 (clone CD28.2; BD Biosciences; 1µgl/ml) antibodies using the cytometric bead array (CBA) (eBiosciences, San Diego, CA), carried out according to the manufacturer's protocol. The characteristics of the subsets, as assayed by cytokine secretion, is shown in Figure S1.

T cell library construction and screening

T cell libraries were established as described before [22]. Cells were grown in complete media (CM) comprising RPMI-1640 supplemented with 2 mM glutamine, 1% v/v non-essential amino acids, 1% v/v sodium pyruvate, 0.1% v/v 2-mercaptoethanol, penicillin (50 U/mL) and streptomycin (50 µg/mL) (Gibco,

Table 1. Streptococcal strains used in this study.

Strains	Description	Source
S. mitis		
SK575 (62644)	*Corresponds to CCUG 62644*	CCUG*
SK579 (62641)	*Corresponds to CCUG 62641*	CCUG
CCUG 31611^T	Wild type S. mitis biovar 1 type strain; corresponds to NCTC12261	CCUG
S. mitis Δ*cps*; MI016	CCUG31611^T cps::*kan*; Kan^R	
S. mitis$_{TIGR4}$; MI030	CCUG31611^T Ω TIGR4 cps locus; Kan^R, Erm^R	
S. pneumoniae		
D39	Corresponds to NCTC 7466	NCTC**
Serotype 1	Corresponds to sequence type 306	Clinical isolate, Norwegian Institute of Public Health
TIGR4	Wild type serotype 4, transformable strain, sequenced genome	
S. pneumoniae Δ*cps*; SP011	TIGR4 cps::*erm*; Erm^R	
S. salivarius		
JIM8777		

*CCUG: Culture collection, University of Göteborg.
**NCTC: National cultures of Type Cultures.

Carlsbad, CA), and 5% v/v human serum (Swiss Blood Center), unless stated otherwise. Memory Th cell subsets obtained by cell sorting as described above, were plated in 96-well U-bottom plates (2000 cells/well) and polyclonally stimulated with 1 µg/mL PHA (Sigma-Aldrich), in the presence of irradiated (45 Gy) allogeneic PBMCs and 500 U/mL IL-2. After 7d, the cells were transferred to 24-well plates for further expansion of total 20d. Half of the volume of the medium was changed every other day. For stimulation, the cultures were washed three times in RPMI-1640 with HEPES (Gibco) and 1% v/v FCS, before each well was tested for streptococcal antigen-reactivity by 3d co-culture of 2.5×10^5 T cells and 2.0×10^4 irradiated (45 Gy) autologous monocytes, pulsed with whole cell UV-inactivated bacteria (MOI: 100:1) for 5 h. At day 3 of the co-culture, [^{3}H]-thymidine was added and proliferation was measured on a beta-counter after 18 h.

Cross reactivity assay

Wells containing Th17 cells reactive to *S. mitis* and *S. pneumoniae* were cloned by limiting dilution. First, T cells (2.5×10^5) were stained with CFSE and co-cultured with irradiated (45 Gy) autologous monocytes pulsed with whole cell UV-inactivated bacteria for 5 h. At day 7 of co-culture, CFSE-low proliferating cells were sorted and plated at 0.5 cells/well, stimulated with 1 µg/mL PHA and 0.5×10^4 irradiated allogeneic PBMCs/well in CM supplemented with 500 U/mL IL-2 in 384-well plates. During 20 d of expansion, proliferating wells were transferred to 96-well U-bottom plates and further to 24-well plates before re-stimulating with whole-cell UV-inactivated bacteria as described above.

Inhibition assay

Tetanus toxoid (TT)-reactive Th17 memory T cells were sorted and cloned as described above. 2.5×10^4 T cells were co-cultured with a 2-fold dilution series of irradiated monocytes, ranging from 4×10^4 to 1.25×10^3 monocytes/well, and 5 µg/mL TT alone or in the presence of whole cells from *S. mitis* or *S. pneumoniae* (MOI: 100:1). After 3 d in culture, [^{3}H]-thymidine was added and proliferation was determined by [^{3}H]-thymidine incorporation after 18 h.

Cytometric bead array (CBA)

To quantify IFN-γ, IL-17A and IL-22, supernatants of CCR6$^+$ Th1 and Th17 cells stimulated with *S. mitis* 31611T and *S. pneumoniae* TIGR4 were analyzed using the cytometric bead array (CBA) (eBiosciences, San Diego, CA), carried out according to the manufacturer's protocol.

Statistical analysis

Student t tests were used to assess differences in cytokine secretion. P values of lower than 0.05 were considered to indicate statistically significant.

Results

Circulating T helper memory cells show a heterogeneous signature after stimulation with *S. mitis*, similar to that obtained with *S. pneumoniae*

Five CD4$^+$ memory Th cell subsets from PBMCs of healthy donors were isolated according to the expression of chemokine receptors as described before [22]. For each CD4$^+$ T cell subset in each donor, 48 cell lines were established and polyclonally expanded for 16–20 days prior to screening. Each T cell line was then screened for reactivity against autologous monocytes

pulsed with three *S. mitis* strains (62644, 62641, 31611T) and responding T cells were detected by [^{3}H]-thymidine incorporation. Cultures containing proliferating T cells were identified by incorporation of [^{3}H]-thymidine and precursor frequencies were calculated based on the number of negative wells, according to the Poisson distribution and expressed per million cells [23]. A representative example obtained from one of the donors is shown in Figure 1 and the distribution of responding T cells in the different subsets for the 6 donors analyzed is summarized in Figure 2. The raw data and the subset distribution of wells reactive with the streptococcal species for each donor as percentage of the total of all subsets for each strain are shown in Tables S2 and S3, respectively. The frequency of Th17 cells was highest while that of the Th22 cells was lowest for all strains. Intraspecies (*S. mitis* 62644, 62641, 31611T) signatures were similar, but frequencies of memory T cells reactive to *S. mitis* strain 62641 were slightly enhanced in all subsets. The frequencies of Th subsets responsive to the commensal *S. salivarius* were similar to that observed for *S. mitis*.

The signatures were viewed relative to that of *S. pneumoniae*, strains TIGR4, D39, Sero 1, representing serotypes 4, 2, and 1, respectively. The profiles of these three strains were similar in the Th1, Th2 and Th22 subsets but strain D39 displayed a stronger reactivity to the CCR6$^+$ Th1 and Th17 subsets (Figure 2). The frequencies of the *S. pneumoniae*-reactive cells were consistently and markedly higher than those for *S. mitis* and *S. salivarius*.

Capsule expression does not significantly affect the pattern of streptococci-reactive Th cell subset frequencies and relative distribution

S. pneumoniae strains are divided into serotypes according to the polysaccharide composition of their capsules. *S. mitis* strains can also express capsule [21]. Deletion of the *S. mitis* capsule or replacing it with capsule from *S. pneumoniae* TIGR4 did not significantly affect reactivities (Figure 1 and 2). In *S. pneumoniae* TIGR4, capsule deletion had no significant effect on Th cell subset frequencies. Capsule from type 1 *S. pneumoniae* strains, such as strain Sero 1, have zwitterionic characteristics and can activate T cell-dependent immune responses [24]. In the present study, however, no significant difference in frequency of Th reactive with type 1 pneumococcus relative to type 2 (D39) or type 4 (TIGR4) was observed (Figure 2).

S. mitis shows a suppressive effect on T cell responses to unrelated antigen

To investigate if the overall lower Th cell responses observed for *S. mitis* compared to *S. pneumoniae* could be due to antigen-unspecific T cell inhibitory effects of *S. mitis*, tetanus toxoid (TT)-specific Th17 cell clones were co-cultured with autologous monocytes pulsed with TT alone or with TT and *S. mitis* 31611T or *S. pneumoniae* TIGR4. Adding *S. mitis* cells to the co-cultures reduced the ability of the TT-specific T cells to respond to TT, while little effect was observed when *S. pneumoniae* cells were added (Figure 3).

S. mitis and *S. pneumoniae* induce IFN-γ, IL-17 and IL-22 secretion by CCR6$^+$ Th1 and Th17 cells

As shown in Figures 1 and 2, the highest response to the streptococcal strains was observed within the CCR6$^+$ Th1 and Th17 memory cell subsets. For closer characterization, quantities of signature cytokines, *i.e.* IFN-γ, IL-17A and IL-22, were examined by a cytometric bead array (CBA) in supernatants of the T cell lines co-cultured 3 d with monocytes pulsed with *S. mitis*

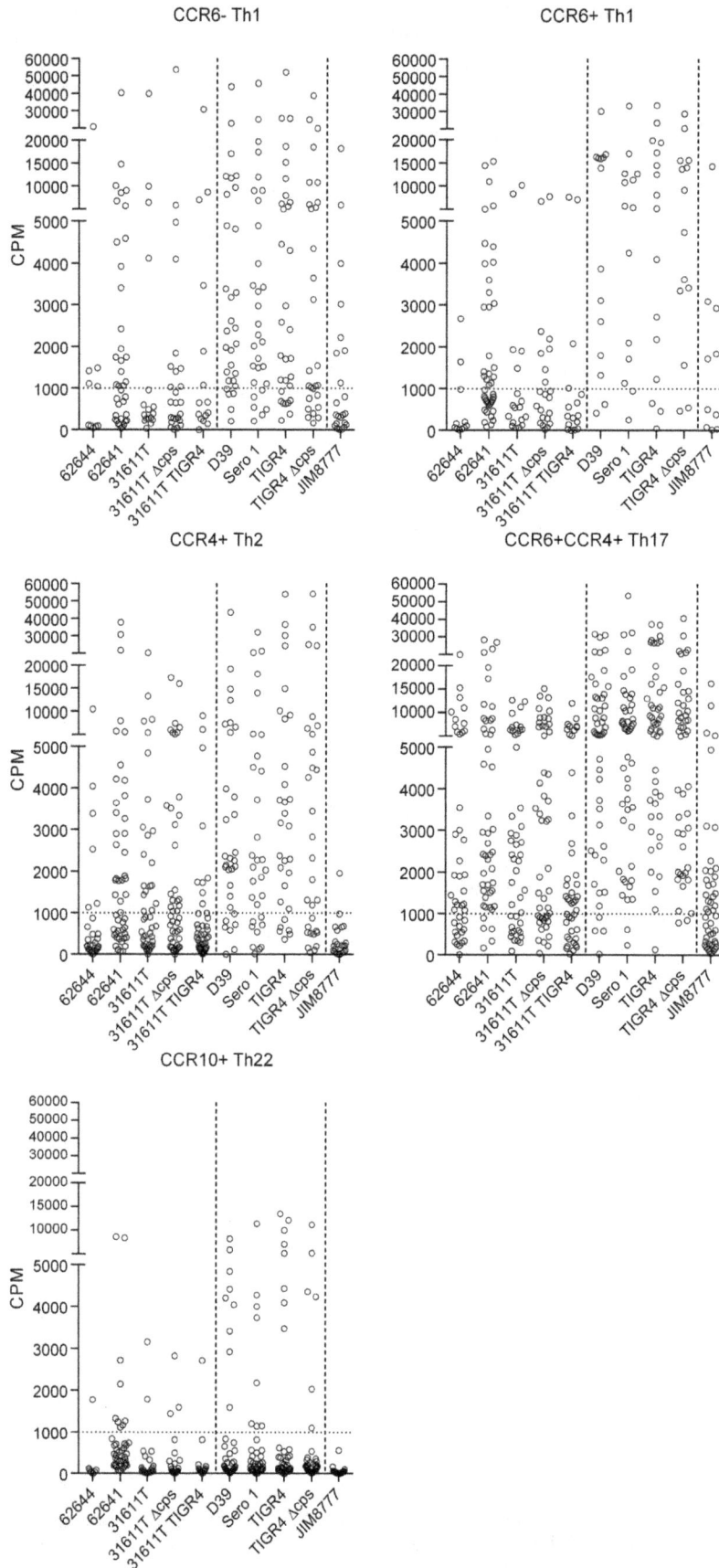

Figure 1. Distribution of antigen-specific memory Th subsets after exposure to streptococcal antigens by autologous monocytes. Raw data of a T cell library of a representative donor screened for reactivity for a panel of ten streptococci. Antigen-specific activity was quantified as a response in increased T cell proliferation determined by thymidine incorporation. Each graph represents the screening of reactivity of one T cell subset to the pane00l of bacteria and each circle represents one well of the respective subset. The dashed line represents lowest counts per minute (CPM) values included in the analysis.

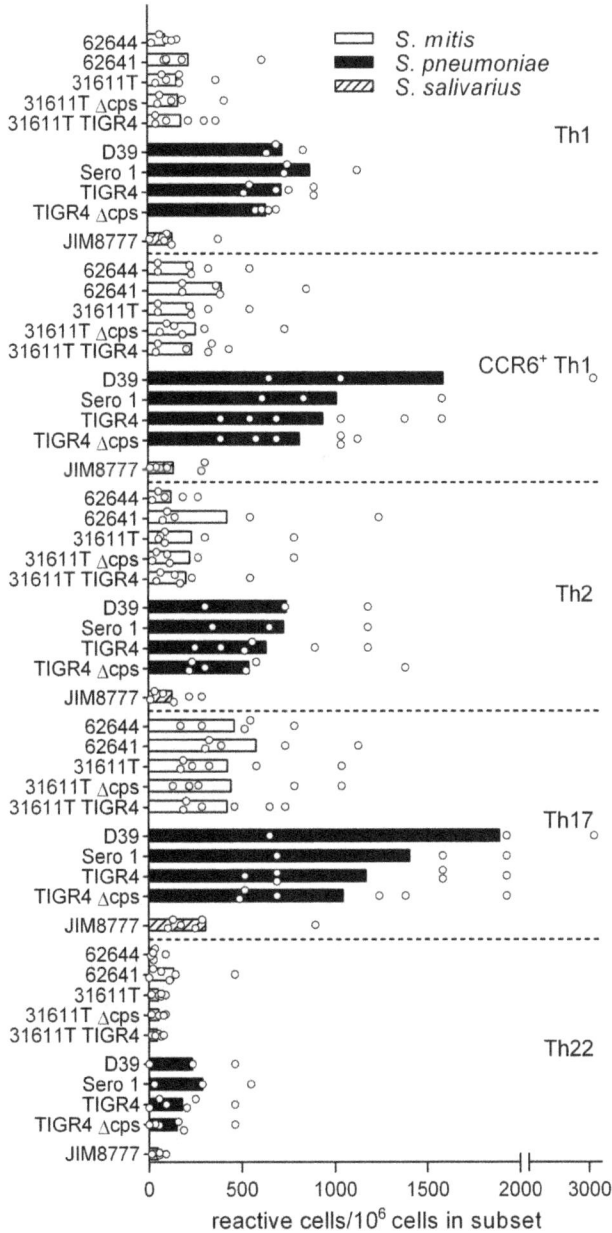

or *S. pneumoniae* wild types. CCR6[+] Th1 cells released more IFN-γ and less IL-17 than the Th17 cells (Figure 4). To evaluate the differences in cytokine secretion between cultures stimulated with either *S. mitis* or *S. pneumoniae*, the donors' cytokine secretion data were averaged within each stimulating strain (3 *S. mitis* and 3 *S. pneumoniae* strains; Figure 4). The means for the *S. mitis* and 3 *S. pneumoniae* stimulations were then compared using Student t tests to reveal differences between the species. No statistically significant differences in cytokine secretion were detected within the CCR6[+] Th1 cells (P>0.05). The Th17 cells stimulated with *S. pneumoniae*, however, released more IFN-γ, IL-17 and IL-22 than those stimulated with *S. mitis* (P<0.05; Figure 4).

Th17 clones show cross-reactivity for *S. mitis* and *S. pneumoniae*

As similar T cell subset patterns were found for *S. mitis* and *S. pneumoniae* and as the library comprised wells that showed reactivity to both *S. mitis* and *S. pneumoniae* strains, we examined whether this could be due to cross-reactive T cells. Cells from

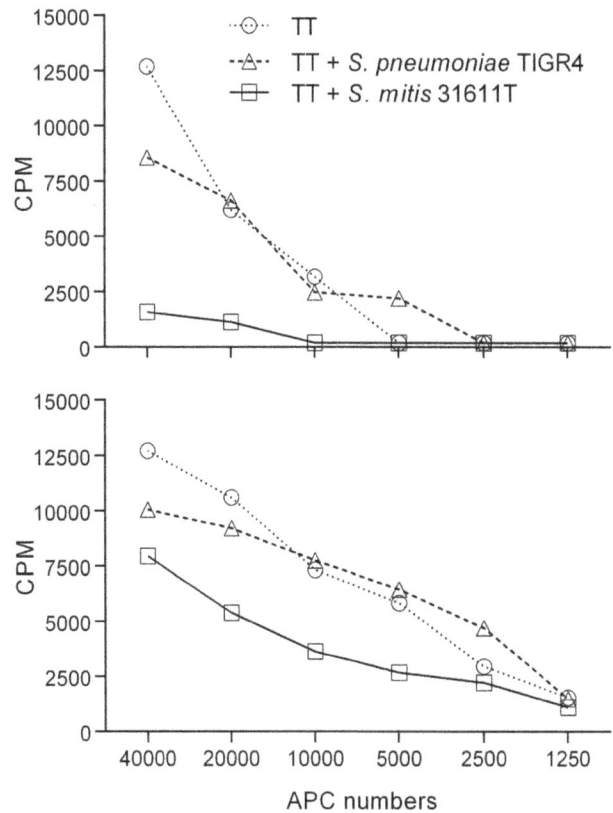

Figure 2. Subset distribution of CD4[+] memory T cells in response to oropharyngeal-associated streptococcal bacteria. Distribution of single donor (circles) (N = 3–6) and mean (bars) frequencies of CD4[+] memory T cells among the CCR6[−] Th1, CCR6[+] Th1, Th2, Th17 and Th22 subsets reactive to streptococcal antigens. Data are presented as reactive cells per one million cells in the respective subsets. Open bars: *S. mitis*; closed bars: *S. pneumoniae*; hatched bars: *S. salivarius*. 62644: *S. mitis* CCUG 62644; 62641: *S. mitis* CCUG 62641; 31611T: *S. mitis* CCUG 31611T; 31611T Δcps: *S. mitis* CCUG 31611T capsule deletion mutant; 31611T TIGR4: *S. mitis* CCUG 31611T mutant with capsule from *S. pneumoniae* TIGR4; D39: *S. pneumoniae* D39; Sero 1: clinical isolate of *S. pneumoniae* serotype 1; TIGR4: *S. pneumoniae* TIGR4; TIGR4 Δcps: *S. pneumoniae* TIGR4 capsule deletion mutant; JIM8777: *S. salivarius* JIM8777.

Figure 3. Response of TT-specific Th17 memory cell clones to native antigen in combination with bacterial cells. Tetanus toxoid (TT)-specific CD4[+] Th17 memory T cell clones were co-cultured with autologous monocytes and either TT alone or TT and *S. mitis* 31611T or *S. pneumoniae* TIGR4 (MOI: 100:1) for 3 d before proliferation was determined by [³H]-thymidine incorporation (A: clone 1, B: clone 2).

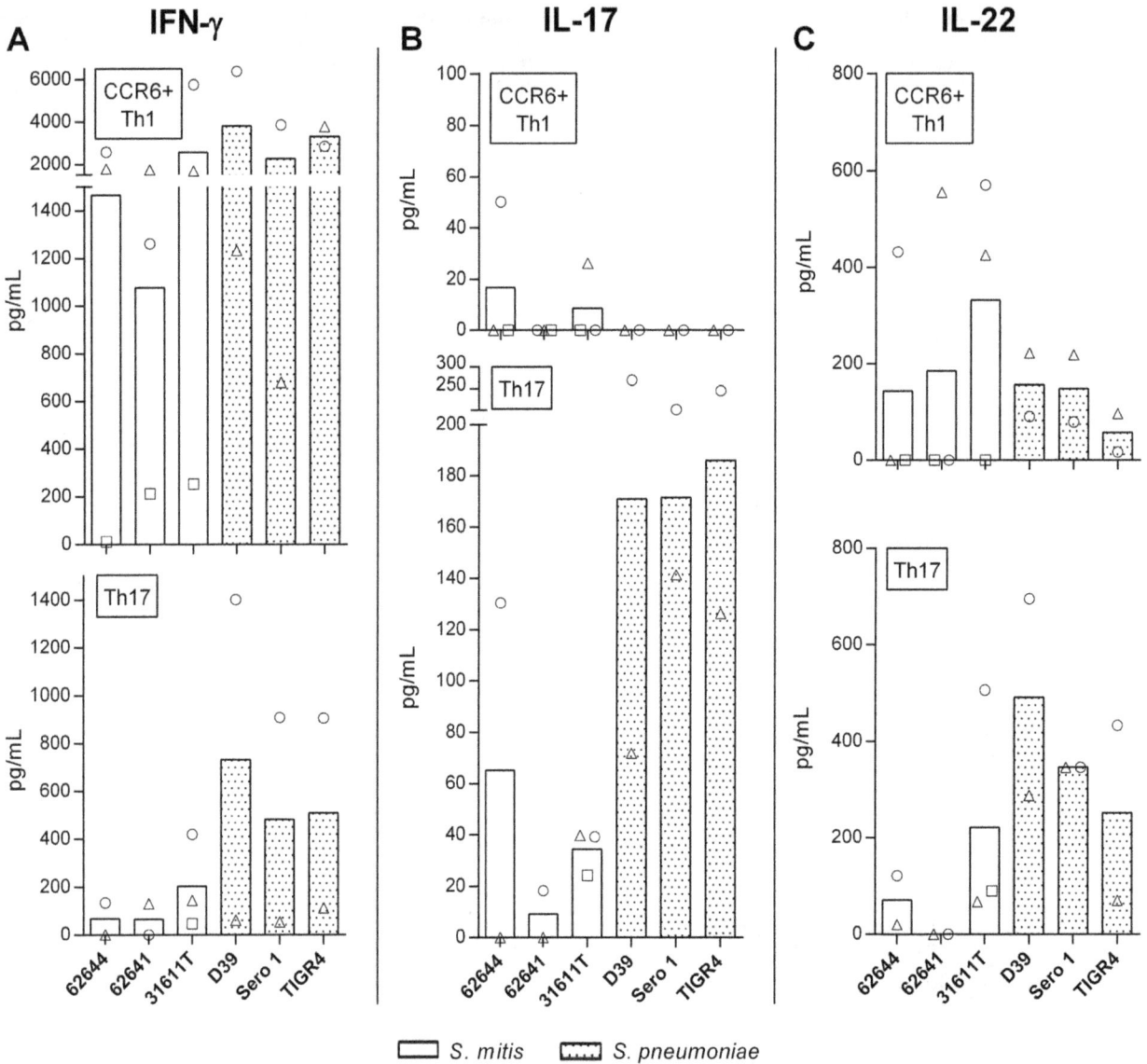

Figure 4. Cytokine production by CCR6+ Th1 and Th17 cells in response to streptococci. Quantities of IFN-γ (A), IL-17A (B) and IL-22 (C) were determined in supernatants of CCR6+ Th1 and Th17 CD4+ memory T cells co-cultured for 3 d with autologous monocytes and whole cell, UV-inactivated *S. mitis* 31611T or *S. pneumoniae* TIGR4 (MOI: 100:1). Bars represent averaged values of different donors (symbols). Th17 cells secreted statistically significantly more IFN-γ, IL-17A and IL-22 when stimulated with *S. pneumoniae* as compared with stimulation with *S. mitis* (Student t test; P < 0.05; see text).

Th17 wells that were reactive with *S. mitis* 62641 or *S. pneumoniae* D39 in the initial stimulation were cloned and re-stimulated with the panel of bacterial strains. Clones initially reactive to *S. mitis* showed both inter- and intraspecies reactivity (Figure 5A), indicating cross-reactivity, while clones initially reactive to *S. pneumoniae* showed considerable cross-reactivity to all *S. mitis* strains (Figure 5B).

Discussion

Little is known about the subsets of Th cells responsive to commensal bacteria [25]. Here, we used a high-throughput T cell library method to map the Th cell signature that recognizes antigens from *S. mitis* and *S. salivarius*. CD4+CD45RA− memory Th cells were sorted into subsets based on differential chemokine

receptor expression. This sorting was based on the knowledge of a co-regulation of effector function and migratory properties during T cell differentiation, a mechanism which ensures selective recruitment of different effector T cells to inflamed tissues in response to inflammatory chemoattractants [26]. Compared with *in vitro* antigen stimulation of unfractionated T cells and subsequent phenotyping, sorting of the cells before stimulation has the advantage of establishing the *in vivo* subsets' identity before the cells are brought into culture, ensuring an "untouched" phenotype. We chose to expose the T cell cultures to whole, UV-inactivated bacterial cells to avoid compromising the integrity of surface molecules by unfavorable thermal or chemical conditions.

The primary aim of this study was to determine the distribution of Th subsets that recognize antigens from the ubiquitous oral commensal *S. mitis* in healthy donors. We found that the numbers

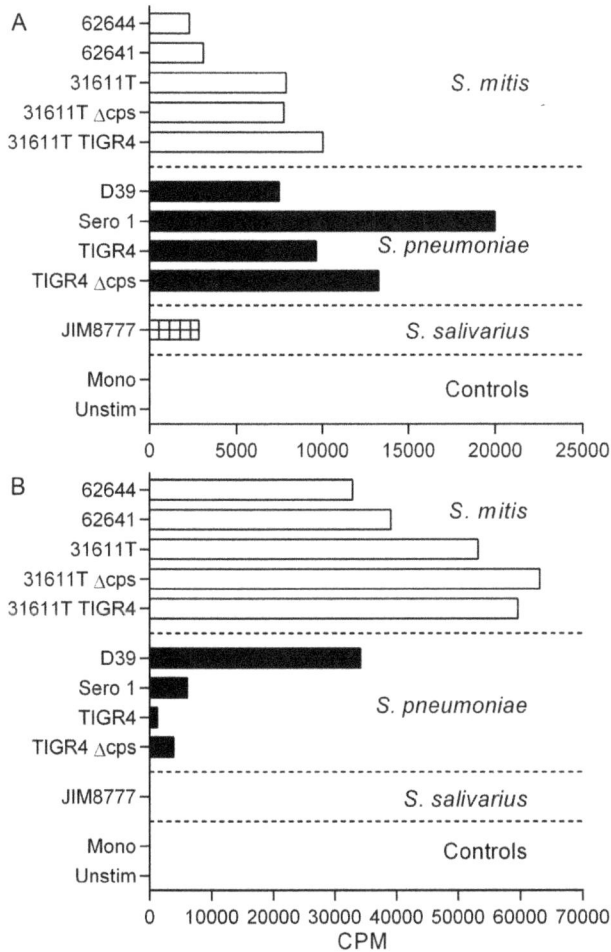

Figure 5. Cross-reactivity of CD4⁺ Th17 memory T cell clones in response to oropharyngeal-associated streptococcal strains. Th17 cells from wells initially reactive to *S. mitis* 62641 (A) and *S. pneumoniae* D39 (B) were cloned by limiting dilution and distribution of intra- and interspecies cross-reactivity was determined by thymidine incorporation. Bars represent single re-stimulation of each clone and data are presented as counts per minute (CPM).

of *S. mitis*- and *S. salivarius*-reactive Th cells were heterogeneously distributed among the five subsets tested, but with a predominance of CCR6⁺ Th1 and Th17 cells. *S. pneumoniae* is genetically closely related to *S. mitis* and was therefore included in the study. As *S. pneumoniae* has a marked pathogenic potential and *S. mitis* seldom causes disease, different distributions of response in the Th subset signature might be expected, but the results obtained showed that the Th response reactive with *S. pneumoniae* is strikingly similar to that of *S. mitis*. The signature and frequencies of responding cells to *S. salivarius* also coincided with that of *S. mitis*. The prominent Th17 response to *S. pneumoniae* is in accordance with studies on human lymphoid tonsillar tissue [27] and bronchoalveolar lavage [28], which show Th1/Th17- and IL-17A-dependent pneumococcal clearance, respectively.

The CCR6⁺ Th1 subset is a recently described Th subset that has characteristics of both Th1 and Th17 subsets. Th1 and Th17 lymphocytes are characterized by specific transcription factors, surface receptors and cytokine secretion (Th1: T-bet, CXCR3, and IFN-γ; Th17: RORC, CCR4/CCR6, and IL-17). Upon

polyclonal stimulation, the intermediate CCR6⁺ Th1 subset can secrete both IL-17 and IFN-γ and express RORC and T-bet ([8,18,29,30]. Expression of the Th17 surface marker CD161 and shared TCR clonality indicate that CCR6⁺ Th1 cells are of Th17 ancestry [29]. Furthermore, Th17 cells exposed to Th1-polarizing conditions convert to the intermediate CCR6⁺ Th1 cells (RORC⁺, T-bet⁺, IL-17⁺ IFN-γ⁺), while Th1 cells exposed to Th17-polarizing conditions remain Th1 cells [29,30]. A proportion of Th1 cells are thought to be of Th17 origin due to expression of factors characteristic for Th17 (RORC, CCR6, CD161) [29]. In contrast to polyclonal stimulation, however, exposure of CCR6⁺ Th1 cells to *Mycobacterium tuberculosis* PPD revealed an antigen-specific response characterized by absence of IL-17 secretion [18]. Our present observation that the CCR6⁺ Th1 cell response to the streptococcal strains tested produced IFN-γ but not IL-17 complies with this observation [18].

The CCR6⁺ Th1 and Th17 subsets presently examined produced a mixture of IFN-γ, IL-17 and IL-22 in response to streptococcal stimulation, effector cytokines that can be involved in the clearance of *S. pneumoniae* in humans. IFN-γ and IL-17 support macrophage and neutrophil defenses, respectively [26]. In a human infection model, carriage of *S. pneumoniae* increased the prevalence of CD4⁺IL-17A⁺TNF⁺IFN-γ⁺ Th cells in lungs and blood, as compared to non-carriers [28]. Another study showed an IFN-γ-dependent but IL-17-independent clearance of invading *S. pneumoniae* [31]. Finally, significant increases in proportions of IFN-γ⁺ CD4⁺ cells were seen in patients with community-acquired pneumonia [32]. IL-22 promotes epithelial proliferation, expression of antimicrobial proteins involved in host defense in the skin, airways and intestine, and production of inflammatory mediators and chemokines from epithelial cells [33]. Knock-out of IL-22 renders mice more susceptible to infection with *S. pneumoniae* than wild type animals [34]. IL-22 by itself has protective and regenerative functions, but together with IL-17, it supports inflammation [33]. Here, we observed that Th17 cells secreted significantly higher amounts of IFN-γ, IL-17 and IL-22 when challenged with *S. pneumoniae* species as compared with *S. mitis*. This suggests that *S. pneumoniae* can induce a more pronounced inflammatory response as compared with *S. mitis*.

A consistently lower frequency of Th cells responsive to *S. mitis* compared to *S. pneumoniae* was observed. The finding that *S. mitis* reduced proliferation of T clones specific for an unrelated antigen (TT) suggests an inhibitory effect of *S. mitis*. This inhibition can either be on the APCs directly by preventing activation and/or antigen presentation, or directly on the memory Th cells by interfering with the APC-T cell interaction. TT-induced T cell proliferation was sustained upon addition of *S. pneumoniae* which indicated that the inhibitory effect is not a shared trait between *S. mitis* and *S. pneumoniae*, but specific for *S. mitis*. Another cause for the higher frequencies of *S. pneumoniae*-specific cells as compared with those for *S. mitis* can be the occurrence of more species-specific immunogenic antigens in the former species.

Expression of capsule is a hallmark of virulence of *S. pneumoniae* and the capsules comprise different serotypes that are important for the species to evade immune responses [35]. Capsule antigens comprise multi-epitopic repetitive carbohydrate units and have been considered as T cell-independent antigens, with exception of that from *S. pneumoniae* type 1 (Sp1) that has zwitterionic properties, and is capable of activating T cells in an MHC class II-dependent manner [24,36]. Recently, *S. mitis* also has been shown to express capsule [21]. We tested isogenic capsule deletion mutants of *S. mitis* and *S. pneumoniae* but little difference in Th cell signatures was observed as compared with wild type strains. Replacing native capsule of *S. mitis* 31611T with capsule of *S. pneumoniae* TIGR4 neither altered the Th cell responses relative to the *S. mitis* wild type. This indicates that other factors than capsule expression are responsible for the raised frequencies of antigen-specific Th cells to *S. pneumoniae* as compared with *S. mitis*. The present human study support previous findings showing that murine splenocytes from animals injected with whole-cell vaccine induce high IL-17 responses, independent of presence or type of capsule [37]. In addition, the lack of differences in Th cell responses to T cell-dependent capsule serotype (Sp1) and T cell-independent capsule serotype (*S. pneumoniae* TIGR4) supports the notion that capsule is not recognized by CD4$^+$ memory T cells *in vivo*.

Heterologous immunity, the immunity that can develop to one pathogen after a host has been exposed to non-identical pathogens, has been closely studied in viral diseases [38], but less is known in bacterial infections. It can be mediated by specific cross-reactive T cells or antibodies, but can also be less specific [38]. We observed many cultures containing Th17 cells reactive for *S. mitis* and *S. pneumoniae* and hypothesized this could be due to cross-reactive cells. Indeed, Th cell clones from cultures responsive to *S. mitis* showed both intra- and inter-species cross-reactivity. Recently, 12 immunogenic Th17 antigens were isolated from soluble fractions of *S. pneumoniae* cell extracts [37]. We inspected the genomes of the three *S. mitis* strains used in this study and this revealed homologues to the 12 prominent T cell antigens from *S. pneumoniae* (90 to 100% identity) in strains 62644 and 62641 (data not shown). In the *S. mitis* type strain 31611T, 11 of the antigens were found. This means that the current cross-reactivity findings can be due to antigens common to *S. mitis* and *S. pneumoniae*. In the present investigation, it is not possible to identify the antigenic origin of any clones, but the existence of Th cell clones cross-reactive for the commensal *S. mitis* and the pathogenic *S. pneumoniae* can mean that immunologic memory induced by exposure to *S. mitis* or other related commensal streptococci can affect both carriage and

clearance of *S. pneumoniae* since it is known that *S. pneumoniae*-specific Th17 cells play a role in these processes [28].

In conclusion, the similar and cross-reactive T memory cell responses against *S. mitis* and *S. pneumoniae* indicate that the species have the potential to influence their mutual colonization. It is possible that carriage distributions of *S. mitis* strains will be shown to affect the performance of future experimental pneumococcal vaccine formulations.

Supporting Information

Figure S1 Cytokine secretion within Th subsets. Th subsets were sorted as described in Material and Methods and cytokine secretion in supernatant was measured by the CBA method after polyclonal stimulation with anti-CD3/anti-CD28 for 24 h. Bars represent averaged values of three samples and flags indicate standard deviation.

Table S1 Overview of surface markers used for sorting of CD45RA$^-$CD4$^+$ Th subsets.

Table S2 Numbers of T cells reactive with streptococci per 1×10^6 T cells per subset per donor.

Table S3 Wells reactive with streptococci as percentage of total number of wells for all subsets within each strain.

Author Contributions

Conceived and designed the experiments: SAE HVR IJB FCP FS KS. Performed the experiments: SAE SB DJ. Analyzed the data: SAE HVR FCP FS KS. Contributed reagents/materials/analysis tools: SAE HVR SB FCP FS KS. Contributed to the writing of the manuscript: SAE FCP FS KS.

References

1. Aas JA, Paster BJ, Stokes LN, Olsen I, Dewhirst FE (2005) Defining the normal bacterial flora of the oral cavity. J Clin Microbiol 43: 5721–32.
2. Dewhirst FE, Chen T, Izard J, Paster BJ, Tanner AC, et al. (2010) The human oral microbiome. J Bacteriol 192: 5002–17.
3. Zaura E, Keijser BJ, Huse SM, Crielaard W (2009) Defining the healthy "core microbiome" of oral microbial communities. BMC Microbiol 9: 259.
4. Brandtzaeg P (2001) Inflammatory bowel disease: clinics and pathology. Do inflammatory bowel disease and periodontal disease have similar immuno-pathogeneses? Acta Odontol Scand 59: 235–43.
5. Donati C, Hiller NL, Tettelin H, Muzzi A, Croucher NJ, et al. (2010) Structure and dynamics of the pan-genome of *Streptococcus pneumoniae* and closely related species. Genome Biol 11: R107.
6. O'Brien KL, Wolfson LJ, Watt JP, Henkle E, Deloria-Knoll M, et al. (2009) Burden of disease caused by *Streptococcus pneumoniae* in children younger than 5 years: global estimates. Lancet 374: 893–902.
7. Granat SM, Ollgren J, Herva E, Mia Z, Auranen K, et al. (2009) Epidemiological evidence for serotype-independent acquired immunity to pneumococcal carriage. J Infect Dis. 200: 99–106.
8. Rapola S, Jäntti V, Haikala R, Syrjänen R, Carlone GM, et al. (2000) Natural development of antibodies to pneumococcal surface protein A, pneumococcal surface adhesion A, and pneumolysin in relation to pneumococcal carriage and acute otitis media. J Infect Dis. 182: 1146–52.
9. Lipsitch M, Whitney CG, Zell E, Kaijalainen T, Dagan R, et al. (2005) Are anticapsular antibodies the primary mechanism of protection against invasive pneumococcal disease? PLoS Med. 2: e15.
10. Lundgren A, Bhuiyan TR, Novak D, Kaim J, Reske A, et al. (2012) Characterization of Th17 responses to *Streptococcus pneumoniae* in humans: Comparisons between adults and children in a developed and a developing country. Vaccine 6; 30: 3897–907.
11. Wirth KA, Bowden GH, Kirchherr JL, Richmond DA, Sheridan MJ, et al. (2008) Humoral immunity to commensal oral bacteria in human infants: evidence that *Streptococcus mitis* biovar 1 colonization induces strain-specific salivary immunoglobulin A antibodies. ISME J 2: 728–38.
12. Kirchherr JL, Bowden GH, Richmond DA, Sheridan MJ, Wirth KA, et al. (2005) Clonal diversity and turnover of *Streptococcus mitis* bv. 1 on shedding and nonshedding oral surfaces of human infants during the first year of life. Clin Diagn Lab Immunol 12: 1184–90.
13. Mosmann TR, Cherwinski H, Bond MW, Giedlin MA, Coffman RL (1986) Two types of murine helper T cell clone. I. Definition according to profiles of lymphokine activities and secreted proteins. J Immunol 136: 2348–57.
14. Langrish CL, Chen Y, Blumenschein WM, Mattson J, Basham B, et al. (2005) IL-23 drives a pathogenic T cell population that induces autoimmune inflammation. J Exp Med 201: 233–40.
15. Duhen T, Geiger R, Jarrossay D, Lanzavecchia A, Sallusto F (2009) Production of interleukin 22 but not interleukin 17 by a subset of human skin-homing memory T cells. Nat Immunol 10: 857–63.
16. Trifari S, Kaplan CD, Tran EH, Crellin NK, Spits H (2009) Identification of a human helper T cell population that has abundant production of interleukin 22 and is distinct from T(H)-17, T(H)1 and T(H)2 cells. Nat Immunol 10: 864–71.
17. Veldhoen M, Uyttenhove C, van Snick J, Helmby H, Westendorf A, et al. (2008) Transforming growth factor-beta 'reprograms' the differentiation of T helper 2 cells and promotes an interleukin 9-producing subset. Nat Immunol 9: 1341–6.
18. Acosta-Rodriguez EV, Rivino L, Geginat J, Jarrossay D, Gattorno M, et al. (2007) Surface phenotype and antigenic specificity of human interleukin 17-producing T helper memory cells. Nat Immunol 8: 639–46.
19. Cosmi L, De Palma R, Santarlasci V, Maggi L, Capone M, et al. (2008) Human interleukin 17-producing cells originate from a CD161+CD4+ T cell precursor. J Exp Med 205: 1903–16.
20. Cosmi L, Maggi L, Santarlasci V, Capone M, Cardilicchia E, et al. (2010) Identification of a novel subset of human circulating memory CD4(+) T cells that produce both IL-17A and IL-4. J Allergy Clin Immunol 125: 222–30.
21. Rukke HV, Hegna IK, Petersen FC (2012) Identification of a functional capsule locus in *Streptococcus mitis*. Mol Oral Microbiol 27: 95–108.
22. Geiger R, Duhen T, Lanzavecchia A, Sallusto F (2009) Human naive and memory CD4+ T cell repertoires specific for naturally processed antigens analyzed using libraries of amplified T cells. J Exp Med 206: 1525–34.

23. Lefkovits I, Waldmann H (1999) Limiting dilution analysis of cells of the immune system. Oxford: Oxford University Press. 285 p.

24. Kalka-Moll WM, Tzianabos AO, Bryant PW, Niemeyer M, Ploegh HL, et al. (2002) Zwitterionic polysaccharides stimulate T cells by MHC class II-dependent interactions. J Immunol 169: 6149–53.

25. Belkaid Y, Bouladoux N, Hand TW (2013) Effector and memory T cell responses to commensal bacteria. Trends Immunol 34: 299–306.

26. Zielinski CE, Corti D, Mele F, Pinto D, Lanzavecchia A, et al. (2011) Dissecting the human immunologic memory for pathogens. Immunol Rev 240: 40–51.

27. Pido-Lopez J, Kwok WW, Mitchell TJ, Heyderman RS, Williams NA (2011) Acquisition of pneumococci specific effector and regulatory Cd4+ T cells localising within human upper respiratory-tract mucosal lymphoid tissue. PLoS Pathog 7: e1002396.

28. Wright AK, Bangert M, Gritzfeld JF, Ferreira DM, Jambo KC, et al. (2013) Experimental human pneumococcal carriage augments IL-17A-dependent T-cell defence of the lung. PLoS Pathog 9: e1003274.

29. Nistala K, Adams S, Cambrook H, Ursu S, Olivito B, et al. (2010) Th17 plasticity in human autoimmune arthritis is driven by the inflammatory environment. Proc Natl Acad Sci U S A 107: 14751–6.

30. Ramesh R, Kozhaya L, McKevitt K, Djuretic IM, Carlson TJ, et al. (2014) Pro-inflammatory human Th17 cells selectively express P-glycoprotein and are refractory to glucocorticoids. J Exp Med 211: 89–104.

31. Glennie SJ, Banda D, Gould K, Hinds J, Kamngona A, et al. (2013) Defective pneumococcal-specific Th1 responses in HIV-infected adults precedes a loss of control of pneumococcal colonization. Clin Infect Dis 56: 291–9.

32. Paats MS, Bergen IM, Hanselaar WE, van Zoelen EC, Verbrugh HA, et al. (2013) T helper 17 cells are involved in the local and systemic inflammatory response in community-acquired pneumonia. Thorax 68: 468–74.

33. Rutz S, Eidenschenk C, Ouyang W (2013) IL-22, not simply a Th17 cytokine. Immunol Rev 252: 116–32.

34. Ivanov S, Renneson J, Fontaine J, Barthelemy A, Paget C, et al. (2013) Interleukin-22 reduces lung inflammation during influenza A virus infection and protects against secondary bacterial infection. J Virol 87: 6911–24.

35. Pletz MW, Maus U, Krug N, Welte T, Lode H (2008) Pneumococcal vaccines: mechanism of action, impact on epidemiology and adaption of the species. Int J Antimicrob Agents 32: 199–206.

36. Velez CD, Lewis CJ, Kasper DL, Cobb BA (2009) Type I Streptococcus pneumoniae carbohydrate utilizes a nitric oxide and MHC II-dependent pathway for antigen presentation. Immunology 127: 73–82.

37. Moffitt KL, Malley R, Lu YJ (2012) Identification of protective pneumococcal T(H)17 antigens from the soluble fraction of a killed whole cell vaccine. PLoS One 7: e43445.

38. Welsh RM, Che JW, Brehm MA, Selin LK (2010) Heterologous immunity between viruses. Immunol Rev 235: 244–66.

20

Cost-Effectiveness of Tenofovir Instead of Zidovudine for Use in First-Line Antiretroviral Therapy in Settings without Virological Monitoring

Viktor von Wyl[1,2]*, Valentina Cambiano[1], Michael R. Jordan[3,4], Silvia Bertagnolio[3], Alec Miners[5], Deenan Pillay[6], Jens Lundgren[7], Andrew N. Phillips[1]

1 University College London, Research Department of Infection and Population Health, London, United Kingdom, 2 CSS Institute for Empirical Health Economics, Lucerne, Switzerland, 3 World Health Organization, Geneva, Switzerland, 4 Tufts University, School of Medicine, Boston, Masschussetts, United States of America, 5 London School of Hygiene and Tropical Medicine, London, United Kingdom, 6 University College London, Division of Infection and Immunity, London, United Kingdom, 7 Copenhagen University Hospital-Rigshospitalet, University of Copenhagen, Copenhagen, Denmark

Abstract

Background: The most recent World Health Organization (WHO) antiretroviral treatment guidelines recommend the inclusion of zidovudine (ZDV) or tenofovir (TDF) in first-line therapy. We conducted a cost-effectiveness analysis with emphasis on emerging patterns of drug resistance upon treatment failure and their impact on second-line therapy.

Methods: We used a stochastic simulation of a generalized HIV-1 epidemic in sub-Saharan Africa to compare two strategies for first-line combination antiretroviral treatment including lamivudine, nevirapine and either ZDV or TDF. Model input parameters were derived from literature and, for the simulation of resistance pathways, estimated from drug resistance data obtained after first-line treatment failure in settings without virological monitoring. Treatment failure and cost effectiveness were determined based on WHO definitions. Two scenarios with optimistic (no emergence; base) and pessimistic (extensive emergence) assumptions regarding occurrence of multidrug resistance patterns were tested.

Results: In the base scenario, cumulative proportions of treatment failure according to WHO criteria were higher among first-line ZDV users (median after six years 36% [95% simulation interval 32%; 39%]) compared with first-line TDF users (31% [29%; 33%]). Consequently, a higher proportion initiated second-line therapy (including lamivudine, boosted protease inhibitors and either ZDV or TDF) in the first-line ZDV user group 34% [31%; 37%] relative to first-line TDF users (30% [27%; 32%]). At the time of second-line initiation, a higher proportion (16%) of first-line ZDV users harboured TDF-resistant HIV compared with ZDV-resistant viruses among first-line TDF users (0% and 6% in base and pessimistic scenarios, respectively). In the base scenario, the incremental cost effectiveness ratio with respect to quality adjusted life years (QALY) was US$83 when TDF instead of ZDV was used in first-line therapy (pessimistic scenario: US$ 315), which was below the WHO threshold for high cost effectiveness (US$ 2154).

Conclusions: Using TDF instead of ZDV in first-line treatment in resource-limited settings is very cost-effective and likely to better preserve future treatment options in absence of virological monitoring.

Editor: Xu Yu, Massachusetts General Hospital, United States of America

Funding: The research leading to these results has received partial funding from the European Community's Seventh Framework Programme (FP7/2007–2013) under the project 'Collaborative HIV and Anti-HIV Drug Resistance Network (CHAIN)' – grant agreement n° 223131. VvW was supported by a Swiss National Science Foundation (SNF) Grant for Prospective Researchers (PBEZP3-125726), and MRJ has received a grant from the National Institutes of Health (NIH K23 AI074423-05). The funders had no role in study design, data collection and analysis, decision to publish, or preparation of the manuscript.

Competing Interests: The authors have declared that no competing interests exist.

* E-mail: viktor.vonwyl@css-institut.ch

Introduction

The public health approach for combination antiretroviral therapy (cART) in resource-limited settings includes the use of one standard first-line and one standard second-line regimen [1]. According to World Health Organization 2010 treatment guidelines, first-line therapy should consist of a non-nucleoside reverse transcriptase inhibitor (NNRTI) and two nucleoside reverse transcriptase inhibitors (NRTI), one of which should be zidovudine (ZDV) or tenofovir (TDF). Second-line ART should consist of a ritonavir-boosted protease inhibitor (PI/r) plus two NRTIs, one of which should be ZDV or TDF, based on what was used in first-line therapy. Ritonavir-boosted atazanavir (ATV/r) or lopinavir/ritonavir (LPV/r) are the preferred PIs. The choice of using TDF or ZDV in first-line treatment is determined at country level. Randomized clinical trials have demonstrated superiority of TDF over ZDV [2,3,4,5] and over stavudine (D4T) [6,7] in combination therapy with regards to virological suppression, as well as a tendency for less toxicity-related discontinuations and improved adherence in industrialized [3] and resource-limited settings [8]. In contrast, the somewhat lower costs favour the use of ZDV, although considerable price reductions for TDF have been achieved more recently so differences are now small [9].

One particular concern regarding the widespread use of TDF in settings without virological monitoring is the potential for development of extensive nucleoside and nucleotide analogue cross-resistance via the emergence of the reverse transcriptase mutation K65R, and possibly also multidrug resistance patterns such as Q151M, although the latter has not been detected in well-controlled clinical trials in resource-rich settings [4,7,10]. Moreover, some in vitro data point to more rapid selection of K65R emergence in subtype C viruses, owing to a specific nucleotide motif at reverse transcriptase position 65 that facilitates the amino acid switch from lysine to arginine [11,12]. Indeed, recent surveys from resource-limited settings suggest a comparatively high prevalence of high-level NRTI cross-resistance resistance associated with K65R (23%) or Q151M (0–19%) amongst patients with clinical or virological treatment failure [13,14].

Previous cost effectiveness analyses have already pointed towards better clinical outcomes of TDF use compared with other NRTIs in industrialized [15] and resource-limited settings [16,17,18,19]. These studies, however, mainly focused on HIV-1 and treatment related morbidities, and did not investigate the impact of the emergence of drug resistance mutations on future therapy options. In the present simulations, we aimed to re-assess the cost effectiveness of TDF over ZDV for settings using the public health approach for ART with one standard first-line and one standard second-line regimen, and without virological monitoring, which is the reality in most resource-poor settings. For this purpose, an established individual-based stochastic model

of HIV transmission and treatment in a resource-limited country was adapted to reflect possible mutation patterns leading to and after first-line treatment failures and to predict costs of treatment for HIV-1 and tuberculosis-(TB) and HIV-related morbidity and mortality [20,21]. We specifically considered the impact of the different resistance patterns generated by the use of TDF or ZDV in first-line cART on efficacy of second-line therapy and subsequent morbidity and mortality.

Methods

Stochastic Simulation

The model presented here corresponds to the version described extensively in [20,21] and the accompanying web appendix (http://links.lww.com/QAD/A113), with deviations in how drug resistance mutations emerge (see below). In brief, the stochastic model, programmed in SAS 9.1, simulates a generalized heterosexual HIV epidemic in a resource-limited country by keeping track of individuals and their health status with regard to HIV and other co-morbidities. Individual characteristics are updated in three month time steps.

A typical simulation run, which is influenced by many random elements, shows the following characteristics: starting in 1989, the population of approximately 25 000 uninfected persons initially contains about 5 HIV infected individuals. The epidemic starts to spread via individuals who acquire HIV through heterosexual contacts with HIV-1 infected short or long term partners. The probability of transmission of HIV depends on whether the partner is undergoing primary infection, on the partner's HIV-RNA viral load (obtained by sampling from the distribution of

Table 1. Selected model input parameters.

	Rates per 3 months	Value for sensitivity analysis	Source
Drug related toxicities (*1.5 times higher in first year)			
Zidovudine (ZDV)			
nausea*	0.1		own estimate
lipodystrophy	0.015		own estimate
anemia*	0.03		[3] and own estimate
Headache*	0.1		own estimate
lactic acidosis	0.001		own estimate
Tenofovir (TDF)			
Nephrotoxicity	0.01		[6] and own estimate.
Antiretroviral treatment adherence			
Adherence benefit of TDF over ZDV	0.03	0	[3]
worse adherence if drug related toxicities	0.1		[40]
Resistance emergence (also see figure 1)			
Emergence of NNRTI mutations in presence of			
Detectable HIV RNA<500 copies/mL	0.4		own estimate
Detectable HIV RNA >500 copies/mL	0.95		own estimate
Emergence of M184V mutations in presence of			
Detectable HIV RNA<500 copies/mL	0.4		own estimate
Detectable HIV RNA >500 copies/mL	0.9		own estimate
Other			
Probability for switch if treatment failure detected	0.8	0.1	[41]

viral load levels found in partnerships formed by HIV-infected people, accounting for gender and age), on the subject's gender and on the presence of other sexually transmitted infections. Each HIV-infected individual experiences HIV RNA levels, CD4 declines and mortality rates that correspond to their specific age and gender, health status with respect to co-morbidities, and to antiretroviral treatment exposure. We assumed that cART became available in 2007 (corresponding to the first availability of TDF in national and regional treatment programs [22,23]), when the HIV prevalence had reached approximately 14%. Treatment either consists of fixed dose, twice daily ZDV+3TC+NVP or once daily TDF+ lamivudine (3TC) and NVP in two tablets, depending on the first-line treatment strategy.

Selected model input parameters are shown in Table 1. In the model, the number of active drugs, adherence and HIV RNA levels affect the probability for suppression of viral replication and the accumulation of resistance mutations. Each individual is assigned a fixed underlying adherence level, which can vary from period to period within certain bounds and can be offset (with an increment) in some circumstances according to specific rules (e.g. worse adherence when drug-related toxic side effects present, table 1). Following these fluctuations in adherence levels to antiretroviral drugs, HIV RNA can rise to detectable levels in individuals who receive ART. The risk for emergence of drug resistance follows an n-shaped relationship with adherence such that resistance risk is highest when adherence is moderate. Further details can be found in the Materials S1. When resistance has emerged, this reduces viral susceptibility to antiretroviral drugs and hence further reduces the probability for suppression of viral replication at the next time step.

Main Assumptions on Setting Characteristics

The setting of the main analysis consists of an HIV-infected population, in which ART has not previously been used. HIV diagnosis became available in 2003 and is either made by voluntary testing of a fixed rate of the population (7.5% chance every three months) or triggered by AIDS defining conditions. CD4 count determinations are performed every 6 months in diagnosed individuals, and if measured CD4 levels drop<200 - cells/mm^3 or a WHO stage 4 event has been diagnosed, ART is initiated.

The definition for treatment failure is based on clinical (new or recurrent WHO stage 4 condition), specific WHO clinical stage 3 conditions (e.g. pulmonary tuberculosis) and immunological criteria (fall of CD4 count to baseline or below, or 50% fall from on-treatment peak value, or persistent CD4 levels below 100 cells/mm3) and CD4 cell measurements occur on a 6-monthly basis. It is also assumed that virological testing is not available and that switching to second-line ART occurs almost immediately after detection of treatment failure at a rate of 80% per 3 months, unless an individual is lost to follow-up.

Second-line ART consists of LPV/r, 3TC, and either ZDV or TDF, whichever has not been used in first-line treatment already. In this hypothetical setting with only two lines of treatment available, individuals who fail second-line therapy remain on the failing regimen.

Treatment Outcomes

Clinical (AIDS-defining conditions, mortality) and treatment outcomes (CD4 cell gain, rates of viral suppression, and treatment failure based on WHO criteria) of the simulation are presented as medians [2.5th–97.5th percentiles] from the distribution of point estimates from all simulation runs per analysis (n = 100). Unless stated otherwise, treatment outcomes were estimated on an intent-

to-continue treatment basis by the Kaplan-Meier method, meaning that study outcomes were still attributed to the respective first-line strategy in spite of possible switches to second-line therapy.

Cost Analyses

Main cost-effectiveness outcomes are average costs (per treated individual) and cumulative costs accrued by year 2022 (15 years after cART became available) for antiretroviral treatment and expenses for management of TB or HIV-related morbidity. In addition, cumulative person-years and quality adjusted life-years (QALY) lived from ART start to death or until 2022, whichever came first, are compared between treatment strategies. On the basis of estimates from [24], we set utilities for estimation of QALY at 0.75 if drug-related toxicities were present, if the individual suffered from AIDS-defining conditions (ADC), or if the individual was infected with TB. Otherwise utility weights were set to 0.8 in HIV-infected individuals [24].

Costs for cART were derived from the Clinton Foundation price list of November 2010 [9]. The price per year of first-line treatment with ZDV/3TC/NVP and TDF/3TC/NVP was set at US$ 140 and US$ 147, respectively. Second-line therapy containing LPV/r and ZDV or TDF was priced at US$ 550. The per 3-month costs for management of TB, ADC, and *Pneumocystis carinii* prophylaxis (PCP) were US$ 50, US$ 200, and US$ 5, respectively. Costs for outpatient visits and laboratory monitoring (e.g. CD4 cell counts) were omitted, because they are the same for both treatment arms. As a measure of cost-effectiveness, incremental cost effectiveness ratios (ICER) were estimated. Incremental cost-effectiveness was defined as the difference in the average treatment costs per ART exposed individual between treatment strategies divided by the difference in average QALY per cART exposed individual between the two therapy strategies (ZDV first or TDF first) since cART became available. Thus, the ICER signifies the magnitude of additional costs incurred by the new treatment strategy to gain one additional QALY. Owing to the repetition of simulations, each model analysis yielded different predictions for QALYs and treatment costs. These results were summarized by calculating the ICER from averages of costs and QALYs over all simulations from the same setting/pathway. We further assessed the uncertainty of our model estimates. Because the simulation yielded no pairing of TDF and ZDV (the estimates for treatment arms were generated in separate simulation runs), we sampled one estimate from the TDF simulation and one estimate from the ZDV simulation to calculate the ICER. By repeating this procedure 1000 times we obtained a distribution of possible ICER outcomes, given the results from the 100 simulations per setting and scenario. We defined uncertainty bounds as the range that included 95% of all sampling repetitions. A health-care cost perspective was applied to the cost-effectiveness analysis, which had a time horizon of 15 years. Costs and life years lived were discounted at 3% per year. Cost effectiveness was determined according to WHO guidelines by comparing ICER estimates with the per capita gross domestic product (GDP; http://www.who.int/choice/costs/CER_levels/en/index.html; *WHO AFRO E region*). According to this definition, incremental cost effectiveness ratios below 3-fold the GDP (US$ 6461) are considered cost effective and ICER below the GDP (*US $2,154*) are very cost effective.

Statistical Analyses of Genotypic Drug Resistance Tests to Derive Input Parameters for Drug Resistance Model

The simulation modelled the emergence of thymidine analogue mutations (TAM), K65R, and Q151M on failing

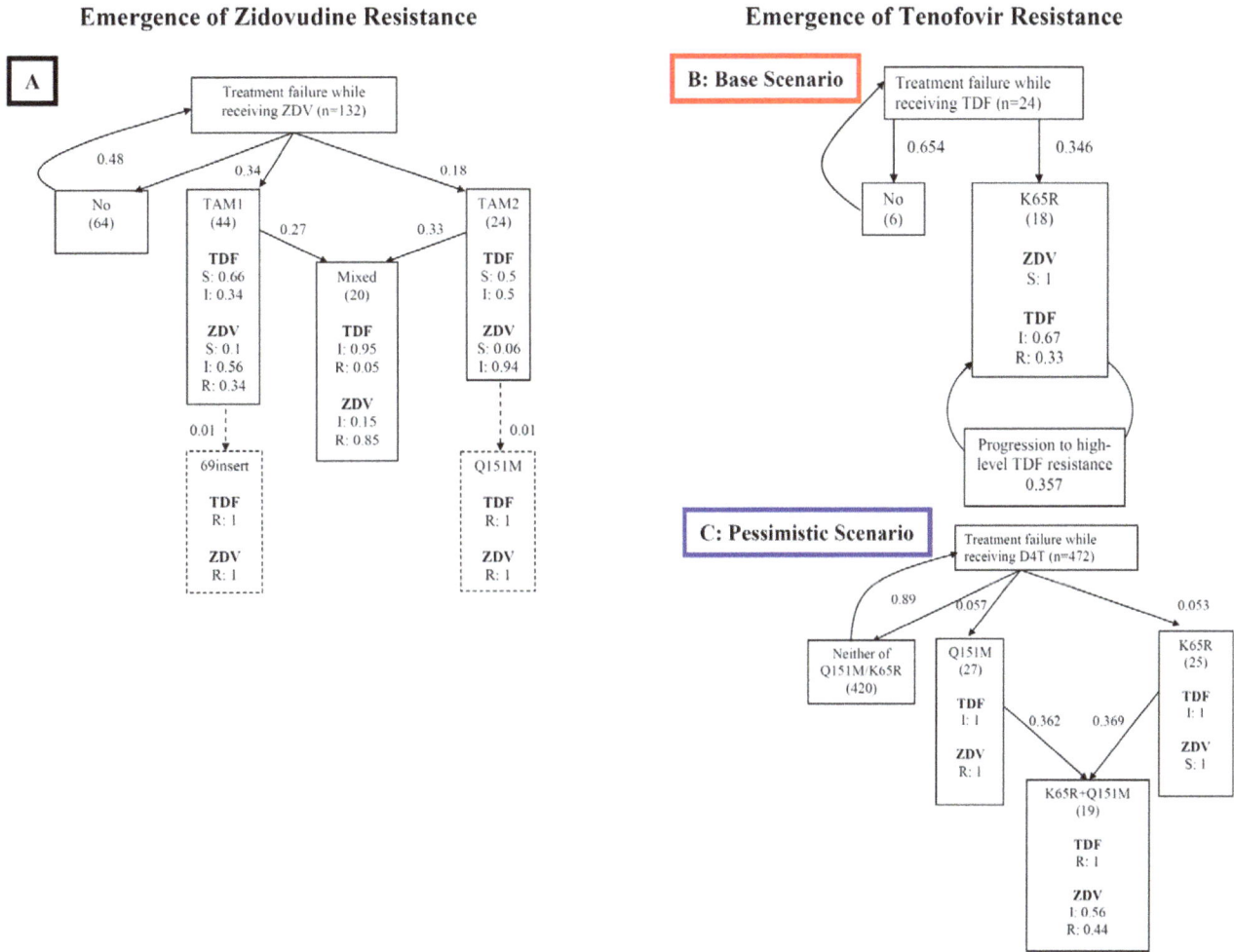

Figure 1. This plots hypothetical pathways of resistance emergence against zidovudine (1A) or tenofovir (1B & 1C) used in this simulation. The transition probabilities given next to arrows are per 3 months spent on a failing treatment with an (unmeasured) HIV RNA >500 copies/mL. Due to scarcity of resistance data of failing tenofovir regimens from developing settings two separate pathways were tested in the simulation. The base scenario (1B) was derived from a limited set of sequences from tenofovir failures and does not include the multidrug resistance pattern Q151M. The pessimistic scenario (1C) is based on estimations from sequences obtained after virological failure with stavudine and allows for extensive multidrug (i.e. Q151M) resistance emergence. Also note that the multidrug resistance patterns in the zidovudine pathway were not observed in the data (enframed by dashed lines), but were assumed to occur at low frequency. Abbreviations: ZDV, Zidovudine; TDF, tenofovir; S, susceptible; I, intermediate resistant; R, fully resistant.

cART. To obtain estimates of rates and order of mutation accumulation of K65R and Q151M, descriptive statistical analyses of six publicly available data sets with genotypic drug resistance test (GRT) data of non-B subtype viruses from Sub-Saharan African settings were performed [13,14,25,26,27,28]. Because the number of data points from first-line TDF use in resource-limited settings was very small (n = 24) in our sample, we additionally approximated rates of K65R and Q151M emergence from individuals failing first-line cART with D4T (along with lamivudine and an NNRTI), since this drug compound is also known to select for K65R and Q151M mutations and more data were available. Therefore, two separate simulations were run: A base scenario (Figure 1B) with mutation rates obtained from the limited set of sequences obtained from first-line TDF treated individuals, and a second scenario (Figure 1C) based on genotypic resistance test data collected after first-line treatment failure with D4T. Contrary to the base scenario, the pessimistic scenario allows for extensive

emergence of the multidrug resistance pattern Q151M, hence it was termed the "pessimistic scenario". Of note, TAM emergence was ignored in these two scenarios, because TDF does not select TAMs.

We constructed mutagenic trees by grouping the GRTs according to mutation patterns with respect to TAM, K65R, and Q151M, and by assuming a specific order for the emergence of these mutations (in Figures 1A, 1B, and 1C) [29]. This tree determines the order of mutation emergence (e.g. high emergence rates suggest early occurrence) as well as the progression of resistance along the tree in a time-dependent manner. Transition probabilities between tree nodes were estimated by counting the number of GRT showing a specific pattern and dividing them by the number of GRTs in the next higher tree node. These probabilities were converted into incidence rates per 3 months on a failing regimen by assuming an average time from virological treatment failure to stop or switch of the failing regimen of 1 year [14,26,27]. In addition, a genotypic sensitivity score (GSS) was

Table 2. Percent of individuals starting partially inactive second-line treatment due to acquired drug resistance during first-line treatment.

Setting	ZDV first	TDF first, base scenario	TDF first, pessimistic scenario
Base			
<2.75 active drugs	16.2 [12.3; 19.3]	0 [0; 0.2]	5.9 [3.7; 8.3]
<2 active drugs	0.7 [0; 1.3]	0	5.0 [3.3; 7.8]
Transmitted Resistance			
<2.75 active drugs	16.3 [13.3; 20.6]	0.2 [0; 0.7]	6.2 [3.6; 8.9]
<2 active drugs	0.8 [0; 1.3]	0	5.4 [3.0; 7.6]
Virological Monitoring			
<2.75 active drugs	6.3 [4.8; 8.9]	0 [0; 0.1]	1.7 [1.0; 3.0]
<2 active drugs	0 [0; 0.5]	0	1.6 [1.0; 2.9]
Switches allowed			
<2.75 active drugs	14.3 [11.2; 18.8]	1.4 [0.4; 2.7]	6.5 [4.4; 8.9]
<2 active drugs	0.9 [0; 2.3]	0.8 [0.2; 1.7]	5.6 [3.1; 8.5]

estimated by applying the Stanford algorithm version 6.0.11 to each GRT that matched the mutation pattern of a specific tree node [30]. This procedure led, for each tree node, to a distribution of GRTs indicating full susceptibility, intermediate resistance, and full resistance to ZDV and TDF. In the stochastic simulation, progression in resistance pathways to the next node, as well as the degree of resistance were determined randomly, but corresponding to the probabilities observed at the respective node of the mutagenic tree.

The estimated 3-month incidence rates for NNRTI and 3TC mutations, which were also derived from genotypic data, are displayed in Table 1.

Sensitivity Analyses

The effect of considering LPV/r worth only 1 drug, of immediate or delayed switching after detection of first-line treatment failure or of the assumed adherence benefit of TDF use on outcomes (and treatment costs in particular), and combinations of these parameters, were subjected to sensitivity analyses by re-running the simulation using predefined parameter values (Table 1). In the base scenario it was assumed that first-line TDF use led to a 3% point higher adherence compared with ZDV use due to better tolerability and once daily dosing [3].

Moreover, simulations were repeated in alternative settings, which included the availability of viral load monitoring, the effect of substituting drug components due to toxic side effects, and by

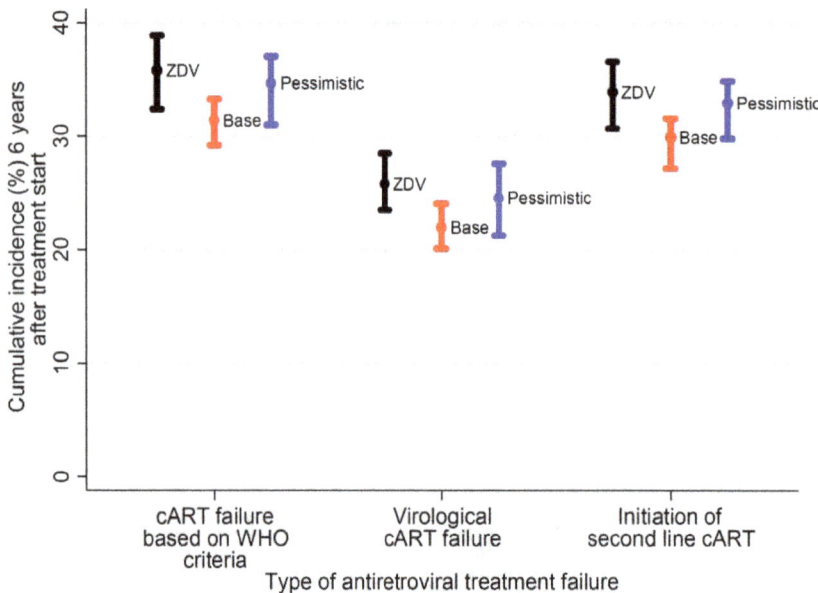

Figure 2. Shows different outcomes of first-line therapy by type of initial combination antiretroviral therapy (either including zidovudine [ZDV] or tenofovir [TDF]). For individuals starting with TDF, resistance emergence was modelled by two different scenarios (also see Figures 1B and 1C): a base scenario (red symbols) and a pessimistic scenario (blue symbols). Abbreviations: cART, combination antiretroviral therapy; WHO, World Health Organization.

introducing ART into a setting where transmitted drug resistance from D4T/3TC/nevirapine was present (for details see Materials S1) [31].

Results

Analysis of Observed and Predicted Drug Resistance Data

A total of 605 genotypic sequences obtained after first line treatment failure with either 3TC+ZDV+NNRTI (n = 133), 3TC+TDF+NNRTI (n = 24) or 3TC+D4T+NNRTI (n = 472) were analyzed. Given the small number of individuals who have received TDF in first-line treatment, rates of K65R and Q151M mutation emergence were also estimated from the D4T data and applied to a separate simulation representing an alternate, "pessimistic" scenario. The distribution of viral subtypes was as follows: C 53% (n = 320); G 16% (n = 97); CRF02_AG 14% (n = 83); and a variety of other non-B subtypes occurring at <4%.

Probabilities for the emergence of resistance upon clinical or immunological treatment failure were calculated as the percentage of genotypic resistance tests showing a specific mutation pattern and are displayed in Figure 1. When analyzing the D4T data, the K65R mutation emerged in 45 of 472 cases, which was considerably lower than what was seen in a limited sample of viral sequences from individuals with TDF treatment failure, where K65R was detected in 75% of 24 available genotypic sequences.

Simulated Study Population at Time of ART Introduction

Out of a population of 4346 [4075; 4618] simulated HIV infected individuals, 2012 [1065; 2501] and 2045 [1536; 2517] individuals ever initiated ART with ZDV or TDF between the years 2007 and 2022 (end of simulation), respectively. The median age at time of cART initiation was 43 years, and 52% were women, irrespective of treatment strategy group. The median follow-up time after initiation of first-line therapy was 6 years. At time of therapy initiation, median values [interquartile range] of HIV RNA measurements were 5.09 [5.06; 5.12] log10 copies/mL, and median [interquartile] CD4 count measurements reached 140 [133; 147] cells/microliter, irrespective of treatment group. Around 7% [6;8] had active TB disease, and 9% [8;11] had experienced AIDS defining conditions.

Differences in first-line therapy outcomes were predicted with respect to CD4 cell count recovery, with a gain of 102 cells/microliter [97; 113] within 1 year in the ZDV group and gains of 114 cells/microliter [107; 121] (base scenario) and 107 cells/microliter [102; 112] (pessimistic scenario) in the TDF group, respectively. Intent to treat viral suppression rates below 50 copies\mL after 1 year were estimated at 64% [62; 67] among ZDV starters and at 68% [66; 71] (base scenario) and 66% [63; 68] (pessimistic scenario), respectively, in the TDF group.

As shown in Figure 2, six years after treatment initiation, corresponding to the median follow-up time after cART initiation, 25.8% [23.5; 28.5] of the ZDV starters had ever experienced a virological treatment failure, and 35.8% [32.4; 38.9] had experienced treatment failure according to the WHO definition based on immunological and clinical criteria. Among individuals who initiated treatment with TDF the proportions of virological and immunological/clinical failures were 22.0% [20.1; 24.1] and 31.4% [29.2; 33.3] respectively for the base scenario and 24.6% [21.3; 27.6] and 34.7% [31.0; 37.1] respectively for the pessimistic scenario. Six years after cART initiation, drug-resistance was predicted to have emerged in 27.9% [25.5; 30.4] of individuals in the ZDV group and in 24.3% [22.7; 26.1] (base scenario) and 26.4% [23.4; 29.8] (pessimistic scenario) of individuals in the TDF group.

Predicted Patterns of Acquired Drug Resistance and Impact on Second-line Therapy

A higher proportion of ZDV starters was predicted to have initiated LPV/r-based second-line therapy within 6 years after antiretroviral treatment initiation (33.9% [30.7; 36.6], median n = 602) when compared with the group of TDF starters (base scenario: 29.9% [27.2; 31.6], median n = 547; pessimistic scenario: 33.0% [29.8; 34.9], median n = 597). Among individuals from the ZDV group who initiated second-line therapy, TAMs were predicted to be present in 28.4% [23.2; 32.5], and none in the two TDF groups. Among individuals who started TDF as first-line therapy, the predicted proportion of K65R was almost 9-fold higher in the base scenario (43.4% [38.8; 48.4]) compared with the pessimistic scenario (4.7% [3.3; 6.7]). In contrast, while there were no Q151M mutations emerging in the base scenario, the prevalence of Q151M was estimated at 5.9% [3.7; 8.3] in the pessimistic scenario. With respect to NNRTI mutations (56–57%) and M184V (62–63%), the simulation yielded almost identical estimates across the three groups (not shown).

Next, we analyzed the potential activity of second-line regimens against a background of different resistance mutations patterns. Previous studies have demonstrated that ritonavir-boosted PIs such as LPV/r have a very high potency to inhibit viral replication and are very robust to the emergence of drug resistance [32,33]. Therefore, we allocated LPV/r a relative activity score of 1.5 in our analyses of second-line treatment outcomes. As shown in Table 2, when considering lopinavir/r as 1.5 active drugs and 3TC use in the presence of the mutation M184V as 0.25 active drugs (owing to the high viral fitness reduction induced by this mutation), 16.2% [12.3; 19.3] of ZDV starters were receiving second-line regimens with less than 2.75 active drugs (corresponding to partially active 3TC, a partially active NRTI, and fully active LPV/r). In contrast, depending on the scenario only 5.9% [3.7; 8.3] (pessimistic) or 0.6% [0; 1.6] (base) among the TDF starters received less than 2.75 fully active drugs. This marked difference was driven by ZDV's potential to induce mutations, and in particular TAMs of group 1, with intermediate to full level cross-resistance to TDF (figure 1A). In contrast, K65R carrying viral strains are known to retain their susceptibility to ZDV [34]. The proportion of individuals with severely compromised second-line treatments with <2 fully active drugs (e.g. fully active LPV/r, partially active 3TC, and no activity of second NRTI) among ZDV starters was 0.7% [0.0; 1.3], but reached 5.0% [3.3; 7.8] when applying the pessimistic TDF scenario, which allows for the emergence of the multidrug resistance pattern Q151M. When translated into absolute numbers (per 1000 individuals starting first-line treatment) and taking into account first-line treatment failure rates, these predictions suggest that, six years after therapy start, 55 from the ZDV group and 19 from the TDF group (pessimistic scenario) will have started partially compromised second-line regimens with <2.75 fully active drugs. However, only 2 per 1000 individuals from the ZDV group, but 17 per 1000 from the TDF group (pessimistic scenario) will have initiated inadequate second-line therapy with <2 fully active drugs due to high-level cross-resistance.

Cost Effectiveness Analysis

For the cost effectiveness analysis, the cumulative treatment costs accrued after therapy start until death or the year 2022 (whichever came first) were compared (table 3). The median observation time was 6 years, over which individuals starting therapy with TDF incurred slightly higher discounted ART-related costs (base scenario: US$ 1070; pessimistic scenario: US$ 1102) than individuals starting first-line treatment with ZDV with US$ 1058.

Table 3. Cost effectiveness analyses.

Scenario	ZDV first, base scenario	TDF first, base scenario	ZDV first, pessimistic scenario	TDF first, pessimistic scenario
Base				
Treatment costs	1058 [904; 1145]	1070 [994; 1140]	1072 [995; 1148]	1102 [997; 1182]
HIV-morbidity related costs	160 [136; 170]	148 [135; 159]	160 [145; 170]	151 [136; 162]
Total costs	1217 [1040; 1314]	1219 [1137; 1292]	1232 [1143; 1314]	1252 [1138; 1338]
Life years lived	4.811 [4.290; 5.100]	4.936 [4.721; 5.172]	4.856 [4.642; 5.062]	4.910 [4.678; 5.125]
QALYs lived	3.719 [3.317; 3.944]	3.869 [3.701; 4.054]	3.753 [3.588; 3.917]	3.846 [3.663; 4.015]
ICER for Treatment costs and				
life years lived		99		540
QALYs lived		83		315
ICER for total costs and				
life years lived		11		377
QALYs lived		9		220
Transmitted Resistance				
Treatment costs	1076 [980; 1162]	1065 [827; 1135]	1070 [998; 1154]	1103 [950; 1177]
HIV-morbidity related costs	161 [151; 175]	149 [120; 159]	161 [145; 174]	152 [134; 162]
Total costs	1237 [1131; 1327]	1213 [948; 1289]	1231 [1146; 1326]	1255 [1085; 1339]
Life years lived	4.856 [4.519; 5.155]	4.895 [4.139; 5.161]	4.832 [4.551; 5.113]	4.891 [4.411; 5.129]
QALYs lived	3.754 [3.492; 3.986]	3.836 [3.244; 4.046]	3.735 [3.518; 3.955]	3.830 [3.454; 4.016]
ICER for Treatment costs and				
life years lived		dominant[a]		551
QALYs lived		dominant[a]		339
ICER for total costs and				
life years lived		dominant[a]		405
QALYs lived		dominant[a]		250
Virological Monitoring				
Treatment costs	1102 [1011; 1170]	1073 [918; 1152]	1112 [997; 1187]	1134 [1056; 1209]
HIV-morbidity related costs	150 [132; 161]	138 [113; 150]	149 [136; 161]	142 [132; 150]
Total costs	1252 [1151; 1325]	1211 [1031; 1295]	1261 [1135; 1339]	1277 [1188; 1355]
Life years lived	4.910 [4.558; 5.174]	4.977 [4.406; 5.243]	4.929 [4.576; 5.178]	4.995 [4.736; 5.241]
QALYs lived	3.800 [3.530; 4.001]	3.905 [3.456; 4.112]	3.815 [3.544; 4.008]	3.915 [3.712; 4.109]
ICER for Treatment costs and				
life years lived		dominant[a]		348
QALYs lived		dominant[a]		229
ICER for total costs and				
life years lived		dominant[a]		243
QALYs lived		dominant[a]		160
Switches allowed				
Treatment costs	1012 [952; 1080]	1021 [937; 1085]	1027 [962; 1087]	1054 [945; 1122]
HIV-morbidity related costs	164 [148; 175]	154 [139; 167]	163 [156; 172]	155 [144; 165]
Total costs	1176 [1104; 1253]	1175 [1084; 1244]	1190 [1126; 1250]	1209 [1091; 1287]
Life years lived	4.803 [4.543; 5.029]	4.908 [4.605; 5.126]	4.855 [4.662; 5.072]	4.884 [4.445; 5.128]
QALYs lived	3.723 [3.524; 3.899]	3.843 [3.606; 4.016]	3.763 [3.611; 3.935]	3.822 [3.477; 4.012]
ICER for Treatment costs and				
life years lived		86		937
QALYs lived		75		453
ICER for total costs and				
life years lived		dominant[a]		663
QALYs lived		dominant[a]		321

Table 3. Cont.

Footnotes:
All costs are in US$.
[a]TDF dominant over ZDV because of lower costs and higher QALYs.

However, less expenditures related to treatment of AIDS defining conditions or tuberculosis were needed in the group of TDF users (base scenario: US$ 148; pessimistic scenario: US$ 151) compared with the ZDV group with US$ 160 per individual on therapy.

Regarding morbidity and life-years lived as outcomes, the three strategies seemed to be comparable: the six year Kaplan-Meier estimates for mortality were 25.9% [22.1; 28.4] for the ZDV group and 23.3% [20.8; 25.9] (base scenario) and 23.6% [21.5; 25.4] (pessimistic scenario) for the TDF groups. The mean number of discounted life years lived since therapy start until death or 2022 per individual looked similar across the three groups (4.9 years, Table 3), but QALY gained were somewhat higher among first-line TDF users compared with the ZDV group (Figure 3A). Costs and QALY measures were then combined into incremental cost effectiveness ratios for different outcomes (Table 3, Figure 3B). When focusing on resistance emergence in the base scenario, our simulation results suggests that TDF use for first-line therapy was a very cost-effective treatment strategy, with an additional quality adjusted life year costing less than US$ 100, and in two scenarios (transmitted resistance present; availability of virological monitoring) even being a dominant strategy because of lower costs and more QALYs gained. However, when considering the pessimistic scenario, which allows for extensive NRTI multidrug resistance, the price for an additional quality adjusted life year rose to up to US$ 450 and TDF use was no longer dominant, although still very cost-effective by WHO standards.

Next, we assessed the robustness of model outcomes in different settings (presence of transmitted resistance, virological monitoring

available, drug switches due to drug toxicities allowed; see Materials S1 for further details) and the reliance on the choice of specific input parameter values, namely the assumed better adherence to TDF compared with ZDV and the impact of delayed switching of drugs after detection of treatment failure. When considering the impact of different settings on model results (Figure 3), we observed that the availability of virological monitoring (i.e. 6-monthly HIV RNA determinations) generally improved cost effectiveness of first-line TDF use relative to the base setting. The other two changes to settings (i.e. presence of transmitted drug resistance or the option to switch drugs in case of toxic side effects) only had a limited effect on cost effectiveness outcomes.

Furthermore, the sensitivity of results to specific parameter values was explored (Table S1 and Table 4). In general, QALY estimates varied notably across the different sensitivity analyses. But overall cost-effectiveness of the TDF strategy over the ZDV strategy was maintained, and generally ICER estimates came to lie below the WHO cost-effectiveness threshold for high cost effectiveness (i.e. ICER < the per capita GDP) in ≥95% of cases (table 4).

Discussion

By using an established stochastic simulation of HIV disease progression and therapy we have explored the impact of using different NRTI drugs (namely ZDV versus TDF) on resistance emergence and its consequences in terms of response to available

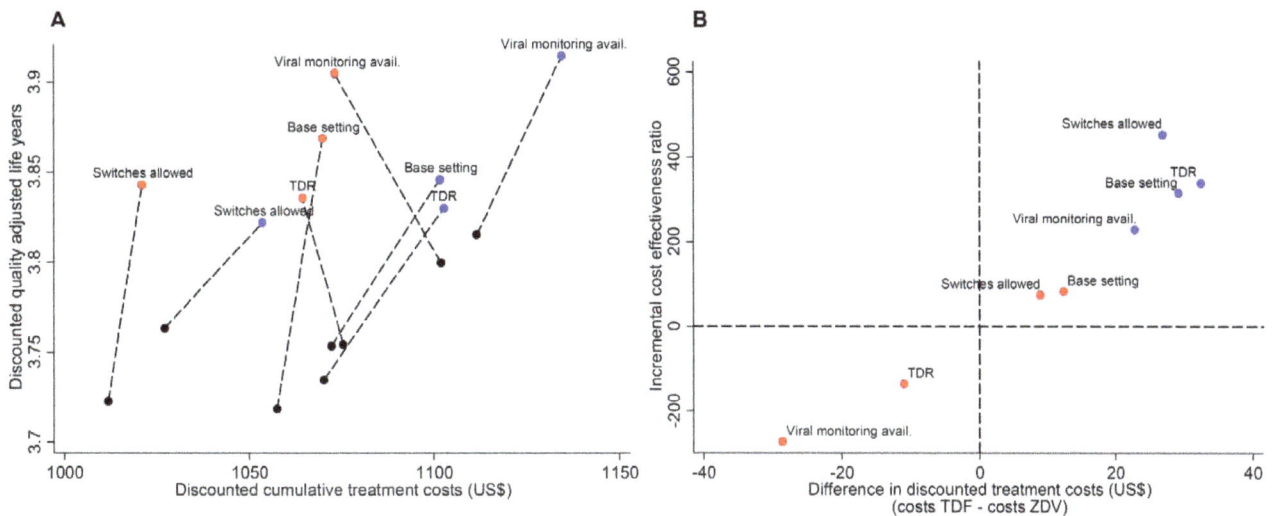

Figure 3. Figure 3A plots the average cumulative costs incurred by first-line tenofovir or zidovudine against quality adjusted life years. The connected dots refer to one set of comparisons between first-line tenofovir (TDF; coloured dots) or zidovudine (ZDV; black dots) using different assumptions regarding scenarios of TDF resistance emergence (red dots: base scenario; blue dots: pessimistic scenario involving the emergence of the Q151M multidrug-resistance complex; see Figure 1 for further details), as well as for alternative settings, which were the availability of 6-monthly HIV RNA determinations; >0% prevalence of transmitted drug resistance (TDR) in the study population; or exchange of ZDV with TDF (and vice versa) due to toxic side effects allowed (see Materials S1 for further details). Figure 3B plots estimates for incremental cost effective ratios against estimates for cumulative cost differences between first-line TDF and ZDV use.

Table 4. Uncertainty bounds of incremental cost effectiveness (ICER) estimates, % of ICER estimates suggesting dominance of the tenofovir (TDF) treatment strategy and % of ICER estimates below the WHO threshold for high cost-effectiveness.

Scenario/Sensitivity analysis	Base Scenario			Pessimistic Scenario		
	Uncertainty bounds of ICER estimates	% TDF strategy dominant	% ICER estimates < WHO threshold	Uncertainty bounds of ICER estimates	% TDF strategy dominant	% ICER estimates < WHO threshold
Base	[−2186; 3269]	27%	97%	[−2439; 2729]	9%	96%
Transmitted Resistance	[−3327; 3353]	32%	95%	[−1347; 2874]	10%	97%
Virological Monitoring	[−5970; 3747]	47%	96%	[−1576; 2683]	14%	97%
Switches allowed	[−1512; 3132]	23%	96%	[−2761; 2676]	6%	97%
LPV worth only 1 drug instead of 1.5	[−2222; 1901]	31%	98%	[−4490; 2133]	19%	98%
Median time to switch 22 months (i.e. 3-month switch probability of 10%)	[−5111; 4950]	32%	95%	[−2981; 3111]	28%	96%
No additional adherence benefit for TDF	[−766; 1807]	5%	98%	[−1240; 2287]	8%	96%
Median time to switch 22 months & no additional adherence benefit for TDF	[−1558; 2406]	13%	97%	[−5426; 5132]	30%	95%

Results were obtained by repeatedly drawing one simulation with TDF as the initial strategy and one simulation with zidovudine (ZDV) in the initial treatment. From this pair of simulations the incremental cost effectiveness ratio was calculated. Dominance was defined by lower costs and higher quality adjusted life year estimates for a specific treatment. By repeating this process 1000 times we obtained an estimate for how frequently the TDF strategy was dominant. Analogous calculations were performed to check how often the ICER estimates were below the WHO threshold for high cost effectiveness (annual per capita gross domestic product of US$ 2154). Uncertainty bounds reflect ranges that include 95% of all ICER estimates.

Abbreviations: ICER, incremental cost effectiveness ratio; TDF, tenofovir; WHO, World Health Organization.

second-line regimens and associated costs. Owing to uncertainty with respect to the influence of prolonged exposure to failing regimens and the effect of non-B subtype infection on NRTI-cross resistance we tested two pathways for resistance emergence while receiving TDF therapy. The base scenario assumed a rapid and frequent emergence of the TDF signature mutation K65R but only a very limited degree of NRTI cross-resistance. The second, pessimistic scenario was derived from analyses of genotypic resistance tests performed after failure of first-line combination treatment with D4T and was characterized by a more limited emergence of K65R, but a considerable risk for NRTI-cross resistance by the emergence of Q151M.

Our analyses suggest that first-line TDF use is a cost-effective treatment strategy compared with first-line ZDV use when considering quality adjusted life years as outcome, although dominance of the TDF strategy was only observed in 11% to 46% of comparisons (table 4). The use of TDF instead of ZDV also led to a reduction in treatment failures on the basis of WHO criteria by approximately 1% (pessimistic scenario) to 4% (base scenario). Consequently, fewer individuals in the TDF group had to switch to more costly second-line therapy compared with ZDV starters, although the magnitude of this difference was dependent on assumptions regarding the TDF resistance pathway. Our study results are in line with those from a modelling analysis by Bendavid et al., who obtained an ICER estimate of US$ 1045 for first-line regimens consisting of TDF, 3TC and NVP when compared with first-line ZDV, 3TC and NVP [19]. Other published cost-effectiveness analyses are not directly comparable to our study, because their reference scenarios involved receiving no cART [16] or receiving D4T [18]. Nevertheless, both studies also reached the conclusion that the TDF first strategy may be cost-effective when compared with the ZDV first strategy because of better tolerability. Further support for this conclusion stems from analyses of antiretroviral treatment programs in southern Africa, which observed fewer drug related toxicity events among first-line TDF users when compared with individuals starting therapy with

ZDV [22,23]. In particular, severe TDF-associated renal toxicity was shown to be rare and often transient, and therefore does not seem to pose a major obstacle for widespread TDF implementation in settings without creatinine clearance monitoring [23,35,36]. In comparison, life-threatening anaemia or lipoatrophy occur frequently in association with ZDV-use, especially in malnourished populations [22,23]. All these are drug side effects, which are not caused by TDF.

Depending on the actual rate of NRTI multidrug resistance emergence, first-line TDF use may increase emergence of extensively NRTI class-resistant HIV by 8.5-fold (17/1000 first-line TDF users in the pessimistic scenario compared with 2/1000 first-line ZDV users). Observational studies have reported associations of K65R mutations with Q151M, possibly pointing towards a co-selection of these mutations [37,38]. However, these studies were performed among patients with extensive antiretroviral drug histories-including exposure to D4T or didanosine, but not necessarily TDF-, and the drugs responsible for selection of K65R and Q151M could not be determined with certainty. In contrast, currently available resistance data from individuals undergoing long-term therapy with TDF support the more optimistic scenario [10,14,39]. If true, the limited degree of cross-resistance even after extended exposure to failing treatment would make TDF a valid option for second-line therapy, in which EFV is replaced by LPV/r. A recent observational study suggests that in salvage settings staying on TDF may be preferable over switching to ZDV due to better tolerability and similar viral load reductions [34].

Some limitations should be noted about this study. Like any model, our simulation involves simplifications of reality and is based on assumptions regarding input parameters. In particular, given the lack of real data we had to make assumptions regarding rates and extent of drug resistance following immunological failures in resource-limited settings, as shown in Figure 1. Given these limitations, we subjected several important parameters to sensitivity analyses and repeated the simulation for different settings. We observed that the pessimistic simulation scenario with regards to drug resistance emergence reduces TDF cost-effectiveness, and so did changes to settings or other input parameters of interest (adherence levels, switch rates, and potency of LPV/r). But these results did not alter our conclusions, because TDF remained very cost effective by WHO standards (table 4). These analyses further revealed that a strategy of first-line TDF use in settings with virological monitoring would further enhance cost effectiveness relative to first-line ZDV use (Table 3 and Figure 3). It should also be noted that measures of treatment outcomes in our analysis such as the proportion of individuals with undetectable viral loads or the increase in CD4 cell counts from baseline tend to be somewhat lower than those observed in clinical trials and observational studies, although this finding has no direct impact on the cost-effectiveness analyses.

In summary, taking into account the possibility of more extensive drug resistance or possible long term renal toxicity by TDF use we conclude that first-line TDF use is likely to be a very cost-effective treatment strategy in resource-limited settings even in the absence of virological monitoring, because of the better tolerability and the small cost difference.

Acknowledgments

The authors wish to thank the two anonymous reviewers for their constructive comments.

Author Contributions

Conceived and designed the experiments: VvW VC MRJ SB ANP. Performed the experiments: VvW. Analyzed the data: VvW VC MRJ SB AM DP JL ANP. Wrote the paper: VvW ANP. N/A.

References

1. (2010) Wold Health Organization (WHO). Antiretroviral therapy for HIV infection in adults and adolescents-2010 revision.
2. Pozniak AL, Gallant JE, DeJesus E, Arribas JR, Gazzard B, et al. (2006) Tenofovir disoproxil fumarate, emtricitabine, and efavirenz versus fixed-dose zidovudine/lamivudine and efavirenz in antiretroviral-naive patients: virologic, immunologic, and morphologic changes-a 96-week analysis. J Acquir Immune Defic Syndr 43: 535–540.
3. Gallant JE, DeJesus E, Arribas JR, Pozniak AL, Gazzard B, et al. (2006) Tenofovir DF, emtricitabine, and efavirenz vs. zidovudine, lamivudine, and efavirenz for HIV. N Engl J Med 354: 251–260.
4. Margot NA, Enejosa J, Cheng AK, Miller MD, McColl DJ (2009) Development of HIV-1 drug resistance through 144 weeks in antiretroviral-naive subjects on emtricitabine, tenofovir disoproxil fumarate, and efavirenz compared with lamivudine/zidovudine and efavirenz in study GS-01-934. J Acquir Immune Defic Syndr 52: 209–221.
5. Arribas JR, Pozniak AL, Gallant JE, Dejesus E, Gazzard B, et al. (2008) Tenofovir disoproxil fumarate, emtricitabine, and efavirenz compared with zidovudine/lamivudine and efavirenz in treatment-naive patients: 144-week analysis. J Acquir Immune Defic Syndr 47: 74–78.
6. Gallant JE, Staszewski S, Pozniak AL, DeJesus E, Suleiman JM, et al. (2004) Efficacy and safety of tenofovir DF vs stavudine in combination therapy in antiretroviral-naive patients: a 3-year randomized trial. JAMA 292: 191–201.
7. Margot NA, Lu B, Cheng A, Miller MD (2006) Resistance development over 144 weeks in treatment-naive patients receiving tenofovir disoproxil fumarate or stavudine with lamivudine and efavirenz in Study 903. HIV Med 7: 442–450.
8. Charurat M, Oyegunle M, Benjamin R, Habib A, Eze E, et al. (2010) Patient retention and adherence to antiretrovirals in a large antiretroviral therapy program in Nigeria: a longitudinal analysis for risk factors. PLoS One 5: e10584.
9. (2010) Clinton Health Access Initiative. Antiretroviral (ARV) Price List-Version November 2010.
10. Chappell BJ, Margot NA, Miller MD (2007) Long-term follow-up of patients taking tenofovir DF with low-level HIV-1 viremia and the K65R substitution in HIV-1 RT. AIDS 21: 761–763.
11. Brenner BG, Oliveira M, Doualla-Bell F, Moisi DD, Ntemgwa M, et al. (2006) HIV-1 subtype C viruses rapidly develop K65R resistance to tenofovir in cell culture. AIDS 20: F9–13.
12. Miller MD, Margot N, McColl D, Cheng AK (2007) K65R development among subtype C HIV-1-infected patients in tenofovir DF clinical trials. AIDS 21: 265–266.
13. Hosseinipour MC, van Oosterhout JJ, Weigel R, Phiri S, Kamwendo D, et al. (2009) The public health approach to identify antiretroviral therapy failure: high-level nucleoside reverse transcriptase inhibitor resistance among Malawians failing first-line antiretroviral therapy. AIDS 23: 1127–1134.
14. Hawkins CA, Chaplin B, Idoko J, Ekong E, Adewole I, et al. (2009) Clinical and genotypic findings in HIV-infected patients with the K65R mutation failing first-line antiretroviral therapy in Nigeria. J Acquir Immune Defic Syndr 52: 228–234.
15. Sanchez-de la Rosa R, Herrera L, Moreno S (2008) Cost-effectiveness analysis of emtricitabine/tenofovir versus lamivudine/zidovudine, in combination with efavirenz, in antiretroviral-naive, HIV-1-infected patients. Clin Ther 30: 372–381.
16. Bender MA, Kumarasamy N, Mayer KH, Wang B, Walensky RP, et al. (2010) Cost-effectiveness of tenofovir as first-line antiretroviral therapy in India. Clin Infect Dis 50: 416–425.
17. Rosen S, Long L, Fox M, Sanne I (2008) Cost and cost-effectiveness of switching from stavudine to tenofovir in first-line antiretroviral regimens in South Africa. J Acquir Immune Defic Syndr 48: 334–344.
18. Jouquet G, Bygrave H, Kranzer K, Ford N, Gadot L, et al. (2011) Cost and cost-effectiveness of switching from d4T or AZT to a TDF-based first-line regimen in a resource limited setting in rural Lesotho. J Acquir Immune Defic Syndr.
19. Bendavid E, Grant P, Talbot A, Owens DK, Zolopa A (2011) Cost-effectiveness of antiretroviral regimens in the World Health Organization's treatment guidelines: a South African analysis. AIDS 25: 211–220.
20. Phillips AN, Pillay D, Miners AH, Bennett DE, Gilks CF, et al. (2008) Outcomes from monitoring of patients on antiretroviral therapy in resource-limited settings with viral load, CD4 cell count, or clinical observation alone: a computer simulation model. Lancet 371: 1443–1451.
21. Phillips AN, Pillay D, Garnett G, Bennett D, Vitoria M, et al. (2011) Effect on transmission of HIV-1 resistance of timing of implementation of viral load monitoring to determine switches from first to second-line antiretroviral regimens in resource-limited settings. AIDS 25: 843–850.
22. Bygrave H, Ford N, van Cutsem G, Hilderbrand K, Jouquet G, et al. (2011) Implementing a tenofovir-based first-line regimen in rural Lesotho: clinical outcomes and toxicities after two years. J Acquir Immune Defic Syndr 56: e75–78.
23. Chi BH, Mwango A, Giganti M, Tambatamba-Chapula B, et al. (2010) Early clinical and programmatic outcomes with tenofovir-based antiretroviral therapy in Zambia. J Acquir Immune Defic Syndr 54: 63–70.
24. Kauf TL, Roskell N, Shearer A, Gazzard B, Mauskopf J, et al. (2008) A predictive model of health state utilities for HIV patients in the modern era of highly active antiretroviral therapy. Value Health 11: 1144–1153.
25. Wallis CL, Mellors JW, Venter WD, Sanne I, Stevens W (2010) Varied patterns of HIV-1 drug resistance on failing first-line antiretroviral therapy in South Africa. J Acquir Immune Defic Syndr 53: 480–484.
26. Ndembi N, Goodall RL, Dunn DT, McCormick A, Burke A, et al. (2010) Viral rebound and emergence of drug resistance in the absence of viral load testing: a randomized comparison between zidovudine-lamivudine plus Nevirapine and zidovudine-lamivudine plus Abacavir. J Infect Dis 201: 106–113.
27. Marconi VC, Sunpath H, Lu Z, Gordon M, Koranteng-Apeagyei K, et al. (2008) Prevalence of HIV-1 drug resistance after failure of a first highly active antiretroviral therapy regimen in KwaZulu Natal, South Africa. Clin Infect Dis 46: 1589–1597.
28. Koyalta D, Charpentier C, Beassamda J, Rey E, Si-Mohamed A, et al. (2009) High frequency of antiretroviral drug resistance among HIV-infected adults receiving first-line highly active antiretroviral therapy in N'Djamena, Chad. Clin Infect Dis 49: 155–159.
29. Scherrer AU, von Wyl V, Gotte M, Klimkait T, Cellerai C, et al. (2012) Polymorphic Mutations Associated With the Emergence of the Multinucleoside/Tide Resistance Mutations 69 Insertion and Q151M. J Acquir Immune Defic Syndr 59: 105–112.
30. Rhee SY, Gonzales MJ, Kantor R, Betts BJ, Ravela J, et al. (2003) Human immunodeficiency virus reverse transcriptase and protease sequence database. Nucleic Acids Res 31: 298–303.
31. Hamers RL, Wallis CL, Kityo C, Siwale M, Mandaliya K, et al. (2011) HIV-1 drug resistance in antiretroviral-naive individuals in sub-Saharan Africa after

rollout of antiretroviral therapy: a multicentre observational study. Lancet Infect Dis.

32. von Wyl V, Yerly S, Boni J, Burgisser P, Klimkait T, et al. (2007) Emergence of HIV-1 drug resistance in previously untreated patients initiating combination antiretroviral treatment: a comparison of different regimen types. Arch Intern Med 167: 1782–1790.

33. von Wyl V, Yerly S, Boni J, Shah C, Cellerai C, et al (2012). Incidence of HIV-1 Drug Resistance Among Antiretroviral Treatment-Naive Individuals Starting Modern Therapy Combinations. Clin Infect Dis 54: 131–140.

34. Grant PM, Taylor J, Nevins AB, Calvez V, Marcelin AG, et al. (2010) International cohort analysis of the antiviral activities of zidovudine and tenofovir in the presence of the K65R mutation in reverse transcriptase. Antimicrob Agents Chemother 54: 1520–1525.

35. Bygrave H, Kranzer K, Hilderbrand K, Jouquet G, Goemaere E, et al. (2011) Renal safety of a tenofovir-containing first line regimen: experience from an antiretroviral cohort in rural Lesotho. PLoS One 6: e17609.

36. Cooper RD, Wiebe N, Smith N, Keiser P, Naicker S, et al. (2010) Systematic review and meta-analysis: renal safety of tenofovir disoproxil fumarate in HIV-infected patients. Clin Infect Dis 51: 496–505.

37. Trotta MP, Bonfigli S, Ceccherini-Silberstein F, Bellagamba R, D'Arrigo R, et al. (2006) Clinical and genotypic correlates of mutation K65R in HIV-infected patients failing regimens not including tenofovir. J Med Virol 78: 535–541.

38. Boucher S, Recordon-Pinson P, Ragnaud JM, Dupon M, Fleury H, et al. (2006) HIV-1 reverse transcriptase (RT) genotypic patterns and treatment characteristics associated with the K65R RT mutation. HIV Med 7: 294–298.

39. Lyagoba F, Dunn DT, Pillay D, Kityo C, Robertson V, et al. (2010) Evolution of drug resistance during 48 weeks of zidovudine/lamivudine/tenofovir in the absence of real-time viral load monitoring. J Acquir Immune Defic Syndr 55: 277–283.

40. Ammassari A, Murri R, Pezzotti P, Trotta MP, Ravasio L, et al. (2001) Self-reported symptoms and medication side effects influence adherence to highly active antiretroviral therapy in persons with HIV infection. J Acquir Immune Defic Syndr 28: 445–449.

41. Keiser O, Tweya H, Boulle A, Braitstein P, Schecter M, et al. (2009) Switching to second-line antiretroviral therapy in resource-limited settings: comparison of programmes with and without viral load monitoring. AIDS 23: 1867–1874.

21

Augmentation of the Antibody Response of Atlantic Salmon by Oral Administration of Alginate-Encapsulated IPNV Antigens

Lihan Chen[1]*, Goran Klaric[2,3]*, Simon Wadsworth[2], Suwan Jayasinghe[3], Tsun-Yung Kuo[4], Øystein Evensen[1], Stephen Mutoloki[1]*

1 Department of Basic Sciences and Aquatic Medicine, Norwegian University of Life Sciences, Oslo, Norway, **2** EWOS Innovation AS, Sandnes, Norway, **3** Department of Mechanical Engineering, University College London, London, United Kingdom, **4** Department of Animal Science/Institute of Biotechnology, National Ilan University, Taipei, Taiwan

Abstract

The objective of the present study was to assess the effect of alginate-encapsulated infectious pancreatic necrosis virus antigens in inducing the immune response of Atlantic salmon as booster vaccines. One year after intraperitoneal injection with an oil-adjuvanted vaccine, post-smolts were orally boosted either by 1) alginate-encapsulated IPNV antigens (ENCAP); 2) soluble antigens (UNENCAP) or 3) untreated feed (control). This was done twice, seven weeks apart. Sampling was done twice, firstly at 7 weeks post 1st oral boost and the 2nd, at 4 weeks after the 2nd oral boost. Samples included serum, head kidney, spleen and hindgut. Serum antibodies were analyzed by ELISA while tissues were used to assess the expression of IgM, IgT, CD4, GATA3, FOXP3, TGF-β and IL-10 genes by quantitative PCR. Compared to controls, fish fed with ENCAP had a significant increase ($p < 0.04$) in serum antibodies following the 1st boost but not after the 2nd boost. This coincided with significant up-regulation of CD4 and GATA3 genes. In contrast, serum antibodies in the UNENCAP group decreased both after the 1st and 2nd oral boosts. This was associated with significant up-regulation of FOXP3, TGF-β and IL-10 genes. The expression of IgT was not induced in the hindgut after the 1st oral boost but was significantly up-regulated following the 2nd one. CD4 and GATA3 mRNA expressions exhibited a similar pattern to IgT in the hindgut. IgM mRNA expression on the other hand was not differentially regulated at any of the times examined. Our findings suggest that 1) Parenteral prime with oil-adjuvanted vaccines followed by oral boost with ENCAP results in augmentation of the systemic immune response; 2) Symmetrical prime and boost (mucosal) with ENCAP results in augmentation of mucosal immune response and 3) Symmetrical priming and boosting (mucosal) with soluble antigens results in the induction of systemic immune tolerance.

Editor: James P. Stewart, University of Liverpool, United Kingdom

Funding: This work was funded by the Research Council of Norway (FUGE project no. 187848). ØE and SW were the grant recipients. The funders had no role in study design, data collection and analysis, decision to publish, or preparation of the manuscript. Goran Klaric and Simon Wadsworth are employed by EWOS Innovation AS. EWOS Innovation AS provided support in the form of salaries for authors GK and SW, but did not have any additional role in the study design, data collection and analysis, decision to publish, or preparation of the manuscript. The specific roles of these authors are articulated in the 'author contributions' section.

Competing Interests: The AGK cell line is under license by the Norwegian University of Life Sciences (NMBU), Faculty of Veterinary Medicine and Biosciences and is the exclusive ownership of SBC Biotech, Taiwan, ROC. The cell line is not available to outside researchers but this restriction will not influence anyone's ability to reproduce the findings of this study as other IPNV-permissive cell lines can be used to (e.g. CHSE or RTG-2 cells) followed by post-culture concentration procedures (e.g. R). Roberts (ed.) Fish Pathology 3rd Edition, W.B. Saunders, London, 2001. P220) if needed. This has been highlighted in the Competing Interest statement as well as in the manuscript.

* Email: stephen.mutoloki@nmbu.no

⑨ These authors contributed equally to this work.

Introduction

Infectious pancreatic necrosis is an important disease of salmonids responsible for great economic losses in the aquaculture industry. It is characterized by loss of appetite, darkened skin pigmentation, distended abdomen and mortalities ranging from negligible to almost 100%. Histopathologically, necrosis of pancreatic acinar cells, multifocal hepatic necrosis and acute catarrhal enteritis are commonly observed [1,2]. The causative agent is infectious pancreatic necrosis virus (IPNV), a double stranded RNA virus belonging to the family *Birnaviridae* and genus *Aquabirnavirus* where it is the type species.

Control of IPN is by vaccination and oil-based vaccines have earned their place in the market mainly because of their contribution to the control of bacterial diseases in the late 80s and early 90s in Norway. The efficacy of these vaccines against diseases caused by intracellular pathogens such as viruses however remains equivocal, thus the need for the continued search for more effective vaccines.

The most desirable vaccines for higher vertebrates and even more so for fish are those delivered orally because of the ease with which they are administered; are stress-free; applicable to smaller fish and are less labour-intensive [3]. Their usage in the aquaculture industry has however been under-exploited because of their poor performance in comparison with injectable and immersion counterparts. Some of the challenges associated with orally delivered vaccines include poor antigen delivery and uptake, degradation during passage through the digestive tract and induction of tolerance [4,5]. Nevertheless, a report of good protection in fish vaccinated with encapsulated DNA plasmids has recently been published [6]. Unfortunately, legislation in most countries at the moment precludes the use of DNA vaccines in food animals [7,8].

One of the challenges faced by vaccination of fish is the duration of protection conferred by different preparations. As already mentioned, oil-based vaccines induce long lasting protection against several bacterial pathogens but this could be at the cost of severe side effects [9]. For viral diseases including IPN, most products on the market do not give satisfactory protection probably because of their failure to induce sufficiently high antibody titers required prior to challenge [10]. Boosting is a good alternative for enhancing or extending protection as shown for lactococcosis [11]. The effect of boosting against IPNV in particular and oral vaccination in general is however not well understood. The main purpose of the present study therefore was to assess the effect of alginate-encapsulated IPNV in stimulating the immune system of Atlantic salmon as a booster vaccine.

Results

Intake of oral boost feeds and IPNV antigen dose

The average weight of the fish during the primary and secondary oral boost feeding, the feed intake and antigen dose are shown in Table 1. As targeted, the average antigen dose administered during each of the boost periods was about 1×10^9 $TCID_{50}$/fish. However, due to the doubling in the fish weight between the two boost periods, the dose per kg of fish body weight during the second boosting was almost half that during the first (Table 1).

Antigen retention in head kidneys and hindguts

To estimate the amount of antigen taken up and retained both locally and systemically in each group, qPCR was used targeting hindgut and head kidneys tissues to examine retained antigens at the time of sampling (7 weeks and 4 weeks following the 1st and 2nd boosts, respectively). The head kidney was used to represent the

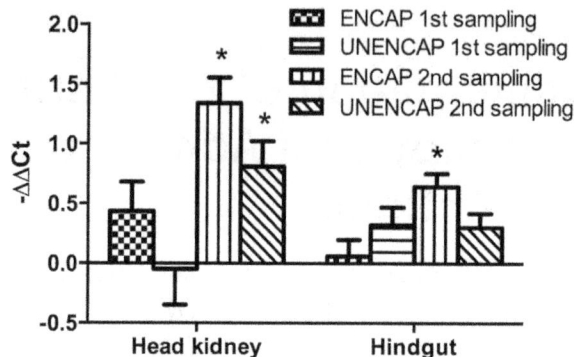

Figure 1. Infectious pancreatic necrosis virus (IPNV) mRNA expressed by real time RT-PCR in selected organs of Atlantic salmon following oral boost with different antigen preparations. This assay was used as a surrogate marker of retained formalin-inactivated IPNV antigens in the present study. All fish were vaccinated with an oil-based vaccine one year prior to the start of this study. The control fish received no booster oral antigens. n = 30; *statistically significant p<0.05.

systemic compartment since this is one of the main antigen trapping organ for blood-borne antigens in fish [12].

The results show that more mRNA of IPNV (used as a surrogate of antigens) were retained in the encapsulated (ENCAP) versus unencapsulated (UNENCAP) groups at both time points (Fig. 1). In the head kidney, a significant increase in antigens retained from the 1st to the 2nd sampling was observed in both groups. A similar trend in the ENCAP group was observed in hindgut while for the UNENCAP group, no difference between sampling times was observed (Fig. 1).

Oral boosting with alginate-based antigens induces a systemic but transient IgM antibody response

Since all experimental fish had previously been vaccinated with an oil-based vaccine that contained IPNV antigens, all the fish had relatively high specific background antibodies as expected. The un-boosted group (control) was used as the baseline for comparison with boosted groups.

In general, the response of antibodies in boosted groups showed a reverse trend over time compared to that of antigens (Fig. 1&2). In the group boosted with ENCAP, the antibody response was significantly higher (p<0.04) than the control following the 1st

Table 1. Fish size in unit of mass (g), Weekly feed intake (FI) per fish, weekly IPNV antigen dose per fish and weekly IPNV antigen (Ag) dose per unit of fish mass (dose/kg).

Period	Group	Feed	Fish size (g) ±SD	Feed intake (g/fish/week) ±SD	IPNV Ag dose (TCID50/fish/week) ±SD	IPNV Ag dose (TCID50/kg/week) ±SD
Primary boost	Control	CF-1	395±92	24.7±0.4	0.00	0.00
	Unencap	OBF-1	375±82	23.9±2.4	$9.6 \times 10^8 \pm 1 \times 10^8$	$2.6 \times 10^9 \pm 6 \times 10^8$
	Encap	OBF-2	426±121	23.1±0.9	$9.3 \times 10^8 \pm 4 \times 10^7$	$2.2 \times 10^9 \pm 6 \times 10^8$
Second boost	Control	CF-2	846±135	39.6±0.4	0.00	0.00
	Unencap	OBF-4	796±126	37.3±3.9	$1.1 \times 10^9 \pm 1 \times 10^8$	$1.4 \times 10^9 \pm 3 \times 10^8$
	Encap	OBF-5	782±105	38.0±1.3	$1.1 \times 10^9 \pm 4 \times 10^7$	$1.5 \times 10^9 \pm 2 \times 10^8$

boost (Fig. 2). At 4 weeks following the 2nd boost however, the antibodies had returned to background levels. In the UNENCAP group, no difference was observed compared to unboosted controls during the 1st sampling while the antibodies were significantly suppressed (p<0.02) following the 2nd boost (Fig. 2).

The systemic immune response is predominantly Th2

The induction of antibodies in the ENCAP group was suggestive of a predominantly humoral response. Thus to verify this, we examined the expression of CD4 and GATA-3 genes that are known to be associated with Th2 responses, in the head kidney and spleen.

At both 7 weeks post primary- and 4 weeks post-secondary boost, the ENCAP group had significantly higher CD4 expression (p<0.04) in both the head kidney and spleen compared to other groups (Fig. 3a). In contrast, this gene was suppressed in the UNENCAP group at the 1st sampling albeit non-significantly. At the 2nd sampling, this gene was significantly suppressed (p<0.01) in this group. In the ENCAP group, the expression of GATA3 was significantly up-regulated (p<0.04) at both time points in the head kidney and spleen, consistent with the results of CD4 while in the UNENCAP group, these genes were not induced (Fig. 3b).

The gut mucosal response is also Th2 and is primarily primed by the oral route

To assess the gut mucosal response, we examined the expression of IgT mRNA since antibodies are not available to us. In addition, mRNA expression of IgM, CD4 and GATA3 genes were also assessed.

After the 1st oral boost, marginal but non-significant inductions of IgT were observed in both the ENCAP and UNENCAP groups compared to the control (Fig 3c). At 4 weeks following the 2nd boost, the expression increased in both groups but more significantly (p<0.01) in the ENCAP compared to UNENCAP group. Interestingly, CD4 and GATA3 expression in this organ had a similar pattern to IgT (Fig. 3a&b), especially for the ENCAP group. Conversely, CD4 and GATA3 expression of the UNEN-CAP group were generally not induced at both time points. The expression of IgM in the hindgut was not differentially expressed in all groups at all-time points examined (Fig. 3d).

The assessment of IgT expression was extended to the head kidney and spleen where at all-time points and in all groups, this gene was not differentially expressed. The only exception was in

the head kidney of the ENCAP group, at 4 weeks following 2nd boost (Fig. 3c), where it was significantly up-regulated (p<0.03).

Repeated oral administration of IPNV antigens results in decreased serum antibodies but not in the hindgut of Atlantic salmon

The reduction in serum antibodies following administration of antigens can be due to consumption [10,13]. Thus in order to check whether this was the case in the present study, we examined the transcript levels of IgM. Fig. 3d shows significant down-regulation of B cell IgM transcripts both in the kidneys (p<0.01) and spleen (0.001) of the UNENCAP group from the 1st to the 2nd samplings. A similar change was observed in the spleen of the ENCAP group (p<0.01) but without any differential regulation in the kidney.

In order to gain insight into the suppression of antibody production by B cells in the UNENCAP group, we examined the expression of forkhead box protein 3 (FOXP3), TGF-β and IL-10.

Consistent with the reduction/suppression of antibodies in the UNENCAP group at 4 weeks following 2nd boost, the expression of FOXP3, TGF-β and IL-10 were all significantly up-regulated (p<0.003, 0.035 and 0.0048, respectively) in the kidneys of this group (Fig. 4a–c). In contrast, no differential expressions of either of these genes were observed in any of the groups after the 1st boost or in the spleen.

In the hindgut, FOXP3 was only induced in the UNENCAP group after the 2nd boost (Fig. 4a) while both TGF-β and IL-10 were significantly induced in both ENCAP and UNENCAP groups (p<0.02 and 0.01 for TGF-β and p<0.01 and 0.01 for IL-10, respectively).

Discussion

The findings of the present study demonstrate that oral boosting of Atlantic salmon following parenteral injection with alginate encapsulated IPNV antigens induces both systemic and mucosal (gut) humoral responses. The significant up-regulation of CD4 (p< 0.02) and GATA-3 (p<0.04) genes in the head kidneys and spleens of the ENCAP group (Fig. 3) fit very well with the induction of serum antibodies and point towards a predominantly T-helper 2 (T$_H$2) response. In higher vertebrates, the intestinal mucosa contains high basal levels of IL-4, IL-10 and TGFβ that are induced shortly after oral vaccination [14]. This micro-environment is thought to tip responses of oral vaccines towards T$_H$2 [4]. Furthermore, the main mechanism of action of alginate encapsulated antigens has been proposed to be biased towards T$_H$2 responses [15–18]. These findings are consistent with reports of others using different antigens [19,20] and suggest that oral boosting with alginate encapsulated antigens holds promise as a means of augmenting immune responses against IPN. One limitation of this study is that the fish were not challenged following vaccination and therefore the protective effects of the responses could not be tested but should be a subject for future studies.

There are conflicting reports when it comes to protection against disease using orally administered vaccines, with some reporting success [6,11,20] while others found little or no difference from controls [17]. Several reasons can be attributed to these variations including the nature of antigens used, formulation of oral preparations, immune response generated versus that desired etc. In the present study, the fish were not challenged following vaccination owing to logistical constraints. While this should be a subject for further studies, it is known from a previous study that high antibody titers against IPNV at the

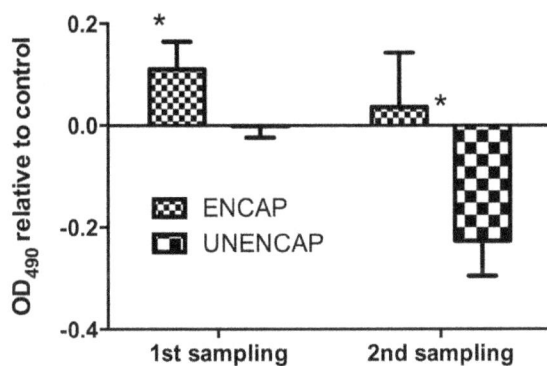

Figure 2. Infectious pancreatic necrosis virus-specific serum antibody levels in orally boosted groups of Atlantic salmon relative to un-boosted controls. Antibodies were assessed by ELISA and the results were obtained by using a plate reader (TECAN, Genios) at a wavelength of 492 nm. n = 30; *statistically significant p<0.05.

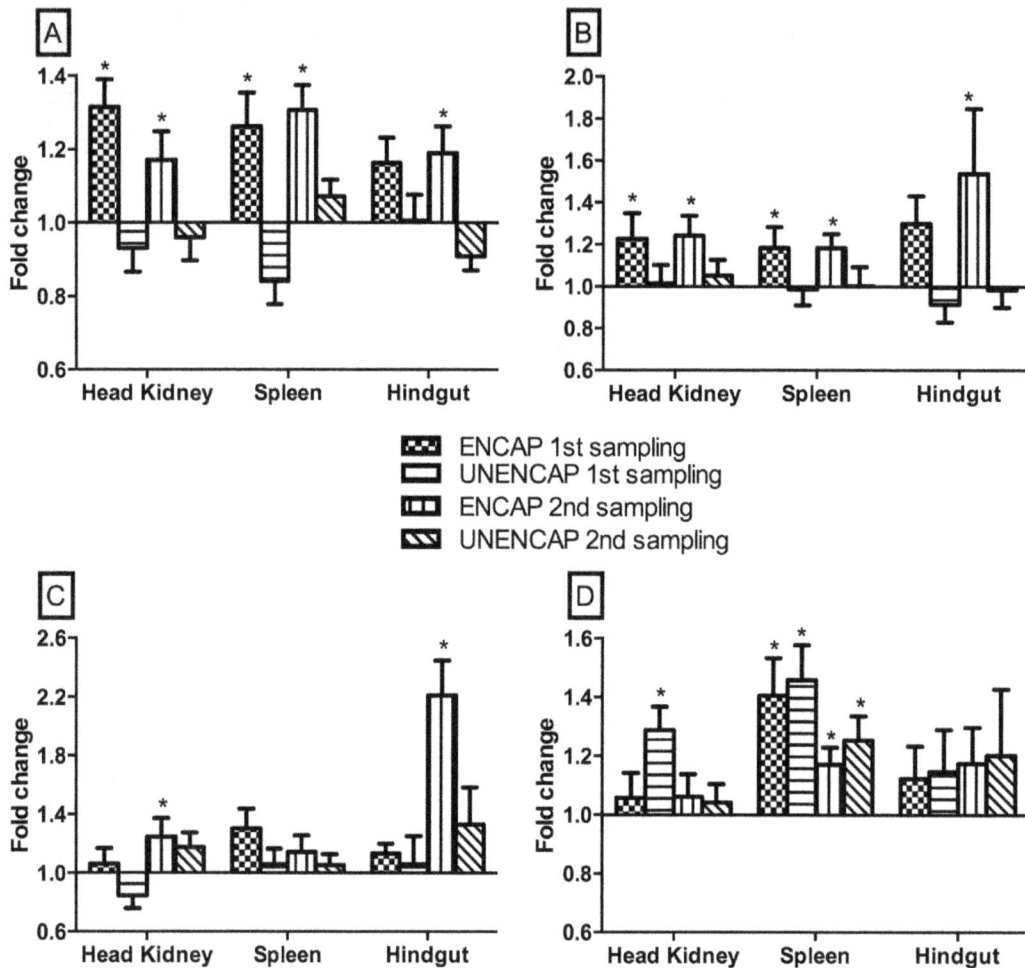

Figure 3. Mean relative expression of A) CD4; B) GATA3; C) IgT; and D) IgM genes of fish orally boosted with different antigen preparations compared to un-boosted controls. Real-time RT-PCR. n = 30; *statistically significant p<0.05.

onset of challenge correlate with protection of the fish [10]. It is not unlikely therefore that the augmentation of the immune response in the present study may have been associated with protection.

It has previously been reported that oral vaccination results in transient antibody response lasting typically 3 weeks post vaccination [20–22], and most of the studies address parenteral/oral combinations or vice-versa. However, very few studies have examined the effect of repeated oral vaccination. In the present study, reductions in serum antibodies following two oral vaccination (7 weeks apart) was observed in the both the ENCAP and UNENCAP groups after the second oral boost. This is consistent with the findings of others who used a similar administration regime (5 days of oral vaccine administration per month) [17]. In the same study however, administering the oral vaccine at a rate of 3 days/week for 2 months resulted in progressive increase in antibody titers over time. Together, these findings suggest that modality by which oral vaccines are administered can determine whether a booster effect or tolerance ensues. The low CD4 expression in the UNENCAP group in the kidney and also its decline in the ENCAP group concurrent with the lack of induction of GATA3 and IgM expression in the present study is however intriguing. It is tempting to speculate that this could point towards anergy as discussed further below.

The induction of the systemic response as measured from serum antibodies and immune gene expression in the kidney of the ENCAP group following the 1st oral boost is in line with previous reports [20,22]. The fact the 1st oral boost did not induce a corresponding change in the mucosal response as measured by gene expression in the hindgut suggests that injection vaccination does not activate mucosal immunity, in common with findings of others [20]. Furthermore, these results (Fig. 3a–c) suggest that in this study, the 1st oral boost served as a "prime" to the mucosal response while the 2nd one "boosted" it. Interestingly, oral boosting had no effect on the IgM expression in the hindgut, a difference from what others have observed assessing mucosal antibodies [20]. The ability of orally administered antigens to stimulate both systemic and mucosal immune responses on one hand and parenteral vaccination inducing only a systemic response demonstrate asymmetrical responses of immune induction as previously observed in mice [23].

One of the challenges of oral vaccination in fish is the induction of tolerance. This has been shown to be easily induced with soluble antigens [21]. In the present study, tolerance was induced by two booster administration of encapsulated IPNV antigen (UNENCAP) feeds (Fig. 2). In higher vertebrates, tolerance is the default immune pathway in mucosal surfaces and is related to the dose of antigens given, i.e. high doses lead to anergy/deletion while the

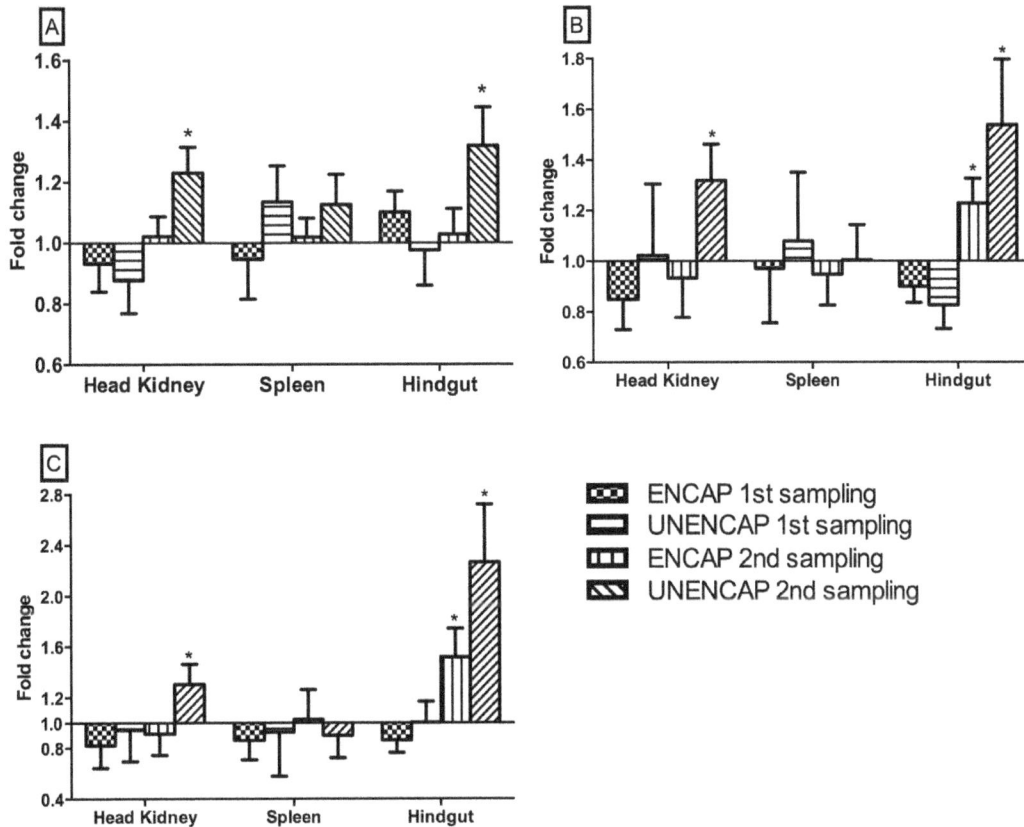

Figure 4. Mean relative expression of A) FOXP3; B) TGF-β and C) IL-10 genes in fish orally boosted with different antigen preparations compared to un-boosted controls. Real-time RT-PCR. n = 30; *statistically significant p<0.05.

opposite leads to regulatory T cells (Treg) induction [24]. The suppression of antibodies in the present study coupled with the induction of FoxP3, TGF-β and IL-10 (Fig. 4) suggests the involvement of both mechanisms. In higher vertebrates, FOXP3 is a key transcription factor of regulatory T cells (Tregs) while TGF-β is known to induce T cells including Tregs [24,25]. IL-10 on the other hand is an anti-inflammatory cytokine that has been shown to contribute towards the induction of immune tolerance [24]. These genes have also been described in fish although their functions relative to immune tolerance remain to be characterized.

While the induction of tolerance may be testimony that much of the un-encapsulated IPNV antigens were taken up, meaning they survived the hostile acidic environment in the stomach, this finding underlines the importance of encapsulation as an aid to stimulating the immune response of fish. It is noteworthy that the doses of vaccines administered during the 2nd boost were lower per body weight of fish compared to the 1st boost since the fish had gained weight by the time they received the second boost. The effect of this was not addressed but should be a subject of future studies.

Finally, the findings of the present study can be summarized as follows: 1) Parenteral prime with oil-adjuvanted vaccine followed by oral boost with ENCAP results in a the augmentation of both the systemic and mucosal immune responses; 2) Mucosal (gut) immunity is primarily primed by oral administration of antigens; 3) Oral prime and boost with ENCAP results in transient augmentation of mucosal immune responses and 4) Oral priming and boosting with UNENCAP results in the induction of tolerance.

Materials and Methods

This study was approved by the Norwegian Animal Research Authority. Prior to sampling, the fish was anaesthetised with Finquel (Scanvacc) at 100 mg/L in order to prevent suffering.

Cell culture

Asian grouper strain K (AGK) cells and Chinook salmon embryo cells (CHSE-214; ATCC CRL-1681) [26] were maintained with L-15 medium (Invitrogen) supplemented with 10% L-glutamine and 1 µl/ml of gentamicin. In addition the medium used with the former also contained 7.5% fetal bovine serum (FBS) and these cells were kept at 28°C while the medium for CHSE cells contained 10% FBS and the cells were maintained at 20°C.

Fish

The experiment was conducted at EWOS Innovation AS facilities in Dirdal, Norway. Healthy Atlantic salmon growers reared in sea water were used. The fish had been vaccinated with ALPHA JECT micro 6 (PHARMAQ) about a year prior to the first boost treatment and were kept at a water temperature of 12°C throughout the experimental duration.

Vaccine preparations

Antigen preparation. A recombinant Sp strain of IPNV (rNVI-15PTA) [10] was used and was prepared as reported previously (Chen et al., 2013). Briefly, approximately 80% confluent AGK cells maintained in L15 media as described above but with 2% FBS were inoculated with IPNV using MOI = 0.1

followed by incubation at 15°C. Note: CHSE or RTG-2 cells can be used as alternatives in the absence of AGK cells, with post-culturing concentration to increase virus amounts if necessary. The virus was harvested following full CPE by centrifugation of the suspension at 2500×g followed by recovery of the supernatant. Titration of the virus was by end point dilution and the titer measured using the Spearman–Karber's 50% tissue culture infectious dose ($TCID_{50}$) in CHSE-214 cells.

The virus was inactivated with formalin (0.5% final concentration equal to 0.2% formaldehyde) at room temperature for 48 hours with continuous stirring using a magnetic stirrer. Thereafter formalin was removed by dialysis. Inactivation was confirmed by inoculating confluent CHSE-214 cells while formalin residual effects were tested by incubating cells with excessive inactivated virus and assessing for toxicity.

Antigen encapsulation and feed preparation. The treatment groups of this study comprised either of the following feeding regimes: 1) untreated feed (control); 2) feed containing unencapsulated IPNV (in suspension); 3) feed containing alginate-encapsulated IPNV antigens.

Oral boost feeds (OBFs) were prepared by applying an oil mixture (OM) to Ewos Opal 200 base pellet (BP) in a vacuum infusion coating process. OMs were formulated by mixing IPNV Ag suspension (10^9 $TCID_{50}$/g), phosphate buffered saline (PBS), ($2.70×10^{10}$ $TCID_{50}$/g) with fish oil. Mixing was performed by using a high-performance disperser (Model T25, IKA Werke GmbH & Co., Germany) at ambient temperature. The OBF were composed with the aim of generating feeds with an antigen level of $4.01×10^7$ $TCID_{50}$/g. This level was selected due to an expected daily feed intake of 3.56 g/fish during the first oral boost period. For the same reason, the targeted antigen level in the second OBF was $2.99×10^7$ $TCID_{50}$/g. Control feeds were produced by mixing PBS with fish oil in advance of applying to BP in the vacuum infusion coating process.

Trial design and oral boosting

As part of a larger study examining responses of Atlantic salmon to different alginate formulations, 360 healthy Atlantic salmon weighing approximately 200 g each were distributed by dip netting and sequential allocation into 9 circular 500 L tanks containing sea water 10 weeks prior to the start of the primary oral boost. A description of the fish is given in section 4.2. The tanks were randomly divided into three groups (Unencap, Encap, and Control), with three tanks being assigned to each group (Figure 5).

The fish were fed with Ewos Opal 200 diet for 10 weeks prior to the first boost and also until the second boost. All fish groups were fed ad-libitum. During primary boosting, normal feed was replaced by OBFs for 7 days. After 7 weeks, the fish were sampled. Sampling was performed on 10 fish from each tank by first anaesthetizing the fish with Finquel (Argent Laboratories) at 100 mg/L. The following samples were collected, blood in heparin tubes for serum extraction; head kidney, spleen and hind gut in both RNAlater (Invitrogen) and formalin.

Following sampling, a secondary boost was performed as described above. From then on, the fish were fed with Ewos Opal 500. The second sampling was done 4 weeks after the secondary boost.

Feed intake assessment

Unconsumed feed was collected during both boost periods to calculate feed intake. Uneaten pellets were spilled out of the tanks within 10 min post feeding and filtered off from the outlet water using an automatic collection system. Residual pellets were removed from the filters and put into a drying cabinet for 24 h

at 70°C. Amount of feed consumed was calculated as the difference between the dry weight of the feed served and the dry weight of unconsumed feed, expressed as the mass of feed per week per fish.

Enzyme-linked immunosorbent assay (ELISA)

Blood samples were centrifuged at 2500×g for 10 min immediately after sampling. Thereafter, the serum was aspirated and transferred to new tubes that was the kept at -80°C until required.

ELISA was done as previously described [26] with minor modifications. Briefly, the wells of ELISA plates (Immunoplates, Nunc Maxisorb, Denmark) were coated with 100 μl of polyclonal anti-IPNV [27] diluted 1:2000 in coating buffer (0.1 M Carbonate buffer pH 9.6) and then incubated at 4°C overnight. The plates were washed prior to the incubation of 200 μl of 5% dry milk per well for 2 hrs at room temperature. All washing steps were done in triplicate with 200 μl PBST/well, all dilutions were with 1% dry milk and all incubation was at room temperatures unless otherwise stated. After washing, the wells were incubated with 100 μl of IPNV supernatant (10^8 $TCID_{50}$/ml) for 2 hours. Following another washing step, serum samples diluted 1:40 were then added to the wells and then incubated at 4°C overnight. After washing, 100 μl of mouse antibody against rainbow trout IgM [28] diluted in 1:5000 was incubated for 2 hours. Following another wash, 100 μl of a 1:1000 dilution of peroxydase conjugated anti-mouse Ig (DAKO, Denmark) was incubated in each well for 1 hour. 100 μl of OPD substrate (O-phenylenediamine dihydrochloride, DAKO) diluted in water was added to each well after washing. This reaction was incubated for 15 min following which the reaction was stopped by the addition of 50 μl/well 1 M H_2SO_4. Results were analyzed by using an ELISA reader (TECAN, Genios) at 492 nm.

RNA isolation and quantitative real-time RT-PCR

Total RNA was isolated by using the RNeasy Plus minikit (Qiagen) according to the manufacturer's instructions, and the concentration of RNA was determined by using the Nanodrop ND1000 (NanoDrop Technologies).

Quantitative PCR was performed by using QuantiFast SYBR Green RT-PCR Kit (Qiagen) and the LightCycler 480 system (Roche). For each gene, 50 ng of RNA was used as a template in a mixture of specific primers (250 μM) (Table 2) and QuantiFast SYBR Green RT-PCR master mix in a total volume of 20 μl. The mixtures were first incubated at 50°C for 10 min, then 95°C for 5 min, followed by 40 amplification cycles (10 s at 95°C; 30 s at 60°C and 8 s at 72°C). The sequences of primers used are given in Table 2.

The $2^{-\Delta\Delta CT}$ method was used to calculate the gene products as described elsewhere [29] and is the relative mRNA expression representing the fold induction over the control group. All quantifications were normalized to β-actin.

Statistical analysis

The amount of feed intake for the three groups, gene expression and Elisa results were analyzed using Student's t test. F test was used to determine if the variances of population were equal or not. The threshold for significance was $p < 0.05$ for both Student's t test and F test.

Author Contributions

Conceived and designed the experiments: LC GK SW SJ TYK ØE SM. Performed the experiments: LC GK SM. Analyzed the data: LC GK SW

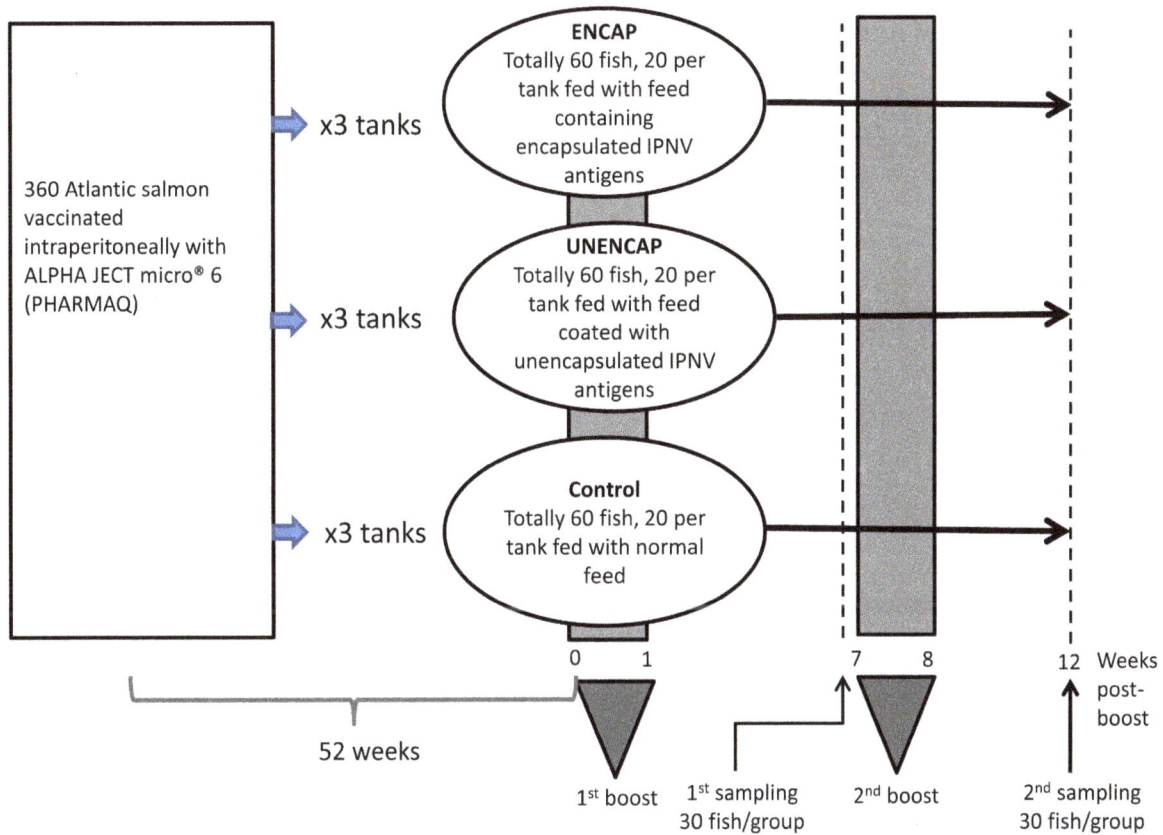

Figure 5. Schematic illustration of the trial plan used in the present study. Atlantic salmon growers previously (1 year) vaccinated against IPNV were split into three groups. Each group was further divided into three replicates (tanks) that were boosted twice orally for one week. Sampling was at 7 weeks post primary boost (a day before the second boost) and at the end of the trial. Ten fish from each tank (30 fish per group) were sampled at each time point.

Table 2. Sequences of primers used in this study.

Genes	Accession number	Primer sequence 5′-3′	D*
β-actin	BT047241.2	CCAGTCCTGCTCACTGAGGC	F
		GGTCTCAAACATGATCTGGGTCA	R
IgT	HQ379938.1	AGAGGTGAAGACACACCGGTCATT	F
		ACGGAGTAGTTGCCTTTCTGGGTT	R
CD4	DQ867019.1	GAGTACACCTGCGCTGTGGAAT	F
		GGTTGACCTCCTGACCTACAAAGG	R
GATA3	NM001171800.1	CCCAAGCGACGACTGTCT	F
		TCGTTTGACAGTTTGCACATGATG	R
IgM	AF228580.1	TGAGGAGAACTGTGGGCTACACT	F
		TGTTAATGACCACTGAATGTGCAT	R
FOXP3	HQ270469	AGCTGGCACAGCAGGAGTAT	F
		CGGGACAAGATCTGGGAGTA	R
TGF-β	BT059581.1	AGTTGCCTTGTGATTGTGGGA	F
		CTCTTCAGTAGTGGTTTGTCG	R
IL-10	AB118099.1	CGCTATGGACAGCATCCT	F
		AAGTGGTTGTTCTGCGTT	R
IPNV	NC_001915.1	ATGCCAAGATGATCCTGTCCCACA	F
		TGCCTTTGAGGTTGGTAGGTCACT	R

D* direction of primer.

SJ ØE SM. Contributed reagents/materials/analysis tools: ØE SW SJ TYK. Wrote the paper: LC GK SM ØE SW.

References

1. Taksdal T, Strangeland K, Dannevig B (1997) Induction of infectious pancreatic necrosis (IPN) in Atlantic salmon *Salmo salar* and brook trout *Salvelinus fontinalis* by bath challenge of fry with infectious pancreatic necrosis virus (IPNV) serotype SP. Dis Aquat Org 28: 39–44.

2. McKnight IJ, Roberts RJ (1976) The pathology of infectious pancreatic necrosis. I. The sequential histopathology of the naturally ocurring condition. Br Vet J 132: 76–85.

3. Adelmann M, Kollner B, Bergmann SM, Fischer U, Lange B, Weitschies W, Enzmann PJ, Fichtner D (2008) Development of an oral vaccine for immunisation of rainbow trout (Oncorhynchus mykiss) against viral haemorrhagic septicaemia. Vaccine 26: 837–844.

4. Weiner HL (2001) Oral tolerance: immune mechanisms and the generation of Th3-type TGF-beta-secreting regulatory cells. Microbes Infect 3: 947–954.

5. Rombout JH, Lamers CH, Helfrich MH, Dekker A, Taverne-Thiele JJ (1985) Uptake and transport of intact macromolecules in the intestinal epithelium of carp (Cyprinus carpio L.) and the possible immunological implications. Cell Tissue Res 239: 519–530.

6. de las Heras AI, Rodriguez Saint-Jean S, Perez-Prieto SI (2010) Immunogenic and protective effects of an oral DNA vaccine against infectious pancreatic necrosis virus in fish. Fish Shellfish Immunol 28: 562–570.

7. Biering E, Salonius K (2014) DNA Vaccines. In: Gudding RLA, Evensen O, editors. Fish Vaccination. John Wiley & Sons. pp. 47–55.

8. Holm A, Rippke BE, Noda K (2014) Legal Requirements and Authorization of Fish Vaccines. In: Gudding RLA, Evensen O, editors. Fish Vaccination. John Wiley & Sons. pp. 128–139.

9. Evensen Ø, Brudeseth B, Mutoloki S (2004) The vaccine formulation and its role in inflammatory processes in fish - effectc and adverse effects. Dev Biol Stand 121: 117–125.

10. Munang'andu HM, Fredriksen BN, Mutoloki S, Dalmo RA, Evensen O (2013) Antigen dose and humoral immune response correspond with protection for inactivated infectious pancreatic necrosis virus vaccines in Atlantic salmon (Salmo salar L). Vet Res 44: 7.

11. Romalde JL, Luzardo-Alvarez A, Ravelo C, Toranzo AE, Blanco-Wendez J (2004) Oral immunization using alginate microparticles as a useful strategy for booster vaccination against fish lactoccocosis. Aquaculture 236: 119–129.

12. Espenes A, Press CM, Reitan LJ, Landsverk T (1996) The trapping of intravenously injected extracellular products from *Aeromonas salmonicida* in head kidney and spleen of vaccinated and nonvaccinated Atlantic salmon, *Salmo salar* L. Fish Shellfish Immunol 6: 413–426.

13. Munang'andu HM, Sandtro A, Mutoloki S, Brudeseth BE, Santi N, et al. (2013) Immunogenicity and cross protective ability of the central VP2 amino acids of infectious pancreatic necrosis virus in Atlantic salmon (Salmo salar L.). Plos One 8: e54263.

14. Gonnella PA, Chen Y, Inobe J, Komagata Y, Quartulli M, et al. (1998) In situ immune response in gut-associated lymphoid tissue (GALT) following oral antigen in TCR-transgenic mice. J Immunol 160: 4708–4718.

15. Sarei F, Dounighi NM, Zolfagharian H, Khaki P, Bidhendi SM (2013) Alginate Nanoparticles as a Promising Adjuvant and Vaccine Delivery System. Indian J Pharm Sci 75: 442–449.

16. Salvador A, Igartua M, Hernandez RM, Pedraz JL (2012) Combination of immune stimulating adjuvants with poly(lactide-co-glycolide) microspheres enhances the immune response of vaccines. Vaccine 30: 589–596.

17. Maurice S, Nussinovitch A, Jaffe N, Shoseyov O, Gertler A (2004) Oral immunization of Carassius auratus with modified recombinant A-layer proteins entrapped in alginate beads. Vaccine 23: 450–459.

18. Mutwiri G, Bowersock T, Kidane A, Sanchez M, Gerdts V, et al. (2002) Induction of mucosal immune responses following enteric immunization with antigen delivered in alginate microspheres. Vet Immunol Immunopathol 87: 269–276.

19. Thinh NH, Kuo TY, Hung LT, Loc TH, Chen SC, et al. (2009) Combined immersion and oral vaccination of Vietnamese catfish (Pangasianodon hypophthalmus) confers protection against mortality caused by Edwardsiella ictaluri. Fish Shellfish Immunol 27: 773–776.

20. Tobar JA, Jerez S, Caruffo M, Bravo C, Contreras F, et al. (2011) Oral vaccination of Atlantic salmon (Salmo salar) against salmonid rickettsial septicaemia. Vaccine 29: 2336–2340.

21. Rombout JHWM, van den Berg AA, van den Berg CTGA, Witte P, Egberts E (1989) Immunological importance of the second gut segment of carp. III. Systemic and/or mucosal immune responses after immunization with soluble or particulate antigen. J Fish Biol 35: 179–186.

22. Joosten PHM, Tiemersma E, Threels A, CaumartinDhieux C, Rombout JHWM (1997) Oral vaccination of fish against Vibrio anguillarum using alginate microparticles. Fish Shellfish Immunol 7: 471–485.

23. Berzofsky JA, Ahlers JD, Derby MA, Pendleton CD, Arichi T, et al. (1999) Approaches to improve engineered vaccines for human immunodeficiency virus and other viruses that cause chronic infections. Immunol Rev 170: 151–172.

24. Weiner HL, da Cunha AP, Quintana F, Wu H (2011) Oral tolerance. Immunol Rev 241: 241–259.

25. Matsuo A, Oshiumi H, Tsujita T, Mitani H, Kasai H, et al. (2008) Teleost TLR22 recognizes RNA duplex to induce IFN and protect cells from birnaviruses. J Immunol 181: 3474–3485.

26. Munang'andu HM, Fredriksen BN, Mutoloki S, Brudeseth B, Kuo TY, et al. (2012) Comparison of vaccine efficacy for different antigen delivery systems for infectious pancreatic necrosis virus vaccines in Atlantic salmon (Salmo salar L.) in a cohabitation challenge model. Vaccine 30: 4007–4016.

27. Evensen O, Rimstad E (1990) Immunohistochemical identification of infectious pancreatic necrosis virus in paraffin-embedded tissues of Atlantic salmon (Salmo salar). J Vet Diagn Invest 2: 288–293.

28. Thuvander A, Fossum C, Lorenzen N (1990) Monoclonal antibodies to salmonid immunoglobulin: characterization and applicability in immunoassays. Dev Comp Immunol 14: 415–423.

29. Livak KJ, Schmittgen TD (2001) Analysis of relative gene expression data using real-time quantitative PCR and the 2(-Delta Delta C(T)) Method. Methods 25: 402–408.

22

Clinical Validation and Implications of Dried Blood Spot Sampling of Carbamazepine, Valproic Acid and Phenytoin in Patients with Epilepsy

Sing Teang Kong[1], Shih-Hui Lim[2,3,4], Wee Beng Lee[1], Pasikanthi Kishore Kumar[1], Hwee Yi Stella Wang[2], Yan Lam Shannon Ng[2], Pei Shieen Wong[2], Paul C. Ho[1]*

1 Department of Pharmacy, National University of Singapore, Singapore, Singapore, **2** Department of Neurology, Singapore General Hospital, Singapore, Singapore, **3** Department of Neurology, National Neuroscience Institute, Singapore, Singapore, **4** Department of Neurology, Duke – National University of Singapore – Graduate Medical School, Singapore, Singapore

Abstract

To facilitate therapeutic monitoring of antiepileptic drugs (AEDs) by healthcare professionals for patients with epilepsy (PWE), we applied a GC-MS assay to measure three AEDs: carbamazepine (CBZ), phenytoin (PHT) and valproic acid (VPA) levels concurrently in one dried blood spot (DBS), and validated the DBS-measured levels to their plasma levels. 169 PWE on either mono- or polytherapy of CBZ, PHT or/and VPA were included. One DBS, containing ~15 μL of blood, was acquired for the simultaneous measurement of the drug levels using GC-MS. Simple Deming regressions were performed to correlate the DBS levels with the plasma levels determined by the conventional immunoturbimetric assay in clinical practice. Statistical analyses of the results were done using MedCalc Version 12.6.1.0 and SPSS 21. DBS concentrations (C_{dbs}) were well-correlated to the plasma concentrations (C_{plasma}): r = 0.8381, 0.9305 and 0.8531 for CBZ, PHT and VPA respectively, The conversion formulas from C_{dbs} to plasma concentrations were $[0.89 \times C_{dbs}CBZ+1.00]$μg/mL, $[1.11 \times C_{dbs}PHT-1.00]$μg/mL and $[0.92 \times C_{dbs}VPA+12.48]$μg/mL respectively. Inclusion of the red blood cells (RBC)/plasma partition ratio (K) and the individual hematocrit levels in the estimation of the theoretical C_{plasma} from C_{dbs} of PHT and VPA further improved the identity between the observed and the estimated theoretical C_{plasma}. Bland-Altman plots indicated that the theoretical and observed C_{plasma} of PHT and VPA agreed well, and >93.0% of concentrations was within 95% CI (±2SD); and similar agreement (1:1) was also found between the observed C_{dbs} and C_{plasma} of CBZ. As the C_{plasma} of CBZ, PHT and VPA can be accurately estimated from their C_{dbs}, DBS can therefore be used for drug monitoring in PWE on any of these AEDs.

Editor: Jong Rho, Alberta Children's Hospital, Canada

Funding: The authors have no funding or support to report.

Competing Interests: The authors have declared that no competing interests exist.

* Email: phahocl@nus.edu.sg

Introduction

Epilepsy is a neurological disease that requires chronic treatment with antiepileptic drugs (AEDs). To date, the most commonly used AEDs are still carbamazepine (CBZ), phenytoin (PHT) and valproic acid (VPA). These drugs have maximum efficacy and minimum toxicity when their plasma drug levels are within their therapeutic indexes. Hence, routine plasma concentration monitoring is recommended especially during dose adjustments, for compliance check and/or for adverse drug reaction investigation [1]. In current practice, monitoring of plasma AEDs is done using the immunoturbidimetric assay for each individual drug. In this assay, the drug of interest complexes with its specific antibody and becomes insoluble. The turbidity generated from the immune complexes corresponds to the drug concentration in sample and is then measured spectrophotometrically. However, for this assay, there is always a risk that the antibody could cross-react with the metabolites of the drug. This could result in overestimation of the plasma concentrations.

During the course of AEDs therapy, approximately 40% to 50% of people with epilepsy (PWE) will require two or more antiepileptic drugs (AEDs) at one point of their therapy [2–4]. Attempts have therefore been made to monitor a few AEDs levels simultaneously [5–7], with the objective to reduce the workload of the hospital laboratories and the TDM cost borne by the patients.

Various biological matrices including cerebrospinal fluid, tear and saliva have been used for TDM [8–10]. In comparison with DBS as the matrix, the acquisition of blood spot is simple, and does not require the aid of phlebotomist. DBS entails small sampling volume (<100 μL) and can be acquired by patients or their caregivers at home. After drying, it can be mailed to the designated laboratory [11,12]. The patients will be able to save their travelling time to the clinics for submitting their TDM samples. The only caveat for DBS acquisition seems to be the patients' acceptability for the needle-prick.

Earlier studies on concurrent monitoring of multiple AEDs from one DBS were done mostly with high performance liquid chromatography (HPLC) and included whole blood concentrations of AEDs such as carbamazepine, phenytoin, lamotrigine and barbiturates with limited clinical validation [13,14]. Recently, a group in North Ireland published a detailed HPLC ultraviolet method for concurrent determination of carbamazepine (CBZ) and its active metabolite carbamazepine-10,11 epoxide (CBZE), levetiracetam (LEV), lamotrigine (LTG) and phenobarbital (PHB) in DBS of children [15]. Similarly, they did not establish the correlations between the DBS and plasma concentrations of the AEDs involved.

In our population of PWE, CBZ, sodium valproate (VPA) and phenytoin (PHT) are the most popular antiepileptic drugs (AEDs) - used either as mono or polytherapy [4]. This has prompted us to investigate the applicability of monitoring all three AEDs using only one DBS. Considering the volatile nature of VPA and previous success in quantitation of CBZ and PHT using gas chromatography mass spectrometry (GCMS) [16], GCMS was ultimately chosen as the analytical tool for simultaneous determination of these AEDs. This study was conducted with the main objective of comparing the newly developed GCMS assay with the conventional immunoturbimetric assays. The DBS-measured concentrations were validated against their corresponding plasma concentrations as determined by the immunoturbimetric assays performed in hospital laboratory. Since plasma-to-RBC drug partitioning effect in relation to the hematocrit level is known to influence the degree of correspondence between plasma and full blood concentration of AEDs, this effect was also investigated in our study.

Methods

This study has obtained approval from the SingHealth Institutional Review Board (CIRB No. 2011/269/A). Only PWE who had routine plasma CBZ, VPA and/or PHT, blood and liver biochemistry monitoring on the day of visit were approached for written consent prior to blood sampling.

Patient Recruitment

Assuming constant analytical standard deviations, the sample size recommended for method validation was suggested to be at least 41 per AED based on the following information: range ratio = 2, $\alpha = 5\%$, power = 90%, standardized slope deviation of 4 [17,18]. PWE who were on either CBZ, VPA or/and PHT were recruited from October 2011 to August 2012 at neurology specialist clinic of a tertiary referral hospital. This study had obtained the local ethics committee approval. Only PWE who had routine plasma CBZ, PHT and/or VPA, blood and liver biochemistries monitoring on the day of visit were included. Informed consent was obtained prior to blood sampling. PWE characteristics and biochemistry results were retrieved from clinical records and hospital information system. Each PWE was interviewed for the time of his/her last AED dose taken. Drug responses were categorized in accordance to the recent International League Against Epilepsy (ILAE) recommendations [19].

Sampling

Venous whole blood samples were collected in EDTA tubes. Two drops of blood from the withdrawn blood, ~30 μL each, were spotted onto 903 cards (903 Neonate Blood Collection Cards, Whatman GmbH, Dassel, Germany) and dried at room temperature, 25°C for at least 3 hours. The rest of the whole blood was sent to hospital laboratory for plasma AED quantitations as per routine protocols. To maintain direct comparability with plasma levels, DBS samples were stored at −80°C until the day of analysis. The 3 AEDs were proven to be stable at −20°C and

25°C for at least 10 days at concentrations ranging from 0.5 mg/L to 100 mg/L (Table S1).

Plasma AEDs Quantification

The routine plasma AEDs quantifications were done in the hospital laboratory using particle enhanced turbidimetric inhibition immunoassays (Beckman Coulter Inc. Unicel DxC800, USA). The imprecisions in CV% (mean level, SD) for low, medium and high concentrations based on 21 data points over a period of typically 10 days are as following: i) Carbamazepine [range 2.0–20.0 mg/L] between run = 9.2% (4.2 mg/L, 0.39), 7.6% (10.79 mg/L, 0.82), 5.9% (15.24 mg/L, 0.93) and within run = 3.9% (3.92 mg/L, 0.15), 2.7% (10.41 mg/L, 0.28, 2.8% (15.24 mg/L, 0.43) ii) Phenytoin [2.5–40 mg/L] between run = 8.0% (5.18 mg/L, 0.42), 5.8% (15.03 mg/L, 0.83), 4.5% (30.40 mg/L, 1.36) and within run = 2.1% (5.00 mg/L, 0.11), 1.5% (13.76 mg/L, 0.20), 2.9% (28.19 mg/L, 0.80) iii) Valproic acid [10.0–150.0 mg/L] between run = 7.8% (33.26 mg/L, 2.59), 7.5% (75.90 mg/L, 5.68), 7.6% (125.70 mg/L, 9.55) and within run = 2.5% (33.03 mg/L, 0.82), 1.0% (67.99 mg/L, 0.70), 3.6% (112.83 mg/L, 4.09).

DBS Samples Processing

Quantitation was based on one 6-mm diameter DBS punch from the centre of the spot, containing approximately 15 μL of blood. AEDs extraction was performed using 500 μL of analytical grade (99%) acetonitrile (Prime Products Pte. Ltd., Singapore) and 1 molar sodium hydroxide (JT Baker, Phillipsburg, NJ, USA) at a ratio of 24:1, v/v with 1 μg/mL 5-(p-methylphenyl)-5-phenylhydantoin (5MP) (Sigma Aldrich, St Louis, MO) as internal standard. The extraction procedure involved 1 min of vortexing and 5 min of sonication. Then, the mixture was centrifuged for 15 min at 6000 g. 400 μL of supernatant was transferred into 15 mL Kimble glass tube (Gerresheimer Co. Glass, Germany) for evaporation under nitrogen gas for 15 mins at 40°C. After addition of 100 μL of toluene to the dried sample, second drying phase under similar condition was carried out. Subsequently, derivatization was attained using 50 μL of N-methyl-N-trimethylsilyltrifluoroacetamide with 1% trimethylchlorosilane (Thermo Scientific Pte. Ltd., Waltham, Massachusetts, USA) incubated at an optimum 70°C for 50 min. Derivatised samples were cooled to room temperature and diluted with 50 μL of heptane before vortexing for 1 min. Finally, 80 μL of mixture was transferred into a 200 μL conical base inert glass insert placed in a 2 mL amber glass vial (Agilent Technologies, Santa Clara, California, USA).

Gas Chromatography Mass Spectrometry settings

The analytical assay was developed and validated with a GC-MS system that comprised of GC 2010 Shimadzu GC coupled to a GCMS-QP2010 Plus quadrupole MS (Shimadzu Corporation, Nishinokyo-Kuwabara-cho, Nakagyo-ku, Kyoto, Japan). GCMSsolution (version 2.0), was utilized for data acquisition and peak area computation. DB5 ms (30 m×0.25 mm×0.25 μm) supplied by Agilent Technologies J&W, Inc. was used as the capillary column. Injector temperature was set at 250°C, while ion source at 220°C. Injection volume of 1 μL was subjected to split ratio of 1:5 and column flow was set at 1.9 mL/min. Column temperature began at 90°C with a 0.2-min isothermal hold. Temperature was then ramped at 4 different rates: i) 10°C/min to 120°C, held for 0.5 min ii) 65°C/min to 285°C, held for 0.5 min iii) 10°C/min to 291°C, held for 0.2 min and iv) 60°C/min to 300°C for a final isothermal hold of 5 min. Selective ion monitoring (SIM) mode was used for detection of the target

Table 1. Tabulation of selective ion monitoring (SIM) attributes and the ions monitored for the respective analytes.

Analytes	Retention Time	Quantifying Ion	Qualifying Ions
Valproic Acid	3.453 min	201	129, 145
Phenytoin	7.068 min	281	165, 176, 253
Carbamazepine	7.166 min	193	194, 293
5-methylphenylhydantoin	7.245 min	267	290, 395

analytes at their respective retention times and are tabulated in Table 1.

Bioanalysis

Calibration and quality control standards were prepared in blood and spotted onto the 903 cards at 30 µL each. One 6-mm diameter disc was punched out from each DBS and used for analysis. The assay was validated over a range of 0.5–120 µg/mL for all three AEDs. Accuracy ranged from 100–110% and imprecision was <10%. The calculated limit of detection was 0.05 µg/mL for VPA and approximately 0.07 µg/mL for both PHT and CBZ. The recoveries of analytes were relatively high (75%–97%) and consistent (SD≤8.2%). Although the inconsistency increased to 11% at the lower limit of quantitation for CBZ, it was still within the FDA acceptable lower limit of quantification (< 20%) (Table S2).

Statistical Analysis

DBS concentrations (C_{dbs}) and plasma concentrations (C_{plasma}) determined by the respective methods were directly compared. Theoretical C_{plasma} was calculated using a formula which accounts for the individual hematocrit values and red blood cell-to-plasma partition (RBC/plasma) ratio [20,21].

$$\text{Theoretical } C_{plasma} = \frac{C_{dbs}}{[1 - Hct(1 - K)]}$$

where Hct is the individual hematocrit value and K is the RBC/plasma ratio of the AEDs. To ease clinical applicability, K was fixed at literature values of 0.29 [22] and 0.43 for PHT [20] and 0.04 [23] and 0.20 [24] for VPA. As for CBZ, its theoretical plasma concentration approaches that of C_{dbs}, rendering the effect of Hct on computation of theoretical C_{plasma} to be negligible. Moreover, the K for CBZ had been reported to be approximately equal to 1 [25].

Statistical analyses were done using SPSS 21 and MedCalc Version 12.6.1.0. Simple Deming regression was utilized to compare the 2 methods. The differences between methods were assessed using paired sample t-test. Bland-Altman plots were subsequently compiled using the theoretical C_{plasma} and observed C_{plasma}. Outliers were confirmed using standardized score and removal was considered if the score exceeded 2.5.

Results

Patients

A total of 181 PWE were recruited but only 165 PWE who provided DBS were included in the final analyses. Fourteen PWE were excluded due to undetectable C_{plasma} (<2 µg/mL), and 2 PWE were excluded as outliers. Characteristics of PWE within each AED group are tabulated in Table 2. Some PWE contributed 2 AED concentrations, resulting in a total DBSs of

more than 165. No significant elevation in biochemistry results was noted. The median hematocrit of the venous samples was 41.3 (range 29.8–51). The average daily doses of CBZ, PHT and VPA used in this population were 870.5±413.22 mg, 284.1±71.33 mg and 934.0±317.89 mg, respectively.

DBS and plasma concentrations

Figure 1 illustrates the relationships between the C_{dbs} and C_{plasma} for the three AEDs. Good correlations were demonstrated for all three AEDs, with correlation coefficients of $r = 0.8381$, 0.9305 and 0.8531 for CBZ, PHT and VPA, respectively. C_{dbs} and C_{plasma} of CBZ were almost identical with the slope converging with line of unity. In contrast, C_{dbs} of PHT and VPA were found consistently lower than their corresponding C_{plasma}, averaging at 2.8±1.89 µg/mL (29.7±13.59%) and 28.3±12.73 µg/mL (49.5±22.3%), respectively ($p<0.005$). Moreover, 95% CI for the slopes of PHT and VPA diverge anticlockwise from the line of unity and did not cross the value 1. This signifies that there was at least a proportional increase in correlation between C_{plasma} and C_{dbs} of the two AEDs.

When regressed against the theoretical C_{plasma}, definite improvements in fit between data points from the turbimetric assay and DBS assay were observed. The lines of regression for respective AEDs rotated closer to the line of unity and data points clustered in greater proximity along the identity line, albeit marginal decrease in correlation coefficients for PHT and VPA (**Figure 2**). The theoretical C_{plasma} of PHT was found to be comparable to its observed C_{plasma} (**Figure 2**, top). However, the regression line drawn using the theoretical C_{plasma} of PHT obtained using K of 0.29 produced a better fit with 95% CI of the slope of 1 (**Figure 2**, top left) than the one obtained using K of 0.43 (**Figure 2**, top right). As for VPA, the observed C_{plasma} was still higher than both theoretical C_{plasma} calculated using K of 0.20 (**Figure 2**, bottom left) and 0.042 (**Figure 2**, bottom right), but at the constant values of their intercepts.

Figure 3 shows the Bland-Altman plots of all three AEDs using their respective theoretical C_{plasma}. The concentration used for CBZ was C_{dbs} while for PHT and VPA, the theoretical C_{plasma} was used in comparison with their observed C_{plasma}. The mean difference between the concentrations from the proposed new method and conventional plasma immunoassay was −0.1 µg/mL for CBZ. For the theoretical PHT C_{plasma} calculated using K = 0.43, the mean difference was −0.7 µg/mL while with K = 0.29, the mean difference was zero. As for VPA, the differences were −13.7 and −8.1 µg/mL with K of 0.20 and 0.042, respectively. Since most of these differences fell within the acceptable limit of ±1.96 SD for all three AEDs, it is safe to assume that the theoretical C_{plasma} derived from C_{dbs} corresponded well with the observed C_{plasma}. Based on the preceding discussion, the theoretical C_{plasma} of VPA estimated from K = 0.04 and PHT estimated from K = 0.29 yielded better fit with

Table 2. Characteristics of the people with epilepsy (PWE) grouped according to the type of antiepileptic drug.

Characteristics	Valproic Acid (n = 92)	Phenytoin (n = 49)	Carbamazepine (n = 108)
Number of Eligible DBS	85	43	101
Number of Excluded DBS	7	6	7
Number of Subjects	84	41	100
Male	48 (57.1%)	22 (53.7%)	48 (48%)
Age, Median (Range)	44.3 (19–78)	50.6 (18–72)	42.9 (20–78)
Ethnic, No. Subjects (%)			
Chinese	74 (88.1%)	37 (90.2%)	89 (89%)
Malay	5 (6.0%)	3 (7.3%)	5 (5%)
Indian	3 (3.6%)	nil	6 (6%)
Others	2 (2.3%)	1 (2.4%)	nil
Concurrent medications, No. Subjects (%)			
None	7 (8.3%)	22 (53.7%)	22 (22%)
Valproic Acid	-	10 (24.4%)	46 (46%)
Phenytoin	10 (11.9%)	-	nil
Carbamazapine	46 (54.8%)	nil	-
Other AEDs	21 (25.0%)	9 (21.9%)	32 (32%)
Blood Chemistry, Median (range)			
Hematocrit (%)	41.6 (30.7–51)	42.7 (33.3–49.2)	41.3 (29.8–49.7)
Hemoglobin (g/dL)	13.9 (9.8–16.8)	14.0 (10.5–16.4)	13.6 (9.2–16.8)
Liver Function Test	Median (range)		
Albumin (g/L)	40 (31–46)	41 (31–47)	41 (31–46)
ALT (U/L)	20 (8–109)	24 (12–79)	19 (9–43)
AST (U/L)	22 (12–59)	22 (16–78)	21 (12–59)
GGT (U/L)	53 (9–333)	84 (27–417)	50 (21–213)
Drug Monitoring (μg/mL), Mean (standard deviation)			
Mean plasma levels	57.1 (22.35)*	9.7 (4.67)*	8.4 (2.32)
Mean DBS levels	29.2 (14.67)*	6.9 (3.92)*	8.3 (2.56)
Mean predicted plasma levels	57.1 (20.31)	9.7 (4.60)	8.4 (2.27)
Average dose (mg), Mean (standard deviation)			
	870.5 (413.22)	934.0 (317.89)	284.1 (71.33)
ILAE Classification of Drug Response			
Drug Responsive	28 (33.3%)	21 (51.2%)	31 (31%)
Drug Resistant	31 (36.9%)	9 (22.0%)	38 (38%)
Undefined	25 (29.8%)	11 (26.8%)	31 (31%)

Total recruited PWE were 183. Only 169 were included in the analysis. The remaining 14 subjects were excluded due to missing plasma levels from hospital laboratory system. (Note: Some recruited PWE contributed to the levels of two AEDs).

convergence to the line of unity and were therefore, recommended for clinical use.

Discussion

In line with a presumed K of 1.06 from literatures, the RBC dilutional effect on C_{dbs} of CBZ was found to be negligible [21,25]. Since CBZ partitions between RBC and plasma to a similar extent, the concentrations measured in whole blood were approximately the same as the plasma concentrations. This enables a direct comparison between C_{dbs} and C_{plasma} of CBZ in this study, giving a conversion factor of about 0.9.

Contrasting to CBZ, the C_{dbs} of VPA was found to be constantly lower than its C_{plasma}. Similar finding were previously observed by Vermeij and Edelbroek in their study. They found a conversion factor of 1.46 from C_{dbs} to C_{plasma}, which implied that the C_{plasma} of VPA was 46% higher than its C_{dbs} [13]. The lower concentrations measured from DBS could be attributed to a combination of factors. Firstly, RBC accounted for 99% of cellular space of blood and its presence may serve to dilute the VPA concentrations compared to those measured in plasma alone [26]. Secondly, for drugs with whole blood-to-plasma concentration ratio of less than (1–Hct), such as VPA, they should not partition into RBC significantly [21]. The inclusion of RBC in DBS will produce a dilution effect upon total drug concentration. It is projected that only the unbound drugs can partition into RBCs [27,28] and that this partition is consistent at varying concentra-

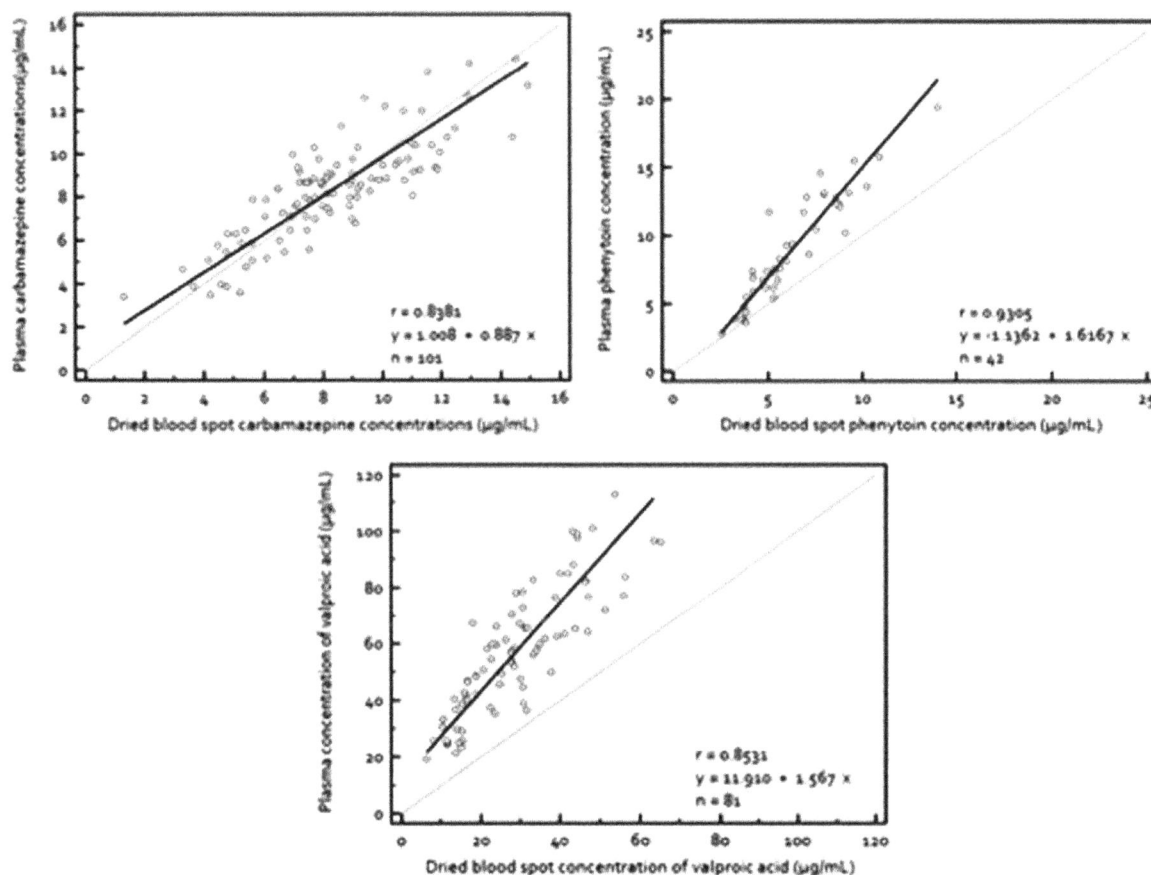

Figure 1. Correlation of plasma concentrations of AEDs with their corresponding dried blood spot concentrations. Plasma concentrations of (**top left**) carbamazepine (**top right**) phenytoin and (**bottom**) valproic acid regressed against their dried blood spot concentrations using Deming regression. The broken line is the line of unity while the continuous line is the line of regression. The (**top left**) slope is 0.84 (95% CI, 0.76 to 1.00) and the intercept is 1.00 (95% CI, 0.04 to 1.97) for carbamazepine, (**top right**) slope is 1.61 (95% CI, 1.39 to 1.84) and the intercept is −1.14 (95% CI, −2.40 to 0.12) for phenytoin and (**bottom**) slope is 1.57 (95% CI, 1.33 to 1.81) and the intercept is 11.91 (95% CI, 5.73 to 18.09) for valproic acid.

tions [29,30]. VPA has been shown to partition into the RBC from the plasma at ratios ranging from 0.04 to 0.20 [23,24,29]. Since most of our patients had plasma VPA concentrations within the therapeutic ranges, and normal albumin levels, the K was presumably to be constant [29]. Hence, the relatively small amount of VPA in RBC was less likely to contribute substantial value towards the overall C_{dbs}. Thirdly, due to its lipophilic nature, VPA could dissolve and detach from RBC during centrifugation of whole blood to obtain the plasma and resulted in the relatively higher concentrations observed in the plasma [31,32]. Alternatively, despite the extraction yield of >80% (RSD<6.0%) between 1 to 250 mg/L (Table S2), the binding of VPA to 903 cards may have some effect affecting the lower C_{dbs}.

After incorporating the hematocrit and K values, definitive improvement was achieved for the computation of the theoretical C_{plasma} of VPA. Yet, the theoretical C_{plasma} derived from C_{dbs} remained consistently lower than C_{plasma}. The most probable explanations include the domination of RBC dilutional effect and VPA binding to 903 cards. In clinical practice, however, the potential consequence of the difference in calculated C_{plasma} from C_{dbs} may not be obvious. An example of a worst case prediction would be, for an actual C_{plasma} of 60 µg/mL, the predicted C_{plasma} could either be 48 or 72 µg/mL. Regardless of the variation in the predicted C_{plasma}, physicians are likely to increase the dose if the

PWE has uncontrolled seizure, hence arriving at the similar clinical decisions. Therefore, the clinical decisions premised upon C_{dbs} will be no different from the clinical decisions made using C_{plasma}.

On the other hand, PHT is readily partitions into and dissociates from the RBC, with a K reported to be approximately 0.29 [22] and 0.43 in healthy patients [20]. Its whole blood-to-plasma concentration was approximately 1.33 in both studies, which was comparable to 1.14 and 1.23, before and after corrected for Hct and K, found in this study. PHT binds to hemoglobin in RBCs [33] and was shown to be released disproportionally *in vivo* [22]. For drugs with high partition ratio into RBC such as thioridazine and derivatives, the RBC concentrations tend to have better association with treatment outcomes as compared to their plasma concentrations [34]. Therefore, obtaining an overall concentration from whole blood might provide insights into uncontrolled seizure despite having optimal plasma PHT concentration.

Effect of hematocrit and compound specific red blood cell-to-plasma ratios

In this study, we demonstrated that compound-specific RBC-to-plasma binding and individual hematocrit level could explain the difference in concentrations detected from DBS and plasma. It

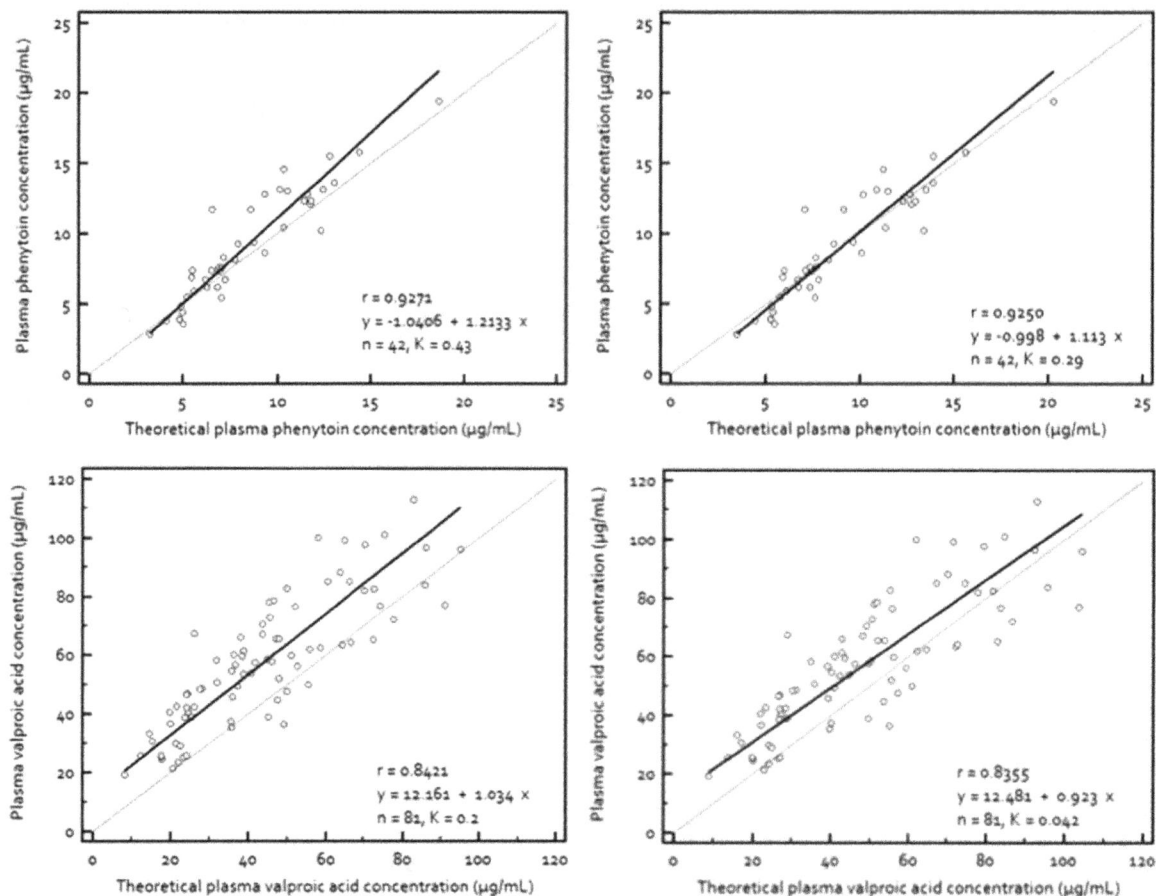

Figure 2. Identity of the plasma concentrations of phenytoin and valproic acid with the theoretical plasma concentrations derived from their dry blood spot concentrations. Plasma concentrations of (**top**) phenytoin and (**bottom**) valproic acid regressed against their theoretical plasma concentrations estimated from dried blood spot concentrations using Deming regression. [Theoretical plasma concentrations = - Dried blood spot concentrations/1–Hct×(1–K)], where Hct is hematocrit and K is the RBC/plasma partition ratio. The broken line is the line of unity while the continuous line is the line of regression. The (**top left**) slope is 1.21 (95% CI, 1.04 to 1.38) and the intercept is -1.04 (95% CI, -2.32 to 0.24) for phenytoin with K=0.43, (**top right**) slope is 1.11 (95% CI, 0.95 to 1.27) and the intercept is -1.00 (95% CI, -2.28 to 0.29) for phenytoin with K=0.29, (**bottom left**) slope is 1.03 (95% CI, 0.87 to 1.20) and the intercept is 12.16 (95% CI, 5.95 to 18.37) for valproic acid with K=0.2 and (**bottom right**) slope is 0.92 (95% CI, 0.77 to 1.07) and the intercept is 12.48 (95% CI, 6.15 to 18.81) for valproic acid with K=0.042.

seems that as RBC-to-plasma partitioning approaches 1, e.g. 1.06 for CBZ, the closer the C_{dbs} is to its C_{plasma} and hematocrit level will have no dilution effect. Conversely, as RBC-to-plasma partitioning approaches 0, the dilution effect of hematocrit level becomes prominent and higher hematocrit levels lower C_{dbs}. DBS does seem to equate the whole blood characteristics which were demonstrated in previous studies [21,30]. For lipophilic drugs such as AEDs, RBC is an important and useful transporter with high capacity but low affinity to the drugs. RBC readily releases the drug it carries and equilibrates with surrounding tissues in capillary system. Although C_{plasma} is an optimal representation of tissue concentration, RBC concentration of drug may function similarly. The constant ratios of RBC/plasma water over a wide range of AEDs concentrations proved that RBC is not a saturable system [22,29]. Therefore, RBC concentration of drug may be negligible at low concentration, but will definitely gain importance as the concentration increases.

At clinically relevant blood and liver biochemistry variations, correcting the C_{dbs} to hematocrit and K improved the theoretical prediction of C_{plasma} for PHT and VPA. Nevertheless, this study catered for the investigation of PWE with AED binding to the red blood cells and albumin in the normal ranges. It is reasonable to

assume that the effects of AED binding to blood cells and albumin should not fluctuate significantly. For the former effect, the Ks were fixed at 2 values for PHT and VPA. As evidenced by the improved graphical fit, correspondence with the actual C_{plasma} was improved with the inclusion of K. Similarly, a constant K value has also been used to enhance the clinical applicability and harmonize the analytical process of PHT and VPA in whole blood samples [22,29],.

The PWE recruited in this study represented the typical population of PWE who required the routine therapeutic drug monitoring. However, there were no inclusion of children, critically ill patients nor subjects who have just started the AED/s treatment. Hence, the applicability of this DBS quantitation method for dose titration for these cohorts of subjects remains unknown. These subjects could have a more fluctuating Hct and/or drug levels. Their theoretical C_{plasma} would be more challenging to be determined from the corresponding C_{dbs} levels. The applicability of C_{dbs} as a surrogate to C_{plasma} and even seizure control in these subjects need to be established in the future studies.

It is noteworthy that on this study, the DBS was obtained from venous source. Theoretically, there could be some differences between capillary and venous concentrations but the differences

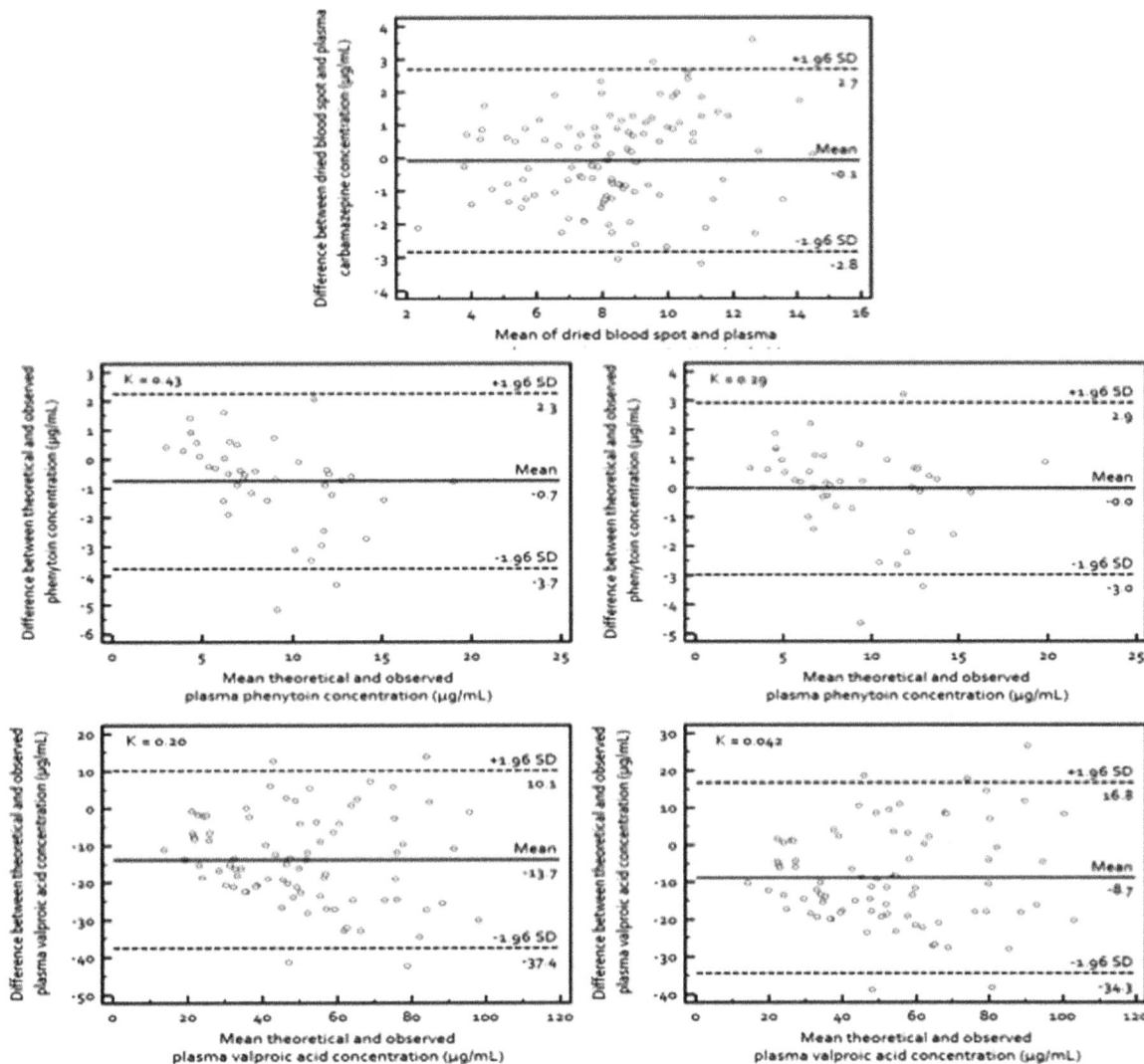

Figure 3. Agreement between the plasma concentrations of carbamazepine and its dried blood spot concentration; and between the plasma concentrations of phenytoin and valproic acid and the theoretical plasma concentrations derived from their dried blood spot concentrations. Bland Altman plots for plasma concentrations of (**top**) carbamazepine, (**middle left**) phenytoin, K = 0.43, (**middle right**) phenytoin, K = 0.29, (**bottom left**) valproic acid, K = 0.20 and (**bottom right**) valproic acid, K = 0.042. The broken lines represent the 95% CI (±1.96 SD) and the continuous line is the mean.

for a majority of xenobiotics were proven not to be obvious, especially after the distribution phase [35–37]. Therefore, at steady state drug concentrations, the difference between capillary and venous concentrations should be negligible. Blood concentrations from either source could be used interchangeably for estimating the AEDs C_{plasma} [37]. In conclusion, the theoretical C_{plasma} can be estimated through the equations below for the respective AEDs:

$$C_{plasma}\,CBZ = (0.89 \times C_{dbs}CBZ) + 1.00 \mu g/mL$$

$$C_{plasma}PHT = (1.11 \times \frac{C_{dbs}PHT}{1-(0.71 \times Hct)}) - 1.00 \mu g/mL$$

$$C_{plasma}\,VPA = (0.92 \times \frac{C_{dbs}VPA}{1-(0.96 \times Hct)}) - 12.48 \mu g/mL$$

where Hct represents the individual hematocrit value, C_{plasma} CBZ, C_{plasma} PHT and C_{plasma} VPA represents the plasma concentrations of CBZ, PHT and VPA, respectively, while C_{dbs} CBZ, C_{dbs} PHT and C_{dbs} VPA represents the dried blood spot concentrations of CBZ, PHT and VPA, respectively For the theoretical C_{plasma} of PHT and VPA, the conversion factors, K = 0.29 and K = 0.04, were respectively recommended due to its proximity to the line of unity.

Conclusion

In view of the good agreement between the theoretical C_{plasma} estimated from the C_{dbs} levels and the observed C_{plasma} for PHT and VPA, and also between the C_{dbs} and the observed C_{plasma} for CBZ, DBS is deemed suitable as an alternative matrix to the conventional plasma samples for TDM of AEDs in the adult population of PWE. Further studies that investigate the pharmacokinetic parameters such as clearance and apparent volume of distribution using the C_{dbs} levels and then correlate these concentrations to the treatment outcomes are warranted.

Supporting Information

Table S1 Stability of quality control samples for carbamazepine (CBZ), phenytoin (PHT) and valproic acid (VPA) under different storage conditions on Day 5 and Day 10. Benchtop represents 25°C while Freezer represents −20°C. QC denotes quality control.

Table S2 Percentage of mean extraction recovery of analytes along with their respective residual standard deviation (RSD) at different concentrations in spiked blood. The consistent and high recovery (>70%) of the analytes allowed for reliable quantitative studies.

Acknowledgments

Previous presentation: Poster presentation of partial results at 10th European Congress on Epileptology, London, 30 September – 4 October 2012.

Author Contributions

Conceived and designed the experiments: STK PCH. Performed the experiments: STK WBL HYSW YLSN PSW. Analyzed the data: STK WBL PKK. Contributed reagents/materials/analysis tools: PCH. Contributed to the writing of the manuscript: STK. Technical advice: SHL. Patients' recruitment: SHL.

References

1. Patsalos PN, Berry DJ, Bourgeois BF, Cloyd JC, Glauser TA, et al. (2008) Antiepileptic drugs–best practice guidelines for therapeutic drug monitoring: a position paper by the subcommission on therapeutic drug monitoring, ILAE Commission on Therapeutic Strategies. Epilepsia 49: 1239–1276.
2. Froscher W, Rosche J (2013) [Combination therapy for epilepsy]. Fortschr Neurol Psychiatr 81: 9–20.
3. Tan WW, Kong ST, Chan DW, Ho PC (2012) A retrospective study on the usage of antiepileptic drugs in Asian children from 2000 to 2009 in the largest pediatric hospital in Singapore. Pharmacoepidemiol Drug Saf 21: 1074–1080.
4. Lim SH, See SJ, Wong PS, Lim SH (2012) Cost of antiepileptic drug monotherapies and combination therapies at a tertiary referral hospital in Singapore. Epilepsia 53: 194.
5. Tai SS, Yeh CY, Phinney KW (2011) Development and validation of a reference measurement procedure for certification of phenytoin, phenobarbital, lamotrigine, and topiramate in human serum using isotope-dilution liquid chromatography/tandem mass spectrometry. Anal Bioanal Chem 401: 1915–1922.
6. Serralheiro A, Alves G, Fortuna A, Rocha M, Falcao A (2013) First HPLC-UV method for rapid and simultaneous quantification of phenobarbital, primidone, phenytoin, carbamazepine, carbamazepine-10,11-epoxide, 10,11-trans-dihydroxy-10,11-dihydrocarbamazepine, lamotrigine, oxcarbazepine and licarbazepine in human plasma. J Chromatogr B Analyt Technol Biomed Life Sci 925: 1–9.
7. Shibata M, Hashi S, Nakanishi H, Masuda S, Katsura T, et al. (2012) Detection of 22 antiepileptic drugs by ultra-performance liquid chromatography coupled with tandem mass spectrometry applicable to routine therapeutic drug monitoring. Biomed Chromatogr 26: 1519–1528.
8. Piredda S, Monaco F (1981) Ethosuximide in tears, saliva, and cerebrospinal fluid. Ther Drug Monit 3: 321–323.
9. Patsalos PN, Berry DJ (2013) Therapeutic drug monitoring of antiepileptic drugs by use of saliva. Ther Drug Monit 35: 4–29.
10. Monaco F, Mutani R, Mastropaolo C, Tondi M (1979) Tears as the best practical indicator of the unbound fraction of an anticonvulsant drug. Epilepsia 20: 705–710.
11. Edelbroek PM, van der Heijden J, Stolk LM (2009) Dried blood spot methods in therapeutic drug monitoring: methods, assays, and pitfalls. Ther Drug Monit 31: 327–336.
12. Li W, Tse FL (2010) Dried blood spot sampling in combination with LC-MS/MS for quantitative analysis of small molecules. Biomed Chromatogr 24: 49–65.
13. Vermeij T, Edelbroek P (2011 Personal Communication) Determination of Anticonvulsant Blood Levels Using the Blood Spot Method.
14. Deglon J, Versace F, Lauer E, Widmer C, Mangin P, et al. (2012) Rapid LC-MS/MS quantification of the major benzodiazepines and their metabolites on dried blood spots using a simple and cost-effective sample pretreatment. Bioanalysis 4: 1337–1350.
15. Shah NM, Hawwa AF, Millership JS, Collier PS, Ho P, et al. (2013) Adherence to antiepileptic medicines in children-A multiple-methods assessment involving dried blood spot sampling. Epilepsia.
16. Rani S, Malik AK (2012) A novel microextraction by packed sorbent-gas chromatography procedure for the simultaneous analysis of antiepileptic drugs in human plasma and urine. J Sep Sci 35: 2970–2977.
17. Linnet K (1999) Necessary sample size for method comparison studies based on regression analysis. Clin Chem 45: 882–894.
18. Krouwer JS (2010) Method comparison and bias estimation using patient samples: approved guidelines. Wayne, Pa: Clinical and Laboratory Standards Institute. xx, 56 p.
19. Kwan P, Arzimanoglou A, Berg AT, Brodie MJ, Allen Hauser W, et al. (2010) Definition of drug resistant epilepsy: consensus proposal by the ad hoc Task Force of the ILAE Commission on Therapeutic Strategies. Epilepsia 51: 1069–1077.
20. Ehrnebo M, Odar-Cederlof I (1975) Binding of amobarbital, pentobarbital and diphenylhydantoin to blood cells and plasma proteins in healthy volunteers and uraemic patients. Eur J Clin Pharmacol 8: 445–453.
21. Hinderling PH (1997) Red blood cells: a neglected compartment in pharmacokinetics and pharmacodynamics. Pharmacol Rev 49: 279–295.
22. Driessen O, Treuren L, Meijer JW, Hermans J (1989) Distribution of drugs over whole blood: II. The transport function of whole blood for phenytoin. Ther Drug Monit 11: 390–400.
23. Han S, Kim Y, Jeon J-Y, Hwang M, Im Y-J, et al. (2012) Rapid and Sensitive Analysis of Valproic Acid in Human Red Blood Cell by LC-MS/MS. Bulletin of the Korean Chemical Society 33: 1681–1685.
24. Shirkey RJ, Jellett LB, Kappatos DC, Maling TJ, Macdonald A (1985) Distribution of sodium valproate in normal whole blood and in blood from patients with renal or hepatic disease. Eur J Clin Pharmacol 28: 447–452.
25. Bonneton J, Genton P, Mesdjian E (1992) Distribution of carbamazepine and its epoxide in blood compartments in adolescent and adult epileptic patients. Biopharm Drug Dispos 13: 411–416.
26. Diem K, Lentner C (1975) Documenta Geigy Scientific Tables. Geigy Pharmaceuticals (Ciba-Geigy Ltd.). 617–618 p.
27. Kurata D, Wilkinson GR (1974) Erythrocyte uptake and plasma binding of diphenylhydantoin. Clin Pharmacol Ther 16: 355–362.
28. Hinderling PH (1984) Kinetics of partitioning and binding of digoxin and its analogues in the subcompartments of blood. J Pharm Sci 73: 1042–1053.
29. Driessen O, Treuren L, Meijer JW (1989) Distribution of drugs over whole blood: I. The transport function of whole blood for valproate. Ther Drug Monit 11: 384–389.
30. Highley MS, De Bruijn EA (1996) Erythrocytes and the transport of drugs and endogenous compounds. Pharm Res 13: 186–195.
31. Schanker LS, Johnson JM, Jeffrey JJ (1964) Rapid Passage of Organic Anions into Human Red Cells. Am J Physiol 207: 503–508.
32. Holder LB, Hayes SL (1965) Diffusion of sulfonamides in aqueous buffers and into red cells. Mol Pharmacol 1: 266–279.
33. Hilzenbecher C (1972) Die bindung von pharmaka an human haemoglobin. [Dissertation]. Munich: Ludwig Maximilian University.
34. Svensson C, Nyberg G, Axelsson R, Martensson E (1986) Concentrations of thioridazine and thioridazine metabolites in erythrocytes. Psychopharmacology (Berl) 89: 291–292.
35. Mohammed BS, Cameron GA, Cameron L, Hawksworth GH, Helms PJ, et al. (2010) Can finger-prick sampling replace venous sampling to determine the pharmacokinetic profile of oral paracetamol? Br J Clin Pharmacol 70: 52–56.
36. Graves NM, Holmes GB, Leppik IE, Galligher TK, Parker DR (1987) Quantitative determination of phenytoin and phenobarbital in capillary blood by Ames Seralyzer. Epilepsia 28: 713–716.
37. Haidukewych D, Splane ML, Vasos B (1986) Enzyme immunochromatographic assay of phenytoin in capillary and venous blood compared with fluorescence polarization immunoassay of plasma from epileptic patients. Clin Chem 32: 204.

23

A Novel Glycated Hemoglobin A1c-Lowering Traditional Chinese Medicinal Formula, Identified by Translational Medicine Study

Hsin-Yi Lo[1,9], **Chien-Yun Hsiang**[2,9], **Tsai-Chung Li**[3], **Chia-Cheng Li**[4], **Hui-Chi Huang**[5], **Jaw-Chyun Chen**[6], **Tin-Yun Ho**[1]*

1 Graduate Institute of Chinese Medicine, China Medical University, Taichung, Taiwan, 2 Department of Microbiology, China Medical University, Taichung, Taiwan, 3 Graduate Institute of Biostatistics, China Medical University, Taichung, Taiwan, 4 Graduate Institute of Cancer Biology, China Medical University, Taichung, Taiwan, 5 Department of Chinese Pharmaceutical Sciences and Chinese Medicine Resources, China Medical University, Taichung, Taiwan, 6 Department of Medicinal Botany and Healthcare, Da-Yeh University, Changhua, Taiwan

Abstract

Diabetes is a chronic metabolic disorder that has a significant impact on the health care system. The reduction of glycated hemoglobin A1c is highly associated with the improvements of glycemic control and diabetic complications. In this study, we identified a traditional Chinese medicinal formula with a HbA1c-lowering potential from clinical evidences. By surveying 9,973 diabetic patients enrolled in Taiwan Diabetic Care Management Program, we found that Chu-Yeh-Shih-Kao-Tang (CYSKT) significantly reduced HbA1c values in diabetic patients. CYSKT reduced the levels of HbA1c and fasting blood glucose, and stimulated the blood glucose clearance in type 2 diabetic mice. CYSKT affected the expressions of genes associated with insulin signaling pathway, increased the amount of phosphorylated insulin receptor in cells and tissues, and stimulated the translocation of glucose transporter 4. Moreover, CYSKT affected the expressions of genes related to diabetic complications, improved the levels of renal function indexes, and increased the survival rate of diabetic mice. In conclusion, this was a translational medicine study that applied a "bedside-to-bench" approach to identify a novel HbA1c-lowering formula. Our findings suggested that oral administration of CYSKT affected insulin signaling pathway, decreased HbA1c and blood glucose levels, and consequently reduced mortality rate in type 2 diabetic mice.

Editor: Xiaoying Wang, Massachusetts General Hospital, United States of America

Funding: This work was supported by grants from National Research Program for Biopharmaceuticals (NSC101-2325-B-039-007, NSC102-2325-B-039-007, and MOST103-2325-B-039-002), Ministry of Science and Technology (NSC101-2320-B-039-034-MY3, NSC101-3114-Y-466-002, NSC102-2632-B-039-001-MY3, and MOST103-2815-C-039-044-B), Council of Agriculture (103AS-14.3.2-ST-a1), China Medical University (CMU101-S-21, CMU101-AWARD-09, CMU102-NSC-04, and CMU103-SR-44), and CMU under the Aim for Top University Plan of the Ministry of Education, Taiwan. The funders had no role in study design, data collection and analysis, decision to publish, or preparation of the manuscript.

Competing Interests: The authors have declared that no competing interests exist.

* Email: cyhsiang@mail.cmu.edu.tw

⑨ These authors contributed equally to this work.

Introduction

Diabetes is a major global health concern with a significant rise in prevalence. The diabetic population worldwide is increased dramatically from 153 million in 1980 to 347 million in 2008 [1]. In addition to prevalence, the economic cost for diabetes is also increased. The National Diabetes Information Clearinghouse estimates that diabetes costs $132 billion in United States in 2002 and the cost exceeds $245 billion in 2012 [2]. Therefore, diabetes has a significant impact on the health care system.

Based on the pathogenesis, diabetes is classified into two major categories: type 1 and type 2. Approximately 90–95% of the diabetic cases is type 2 diabetes. Moreover, increasing obesity and reduced activity levels lead to the rapid increased prevalence of type 2 diabetes. Type 2 diabetes displays the phenotype of hyperglycemia which results from insulin resistance and impaired insulin secretion. In addition to hyperglycemia, diabetes leads to both microvascular complications, such as retinopathy, nephrop-athy and neuropathy, and macrovascular complications, such as myocardial infarction and stroke [3–5].

It has been proved that improvement of glycemic control reduces or slows the progression of diabetic complications. For examples, the Diabetes Control and Complications Trial [6] proves that improvement of glycemic control reduces and prevents many of the early diabetic complications, such as retinopathy, microalbuminuria, nephropathy, and neuropathy. In addition, their results predict that individuals with the intensive diabetes management would gain an additional 5.1 years of life expectancy. Glycated hemoglobin A1c (HbA1c) is considered as the gold standard for monitoring glycemic control. A higher amount of HbA1c level indicates a poorer control of blood glucose and a higher prevalence of diabetic complications. Moreover, a regular assessment of HbA1c level in diabetic patients allows the adjustment of patients' drugs or dosages [7,8]. With the increasing use of combination therapy with synthetic drugs and Chinese medicinal formulae in diabetic patients in Taiwan, we proposed that some Chinese medicinal formulae might exhibit HbA1clowering potentials in clinics. Therefore, we applied a translational medicine study to prove our speculation. By surveying the clinical evidences from diabetic patients enrolled in Diabetes Care Management Program, we found that Chu-Yeh-Shih-Kao-Tang (CYSKT) exhibited a HbA1c-lowering potential. The effects of CYSKT on the regulation of HbA1c and blood glucose in type 2 diabetic mice were further elucidated in this study.

Materials and Methods

Materials

Chinese medicinal formula CYSKT was purchased from the GMP pharmaceutical company (Sun Ten Pharmaceutical Co., Taipei, Taiwan). CYSKT was composed of seven ingredients: bamboo leaves (5.1%), gypsum (41%), pinellia rhizome (10.3%), ginseng root (7.7%), licorice root (5.1%), rice (15.4%), and ophiopogon tuber (15.4%). The ethanolic extract of CYSKT was analyzed by high-performance liquid chromatography using glycyrrhizin (Sigma, St. Louis, MO, USA) as a reference standard (Figure S1). The details of high-performance liquid chromatography is described in Text S1. Each gram of freeze-dried extract of CYSKT contained 90 mg of glycyrrhizin.

Study Participants

The clinical data analyzed in this study were obtained from Diabetes Care Management Program, which was launched by Taiwan National Health Insurance Administration. Study participants were patients diagnosed as diabetes with International Classification of Diseases, Nine Revision, Clinical Modification code ICD-9-CM250. A total of 64,878 diabetic patients was enrolled in Diabetes Care Management Program between 2001 and 2004. The selection criteria for this study was that patients had follow-up records for at least one year. A total of 9,973 participants who met the aforementioned criteria was selected in this study. We applied a retrospectic cohort study. The independent variables were patient's age, gender, family, history, health behavior, complications, comorbidities, and Chinese medicinal formula usage. The dependent variable was the change of HbA1c value between baseline and one-year follow-up records of patients. This study was approved by Ethics Review Board of China Medical University Hospital (Permit No. DMR97-IRB-272). Patient records and information were anonymized and de-identified prior to analysis.

Animal Experiments

BALB/c mice were obtained from National Laboratory Animal Center (Taipei, Taiwan). Mouse experiments were conducted under ethics approval from China Medical University Animal Care and Use Committee (Permit No. 101-188-N). Mice were maintained under a 12:12 light-dark cycle with free access to water and food unless indicated.

Mice with type 2 diabetes were generated by a combination of high-fat diet-induced insulin resistances and low-dose streptozotocin-induced defects in insulin secretion [9,10]. Briefly, 4-week-old male BALB/c mice were fed with high-fat diet (TestDiet, St. Louis, MO, USA), in which 60% of energy was from fat. Three weeks later, mice were intraperitoneally injected once with 100 mg/kg streptozotocin and fed with high-fat diet for another 3 weeks. At 10 weeks of age, mice were bled via tail veins after 4 h starvation and blood glucose levels were measured by a glucose oxidase method using a glucometer (ACCU-CHEK Advantage, Roche Diagnostics, Basel, Switzerland). High-fat diet- and streptozotocin-induced mice with fasting blood glucose levels $\geq$ 230 mg/dL were selected and then divided randomly into mock,

CYSKT, TZD, and CYSKT/TZD groups. Normal mice were divided randomly into mock and CYSKT groups. Glucose tolerance test was performed as described previously [11]. Data were expressed as area under the curve (AUC). Serum renal function indexes, such as blood urea nitrogen (BUN) and creatine, were measured using an autoanalyzer (COBAS Mira Plus, Roche Diagnostics, Basel, Switzerland).

Microarray Analysis

Type 2 diabetic mice were given orally with 200 mg/kg CYSKT for 30 consecutive days. Total RNAs were extracted from muscle tissues using RNeasy Mini kit (Qiagen, Valencia, CA, USA) and analyzed for RNA integrity by Agilent 2100 bioanalyzer (Agilent Technologies, Santa Clara, CA, USA). Microarray analysis was performed as described previously [12,13]. Briefly, fluorescence-labeled RNA targets were hybridized to the Mouse Whole Genome OneArray (Phalanx Biotech Group, Hsinchu, Taiwan) and fluorescent signals on the array were scanned by an Axon 4000 scanner (Molecular Devices, Sunnyvale, CA, USA). The fluorescent intensity of each spot was analyzed by genepix 4.1 software (Molecular Devices, Sunnyvale, CA, USA) and normalized by R program in the limma package using quantile normalization. For pathway analysis, normalized data were analyzed using the "geneSetTest" function implemented in the limma package to detect groups of genes in Kyoto Encyclopedia of Genes and Genomes pathways (http://www.genome.jp/kegg/pathway.html). This function computes a p-value to test the hypothesis that the selected genes in the pathway tend to be differentially expressed. For diseases analysis, we built 735 disease-gene sets from genetic association database according to Medical Subject Headings (MeSH) terms (http://www.nlm.nih.gov/mesh/meshhome.html) [14]. We applied "geneSetTest" function to detect groups of genes in MeSH disease terms. This function computes a p-value to test the hypothesis that the selected genes tend to be upregulated or downregulated. Microarray data are MIAME compliant and raw data have been deposited in the Gene Expression Omnibus (Accession number: GSE53119). Number of replicate was three.

Cell Culture and Insulin Receptor (IR)-Binding Assay

HepG2 cells were maintained in Dulbecco's modified Eagle's medium (DMEM) (Invitrogen, Carlsbad, CA, USA) supplemented with 10% fetal bovine serum (Hyclone, Logan, UT, USA). HepG2 cells were cultured in 25-cm^2 flasks at 37°C. After a 24-h incubation, cells were treated with various amounts of CYSKT in DMEM, incubated at 37°C for 10 min, and then solubilized by lysis buffer (1% NP-40, 20 mM Tris-HCl, pH 8.0, 137 mM NaCl, 10% glycerol, 2 mM EDTA, 1 mM sodium orthovanadate, 10 µg/mL aprotinin, 10 µg/mL leupeptin). Cell lysates were centrifuged at 2,000×g for 5 min at 4°C, supernatants were collected, and protein concentrations in supernatants were quantified using a Bradford method (Bio-Rad, Hercules, CA, USA). For in vivo experiment, BALB/c mice were fasted for 18 h and then given orally with various amounts of CYSKT. One hour later, mice were sacrificed, and livers were collected and solubilized by lysis buffer. IR-binding assay was performed using Phospho-IR set (R&D Systems, Minneapolis, MN). The amount of phosphorylated IR was quantified by sandwich enzyme-linked immunosorbent assay (ELISA). The absorbance at 450 nm was measured in an ELISA plate reader.

Immunohistochemical Staining (IHC)

Parafilm-embedded muscle tissues were cut into 5-µm sections, deparaffinized in xylene, and then rehydrated in graded alcohol.

Endogenous peroxidase was quenched with 3% hydrogen peroxide in methanol and the nonspecific binding was blocked with 1% bovine serum albumin. Sections were incubated with rabbit polyclonal antibody against glucose transporter 4 (GLUT-4) (Chemicon, Temecula, CA, USA) at 1:200 dilution overnight at 4°C and then incubated with biotinylated secondary antibody (Zymed Laboratories, South San Francisco, CA, USA) at room temperature for 20 min. Finally, slides were incubated with avidin-biotin complex reagent and stained with 3,3'-diaminobenzidine according to manufacturer's protocol (Histostain-Plus, Zymed Laboratories, South San Francisco, CA, USA). GLUT-4 positive areas were measured using Image-Pro Plus (Media Cybernetics, Bethesda, MD, USA) to quantify the expression of GLUT-4. The proportions of GLUT-4 area (%) were calculated as area occupied with brown color/area of whole field.

Statistical Analysis

Differences in HbA1c values and CYSKT usage were assessed using χ^2 test and further analyzed by multiple linear regression analysis and multiple logistic regression. All analyses were conducted using SAS statistical software version 9.1 (SAS Institute Inc., Cary, NC, USA). Data from cellular and animal experiments were presented as mean ±standard deviation (SD). Student's t test was used for comparisons between two experiments. Results were considered statistically significant if 2-tailed p values were less than 0.05.

Results

Characteristics of Study Participants

A total of 64,878 diabetic patients was enrolled in Diabetic Care Management Program between 2001 and 2004, and a total of 9,973 patients who had follow-up records for at least one year was selected in this study. Details of demographic distribution of participants are shown in Table 1. The average age of participants was 60.52±11.62 years old. The majority (96.72%) of study participants was type 2 diabetes. The average value of HbA1c among all participants was 8.11±1.86% (65±20.3 mmol/mol).

By analyzing the types of medical care of 9,973 patients, we found that 9,444 patients (94.7%) used synthetic drugs alone and 529 patients (5.3%) used both synthetic drugs and medicinal formulae for the treatment of diabetes. The top ten most commonly used Chinese medicinal formulae are shown in Table S1. We further analyzed the relationship between medicinal formula usage and HbA1c levels in type 2 diabetic patients who used both synthetic drugs and medicinal formulae. The HbA1c values of patients taking with CYSKT were significantly reduced in comparison with those taking without CYSKT by multiple linear regression analysis (1.1% vs. 0.14%, $p = 0.0025$). The odds ratio of reduction in HbA1c levels in patients taking with CYSKT was significantly higher (3.55-fold, $p = 0.0036$, 95% confidence intervals) than those taking without CYSKT by multiple logistic regression. Synthetic drugs used in patients taking with CYSKT and the duration of CYSKT administration are shown in Table S2 and Figure S2. These findings suggested that administration of CYSKT might reduce the HbA1c levels in diabetic patients. Therefore, the effects of CYSKT on the regulation of HbA1c and blood glucose levels were analyzed in type 2 diabetic mice.

Effects of CYSKT on HbA1c and Blood Glucose Levels in Type 2 Diabetic Mice

Type 2 diabetic mice were given orally with 200 mg/kg CYSKT for 30 consecutive days and blood samples were collected every 10 days. As shown in Figure 1A, HbA1c levels of mock mice

were approximately 7% (53 mmol/mol). CYSKT significantly lowered the HbA1c levels and the reduction displayed a time-dependent manner. The fasting blood glucose levels were also measured every 10 days and the glucose tolerance test was performed on the 30th day. As shown in Figure 1B, in comparison with mock, CYSKT significantly lowered the fasting blood glucose levels measured on the 10th, 20th, and 30th days. Glucose tolerance test showed that mock group displayed a very poor glucose clearance ability, while oral administration of CYSKT displayed a rapid clearance of glucose (Figure 1C). AUC values were also significantly decreased by CYSKT, in comparison with mock (36360±8104.4 mg/dL·min vs. 70687.5±711.7 mg/dL·min, $p = 0.001865$). In addition to diabetic mice, normal mice were given orally with various amounts (10, 100, and 200 mg/kg) of CYSKT. As shown in Figure 2, the fasting blood glucose level was approximately 70 mg/dL and the blood glucose concentration reached a maximal level at 60 min after glucose challenge. Mock group displayed a poor glucose clearance. Oral administration of CYSKT significantly stimulated the blood glucose clearance and the stimulation displayed a dose-dependent manner. These data indicated that CYSKT alone exhibited HbA1c-lowering and hypoglycemic effects in normal and type 2 diabetic mice.

Analysis of HbA1c-Lowering and Hypoglycemic Mechanisms of CYSKT in Type 2 Diabetic Mice

To elucidate the hypoglycemic mechanism of CYSKT, we collected muscle tissues from type 2 diabetic mice given orally with 200 mg/kg CYSKT for 30 consecutive days, extracted RNA samples from muscle tissues, and performed microarray analysis. In a total of 29,922 transcripts, 283 transcripts with fold change ≥

Table 1. Demographic information of participants in this study.

Variable	Population ($n=9,973$)	
	Number	Percentage
Age intervals		
<40 y	389	3.90
40–50 y	1,299	13.03
50–60 y	2,603	26.10
60–70 y	3,297	33.06
>70 y	2,385	23.91
Type of diabetes		
Type 1	162	1.62
Type 2	9,646	96.72
Other	71	0.71
Loss	94	0.95
HbA1c value		
<7% (53 mmol/mol)	3,050	30.58
≥7% (53 mmol/mol)	6,844	68.63
Loss	79	0.79
History intervals		
0–10 y	7,139	71.58
>10 y	2,781	27.89
Loss	53	0.53

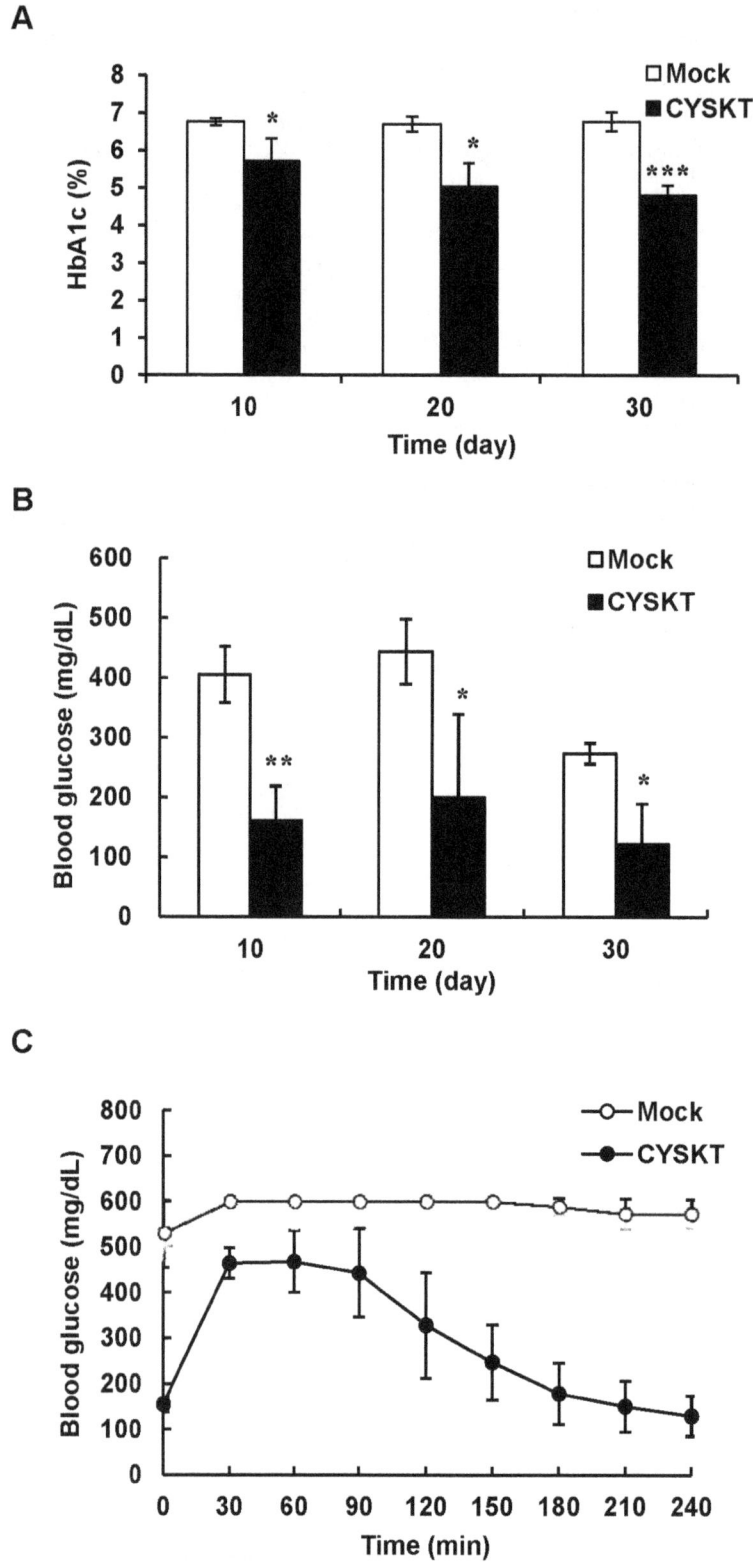

Figure 1. Effects of CYSKT on the levels of HbA1c and blood glucose in type 2 diabetic mice. Type 2 diabetic mice were administered orally 200 mg/kg CYSKT for 30 consecutive days. Blood samples were collected every 10 days and measured for HbA1c levels (A) and fasting blood glucose levels (B). Glucose tolerance test was performed on 30th day after CYSKT administration. Mice were fasted for 4 h, glucose (1 g/kg) was injected intraperitoneally, and the blood glucose levels at intervals were measured (C). Values are mean $\pm$ SD ($n = 5$). *$p < 0.05$, **$p < 0.01$, ***$p < 0.001$, compared with mock.

A

B

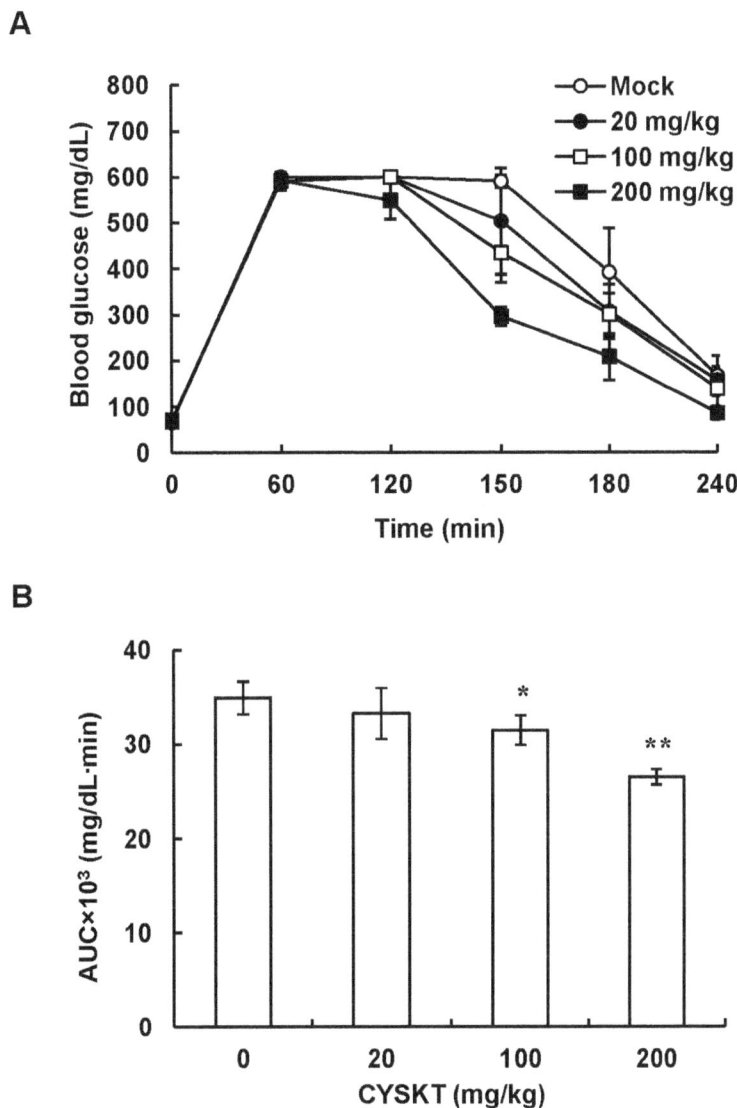

Figure 2. Effect of CYSKT on blood glucose levels in normal mice. Normal mice were administered orally various amounts of CYSKT. Glucose (4 g/kg) was injected intraperitoneally 15 min later, blood samples were collected at intervals, and blood glucose levels were measured by a glucometer (A). (B) AUC of glucose tolerance assay. Values are mean ± SD ($n = 5$). *$p < 0.05$, **$p < 0.01$, compared with mock.

1.5 or ≤ -1.5 were selected for pathway analysis. A total of 69 pathways was significantly regulated by CYSKT and the affected pathways involved in glucose and lipid metabolism are shown in Table 2. CYSKT significantly affected insulin, insulin-like growth factor, peroxisome proliferator-activated receptors (PPAR), free fatty acid, leptin, and adipocytokine signaling pathways. CYSKT also significantly regulated citrate cycle and fatty acid metabolism. These data suggested that CYSKT might regulate HbA1c and blood glucose levels via insulin signaling pathway.

We further analyzed effects of CYSKT on IR activation and GLUT-4 translocation. We treated HepG2 cells, which have been known to express IR on cell membranes, with CYSKT and measured the amounts of phosphorylated IR by ELISA. As shown in Figure 3A (left panel), insulin significantly increased the levels of phosphorylated IR. CYSKT also stimulated the phosphorylation of IR and the maximal induction was achieved by 5 µg/mL CYSKT. In addition to HepG2 cells, we also analyzed the amounts of phosphorylated IR in livers of normal mice. As shown

in Figure 3A (right panel), the amounts of phospho-IR in livers were significantly increased by CYSKT in a dose-dependent manner. These data suggested that CYSKT might interact physically with IR and stimulate the phosphorylation of IR. Buts et al [15] indicate that enterocytes of rodents express IR. Because CYSKT was administered orally and we proposed that CYSKT might activate IR signaling pathway, we chose small intestinet for the IR phosphorylation experiment. In addition, oral administration of 200 mg/kg CYSKT for 30 days also significantly increased the levels of phosphorylated IR in intestines and muscles of type 2 diabetic mice (Figure 3B). These findings suggested that CYSKT activated insulin signaling pathway by stimulating the phosphorylation of IR. Following IR phosphorylation, GLUT-4, an insulin-dependent glucose transporter, is translocated into cell membrane and uptakes blood glucose into cells. We therefore analyzed the translocation of GLUT-4 in muscle by IHC. Figure 3C shows that, in comparison with mock, there were many immuno-reactive cells in CYSKT-treated muscle tissues. The proportions of GLUT-

Table 2. Pathways significantly regulated by CYSKT in type 2 diabetic mice*.

Pathway[†]	p value[‡]
Citrate cycle	1.45×10^{-9}
Insulin signaling pathway	0.000117
Insulin-like growth factor signaling pathway	0.000142
PPAR signaling pathway	0.000311
Fatty acid metabolism	0.000747
Free fatty acid signaling pathway	0.001233
Fatty acid elongation in mitochondria	0.001549
Glycerolipid metabolism	0.008970
Leptin signaling pathway	0.018841
Adipocytokine signaling pathway	0.040090

*Type 2 diabetic mice were given orally with 200 mg/kg CYSKT for 30 consecutive days. Total RNAs were extracted from muscle tissues and analyzed by microarray.
[†]Pathways associated with glucose and lipid metabolism are shown.
[‡]p values were calculated by geneSetTest function implemented in the limma package.

4 area (%) were $27.2 \pm 4.8\%$ in mock group and $84.9 \pm 9.7\%$ in CYSKT group ($p < 0.001$). These data suggested that CYSKT exhibited HbA1c-lowering and hypoglycemic effects by activating the phosphorylation of IR and enhancing the translocation of GLUT-4 to the cell membrane.

Effects of CYSKT on Diabetic Complications and Survival Rate in Type 2 Diabetic Mice

The reduction of HbA1c is highly associated with the improvement of glycemic control and diabetic complications. The effects of CYSKT on diabetic complications were further analyzed by gene expression profiling, renal function indexes, and survival rate. Type 2 diabetic mice were given orally with 200 mg/ kg CYSKT for 30 consecutive days, and RNA samples from muscle and serum samples were collected for microarray and serum biochemical analyzes, respectively. By analyzing the similarity between CYSKT-affected genes and disease-affected genes, we found that 55 terms were significantly affected by CYSKT among 735 tested MeSH disease terms. CYSKT affected genes associated with diabetes (Table 3). It also affected gene sets involved in diabetic complications, such as retinopathy, nephropathy, neuropathy, and cardiovascular disorders. These data indicated that CYSKT might affect the progression of diabetic complications. We further analyzed the levels of BUN and creatinine in sera. CYSKT significantly decreased the levels of BUN and creatinine (Figure 4A), suggesting that CYSKT might improve the diabetic renal complications in type 2 diabetic mice. It is known that the improvement of diabetic complications prolongs the lifespan of diabetic patients [4]. Therefore, we administered type 2 diabetic mice with 200 mg/kg CYSKT for 120 days and observed the number of death daily. As shown in Figure 4B, the survival rate of mock and CYSKT groups were 5/10 and 10/10, respectively, at the end of experiments. In addition, the survival rate of CYSKT treatment was similar to those of thiazolidinedione (TZD) treatment (8/10) and TZD/CYSKT combinatory therapy (9/10). Moreover, in comparison with mock, administration of CYSKT in CYSKT and CYSKT/TZD groups decreased the levels of HbA1c (Figure S3). These data suggested that CYSKT regulated HbA1c and blood glucose values, improved diabetic

complications, and consequently decreased the mortality rate of type 2 diabetic mice.

Discussion

In this study, we performed a translational medicine research on a traditional Chinese medicinal formula CYSKT. By surveying the medical usage of diabetic patients enrolled in Diabetes Care Management Program and analyzing the association between medical usage and HbA1c values, we found that CYSKT exhibited a HbA1c-lowering potential in diabetic patients. We chose the changes of HbA1c values instead of fasting blood glucose levels as the dependent variable because HbA1c is considered as the gold standard for monitoring glycemic control [7,8]. The formation of HbA1c mainly depends on the interaction between blood glucose concentrations and life span of red blood cells. Therefore, HbA1c value represents the average blood glucose level of a patient in past 2 to 3 months [16,17]. In addition, clinical studies indicate that reduction in HbA1c values directly reflects the improvement of diabetic complications. For examples, a 37% reduction in combined microvascular complications, a 21% reduction in diabetes-related deaths, and a 14% decrease in combined fatal and nonfatal myocardial infarction are noted for every 1% reduction in HbA1c value. Moreover, the strict glycemic control and the reduction of HbA1c to 7% (53 mmol/mol) or less lead to a decreased incidence of microvascular and macrovascular complications [18–20].

The increasing use of complementary and alternative medicine among the general public has been noticed [21]. By surveying the medical choice of patients, we also found that, although there are several synthetic drugs available for diabetes, there are 5.3% of study participants used both synthetic drugs and medicinal formulae for the treatment of diabetes. The use of medicinal formulae or herbs has the advantage that they do not cause significant side effects, in comparison with synthetic drugs. For examples, metformin may increase the risk of lactic acidosis and gastrointestinal side effects [22], while sulfonylurea treatment may result in a significant hypoglycemia or weight gain [23]. Chinese medicinal herbs have been used in the clinics for the treatment of diabetes for years. Yeh et al [24] review the clinical researches and find that *Coccinia indica* and American *ginseng* decrease the levels of fasting blood glucose and HbA1c in patients [25,26]. *Gymnema sylvestre*, *Aloe vera*, and *Momordica charantia* also display the clinical effectiveness in patients in nonrandomized trials or short-term metabolic trials [27–29]. Therefore, we tried to figure out the Chinese medicinal formulae with HbA1c-lowering potential from clinical data, and our findings suggested that CYSKT was a candidate because diabetic patients taking with CYSKT showed lower HbA1c levels than those taking without CYSKT.

CYSKT is a traditional Chinese medicinal formula that has been used for the treatment of respiratory diseases and diabetes in China for years. It is comprised of seven ingredients. The major ingredient of CYSKT is gypsum, followed by ophiopogon tuber, rice, pinellia rhizome, ginseng root, bamboo leaves, and licorice root. So far, several ingredients of CYSKT have showed the hypoglycemic effects in diabetic animals or patients. For examples, the polysaccharide from the tuber of *Ophiopogon japonicus* improves glucose tolerance and impaired insulin secretion via phosphatidylinositide 3-kinase (PI3K)/Akt pathway in diabetic animals [30]. It also protects diabetes-caused hepatol and renal injuries via antioxidant ability in rats [31]. Ginseng, the root of *Panax ginseng*, alleviates the hyperglycemia and insulin resistance of type 2 diabetic animals [32]. The anti-diabetic effects of ginseng have also been reported in the clinical trials [33]. Licorice root, the

A

B

C

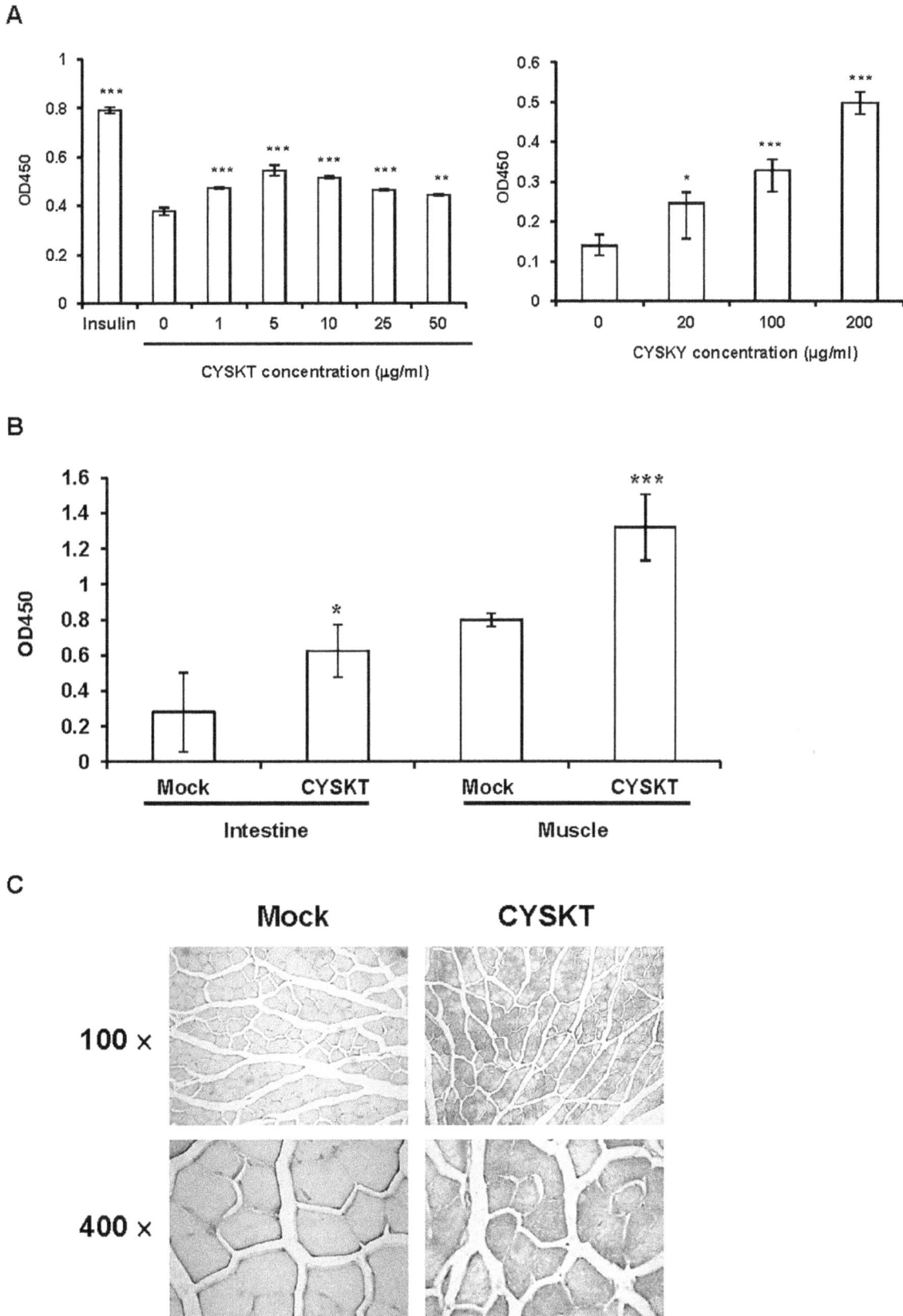

Figure 3. Effects of CYSKT on IR phosphorylation and GLUT-4 translocation. (A) Phospho-IR ELISA. Left panel: HepG2 cells were treated with 0.5 μM insulin or various amounts of CYSKT. Ten minutes later, cellular proteins were collected and the levels of phosphorylated IR were measured by ELISA. Values are mean ± SD (*n* = 6). Right panel: BALC/c mice were given orally with various amounts of CYSKT. One hour later, mice

were sacrificed, and livers were collected for analysis. Values are mean ± SD ($n = 6$). *$p < 0.05$, ***$p < 0.001$, compared with mock. (B) Phospho-IR ELISA. Type 2 diabetic mice were administered orally 200 mg/kg CYSKT for 30 days. Proteins were extracted from intestines and muscles, and the levels of phosphorylated IR were measured by ELISA. Values are mean ± SD ($n = 5$). *$p < 0.05$, **$p < 0.01$, ***$p < 0.001$, compared with mock. (C) IHC. Type 2 diabetic mice were administered orally 200 mg/kg CYSKT for 30 consecutive days. Muscle tissues were collected and the sections were stained by IHC using antibody against GLUT-4 ($100 \times$ and $400 \times$ magnification). Photos are representative images ($n = 5$).

radix of *Glycyrrhiza uralensis*, enhances the insulin-stimulated glucose uptake through PPAR-γ activation in 3T3-L1 cells and improves the glucose tolerance in diabetic animals [34]. In this study, we found that CYSKT steadily decreased the levels of blood glucose and HbA1c in type 2 diabetic mice. The ingredients, such ophiopogon tuber, ginseng root and licorice root, might be responsible for the hypoglycemic effect of CYSKT.

Type 2 diabetes is characterized by both insulin resistance and impaired insulin secretion. Insulin secretagogues like sulfonylureas are used to stimulate insulin secretion by interacting with the ATP-sensitive potassium channel on the pancreatic beta cells. TZDs bind to PPAR-γ nuclear receptor and improve the insulin resistance [35]. In this study, we suggested that CYSKT ameliorated the hypoglycemic status of type 2 diabetic mice by activating the autophosphorylation of IR. IR is a transmembrane protein which exhibits tyrosine kinase activity. Upon binding of insulin to the extracellular domain of IR, the tyrosine kinase is activated and then proceeded the autophosphorylation of IR and

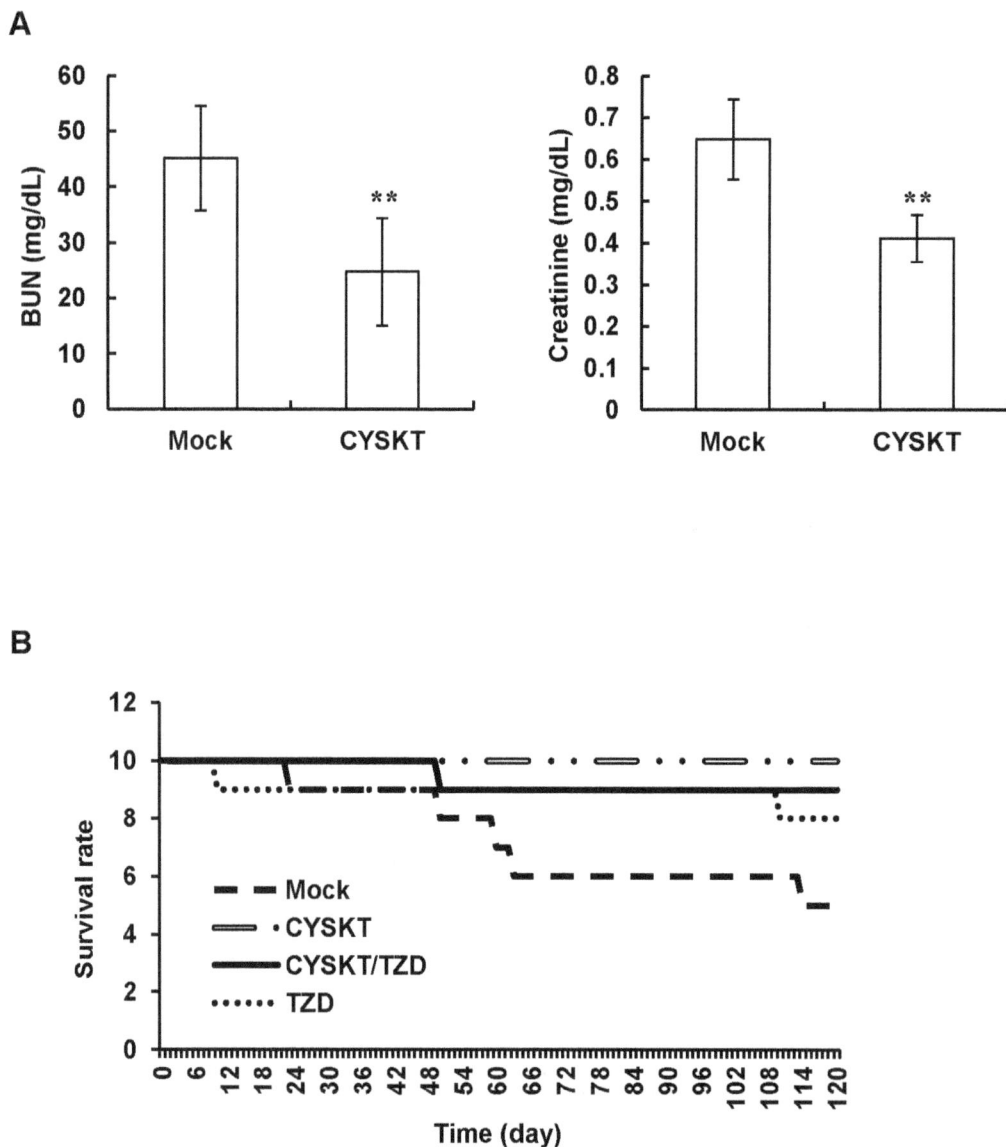

Figure 4. Effects of CYSKT on renal function indexes and survival rate in type 2 diabetic mice. (A) CYSKT (200 mg/kg) was orally given to type 2 diabetic mice for 30 consecutive days. The levels of BUN and creatinine in sera were measured by an autoanalyzer. Values are mean ± SD ($n = 5$). **$p < 0.01$, compared with mock. (B) Long-term survival rate. Type 2 diabetic mice were administered orally with 200 mg/kg CYSKT and/or 20 mg/kg TZD for 120 consecutive days. The number of death was observed daily.

Table 3. Gene-expression connection of CYSKT treatments with disease states*.

MeSH disease term	p value[†]
Diabetes mellitus, type 2	0.0012
Uremia	0.0035
Macular degeneration	0.0045
Diabetic retinopathy	0.0079
Diabetic angiopathies	0.0092
Myocardial ischemia	0.0126
Coronary vasospasm	0.0204
Heart diseases	0.0375

*Type 2 diabetic mice were given orally with 200 mg/kg CYSKT for 30 consecutive days. Total RNAs were extracted from muscle tissues and analyzed by microarray.
[†]p values were calculated by geneSetTest function implemented in the limma package.

cellular proteins, which leads to the activation of PI3K and translocation of GLUT-4 [36]. CYSKT increased the amount of phosphorylated IR and stimulated the translocation of GLUT-4 to cell membrane suggested that CYSKT might bind to IR, activate the phosphorylation of IR, and stimulate the down-stream signaling pathway. In our previous study, we have identified that the protein component from *Momordica charantia* binds to IR, activates the insulin signaling pathway, and lowers the blood glucose levels in diabetic mice [11]. Zhao et al [37] have also found that Chinese medicinal herbs containing berberine exhibit sustained antidiabetic effects via altering hepatic gene expression. We suggested that the chemical or protein constituents of CYSKT might bind to IR and then improve the insulin resistance in type 2 diabetic mice.

In conclusion, we applied a translational medicine study to figure out that CYSKT exhibited the HbA1c-lowering potential by surveying 9,973 patients enrolled in Diabetes Care Management Program. Our data showed that CYSKT indeed was a HbA1c-lowering formula that steadily decreased the levels of HbA1c and blood glucose by activating the insulin signaling

pathway and enhancing the translocation of GLUT-4 to the cell membrane, and consequently reduced the mortality in type 2 diabetic mice.

Supporting Information

Figure S1 HPLC chromatograph of CYSKT using glycyrrhizin as a reference standard. (A) The chromatogram of ethanolic extract of CYSKT. (B) The chromatogram of glycyrrhizin standard. The retention time of glycyrrhizin was 47.3 min. Arrow indicate the peaks representing glycyrrhizin.

Figure S2 The duration of CYSKT administration and HbA1c measurement in diabetic patients. Rectangle represents the duration of CYSKT administration. Triangle represents the time of HbA1c measurement. The number below each triangle represents the HbA1c value (%).

Figure S3 Effects of CYSKT on the HbA1c levels in type 2 diabetic mice. Type 2 diabetic mice were administered orally with 200 mg/kg CYSKT and/or 20 mg/kg TZD for 120 consecutive days. Sixty days after CYSKT administration, blood samples were collected every 30 days and measured for HbA1c levels. Values are mean $\pm$ SD ($n = 5$).

Author Contributions

Conceived and designed the experiments: HYL CYH TYH. Performed the experiments: HYL CCL HCH JCC. Analyzed the data: CYH TCL TYH. Wrote the paper: HYL CYH TYH.

References

1. Danaei G, Finucane MM, Lu Y, Singh GM, Cowan MJ, et al. (2011) National, regional, and global trends in fasting plasma glucose and diabetes prevalence since 1980: systematic analysis of health examination surveys and epidemiological studies with 370 country-years and 2.7 million participants. Lancet 378: 31–40.
2. American Diabetes Association (2013) Economic costs of diabetes in the U.S. in 2012. Diabetes Care 36: 1033–1046.
3. American Diabetes Association (2013) Diagnosis and classification of diabetes mellitus. Diabetes Care 36: S67–74.
4. Hu FB (2011) Globalization of diabetes: the role of diet, lifestyle, and genes. Diabetes Care 34: 1249–1257.
5. Powers AC (2012) Diabetes mellitus. In: Longo DL, Fauci AS, Kasper DL, Hauser SL, Jameson JL, Loscalzo J, editors. Harrison's principles of internal medicine. New York: The McGraw-Hill Companies, Inc. pp. 2275–2304.
6. The Diabetes Control and Complications Trial Research Group (1993) The effect of intensive treatment of diabetes on the development and progression of long-term complications in insulin-dependent diabetes mellitus. N Eng J Med 329: 977–986.
7. Kilpatrick ES (2008) Haemoglobin A1c in the diagnosis and monitoring of diabetes mellitus. J Clin Pathol 61: 977–982.
8. Zhang X, Gregg EW, Williamson DF, Barker LE, Thomas W, et al. (2010) A1C level and future risk of diabetes: a systematic review. Diabetes Care 33: 1665–1673.
9. Luo J, Quan J, Tsai J, Hobensack CK, Sullivan C, et al. (1998). Nongenetic mouse models of non-insulin-dependent diabetes mellitus. Metabolism 47: 663–668.
10. Mu J, Woods J, Zhou YP, Roy RS, Li Z, et al. (2006) Chronic inhibition of dipeptidyl peptidase-4 with a sitagliptin analog preserves pancreatic beta-cell mass and function in a rodent model of type 2 diabetes. Diabetes 55: 1695–1704.
11. Lo HY, Ho TY, Lin C, Li CC, Hsiang CY (2013) *Momordica charantia* and its novel polypeptide regulate glucose homeostasis in mice via binding to insulin receptor. J Agric Food Chem 61: 2461–2468.
12. Chang CT, Ho TY, Lin H, Liang JA, Huang HC, et al. (2012) 5-Fluorouracil induced intestinal mucositis via nuclear factor-κB activation by transcriptomic analysis and *in vivo* bioluminescence imaging. PLoS ONE 7: e31808.
13. Li CC, Lo HY, Hsiang CY, Ho TY (2012) DNA microarray analysis as a tool to investigate the therapeutic mechanisms and drug development of Chinese medicinal herbs. BioMedicine 2: 10–16.
14. Becker KG, Barnes KC, Bright TJ, Wang SA (2004) The genetic association database. Nature Genet 36: 431–432.
15. Buts JP, De Keyser N, Marandi S, Maernoudt AS, Sokal EM, et al. (1997) Expression of insulin receptors and of 60-kDa receptor substrate in rat mature and immature enterocytes. Am J Physiol 273: G217–G226.
16. Bunn HF, Gabbay KH, Gallop PM (1978) The glycosylation of hemoglobin: relevance to diabetes mellitus. Science 200: 21–27.
17. Bunn HF, Haney DN, Kamin S, Gabbay KH, Gallop PM (1976) The biosynthesis of human hemoglobin A1c. Slow glycosylation of hemoglobin *in vivo*. J Clin Invest 57: 1652–1659.

18. United Kingdom Prospective Diabetes Study (UKPDS) Group (1998) Intensive blood-glucose control with sulphonylureas or insulin compared with conventional treatment and risk of complications in patients with type 2 diabetes (UKPDS 33). Lancet 352: 837–853.

19. Stratton IM, Adler AI, Neil HA, Matthews DR, Manley SE, et al. (2000) Association of glycaemia with macrovascular and microvascular complications of type 2 diabetes (UKPDS 35): prospective observational study. BMJ 321: 405–412.

20. Nathan DM, Cleary PA, Backlund JY, Genuth SM, Lachin JM, et al. (2005) Intensive diabetes treatment and cardiovascular disease in patients with type 1 diabetes. N Engl J Med 353: 2643–2653.

21. Frass M, Strassl RP, Friehs H, Müllner M, Kundi M, et al. (2012) Use and acceptance of complementary and alternative medicine among the general population and medical personnel: a systematic review. Ochsner J 12: 45–56.

22. Ali S, Fonseca V (2012) Overview of metformin: special focus on metformin extended release. Expert Opin Pharmacother 13: 1797–1805.

23. Gallwitz B, Rosenstock J, Rauch T, Bhattacharya S, Patel S, et al. (2012) 2-year efficacy and safety of linagliptin compared with glimepiride in patients with type 2 diabetes inadequately controlled on metformin: a randomised, double-blind, non-inferiority trial. Lancet 380: 475–483

24. Yeh GY, Eisenberg DM, Kaptchuk TJ, Phillips RS (2003) Systematic review of herbs and dietary supplements for glycemic control in diabetes. Diabetes Care 26: 1277–1294.

25. Sotaniemi EA, Haapakoski E, Rautio A (1995) Ginseng therapy in non-insulin dependent diabetic patients: effects on psychophysical performance, glucose homeostasis, serum lipids, serum aminoterminalpropeptide concentration, and body weight. Diabetes Care 18: 1373–1375.

26. Kamble SM, Jyotishi GS, Kamlakar PL, Vaidya SM (1996) Efficacy of *Coccinia indica* W.& A in diabetes mellitus. J Res Ayurveda Siddha XVII: 77–84.

27. Leatherdale BA, Panesar RK, Singh G, Atkins TW, Bailey CJ, et al. (1981) Improvement in glucose tolerance due to *Momordica charantia* (karela). Br Med J 282: 1823–1824.

28. Ghannam N, Kingston M, Al-Meshaal IA, Tariq M, Parman NS, et al. (1986) The antidiabetic activity of aloes: preliminary clinical and experimental observations. Horm Res 24: 288–294.

29. Shanmugasundaram ERB, Rajeswari G, Baskaran K, Kumar BRR, Shanmugasundaram KR, et al. (1990) Use of *Gymnema sylvestre* leaf extract in the control of blood glucose in insulin-dependent diabetes mellitus. J Ethnopharmacology 30: 281–294.

30. Wang LY, Wang Y, Xu DS, Ruan KF, Feng Y, et al. (2012) MDG-1, a polysaccharide from *Ophiopogon japonicus* exerts hypoglycemic effects through the PI3K/Akt pathway in a diabetic KKAy mouse model. J Ethnopharmacol 143: 347–354.

31. Chen X, Tang J, Xie W, Wang J, Jin J, et al. (2013) Protective effect of the polysaccharide from *Ophiopogon japonicus* on streptozotocin-induced diabetic rats. Carbohydr Polym 94: 378–385.

32. Liu Z, Li W, Li X, Zhang M, Chen L, et al. (2013) Antidiabetic effects of malonyl ginsenosides from *Panax ginseng* on type 2 diabetic rats induced by high-fat diet and streptozotocin. J Ethnopharmacol 145: 233–240.

33. Vuksan V, Sung MK, Sievenpiper JL, Stavro PM, Jenkins AL, et al. (2008) Korean red ginseng (*Panax ginseng*) improves glucose and insulin regulation in well-controlled, type 2 diabetes: results of a randomized, double-blind, placebo-controlled study of efficacy and safety. Nutr Metab Cardiovasc Dis 18: 46–56.

34. Mae T, Kishida H, Nishiyama T, Tsukagawa M, Konishi E, et al. (2003) A licorice ethanolic extract with peroxisome proliferator-activated receptor-gamma ligand-binding activity affects diabetes in KK-Ay mice, abdominal obesity in diet-induced obese C57BL mice and hypertension in spontaneously hypertensive rats. J Nutr 133: 3369–3377.

35. Stein SA, Lamos EM, Davis SN (2013) A review of the efficacy and safety of oral antidiabetic drugs. Expert Opin Drug Saf 12: 153–175.

36. Saltiel AR, Kahn CR (2001) Insulin signalling and the regulation of glucose and lipid metabolism. Nature 414: 799–806.

37. Zhao HL, Sui Y, Qiao CF, Yip KY, Leung RK, et al. (2012) Sustained antidiabetic effects of a berberine-containing Chinese herbal medicine through regulation of hepatic gene expression. Diabetes 61: 933–943.

24

A *Yersinia pestis tat* Mutant Is Attenuated in Bubonic and Small-Aerosol Pneumonic Challenge Models of Infection but Not As Attenuated by Intranasal Challenge

Joel Bozue[1]*, Christopher K. Cote[1], Taylor Chance[2], Jeffrey Kugelman[3], Steven J. Kern[4], Todd K. Kijek[1], Amy Jenkins[1], Sherry Mou[1], Krishna Moody[1], David Fritz[1], Camenzind G. Robinson[2], Todd Bell[2], Patricia Worsham[1]

1 Bacteriology Division, The United States Army of Medical Research Institute of Infectious Diseases, Fort Detrick, Maryland, United States of America, 2 Pathology Division, The United States Army of Medical Research Institute of Infectious Diseases, Fort Detrick, Maryland, United States of America, 3 Center for Genome Sciences, The United States Army of Medical Research Institute of Infectious Diseases, Fort Detrick, Maryland, United States of America, 4 Office of Research Support, The United States Army of Medical Research Institute of Infectious Diseases, Fort Detrick, Maryland, United States of America

Abstract

Bacterial proteins destined for the Tat pathway are folded before crossing the inner membrane and are typically identified by an N-terminal signal peptide containing a twin arginine motif. Translocation by the Tat pathway is dependent on the products of genes which encode proteins possessing the binding site of the signal peptide and mediating the actual translocation event. In the fully virulent CO92 strain of *Yersinia pestis*, the *tatA* gene was deleted. The mutant was assayed for loss of virulence through various *in vitro* and *in vivo* assays. Deletion of the *tatA* gene resulted in several consequences for the mutant as compared to wild-type. Cell morphology of the mutant bacteria was altered and demonstrated a more elongated form. In addition, while cultures of the mutant strain were able to produce a biofilm, we observed a loss of adhesion of the mutant biofilm structure compared to the biofilm produced by the wild-type strain. Immuno-electron microscopy revealed a partial disruption of the F1 antigen on the surface of the mutant. The virulence of the Δ*tatA* mutant was assessed in various murine models of plague. The mutant was severely attenuated in the bubonic model with full virulence restored by complementation with the native gene. After small-particle aerosol challenge in a pneumonic model of infection, the mutant was also shown to be attenuated. In contrast, when mice were challenged intranasally with the mutant, very little difference in the LD$_{50}$ was observed between wild-type and mutant strains. However, an increased time-to-death and delay in bacterial dissemination was observed in mice infected with the Δ*tatA* mutant as compared to the parent strain. Collectively, these findings demonstrate an essential role for the Tat pathway in the virulence of *Y. pestis* in bubonic and small-aerosol pneumonic infection but less important role for intranasal challenge.

Editor: Mikael Skurnik, University of Helsinki, Finland

Funding: The research described herein was sponsored by the Defense Threat Reduction Agency JSTO-CBD (project number 923698). The funders had no role in study design, data collection and analysis, decision to publish, or preparation of the manuscript.

Competing Interests: The authors have declared that no competing interests exist.

* Email: joel.a.bozue@us.army.mil

Introduction

Yersinia pestis is the causative agent of plague and primarily a disease of rodents, transmitted typically by fleas. Clinical forms of the disease in humans are bubonic, septicemic, and pneumonic. Humans most often become infected by fleabites which manifests in the bubonic form of plague and is characterized by painful local lymphadenopathy, referred to as a bubo. Infection of the lymph node may disseminate throughout the body leading to septicemic plague. *Y. pestis* may also reach the lungs and lead to the pneumonic form of plague which could be spread human-to-human by the respiratory route. Pneumonic plague is the most severe and frequently fatal form of the disease [1,2].

Similar to other bacteria, *Yersinia* species have several mechanisms for the transport and secretion of proteins. The most studied of these mechanisms is the type III secretion system which delivers *Yersinia* outer proteins (Yops) into host cells [3–5]. The general method bacteria, including *Yersinia*, use for secretion is the Sec system which transports proteins across the cytoplasmic membrane in an unfolded state [6]. In contrast to the Sec system, twin arginine translocation (Tat) system delivers folded proteins into the periplasm, using the proton motive force at the membrane [7]. Proteins to be translocated by the Tat system typically have a consensus signal sequence containing twin arginines at the N-terminal signal peptide. The genes encoding the Tat system include *tatA*, *tatB*, *tatC*, and *tatD* which may or may not be associated in an operon, depending on the bacterium. The TatB and TatC proteins possess the primary binding site of the signal peptide of the protein directed for translocation [8–10]; whereas TatA mediates the actual translocation event [11,12]. Recent evidence also suggests that TatE may also play some role in the transport of Tat substrates [13]. Interestingly, the TatD protein is located within the cytoplasm and possesses DNase activity but is not required for Tat translocation of proteins [14].

The Tat system has been shown to be important for virulence in both animal and plant pathogens [15–25], including *Yersinia pseudotuberculosis* [26]. Therefore, the Tat system represents a potential therapeutic target for a wide range of bacterial pathogens. To determine what role this translocation system may play in virulence in *Y. pestis*, we deleted the *tatA* gene from the chromosome of the fully virulent CO92 strain [27] and found several dramatic phenotypic effects.

Materials and Methods

Bacterial strains and medium

The *Escherichia coli* and *Y. pestis* strains and plasmids used in this study are listed in Table 1. All *E. coli* strains were grown at 37°C on Luria-Bertani (LB) plates or in LB broth, and when needed, ampicillin was included at 50 µg/mL. For routine growth, the CO92 strain of *Y. pestis* was maintained on sheep blood agar plates or in heart infusion (HI) broth at 28°C. When grown at 37°C, medium was supplemented with either 2.5 mM $CaCl_2$ or 20 mM $MgCl_2$ and 20 mM sodium oxalate (MOX), as indicated. Selection of *Y. pestis* cointegrants or mutant strains occurred on LB Lennox agar (L2897; Sigma-Aldrich; Saint Louis, MO) plates supplemented with ampicillin (50 µg/mL) or 5% sucrose, as needed. To verify that the mutant retained the *pgm* locus, *Y. pestis* strains were screened on Congo Red agar plates [28]. To confirm that the bacteria isolated following animal challenges was *Y. pestis*, bacteria were screened on *Yersinia* selective agar plates which contains cefsulodin, irgasan, and novobiocin (R01988; Remel, Inc; Lenexa, KS).

USAMRIID is compliant with all federal and Department of Defense regulations pertaining to the use of Select Agents.

Growth assays

Growth assays were performed in HI broth at 28°C or 37°C with either $CaCl_2$ or MOX, as indicated. Assays were performed using an Infinite M200 pro (Tecan; Männedorf, Switzerland)

microplate reader in 96-well microtiter plates. The OD_{600} was measured every 60 min. For all assays, the bacterial strains were grown overnight at 28°C in HI broth and resuspended in fresh HI broth (alone or with $CaCl_2$ or MOX as indicated) at an OD_{600} of ~0.1. The resuspended cultures were diluted 1:1 into the respective HI broth. For the assays performed at 37°C, the cultures were initially incubated at 28°C for 1 h for strain acclimation and then increased to 37°C. All samples were performed in quadruplicate and included medium controls to confirm sterility and for use as blanks to calculate the absorbance of the cultures. Additional well samples were included to monitor the increase of CFUs over the course of the growth study.

Mutant construction

A fragment of DNA containing the *tatA* gene was PCR amplified (Table 2) using Phusion Taq polymerase (New England Biolabs, Inc.; Ipswich, MA) from genomic DNA from the CO92 strain of *Y. pestis*. The PCR product was ligated into pJET1.2 (Fermentas, Inc.; Glen Burnie, Maryland). The *tatA* gene was removed from the plasmid in-frame through inverse PCR (Table 2) while retaining the first and last three nucleotides of the gene. The *Y. pestis* DNA containing the deleted *tatA* gene was excised as an EcoRI fragment and cloned into pWSK30 [29]. The insert was then sub-cloned as a SacI-SalI fragment into vector pCDV422 [30].

Construction of the *Y. pestis* Δ*tatA* mutant was performed by the procedure as previously described [5,31]. Briefly, the pCDV422+Δ*tatA* plasmid was introduced by electroporation into electrocompetent *Y. pestis* [32]. Cointegrates were selected on LB agar plates containing ampicillin. The cointegrate strain was grown overnight in HI broth and plated on LB agar plates containing 5% sucrose to select for allelic exchange recombinants. Deletion mutants of Δ*tatA* were identified by PCR (Table 2). The presence of the *Y. pestis* virulence plasmids was confirmed via PCR (Table 2). The Δ*tatA* mutant strain was next passaged through Swiss Webster mice by subcutaneous challenge, as routinely

Table 1. Strains and Plasmids.

	Relevant Characteristics	Reference/Source
E. coli strains		
DH5α		NEB
TransforMax EC100D	*pir*-116	EPICENTRE
Y. pestis CO92 strains		
wild-type	fully virulent	[27]
Δ*tatA*	*tatA* in-frame deletion mutant	this study
Δ*tatA*/pJET1.2+*tatA*	complemented Δ*tatA* mutant	this study
CO92-C12	F1 antigen negative strain	[57]
CO92 pLcr⁻	pLcr negative strain	USAMRIID collection
Plasmid		
pJET1.2	PCR cloning vector	Fermentas, Inc
pJET1.2+*tatA*	contains DNA fragment of *tatA* gene and flanking sequence	this study
pJET1.2+ Δ*tatA*	deletion of *tatA* from DNA fragment	this study
pWSK30	low copy *E. coli* vector for cloning	[29]
pWSK30+ Δ*tatA*	deletion of *tatA* from DNA fragment	this study
pCDV422	suicide vector containing Amp^R and *sacB*	[30]
pCDV422+Δ*tatA*	vector to introduce in-frame deletion of *tatA* from DNA fragment	this study

Table 2. Primers.

Cloning *tatA*	
tatA 5':	CCGCTCGAGACGCTGTCCCTGCCTCAAGTA
tatA 3'	CGGGATCCCGCGCCGTTTTAATATGGAAGTA
Deleting *tatA*	
tatA inverse 5':	GCTGTGTTCGATATCGGGTTTA
tatA inverse 3':	CATATTACCTACCTCTATTTATA
Screening for mutant	
tatA upstream:	TACACCCGCCCAACACAAGAGA
tatA downstream:	CGCGCCGTTTTAATATGGAAGTA
Screening for pCD1	
lcrV-1:	AGGGTGGAACAACTTACTG
lcrV-2:	GTGCCACTACTAGACAGATGC
Screening for pMT	
Ymt-5'	TTTCGGCCAATCTCCAACAGTA
Ymt-3'	TCCGACCGCCCACATCA
CapAG-5'	AAAAATCAGTTCCGTTATCG
CapAG-3'	CTGCCCGTAGCCAAGAC
Screening for pPst	
Pla-5'	TGGCTTCCGGGTCAGGTA
Pla-3'	AGCCGGATGTCTTCTCACG

practiced by many labs [31,33,34], in order to ensure the genetic stability of the mutant strain after numerous *in vitro* growth steps needed to construct the mutant strain. The *Y. pestis* genome is unstable due to the presence of numerous IS*100* elements [35–37], and the passage of the mutant through an animal decreases the likelihood of a mixed population [2]. Animal passaged isolates of the Δ*tatA* mutant strain were harvested from the spleens of moribund mice following euthanasia.

To demonstrate phenotypes observed for the Δ*tatA* mutant were due specifically to the deletion of the gene, the mutant strain was complemented with an intact functional *tatA* gene present on pJET1.2 *in trans* via electroporation as described above.

Microscopy

Light microscopy. *Y. pestis* strains were grown as indicated and fixed in 4% formaldehyde. The samples were then stained with Wayson stain [38] and observed with an Eclipse E800 fluorescence microscope (Nikon, Inc.; Melville, NY). Images were captured using a Microfire camera and Pictureframe software (Optronics; Goleta, California). Fluorescence microscopy. *Y. pesits* was grown at 37°C in HI broth in the presence of CaCl$_2$ and fixed as described above. The presence of F1 antigen on *Y. pestis* was determined by indirect fluorescence microscopy (IFM) using the mouse monoclonal antibody (mAb) F1-04-A-G1 [39]. Samples were spun onto slides using a Cyto-Spin centrifuge (Thermo Shandon; Pittsburgh, PA), blocked with 7% skim milk in PBS for 30 min, exposed to the primary antibody (1:5,000) in the presence of skim milk in PBS containing 0.1% Tween-20 (PBST) for 1 h, washed three times with PBST, incubated with a secondary antibody (goat-anti mouse antibody conjugated with Texas Red) in the presence of 7% skim milk in PBST for 1 h, washed again, and then observed as described above.

Electron microscopy. Standard methods for transmission electron microscopy (TEM) were employed. *Y. pestis* samples were fixed with 1% glutaraldehyde and 4% formaldehyde in 0.1 M phosphate buffer for several days and sterility was confirmed. Post fixation was performed for 1 h at room temperature in phosphate buffer containing 1% osmium tetroxide and contrasted in ethanolic uranyl acetate before dehydration in a graded series of ethanol rinses and propylene oxide. The samples were embedded into EMbed-812 embedding medium (Electron Microscopy Sciences; Hatfield, PA) overnight at room temperature and the samples were then sectioned into 90-nm sections. These sections were counterstained with uranyl and lead salts. For immuno-EM (IEM) analysis, samples were fixed in 0.1% glutaraldehyde and 4% paraformaldehyde in 0.1 M phosphate buffer for several days and sterility confirmed. Samples were dehydrated using graded ethanol, embedded in LR White resin (Polysciences Inc., Warrington, PA), and heat cured. Sections were cut as described above, blocked, exposed to primary antibody to F1 at a 1:100 dilution, washed, and then incubated with the secondary antibody conjugated with 10 nm gold particles. Sections were counterstained with uranyl and lead salts. All EM samples were examined using a JEOL 1011 transmission electron microscope.

Biofilm assay

Y. pestis strains were tested for biofilm formation and adherence. The methods followed were previously described [40], except that bacteria were grown in HI broth for 24 h and then diluted in 40% HI broth for biofilm measurements in 24-well polystyrene dishes. The bacteria were grown at 200 rpm for approximately 18 h at 26°C. The biofilm was stained with 0.01% crystal violet. The wells were washed three times and bound dye was solubilized with 80% ethanol-20% acetone. The crystal violet was assayed by absorbance. The standard deviation was derived from quadruplicate samples. These data represent three separate experiments.

Protein extraction and analysis

Both whole-cell extracts and supernatants were collected for protein analysis from *Y. pestis* strains grown in HI broth at 28°C or at 37°C (with $CaCl_2$ or MOX, as indicated) as previously described [5]. Briefly, whole-cell extracts from *Y. pestis* were obtained from collecting bacteria from 18 h grown cultures. The cultures were centrifuged, the supernatant fluids collected, and the pellets resuspended in 1 ml of ice-cold water. The cultures were pelleted, suspended in water with MPBio Lysing Matrix B (MP Biomedicals; Solon, OH), bead beat for 40 s with a FastPrep FP120 Cell Disrupter (MP Biomedicals), chilled on ice, bead beat again for 40 s, microfuged for 5 min, and then passed through a 0.2 micron filter. The preparation was then sterility checked by plating a portion of the sample on sheep blood agar plates. The *Y. pestis* supernatants were concentrated by passage through a centrifugal filter device (Amicon Ultra-10K, Millipore; Billerica, MA), heat fixed (95°C for 30 min), and sterility checked. The protein concentrations from all samples were determined using the BCA Protein Assay kit (Pierce; Rockford, IL) per the manufacture's recommendations. Equal protein concentrations of samples were run on 10% Bis-Tris gels (Invitrogen; Carsbland, CA) and stained using the Gel Code Blue kit (Pierce).

For Western analysis, fractionated proteins were transferred onto a PVDF membrane overnight at 4°C in 1× NuPAGE transfer buffer (Invitrogen), 0.35% SDS, and 20% methanol. After transfer, the membranes were blocked with 10% skim milk in PBS containing 0.1% Tween-20. Mouse monoclonal antibodies [anti-F1, anti-GroEL (Enzo-Life Sciences, Plymouth Meeting, PA), or anti-LcrV [41]] were used at a dilution of 1:5,000 and secondary rabbit anti-mouse horseradish peroxidase was used at a dilution of 1:5,000. Bands were visualized using 4-chloronaphthol/3,3'-diaminobenzidine (Pierce). To demonstrate that the bands were the expected respective proteins, recombinant F1, GroEL, or LcrV were also run on the gels for control purposes.

Animal challenges

To determine the LD_{50} values for the wild-type and Δ*tatA* mutant, at least 5 groups of 10 naïve female 6–8-week-old Swiss Webster mice were challenged by the various routes. For all methods of infection, the challenge doses were determined by serial dilutions and plating. Subcutaneous challenge (sub-Q). Frozen *Y. pestis* stocks were streaked onto tryptose blood agar base (Difco Laboratories, Detroit, MI) slants and incubated at 28°C for 2 days. Bacterial cells were harvested from the slants in 10 mM KPBS (potassium phosphate buffered solution), and mice were challenged with 0.2 ml aliquots at various cell concentrations. Aerosol challenge. For aerosol challenges, a suspension of *Y. pestis* prepared from a slant suspension was used to inoculate flasks containing 100 ml of HI broth at an approximate OD_{600} of 0.01. The broth cultures were grown for 24 h in a 30°C shaker at 100 rpm, centrifuged, washed twice with HI broth, adjusted for various challenge doses. Mice were exposed to *Y. pestis* using a dynamic 30-liter humidity-controlled Plexiglas whole-body exposure chamber, as previously described [42]. The calculated inhaled doses were obtained as previously described [42,43]. Intranasal challenge. Mice were anesthetized with 150 μl of ketamine, acepromazine, and xylazine injected intramuscularly. The mice were then challenged by intranasal instillation with 50 μl of *Y. pestis* suspended in KPBS from slant grown cultures as described above. For all challenge experiments, mice were monitored several times each day and mortality rates (or euthanasia when moribund) were recorded. *In vivo* dissemination experiments. For *Y. pestis* dissemination studies after intranasal challenge, approximately equal numbers of either the parental (113,000 CFU) or Δ*tatA*

mutant (76,000 CFU) strains were used to challenge mice as described above. At specified time points after challenge, mice (n = 4–5) were then humanely euthanized within a CO_2 chamber. The lungs and spleens were harvested, rinsed with KPBS, weighed, and then homogenized in 1 ml of KPBS in a tissue grinder (Kendall Healthcare Precision Disposable Tissue Grinder Systems, Covidien; Mansfield, MA). The homogenates were then serially diluted and plated on to sheep blood agar plates.

Challenged mice were observed at least twice daily for 21 days for clinical signs of illness. Humane endpoints were used during all studies, and mice were humanely euthanized when moribund according to an endpoint score sheet. Animals were scored on a scale of 0–12:0–3 = no clinical signs; 4–7 = clinical symptoms; increase monitoring; 8–12 = distress; euthanize. Those animals receiving a score of 8–12 were humanely euthanized by CO_2 exposure using compressed CO_2 gas followed by cervical dislocation. However, even with multiple checks per day, some animals died as a direct result of the infection.

Animal research at The United States Army of Medical Research Institute of Infectious Diseases was conducted and approved under an Institutional Animal Care and Use Committee in compliance with the Animal Welfare Act, PHS Policy, and other Federal statutes and regulations relating to animals and experiments involving animals. The facility where this research was conducted is accredited by the Association for Assessment and Accreditation of Laboratory Animal Care, International and adheres to principles stated in the Guide for the Care and Use of Laboratory Animals, National Research Council, 2011.

Pathology

Postmortem tissues were collected from mice challenged with *Y. pestis*, fixed in 10% neutral buffered formalin, routinely processed, embedded in paraffin, and sectioned for hematoxylin and eosin (HE) staining as previously described [44]. Immunohistochemistry was performed on sections using a primary antibody to the F1 antigen and secondary antibody, a peroxidase-labeled polymer, EnVision Peroxidase kit (Dako Corp., Carpinteria, CA). The slides were stained with substrate-chromogen solution and counter stained with hematoxylin.

Statistics

For comparing data from the biofilm experiments and TTD studies of mouse challenges, statistical significance ($P < 0.05$) was determined by the two-tailed Student t test. LD_{50} analysis was determined by the Bayesian probit analysis. Survival rates were compared between groups by Fisher exact tests with permutation adjustment for multiple comparisons using SAS Version 8.2 (SAS Institute Inc., SAS OnlineDoc, Version 8, Cary, N.C. 2000).

Screening the *Y. pestis* genome for Tat motifs

To scan for additional Tat-like motifs, we developed a script that allows more flexibility at each position in the motif with amino acids in the same basic grouping: non-polar, polar, acidic and basic. For positions with validated variants from multiple groups, we allowed substitution to either group. The script does not calculate total similarity distance from the original sequence allowing for multiple changes in order to give us the most flexibility possible within each grouping at each position. The resulting hits largely agree with the Hidden Markov Model results for the Tat signal motif available at Pfam (PF10518). Model data available at pfam.sanger.ac.uk/family/PF10518/hmm.

Results

Construction of the ΔtatA mutant

In *Y. pestis*, the *tatABCD* genes are clustered very closely together on the chromosome [45]. The *tatA* gene (267 bp) is 4 bp downstream of *tatB* (663 bps). Three bp downstream of *tatB* is the *tatC* gene (777 bp). The *tatD* gene is 540 bp in length and is 14 bp downstream of *tatC*. The *tatA* gene was deleted in-frame from the chromosome of the fully virulent CO92 strain of *Y. pestis*, as described above in the Materials and Methods section. Deletion mutants were screened by PCR using primers outside of the *tatA* cloning region (Table 2). For those clones which reverted back to the wild-type strain, a PCR fragment of 2.1 kb was observed. However, for those mutants deleted of the *tatA* gene, a shift of approximately 250 bp was observed (data not shown).

Growth of the ΔtatA mutant in culture medium is not altered but cell morphology is

Growth curves were performed comparing the wild-type and ΔtatA mutant in HI broth (28°C, 37°C with CaCl₂, and 37°C with MOX) by both optical density (OD_{600}) and CFU counts (Fig. 1). No differences in growth rates were observed between strains as observed by OD (Fig. 1). However, CFU counts at all-time points (even for the starting inoculum at Time 0), were consistently lower in the mutant strain compared to the wild-type strain despite having similar OD measurements. However, the increase in CFU counts of both parent and mutant strains over the time course was still similar.

To determine why the CFU counts between the two strains were different; cells were examined by light microscopy. The mutant displayed an abnormal morphological phenotype at both 28°C (data not shown) and 37°C with CaCl₂ (Fig. 2). The ΔtatA bacteria lost the typical *Yersinia* coccobacillus shape and became more elongated to a pronounced bacillus form, as compared to the wild-type strain (Fig. 2A and B). To further characterize the structural differences of the ΔtatA mutant strain, TEM was performed with the parental and mutant strains grown at 37°C with CaCl₂ (Fig. 2C and D). Again for the ΔtatA mutant, the bacteria displayed an elongated bacillus form. In addition, many of the bacteria appeared to be inhibited in separating from one another during cellular division. This phenomenon is discussed further below; however, our morphological results are in general agreement with *tat* mutations in other bacteria [25,46,47].

The integrity of biofilm in the ΔtatA mutant is affected

In addition to the structural differences observed with the ΔtatA strain, the mutant also demonstrated a defect in biofilm integrity. After overnight growth at 26°C, a bacterial biofilm formed for both the *Y. pestis* wild-type (Fig. 3A) and mutant (Fig. 3B) cultures at the liquid/air interface. The biofilm, however, of the ΔtatA cultures was easily dislodged as compared to the wild-type strain.

To quantitate the adherence defect of the ΔtatA mutant, it was assayed as previously described [40]. As shown in Fig. 3C, the quantity of biofilm detected between wild-type *Y. pestis* and the ΔtatA mutant differed significantly ($P = <0.0001$). As described above, the ΔtatA bacteria were still able to produce biofilm; however, there was a defect in the adherence or integrity of the biofilm to bind to the substrate. In this assay, the biofilm was dislodged during the wash steps and prior to the absorbance readings. To demonstrate this adherence defect was due specifically to the deletion of *tatA*, the mutant was complemented with a functional *tatA* gene. As shown in Fig. 3C, the quantity of measured adherent biofilm for the complemented mutant strain and wild-type CO92 did not differ significantly ($P = 0.09$).

Therefore, providing a functional *tatA* gene was able to restore the adherence/integrity defect of the ΔtatA mutant strain.

The ΔtatA mutant is altered in F1 antigen localization

As the deletion of the *tatA* gene would affect translocated proteins, we examined proteins extracted from both the cell pellet and supernatant fractions of mutant and wild-type bacteria grown in HI broth at 28°C or 37°C containing CaCl₂. As shown in Fig. 4A, the proteins collected from pellets of *Y. pestis* grown at 28°C were separated on a 10% Bis-Tris gels, but no obvious differences were observed in the protein profile between wild-type, ΔtatA, or C12 (F1 antigen/*caf1* mutant) strains. However, when the protein pellets were examined from *Y. pestis* grown at 37°C under high calcium conditions, an intense band at <19 kDa appeared for wild-type CO92 which was not present for the 28°C samples. For proteins extracted for the ΔtatA pellet, this band was also present but not as intense as observed for the wild-type strain. We presumed that this band corresponded to the F1 antigen protein encoded by the *caf1* gene which is expressed by *Y. pestis* at 37°C and has a molecular mass of 15.5 kDa [48–50]. Further demonstrating that this band corresponded to the F1 antigen, it was absent from the protein profile of the C12 strain of *Y. pestis* (Fig. 4A).

Likewise, when pelleting *Y. pestis* cultures after growth at 37°C with calcium, wild-type *Y. pestis* formed a flocculent pellet (data not shown). In contrast, when the ΔtatA mutant was grown similarly, a very tight pellet was formed, similar to pelleted cultures of C12, the F1antigen mutant (data not shown). This defect was due specifically to the loss of the *tatA* gene since a complemented mutant would once again form a flocculent pellet similar to wild-type cultures (data not shown).

When performing Western blot analysis with a monoclonal antibody to the F1 antigen with equal amounts of proteins extracted from the pellets of CO92, ΔtatA, and C12 strains, similar results were obtained (Fig. 4B). A large prominent band was observed for the wild-type strain, a weaker band for the ΔtatA mutant, and no band was apparent for the F1 antigen mutant. Recombinant F1 antigen was also included as a positive control and corresponded in size to the bands observed for the bacterial pellets (Fig. 4B). Similar results were observed with the discrepancy between the amount of F1 antigen observed in the supernatants collected from wild-type and ΔtatA mutant cultures (data not shown). In addition, a control Western blot was performed using the same amount of protein but probing with a monoclonal antibody to GroEL, a 56-kDa molecular chaperone [51]. As shown in Fig. 4C and in contrast to the results observed with the anti-F1 antigen, no difference in the amount of GroEL was observed between strains.

To determine if synthesis or secretion of the V-antigen/LcrV, one of the *Yersinia* Yops which is surface exposed and serves many roles, one being necessary for translocation of the effector Yops [52–54], was also affected by deletion of the *tatA* gene; *Y. pestis* strains were grown at 37°C with MOX to induce expression of the low calcium response [4]. Proteins were collected from cell pellets, ran on SDS-PAGE gels, and tested by Western analysis using a monoclonal antibody to the V-antigen. As shown in Fig. 4D, no differences were observed for the presence of the V-antigen between strains in cell associated proteins, except for the *Y. pestis* strain which lacks the pLcr plasmid. Similar results were observed for proteins from culture supernatants (data not shown).

To attempt to define this defect in the concentration of the F1 antigen for the ΔtatA mutant, *Y. pestis* cells were examined by microscopy using both IFM and IEM. As shown in Fig. 5A, when wild-type CO92 was grown under conditions to promote F1

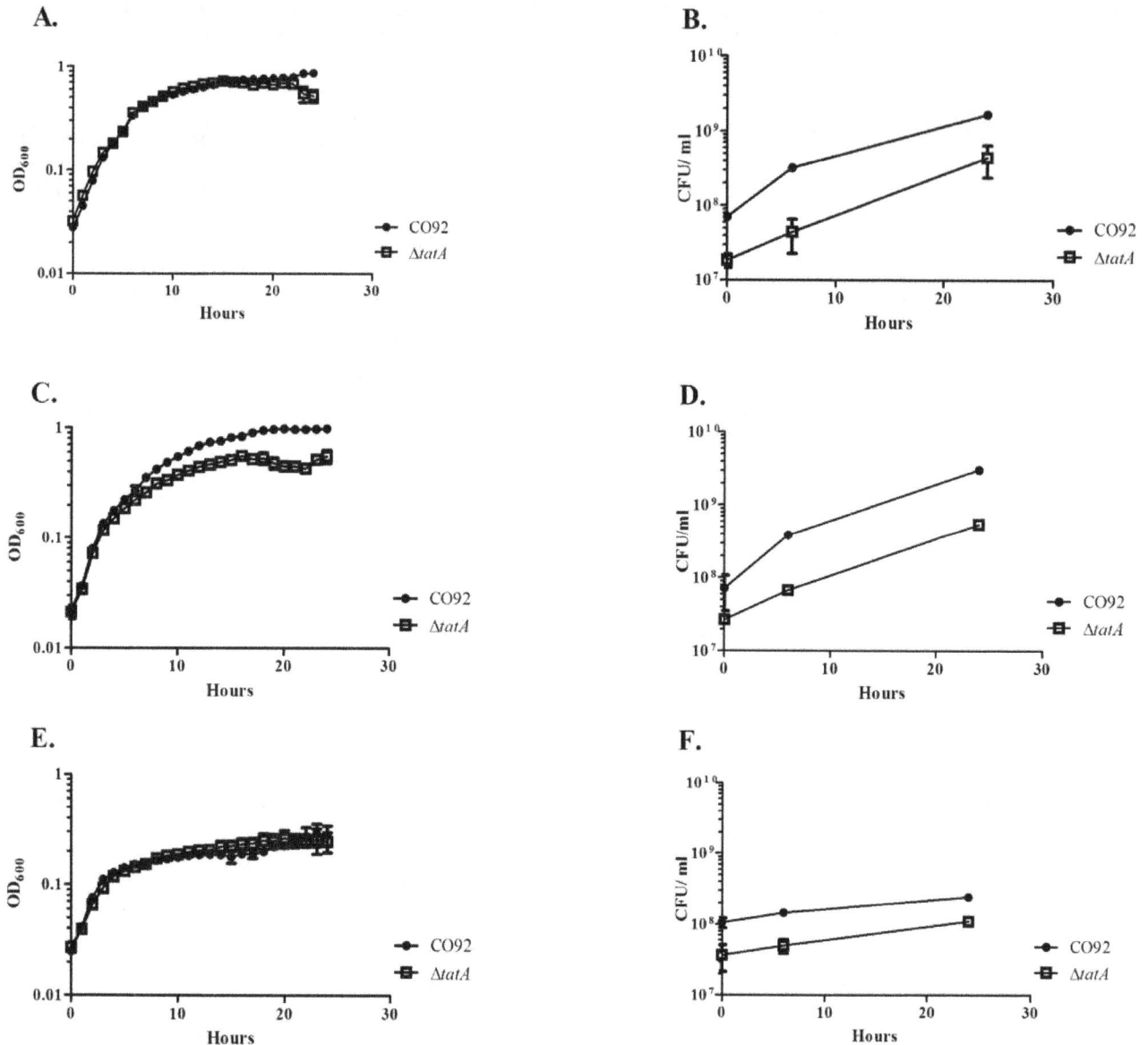

Figure 1. Growth assays. *Y. pestis* wild type and Δ*tatA* mutant strains were grown in HI broth at 28°C (A and B), 37°C with CaCl$_2$ (C and D), or 37°C with MOX (E and F). Growth was monitored by both optical density (A, C, and E) and CFU counts (B, D, and F). OD measurements are based upon quadruplicate samples and bars represent standard deviation. CFU measurements are based upon triplicate samples and bars represent standard deviation. These data represent at least two separate experiments.

antigen synthesis and visualized by IFM using an antibody specific to the F1 antigen, the cells displayed a tight layer of fluorescence that surrounded the cells and in close association to the membrane. The Δ*tatA* mutant was grown under identical conditions but was only slightly fluorescent, indicating the presence of low but still detectable levels of F1 antigen. (Fig. 5B) However, fluorescence was not as intense as observed with the parental strain. In addition, the labeling for the mutant appeared to be more diffuse around the cells and not as tightly associated. To determine if this defect was due specifically to the deletion of the *tatA* gene, we observed the complemented mutant strain by IFM (Fig. 5C). As expected, the fluorescence of the complemented Δ*tatA* strain was restored to the intense fluorescent labeling that was associated with the wild-type bacterial cells. Also included in this study was the C12 strain which lacks the F1 antigen protein

and no fluorescent labeling of this strain was observed (data not shown).

We further confirmed these studies by IEM. As shown in Fig. 5D, wild-type cells were decorated with gold bead labeling, indicating the presence of the F1 antigen, both in contact with the outer bacterial membrane and surrounding the outer area. In contrast, the gold labeling observed with the Δ*tatA* mutant was much less intense than the wild-type strain. The gold beads observed were rarely in association with the membrane but appeared diffuse away from the cell (Fig. 5E). The control for this study to demonstrate specificity of the labeling for the F1 antigen was the C12 strain. As shown in Fig. 5F, no gold beads were found associated with this strain.

A.

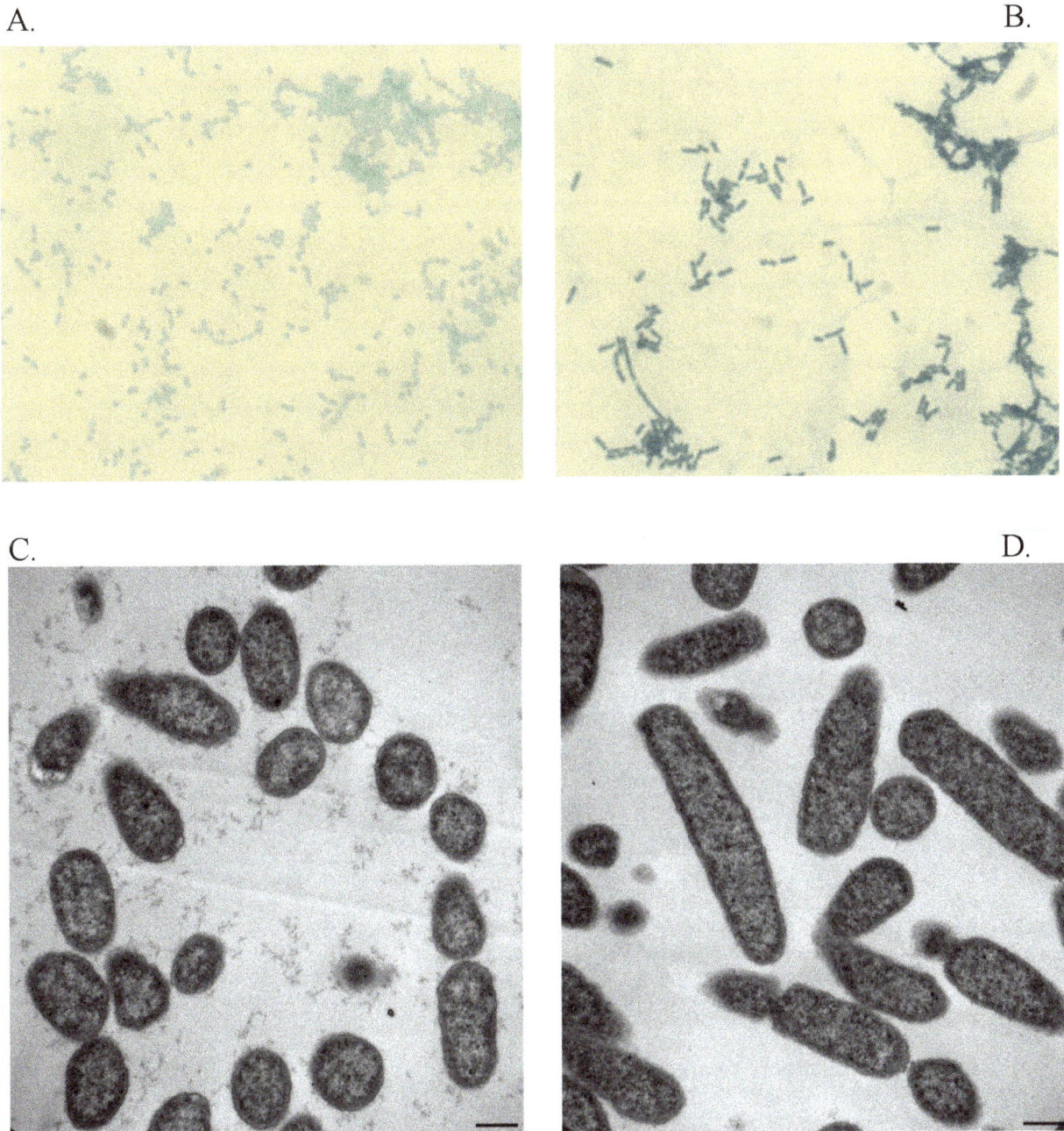

B.

C.

D.

Figure 2. Morphology of *Y. pestis* strains. *Y. pestis* was grown at 37°C in presence $CaCl_2$ and examined by microscopy. The samples, wild-type (A) and Δ*tatA* (B), were fixed, stained with Wayson stain, and examined by microscopy (100×). Additionally, samples, wild-type (C; micron bar = 0.5 μm) and Δ*tatA* (D; micron bar = 0.5 μm), were examined by TEM.

The Δ*tatA* mutant is attenuated in both bubonic and aerosol administered inhalational models of plague infection but not as attenuated following intranasal challenge

The virulence of the Δ*tatA* mutant was assessed and compared to wild-type CO92 challenge through bubonic and pneumonic murine models (small-particle aerosol and intranasal instillation) of plague infection. From these assays, survival following challenge is shown in Fig. 6, and the LD_{50} values were determined for each route and summarized in Table 3.

The LD_{50} for the CO92 wild-type strain by the bubonic challenge route with Swiss Webster mice was determined to be only ~2 CFU (Fig. 6A and Table 3), in general agreement with previous estimates [55]. In contrast, the LD_{50} for Δ*tatA* mutant was calculated to be 1.46×10^7 CFU (Fig. 6B and Table 3). To demonstrate this severe attenuation was due specifically to the deletion of the *tatA* gene, mice were then challenged with the complemented mutant. As expected, the LD_{50} for the complemented Δ*tatA* strain was restored to wild-type levels and determined to be ~1 CFU (Fig. 6C and Table 3).

A.

B.

C.

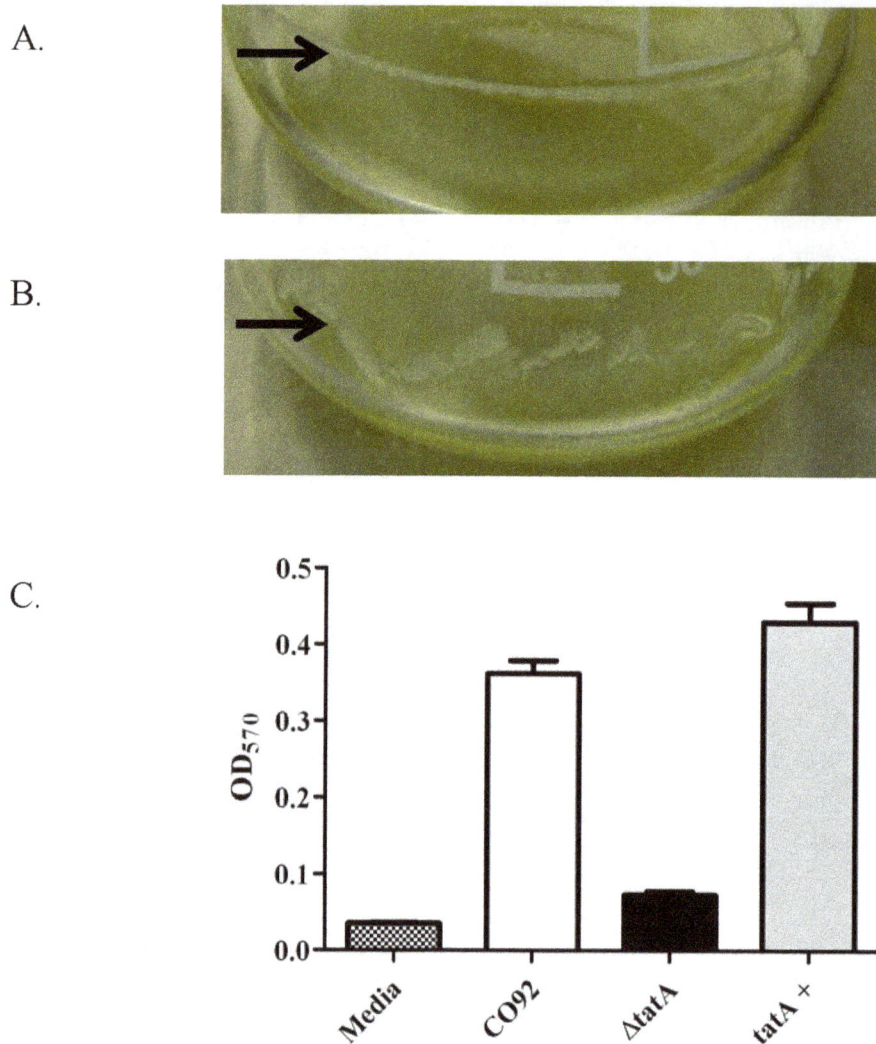

Figure 3. Adherence of *Y. pestis* **biofilm.** The *Y. pestis* A) wild-type CO92 and B) Δ*tatA* mutant cultures were grown in HI broth at 26°C. Arrows indicate biofilm formation. C) To measure biofilm adherence, the biofilm of wild-type CO92, Δ*tatA* mutant, and complemented Δ*tatA* mutant was stained with crystal violet and assayed by absorbance as described in the Materials and Methods. The standard deviation was derived from quadruplicate samples. These data represent three separate experiments.

Next, mice were challenged by aerosol exposure with either the wild-type or Δ*tatA* to determine if the mutant was also attenuated by this model of pneumonic challenge. The LD_{50} for the CO92 strain was calculated to the 6.7×10^4 CFU (Fig. 6D and Table 3), in general agreement with our previously published value of 6×10^4 CFU [31]. In contrast, no mice succumbed to infection when challenged with the aerosolized Δ*tatA* at an estimated inhaled dose up to 9.43×10^5 CFU. When mice were challenged at two additional higher doses (2.65×10^6 and 3.31×10^6), mortality was observed. However, the mice did not succumb to infection in a dose dependent manner (Fig. 6E). Therefore, we were not able to calculate a valid LD_{50} measurement. Regardless, the LD_{50} for the Δ*tatA* mutant would be 9.43×10^5 CFU.

Surprisingly, when performing intranasal challenges as an additional method of pneumonic infection with the wild-type and mutant, little difference was observed between the calculated LD_{50} values between strains, 1.4×10^3 CFU versus 2.4×10^3 CFU, respectively (Figs. 6F,G and Table 3). Likewise, no differences in survival between groups of mice challenged at approximately

equal doses between the two strains were noted except for the $\sim 10^3$ CFU challenge group (Table 4). In contrast, we observed a significant difference in TTD for mice challenged with the Δ*tatA* as compared to the wild-type strain (Table 4). Mice challenged intranasally with Δ*tatA* succumbed to infection at significantly later time points as compared to mice challenged with the wild-type strain at all doses (Table 4).

The course of disease was very different for mice challenged intranasally with the Δ*tatA* mutant as compared to mice challenged with CO92. Whereas wild-type challenged mice succumbed to infection between 3–5 days (Table 4), approximately 1 week post challenge, the mice infected with the Δ*tatA* mutant began to display signs of inner ear infection: holding their head at a tilt and then progressing to whole body spinning. However, within a day or two, some mice clinically improved, even though residual tissue damage was noted during histological evaluation (discussed below). Other mice eventually succumbed to infection or were euthanized when moribund.

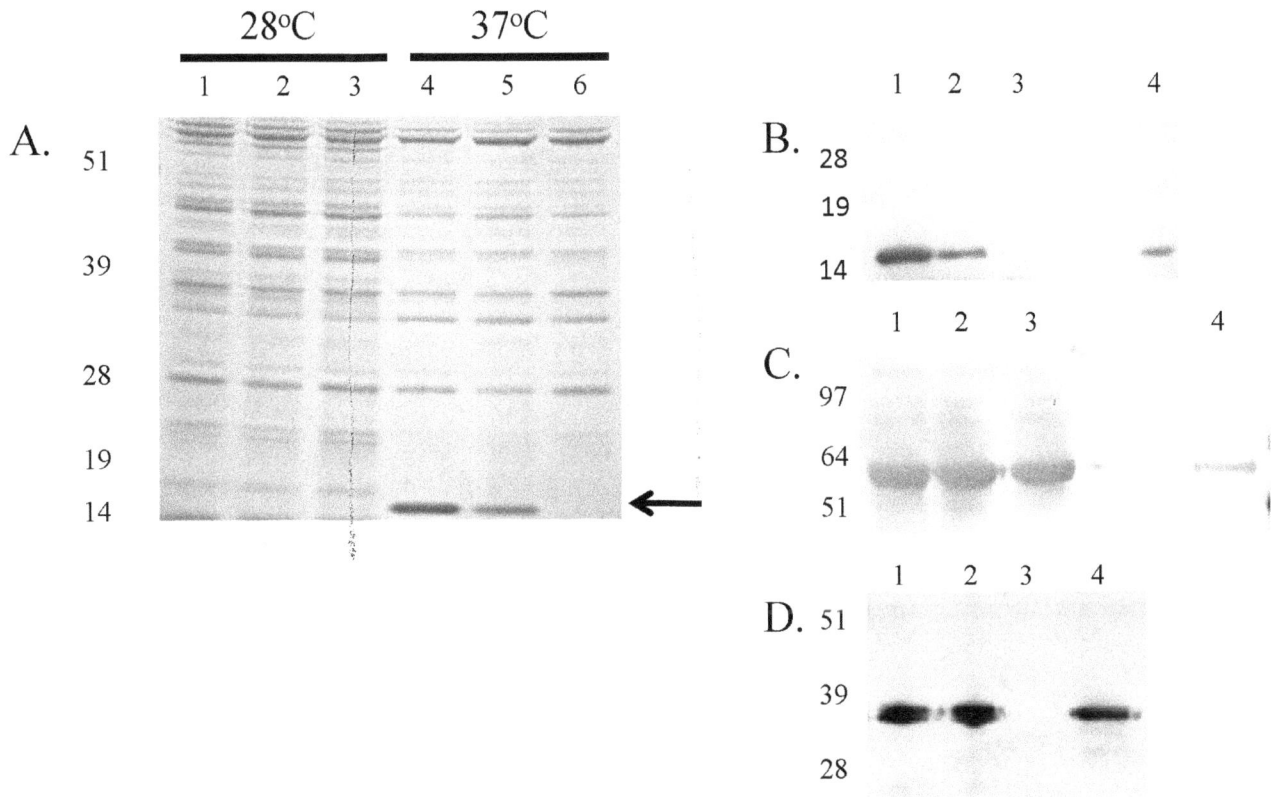

Figure 4. Analysis of *Y. pestis* **proteins.** A) Strains (wild-type, lanes 1 and 4; Δ*tatA*, lanes 2 and 5, and C12, lanes 3 and 6) were grown in HI broth at 28°C or 37°C containing CaCl₂, as indicated. Proteins were extracted and ran on a SDS-PAGE gel at equal concentrations. The arrow indicates a protein band that is synthesized at 37°C for the CO92 and to a lesser extent the Δ*tatA* mutant but not in C12, a F1-antigen mutant strain. Molecular masses are indicated on the left in KDa. Strains were grown in HI broth at 37°C containing CaCl₂ and proteins extracted for Western analysis. Equal concentrations of proteins from *Y. pestis* strains were blotted with a monoclonal antibody to either the F1 antigen (B) or GroEL (C). Lanes: 1, wild-type; 2, Δ*tatA*; 3, C12; and 4, recombinant protein (F1 antigen or GroEL, respectively). Molecular masses are indicated on the left in KDa. D) Strains were grown in HI broth at 37°C in the presence of MOX to create low calcium conditions. Equal concentrations of proteins from *Y. pestis* strains were blotted with an antibody to LcrV Lanes: 1, CO92 wild-type; 2, Δ*tatA*; 3, *Y. pestis* pLcr⁻; and 4, rLcrV protein. Molecular masses are indicated on the left in KDa.

Histologic examination of cranial sections of mice infected intranasally with the Δ*tatA* mutant (Fig. 7A) or the wild-type CO92 strain (Fig. 7C) showed severe middle ear involvement, which was usually bilaterally present. The high incidence of infection/inflammation of the inner and external ear canal was most likely related to the intranasal route of exposure. Lesions were characterized by necrosuppurative inflammation with marked bacterial colonization in the associated bone marrow within the tympanic bulla, inner ear, and/or external ear (Fig. 7A–C). Bacteria were confirmed to be *Y. pestis* through immuno-histochemical (IHC) staining with antibody to the F1 capsule which is specific for *Y. pestis* [56,57] (Fig. 7B).

Histologic examination of many of the mutant challenged mice (8/10) that succumbed to infection revealed moderate meningitis of the ventral meninges of the cerebrum and/or cerebellum. The areas of meningitis were characterized by necrotic debris and neutrophils admixed with fibrin, coccobacilli, and congested vessels (Fig. 7A and B). The meningitis in the ventral aspect of the cerebrum/cerebellum is probably an extension of inflammation/necrosis from the nasopharynx/nasal cavity and/or middle/inner ear through the osseous structures of the cranium. Again, the bacteria were confirmed to be *Y. pestis* through IHC staining with anti-F1 antibody (Fig. 7B). In addition, three of the mice which survived 21 days post challenge with higher doses of the Δ*tatA*

mutant still retained a head tilt and histologic lesions consisted of meningitis characterized by necrosis and neutrophilic inflammation admixed with macrophages and fibrous connective tissue (data not shown).

In the case of CO92-infected mice, disease progression following intranasal instillation was much quicker as compared to challenge with the mutant strain, and the resulting illness was acute. In wild-type exposed mice, the presence of *Y. pestis* in the inner ear did not progress to meningitis because the time from exposure to the succumbing to infection was too short for lesions to develop (Fig. 7C), as opposed to what was observed with mice infected with the Δ*tatA* mutant strain (Fig. 7A). The lungs of the intranasal challenged mice from both the wild-type and the mutant were also examined. Overall, lung lesion development and characteristics were the same between mice challenged with either strain (Figs. 7 D–E).

To determine if the presence of *Y. pestis* bacteria within the inner ear was specific to exposure by the intranasal route, pathology samples were also examined from mice challenged by small particle aerosol with either the wild-type or mutant strain. In contrast to the observations with intranasal challenged mice (Fig. 7A–C), no inflammation or bacterial colonization was observed in the inner ear or meningeal areas for mice challenged via small-particle aerosol delivery for the *Y. pestis* strains (Figs. 8A

A.   B.   C.

D.   E.   F.

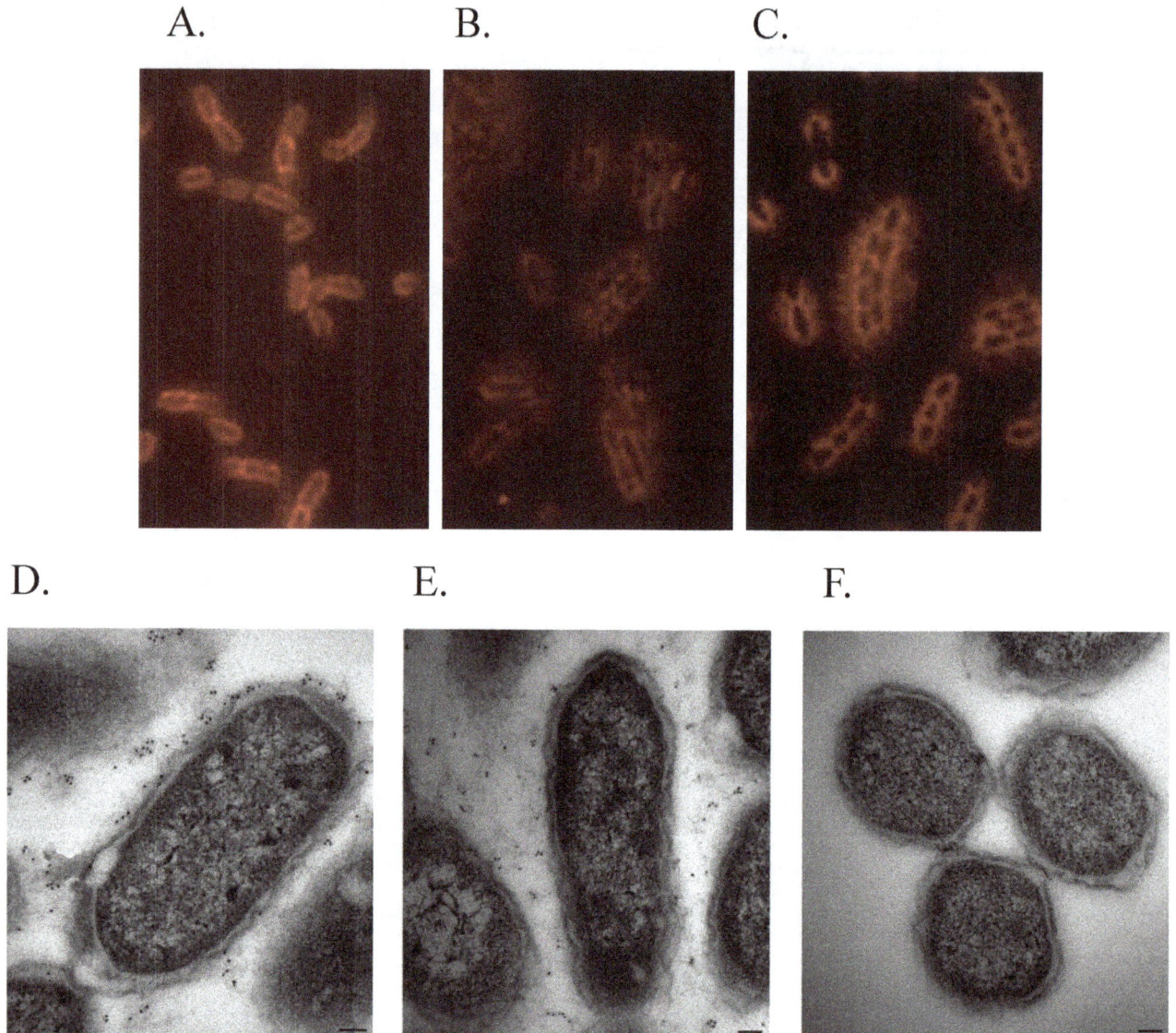

Figure 5. Localizing the F1 capsule by microscopy. *Y. pestis* strains were grown at 37°C in HI broth containing $CaCl_2$ and exposed to an antibody against the F1 capsule. IFM samples: A) wild-type, B) Δ*tatA* mutant, and C) complemented Δ*tatA* mutant. The images (100×) were captured for all samples at identical camera settings to maintain relative fluorescence. IEM samples: D) wild-type (micron bar = 0.1 μm), E) Δ*tatA* mutant (micron bar = 0.1 μm), and F) C12, F1 negative (micron bar = 0.5 μm).

and B). Additionally, lungs were examined from mice challenged by aerosol with each strain (Figs. 8C and D). Again, there was no difference in lung lesion characters or severity in mice challenged between strains.

The recovery and dissemination of the Δ*tatA* mutant is hindered after intranasal challenge

Since there was little difference in the intranasal LD_{50} calculated between strains but a significant increase in TTD for mutant challenged mice, the dissemination of wild-type and mutant bacteria following intranasal challenge was compared. Groups of mice were separately challenged with approximately equal doses of either CO92 (113,000 CFU) or the Δ*tatA* mutant (76,000 CFU). For mice challenged with wild-type CO92, CFU recovery from the lungs showed some progression by day 1 and then increased rapidly for days 3 and 4 for all mice tested

(Fig. 9A). By day 3, only four mice were alive for testing, while the remaining animals had succumbed to infection. For recovery of CFU from the spleen, wild-type bacteria were detected for one mouse by day 1; however, spleens for all mice had increased bacterial burden loads by days 2 and 3 (Fig. 9B).

In contrast, mice challenged intranasally with the Δ*tatA* mutant were severely delayed in progression of bacterial dissemination. Recovery of bacteria from the lungs 2 h postchallenge did not differ greatly between the wild-type and mutant strains (5.8% versus 4.2%, respectively) (Fig. 9A). Therefore, differences in tissue tropism or bacterial adherence to host cells after initial exposure would not appear to be a factor for the delay. However, through day 2, recovery of the Δ*tatA* mutant from the lungs decreased. For the remainder of the study, a slight increase in CFU was detected in the lungs. However, at least one mouse out of the five tested for each time point starting on day 2 had no *Y. pestis* recovered from the lungs (Fig. 9A). A similar delay was observed for trafficking of

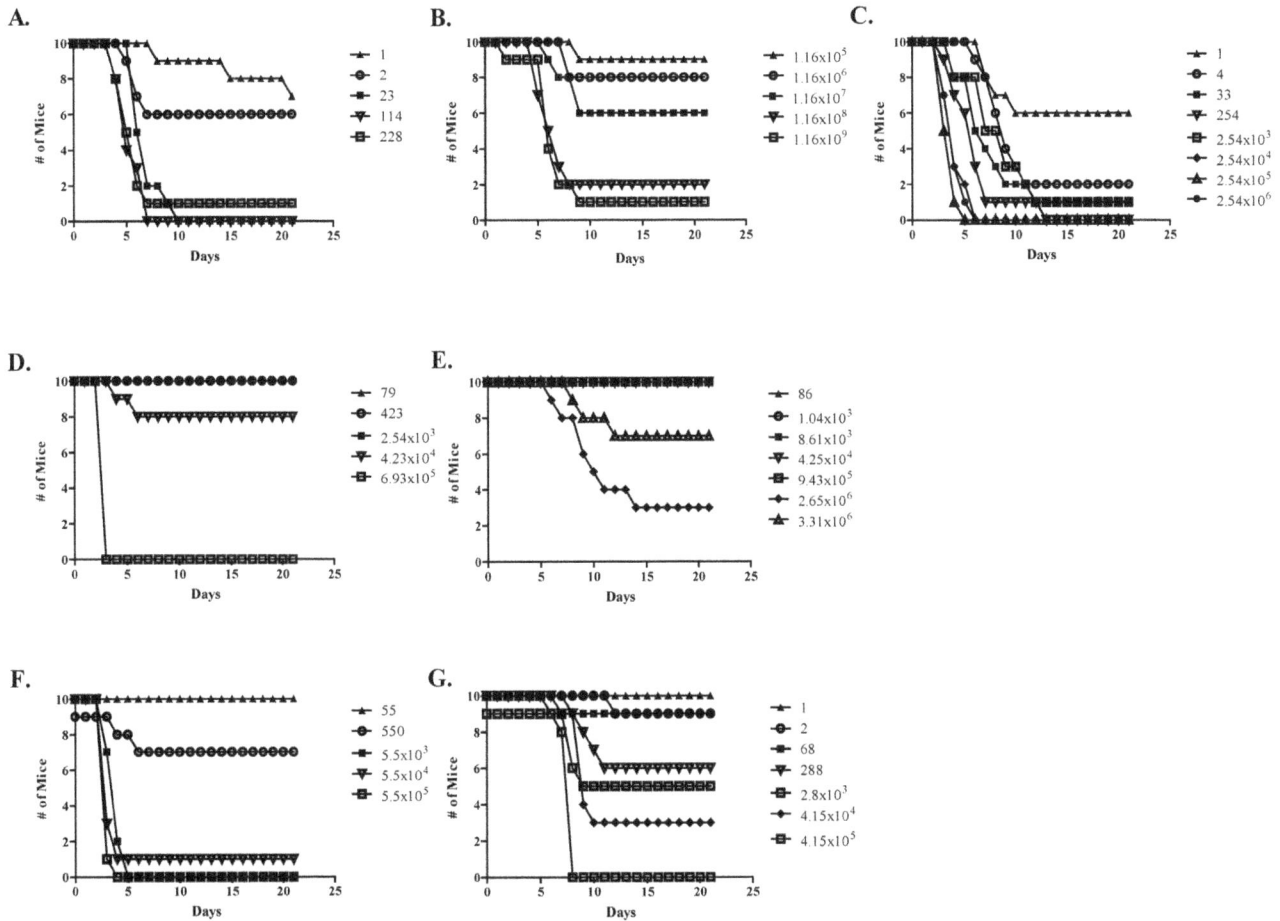

Figure 6. Animal challenge data. Groups of Swiss Webster mice were challenged and survival monitored following various plague models of infection (sub-Q injections A–C; small-particle aerosol D and E; and intranasal F and G) with various strains of *Y. pestis* (wild-type A, D, and F; ΔtatA mutant B, E, and G; and the complemented ΔtatA mutant C). The calculated LD₅₀ values are included in Table 3.

the mutant to spleens (Fig. 9B). On day 4, one mouse did show a high bacterial burden. However, the majority of bacteria were recovered from spleens between days 5–9. As was the case observed for the lungs, at least one mouse for each time point (except for day 7), ΔtatA bacteria were not recovered from the spleens (Fig. 9B).

Screening the *Y. pestis* genome for Tat motifs

To determine how the deletion of the *tatA* gene could affect capsule formation or other known virulence factors, the CO92 *Y. pestis* genome was screened for proteins containing the Tat motif

(SRRXFLK) [7]. A previous study employing the TATFIND computer program identified 19 *Y. pestis* proteins predicted to be secreted via the Tat translocation pathway [58]. None of the proteins identified in this study as Tat secreted proteins appears to be directly linked to defect in capsule, biofilm formation, or other known *Y. pestis* virulence factors. Additionally, there is sufficient evidence to suggest that there is some degree of fluidity in the composition and organization of this domain [59–62]. Therefore, we decided to conduct an *in silico* search allowing more flexibility at each position. Table 5 lists nine proteins which contain Tat-like motifs in the N terminal region, four that are unique to this study.

Table 3. Calculated LD₅₀ for the CO92 wild-type and ΔtatA mutant *Y. pestis* strains.

Strain	LD₅₀ sub-Q.	LD₅₀ aerosol[a]	LD₅₀ intranasal
Wild-type CO92	~2 CFU	6.7×10^4 CFU	1.4×10^3 CFU
ΔtatA	1.46×10^7 CFU	$>9.43 \times 10^5$ CFU	2.4×10^3 CFU
ΔtatA complement	~1 CFU[b]	ND[c]	ND[c]

[a]Calculated inhaled dose.
[b]A significant difference was observed between the LD₅₀ determinations between the ΔtatA mutant and complemented strain (p<0.0001).
[c]Not determined.

Table 4. Survival and TTD comparisons between mice challenged intranasally with the ΔtatA mutant and wild-type Y. pestis strains.

Strain	Dose (CFU)	Total	Alive	% Survival	p value	TTD±SD[a]	p value
CO92	550	9	7	78	0.63	5.00±1.14	0.0402*
ΔtatA	288	10	6	60		9.25±1.71	
CO92	5,500	10	0	0	0.01*	3.90±0.74	<0.0001*
ΔtatA	2,880	9	5	56		8.25±0.50	
CO92	55,000	10	1	10	0.582	3.22±0.44	<0.0001*
ΔtatA	41,500	10	3	30		8.86±0.90	
CO92	550,000	10	0	0	1	3.10±0.32	<0.0001*
ΔtatA	415,000	10	0	0		7.70±0.67	

[a]Time to death ± standard deviation in days.
*Statistical differences were considered significant when $p < 0.05$.

From our search, we identified several proteins that have been associated with the Tat translocation system in other bacteria (TauA, SufI, DmaA and NapA). From the newly identified Tat secreted candidates; we did not establish any direct links to the phenotypes observed for the Y. pestis mutant. However, there were several hypothetical proteins identified that warrant further characterization, such as YPO2150, a LysR regulator.

Discussion

In this study, we examined the role of the Tat translocation system in a fully virulent Y. pestis strain. The disruption of the Tat pathway by the in-frame deletion of the tatA gene led to several interesting phenotypes. The morphology of the mutant bacteria was severely altered and tended to have a more bacillus shape than the typical shape of Y. pestis (Fig. 2). The effect this structural alteration would have specifically on virulence of the ΔtatA strain remains to be determined.

The change in shape of the ΔtatA mutant is likely due to the defect in cell division as was previously described for tat mutations in E. coli, Burkholderia thailandensis, and Helicobacter pylori [25,46,47]. In screening the Y. pestis genome for Tat motifs, the SufI protein sequence contained a putative Tat signal [58]. SufI was previously shown to be transported by the Tat system [60] and to also suppress cell division [63]. However, E. coli mutants in the sufI gene do not show these cell morphology defects [46,63].

In addition to the altered morphology of the bacteria, the ΔtatA bacteria had a defect in biofilm integrity. The mutant strain was able to synthesize a biofilm; however, the adherence of the biofilm to the substrate was weak and could easily be dislodged (Fig. 3). Defects in biofilm formation have been observed in other bacteria when mutated in tat genes [17,20,22,64,65]. Currently, the exact reason for the loss of biofilm adherence in the Y. pestis ΔtatA mutant remains to be determined. For tat mutants in other bacteria, the decrease in biofilm production was due to loss of flagella motility or pili-twitching [20,22]. However, Y. pestis is non-motile due to a mutation within the flhD gene [45].

The distribution and/or localization of the F1 antigen of the ΔtatA mutant was also affected despite the Caf1 or other related proteins not possessing an obvious Tat motif. The F1 antigen is synthesized on the bacterial surface through a chaperone/usher pathway [48,66]. When performing Western analyses with an anti-F1 antibody and proteins of lysed whole cell or supernatants, a band corresponding to the F1 protein was still observed with the ΔtatA mutant, but the intensity was less than with the parenteral strain (Fig. 4A). In addition, when examining these strains by IFM or IEM with an antibody to the F1 protein, both the wild-type and mutant strains were highly labeled. However, the amount of membrane associated F1 antigen detected with the ΔtatA mutant was diminished (Fig. 5).

It appears that the F1 antigen protein was able to be secreted but unable to localize properly to the outer membrane surface of Y. pestis. The protein would then diffuse away from the cell. It has been previously reported that the Caf1A usher is necessary for assembly of F1 antigen onto the surface of the bacteria but not for secretion into the extracellular media [48,67]. Additionally, various novel chaperone/usher loci have been described for Y. pestis that play some role with biofilm and F1 capsule synthesis [68]. Perhaps the initial assembly and anchoring of the F1 protein onto the surface of the Y. pestis ΔtatA mutant is altered due to loss of some chaperone/usher transported by the Tat system.

When examining the Y. pestis ΔtatA for virulence defects, the mutant was severely attenuated in a bubonic model of infection. The LD_{50} for the ΔtatA mutant was 10^7 times higher as compared

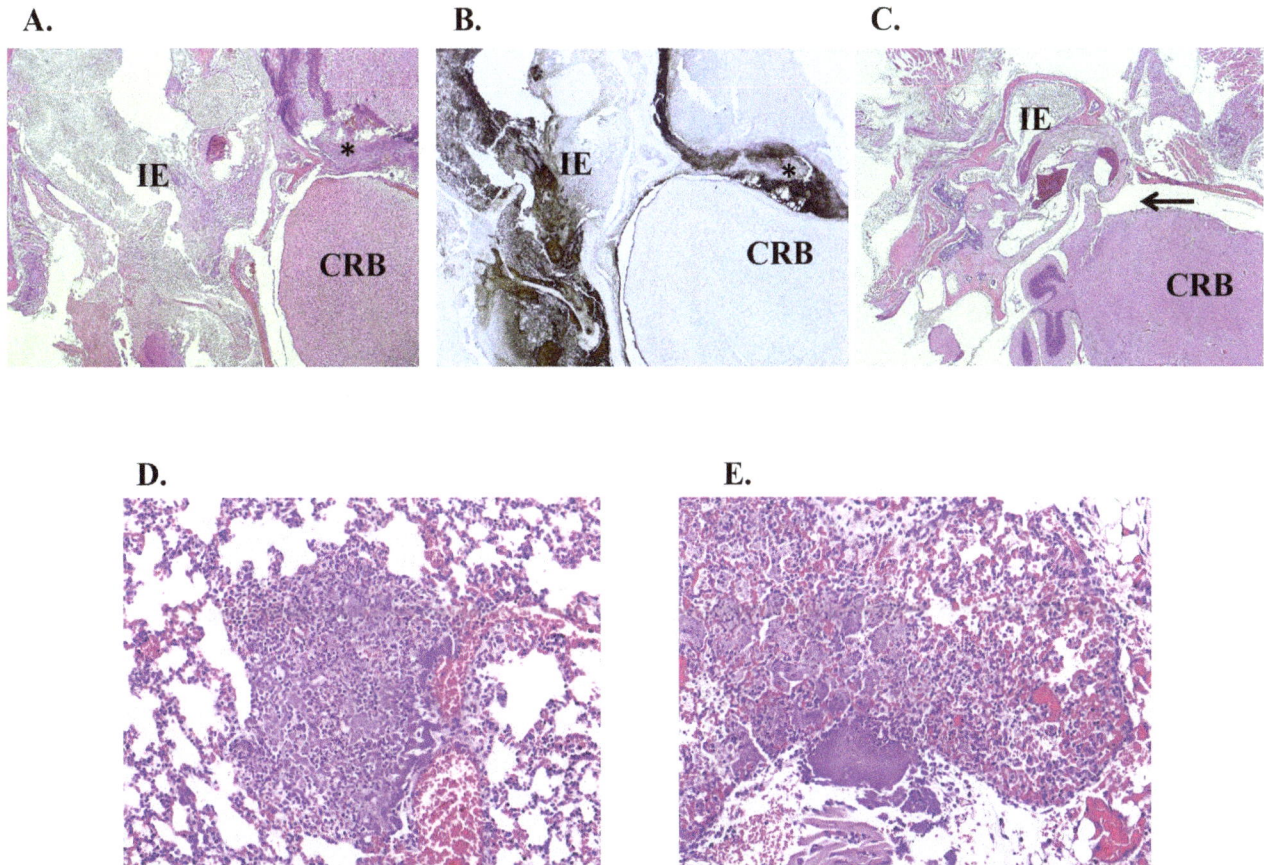

Figure 7. Pathology of mice challenged intranasally with Y. pestis. A and B) Skull sections (4×) of a mouse challenged with the ΔtatA mutant (2,800 CFU). The mouse was moribund and euthanized on day 8 postchallenge. Note inflammation (indicated by *) that extends into the cranial vault and meninges. Panel A shows HE staining, and Panel B shows IHC staining with antibody to the F1 capsule. C) HE stained section from a mouse (2×) challenged with wild-type Y. pestis (5,500 CFU) that succumbed to infection on day 3 post challenge. In contrast to panel A, the inflammation for mice challenged with the wild-type strain, is contained in the inner ear area and did not extend into the brain (arrow). D and E) Lung sections of mice challenged intranasally with Y. pestis. Overall, lung lesion development and character are the same between strains with necrosuppurative inflammation surrounding large colonies of bacteria. Panel D is of a lung section stained with HE (20×) from a mouse challenged with the ΔtatA mutant. Panel E is of a lung section stained with HE (20×) challenged with wild-type Y. pestis. IE = inner ear; CRB = cerebrum.

to the parental strain (Table 3). We demonstrated that this defect was due specifically to the loss of the tatA gene through restoring virulence via complementation. When the ΔtatA mutant was tested in pneumonic models of plague, contrasting results between delivery methods were observed. When whole-body small-particle aerosol challenges were performed, the LD_{50} for the ΔtatA mutant would be greater than 14 times of the wild-type CO92 strain (Table 3). We were not able to calculate a reliable LD_{50} measurement from the survival curve for challenged mice due to a lack of a monotonic response. However, other attenuated strains of Y. pestis have demonstrated a poor dose response in animal models of plague challenge [31,69,70]. Though the mutant was not as attenuated via aerosol challenge as was observed with the bubonic model, this is not unprecedented. Differences in virulence have been observed frequently with other Y. pestis mutants dependent upon the routes of challenge [31,43,55,71–73].

In contrast to the differences in LD_{50} measurements observed with the other models of challenge, the LD_{50} for the ΔtatA mutant was only 1.7 times higher than the wild-type strain by intranasal challenge (Table 3). However, the mutant did display attenuation by other measurements of virulence following intranasal instillation: TTD (Table 4) and delayed dissemination and recovery from

organs following challenge (Fig. 9). Interestingly, the ΔtatA mutant virulence data are very similar to the results previously reported with a Δpla mutant in regards to minimal difference between LD_{50} values but large differences in TTD and CFU recoveries following intranasal challenge [74].

The intranasal challenge model is useful to study pathogenesis of infectious diseases, including pneumonic plague [74–78]. It is possible that the presence of bacteria, both wild-type and ΔtatA mutant, within the inner ear may be due to the delivery method. For wild-type Y. pestis, pneumonic plague and death occurs so rapidly that disease from the inner ear is not able to progress to meningitis. In contrast, infection with the ΔtatA mutant is slowed which allows the bacteria to persist within the inner ear and then eventually reach the brain. Interestingly, a recent article described the ability of Y. pestis to create a localized anti-inflammatory state that creates a protective environment for itself and other non-pathogenic bacteria in the immediate vicinity [79]. Perhaps the ΔtatA mutant, though attenuated by other methods of challenge, becomes an "opportunistic pathogen" when able to gain access for a prolonged time to the inner ear of a mouse and create a suitable environment for it to infect the host.

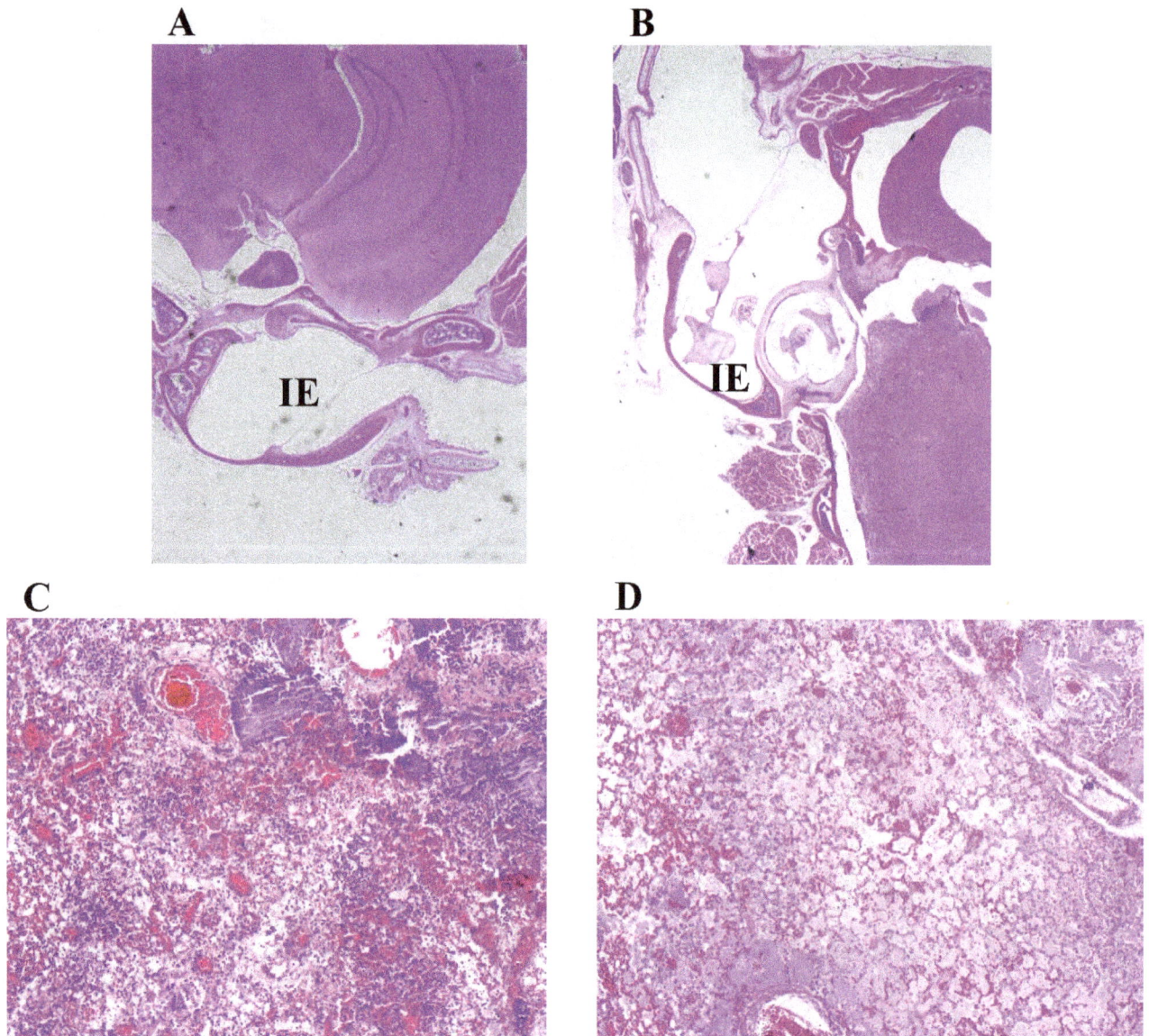

Figure 8. Pathology of mice challenged with *Y. pestis* by small particle aerosol. A and B) HE stained skull sections of aerosol challenged mice. A) Mouse (2×) challenged with wild-type CO92 (6.9×10^5 CFU) that was moribund and euthanized on day 3 postchallenge. B) Mouse (4×) challenged with Δ*tatA* mutant (3.3×10^6 CFU) that was moribund and euthanized on day 7 postchallenge. No inner ear (IE) or meningeal involvement was detected for mice aerosol challenged with either strain of *Y. pestis*. HE stained lung sections (10×) of mice aerosol challenged with CO92 (C) or Δ*tatA* mutant (D). There was no difference in lesion character or severity in mice challenged with either strain.

Challenges by intranasal instillation versus small-particle aerosol differ in many aspects. Namely, the sizes of the particles generated differ between the two routes and would therefore colonize different parts of the lung and body. The smaller particles generated by a whole-body aerosol chamber would be inhaled deeper into the lung. In contrast, the particles from intranasal challenges would by much larger and would infect both the upper and lower respiratory tract and be much more likely to be swallowed and infect the digestive system. Similar to the results from our current study, mice that were challenged by intranasal delivery with *Burkholderia pseudomallei* also showed a high incidence of meningitis [80]. In addition, other studies have shown differences between intranasal or aerosol delivery in dissemination of bacterial pathogens [80,81] or inflammation response to allergens [82] in mice.

It would be tempting to speculate that the loss of virulence associated with the Δ*tatA* mutant is due to the altered F1 antigen. However, it has been shown by others that loss of the *Y. pestis* F1 antigen had little to or no difference in virulence in mice [72,83–87]. In contrast, Sebbane et al. demonstrated that *Y. pestis* deleted of the *caf1M1A1* operon are affected in their ability to cause bubonic plague in mice following flea bites [88]. As the Δ*tatA* mutant was severely hindered following subcutaneous infection and displays an altered F1 antigen, it would be interesting to determine if it would be similarly defective via a flea bite route of infection. In addition, a recent study demonstrated a *caf1* deletion mutant in the CO92 strain of *Y. pestis* was attenuated by bubonic and pneumonic (intranasal) models of infection depending on the strain of mouse [77]. Our current challenge studies with the Δ*tatA* mutant were limited to Swiss Webster mice. It would be of interest

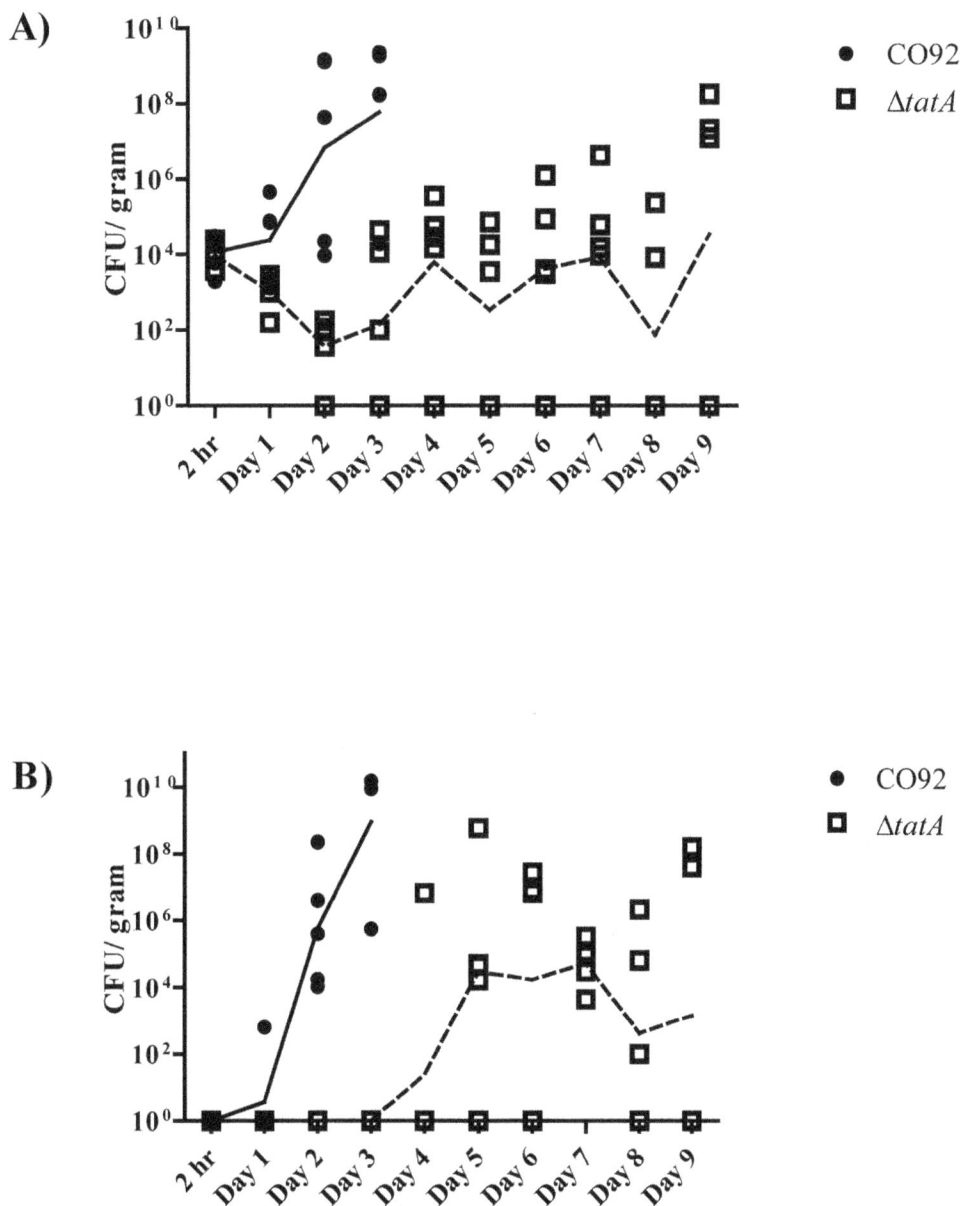

Figure 9. Dissemination studies of mice challenged intranasally with *Y. pestis*. Mice were challenged with CO92 (113,000 CFU) or ΔtatA mutant (76,000 CFU). At set time points, mice were euthanized, and the lungs and spleens were harvested. The A) lungs and B) spleens were homogenized and plated to determine bacterial recovery. For each time point, five mice were assayed, except for day 3 for wild-type challenged mice. Only four mice were tested as the remaining challenged mice had succumbed to infection. The lines (solid = CO92 and hashed = ΔtatA) are connecting at the geometrical means at the data points of CFU recovery from the respective organs are represent the overall trend during the course of infection.

to extend these studies to additional mouse strains as described by Weening at al. [77] to determine if the ΔtatA mutant would be more attenuated by the intranasal challenge model of plague.

Based upon proteomic and bioinformatic analysis of *E. coli* and *B. subtilis*, as much as 5–8% of secreted proteins are translocated by the Tat pathway [89]. A previous study using the TATFIND computer program, identified a total of 19 putative Tat secreted proteins [58]; however, none of the candidates seemed likely to be effectors of the phenotypes observed in the mutant. To identify *Y. pestis* Tat secreted proteins that may be responsible for the loss of virulence, biofilm adherence, or the altered F1 protein, the *Y. pestis* CO92 genome was screened for proteins containing the Tat-

like motifs within the N-terminal portion substituting similar amino acids for the consensus motif sequence. Nine proteins were identified during this screen five of which have homologs demonstrated to be Tat translocation products in other bacterial species [19,63,90,91]. However, many of the identified *Y. pestis* proteins from both of these studies are hypothetical or potential putative proteins of broad function. For instance, YPO2150 is a predicted transcriptional regulator and a member of the LysR family which can regulate capsule, fimbriae, and biofilm production in other bacterial pathogens [92–94]. In addition, novel chaperone/usher loci were recently described for *Y. pestis* [68].

Table 5. *Y. pestis* proteins containing putative Tat motifs.

Motif*	Protein	Product
SRRSFLQ	TauA	taurine transporter substrate binding subunit**
SRRSFLQ	SufI	repressor protein for FtsI**
TRRKFLM	YPO0986	hypothetical protein**
SRRLALL	YPO2150	LysR family transcriptional regulator
SRREFIQ	DmsA	putative dimethyl sulfoxide reductase chain A protein**
SRRDFMK	NapA	nitrate reductase catalytic subunit**
TRRDALA	YadG	putative ABC transporter ATP-binding protein
SRRLAIL	YPO3648	putative 2-hydroxy-3-oxopropionate reductase
TRRIFIL	YPO0009	putative membrane transport protein

*Underlined letters indicate substitution with a similar amino acid from the consensus Tat motif (SRRXFLK).
**Indicates a protein that overlaps with a previous study [58] that identified predicated Tat substrates from the CO92 *Y. pestis* genome.

Perhaps the Tat pathway interacts with these proteins and is able to directly or indirectly affect virulence.

Obviously, other Tat translocated proteins must exist in *Y. pestis* which affect pathogenesis. Recently, other proteins which utilize the Tat system but lack the signal motif were identified [59]. A more thorough examination utilizing more sophisticated methods would need to be pursued to identify *Y. pestis* Tat secreted proteins. It is likely that some of these proteins may be important virulence factors. Finally, this study further demonstrates the possibility of targeting the Tat pathway for novel therapeutics not only for *Y. pestis* but for many other bacterial pathogens.

Acknowledgments

We thank Kathy Kuehl for assistance with the EM samples, and Susan Welkos, Kei Amemiya and Jennifer Dankmeyer for providing the antibodies and recombinant proteins. Opinions, interpretations, conclusions, and recommendations are those of the authors and are not necessarily endorsed by the U.S. Army.

Author Contributions

Conceived and designed the experiments: JB JK PW. Performed the experiments: JB CKC TKK AJ SM KM TB. Analyzed the data: JB TC SJK JK DF CGR TB. Wrote the paper: JB TB.

References

1. Worsham PL, McGovern TW, Vietri NJ, Friedlander AM (2007) Plague. In: Dembek ZF, editor. Medical Aspects of Biological Warfare. Washington, DC: Office of The Surgeon General. 91–119.
2. Perry RD, Fetherston JD (1997) *Yersinia pestis*–etiologic agent of plague. Clin Microbiol Rev 10: 35–66.
3. Cornelis GR, Biot T, Lambert de Rouvroit C, Michiels T, Mulder B, et al. (1989) The *Yersinia yop* regulon. Mol Microbiol 3: 1455–1459.
4. Straley SC (1991) The low-Ca2+ response virulence regulon of human-pathogenic *Yersiniae*. Microb Pathog 10: 87–91.
5. Bozue J, Cote CK, Webster W, Bassett A, Tobery S, et al. (2012) A *Yersinia pestis* YscN ATPase mutant functions as a live attenuated vaccine against bubonic plague in mice. FEMS Microbiol Lett 332: 113–121.
6. Mori H, Ito K (2001) The Sec protein-translocation pathway. Trends Microbiol 9: 494–500.
7. Berks BC (1996) A common export pathway for proteins binding complex redox cofactors? Mol Microbiol 22: 393–404.
8. Buchanan G, de Leeuw E, Stanley NR, Wexler M, Berks BC, et al. (2002) Functional complexity of the twin-arginine translocase TatC component revealed by site-directed mutagenesis. Mol Microbiol 43: 1457–1470.
9. de Leeuw E, Granjon T, Porcelli I, Alami M, Carr SB, et al. (2002) Oligomeric properties and signal peptide binding by *Escherichia coli* Tat protein transport complexes. J Mol Biol 322: 1135–1146.
10. De Leeuw E, Porcelli I, Sargent F, Palmer T, Berks BC (2001) Membrane interactions and self-association of the TatA and TatB components of the twin-arginine translocation pathway. FEBS Lett 506: 143–148.
11. Gohlke U, Pullan L, McDevitt CA, Porcelli I, de Leeuw E, et al. (2005) The TatA component of the twin-arginine protein transport system forms channel complexes of variable diameter. Proc Natl Acad Sci U S A 102: 10482–10486.
12. Porcelli I, de Leeuw E, Wallis R, van den Brink-van der Laan E, de Kruijff B, et al. (2002) Characterization and membrane assembly of the TatA component of the *Escherichia coli* twin-arginine protein transport system. Biochemistry 41: 13690–13697.
13. Baglieri J, Beck D, Vasisht N, Smith CJ, Robinson C (2012) Structure of TatA paralog, TatE, suggests a structurally homogeneous form of Tat protein translocase that transports folded proteins of differing diameter. J Biol Chem 287: 7335–7344.
14. Wexler M, Sargent F, Jack RL, Stanley NR, Bogsch EG, et al. (2000) TatD is a cytoplasmic protein with DNase activity. No requirement for TatD family proteins in sec-independent protein export. J Biol Chem 275: 16717–16722.
15. Bronstein PA, Marrichi M, Cartinhour S, Schneider DJ, DeLisa MP (2005) Identification of a twin-arginine translocation system in *Pseudomonas syringae* pv. tomato DC3000 and its contribution to pathogenicity and fitness. J Bacteriol 187: 8450–8461.
16. Chen L, Hu B, Qian G, Wang C, Yang W, et al. (2009) Identification and molecular characterization of twin-arginine translocation system (Tat) in *Xanthomonas oryzae* pv. oryzae strain PXO99. Arch Microbiol 191: 163–170.
17. Zhang L, Zhu Z, Jing H, Zhang J, Xiong Y, et al. (2009) Pleiotropic effects of the twin-arginine translocation system on biofilm formation, colonization, and virulence in *Vibrio cholerae*. BMC Microbiol 9: 114.
18. Rodriguez-Sanz M, Antunez-Lamas M, Rojas C, Lopez-Solanilla E, Palacios JM, et al. The Tat pathway of plant pathogen *Dickeya dadantii* 3937 contributes to virulence and fitness. FEMS Microbiol Lett 302: 151–158.
19. van Mourik A, Bleumink-Pluym NM, van Dijk L, van Putten JP, Wosten MM (2008) Functional analysis of a *Campylobacter jejuni* alkaline phosphatase secreted via the Tat export machinery. Microbiology 154: 584–592.
20. Ochsner UA, Snyder A, Vasil AI, Vasil ML (2002) Effects of the twin-arginine translocase on secretion of virulence factors, stress response, and pathogenesis. Proc Natl Acad Sci U S A 99: 8312–8317.
21. Voulhoux R, Ball G, Ize B, Vasil ML, Lazdunski A, et al. (2001) Involvement of the twin-arginine translocation system in protein secretion via the type II pathway. EMBO J 20: 6735–6741.
22. De Buck E, Maes L, Meyen E, Van Mellaert L, Geukens N, et al. (2005) *Legionella pneumophila* Philadelphia-1 *tatB* and *tatC* affect intracellular replication and biofilm formation. Biochem Biophys Res Commun 331: 1413–1420.
23. Rossier O, Cianciotto NP (2005) The *Legionella pneumophila tatB* gene facilitates secretion of phospholipase C, growth under iron-limiting conditions, and intracellular infection. Infect Immun 73: 2020–2032.
24. Caldelari I, Mann S, Crooks C, Palmer T (2006) The Tat pathway of the plant pathogen *Pseudomonas syringae* is required for optimal virulence. Mol Plant Microbe Interact 19: 200–212.
25. Wagley S, Hemsley C, Thomas R, Moule MG, Vanaporn M, et al. (2014) The Twin Arginine Translocation System Is Essential for Aerobic Growth and Full Virulence of *Burkholderia thailandensis*. J Bacteriol 196: 407–416.
26. Lavander M, Ericsson SK, Broms JE, Forsberg A (2006) The twin arginine translocation system is essential for virulence of *Yersinia pseudotuberculosis*. Infect Immun 74: 1768–1776.

27. Doll JM, Zeitz PS, Ettestad P, Bucholtz AL, Davis T, et al. (1994) Cat-transmitted fatal pneumonic plague in a person who traveled from Colorado to Arizona. Am J Trop Med Hyg 51: 109–114.

28. Surgalla MJ, Beesley ED (1969) Congo red-agar plating medium for detecting pigmentation in Pasteurella pestis. Appl Microbiol 18: 834–837.

29. Wang RF, Kushner SR (1991) Construction of versatile low-copy-number vectors for cloning, sequencing and gene expression in Escherichia coli. Gene 100: 195–199.

30. Donnenberg MS, Kaper JB (1991) Construction of an eae deletion mutant of enteropathogenic Escherichia coli by using a positive-selection suicide vector. Infect Immun 59: 4310–4317.

31. Bozue J, Mou S, Moody KL, Cote CK, Trevino S, et al. (2011) The role of the phoPQ operon in the pathogenesis of the fully virulent CO92 strain of Yersinia pestis and the IP32953 strain of Yersinia pseudotuberculosis. Microb Pathog 50: 314–321.

32. Conchas RF, Carniel E (1990) A highly efficient electroporation system for transformation of Yersinia. Gene 87: 133–137.

33. Hinchliffe SJ, Isherwood KE, Stabler RA, Prentice MB, Rakin A, et al. (2003) Application of DNA microarrays to study the evolutionary genomics of Yersinia pestis and Yersinia pseudotuberculosis. Genome Res 13: 2018–2029.

34. Anisimov AP, Bakhteeva IV, Panfertsev EA, Svetoch TE, Kravchenko TB, et al. (2009) The subcutaneous inoculation of pH 6 antigen mutants of Yersinia pestis does not affect virulence and immune response in mice. J Med Microbiol 58: 26–36.

35. Fetherston JD, Schuetze P, Perry RD (1992) Loss of the pigmentation phenotype in Yersinia pestis is due to the spontaneous deletion of 102 kb of chromosomal DNA which is flanked by a repetitive element. Mol Microbiol 6: 2693–2704.

36. Fetherston JD, Perry RD (1994) The pigmentation locus of Yersinia pestis KIM6+ is flanked by an insertion sequence and includes the structural genes for pesticin sensitivity and HMWP2. Mol Microbiol 13: 697–708.

37. Buchrieser C, Brosch R, Bach S, Guiyoule A, Carniel E (1998) The high-pathogenicity island of Yersinia pseudotuberculosis can be inserted into any of the three chromosomal asn tRNA genes. Mol Microbiol 30: 965–978.

38. Daly JA, Gooch WM, 3rd, Matsen JM (1985) Evaluation of the Wayson variation of a methylene blue staining procedure for the detection of microorganisms in cerebrospinal fluid. J Clin Microbiol 21: 919–921.

39. Anderson GW Jr, Worsham PL, Bolt CR, Andrews GP, Welkos SL, et al. (1997) Protection of mice from fatal bubonic and pneumonic plague by passive immunization with monoclonal antibodies against the F1 protein of Yersinia pestis. Am J Trop Med Hyg 56: 471–473.

40. Sun YC, Hinnebusch BJ, Darby C (2008) Experimental evidence for negative selection in the evolution of a Yersinia pestis pseudogene. Proc Natl Acad Sci U S A 105: 8097–8101.

41. DiMezzo TL, Ruthel G, Brueggemann EE, Hines HB, Ribot WJ, et al. (2009) In vitro intracellular trafficking of virulence antigen during infection by Yersinia pestis. PLoS One 4: e6281.

42. Glynn A, Roy CJ, Powell BS, Adamovicz JJ, Freytag LC, et al. (2005) Protection against aerosolized Yersinia pestis challenge following homologous and heterologous prime-boost with recombinant plague antigens. Infect Immun 73: 5256–5261.

43. Worsham PL, Roy C (2003) Pestoides F, a Yersinia pestis strain lacking plasminogen activator, is virulent by the aerosol route. Adv Exp Med Biol 529: 129–131.

44. Davis KJ, Vogel P, Fritz DL, Steele KE, Pitt ML, et al. (1997) Bacterial filamentation of Yersinia pestis by beta-lactam antibiotics in experimentally infected mice. Arch Pathol Lab Med 121: 865–868.

45. Parkhill J, Wren BW, Thomson NR, Titball RW, Holden MT, et al. (2001) Genome sequence of Yersinia pestis, the causative agent of plague. Nature 413: 523–527.

46. Stanley NR, Findlay K, Berks BC, Palmer T (2001) Escherichia coli strains blocked in Tat-dependent protein export exhibit pleiotropic defects in the cell envelope. J Bacteriol 183: 139–144.

47. Benoit SL, Maier RJ (2014) Twin-Arginine Translocation System in Helicobacter pylori: TatC, but Not TatB, Is Essential for Viability. MBio 5.

48. Karlyshev AV, Galyov EE, Smirnov O, Guzayev AP, Abramov VM, et al. (1992) A new gene of the f1 operon of Y. pestis involved in the capsule biogenesis. FEBS Lett 297: 77–80.

49. Chen TH, Elberg SS (1977) Scanning electron microscopic study of virulent Yersinia pestis and Yersinia pseudotuberculosis type 1. Infect Immun 15: 972–977.

50. Simpson WJ, Thomas RE, Schwan TG (1990) Recombinant capsular antigen (fraction 1) from Yersinia pestis induces a protective antibody response in BALB/c mice. Am J Trop Med Hyg 43: 389–396.

51. Mehigh RJ, Braubaker RR (1993) Major stable peptides of Yersinia pestis synthesized during the low-calcium response. Infect Immun 61: 13–22.

52. Sarker MR, Neyt C, Stainier I, Cornelis GR (1998) The Yersinia Yop virulon: LcrV is required for extrusion of the translocators YopB and YopD. J Bacteriol 180: 1207–1214.

53. Sarker MR, Sory MP, Boyd AP, Iriarte M, Cornelis GR (1998) LcrG is required for efficient translocation of Yersinia Yop effector proteins into eukaryotic cells. Infect Immun 66: 2976–2979.

54. Pettersson J, Holmstrom A, Hill J, Leary S, Frithz-Lindsten E, et al. (1999) The V-antigen of Yersinia is surface exposed before target cell contact and involved in virulence protein translocation. Mol Microbiol 32: 961–976.

55. Welkos SL, Davis KM, Pitt LM, Worsham PL, Freidlander AM (1995) Studies on the contribution of the F1 capsule-associated plasmid pFra to the virulence of Yersinia pestis. Contrib Microbiol Immunol 13: 299–305.

56. Guarner J, Shieh WJ, Greer PW, Gabastou JM, Chu M, et al. (2002) Immunohistochemical detection of Yersinia pestis in formalin-fixed, paraffin-embedded tissue. Am J Clin Pathol 117: 205–209.

57. Davis KJ, Fritz DL, Pitt ML, Welkos SL, Worsham PL, et al. (1996) Pathology of experimental pneumonic plague produced by fraction 1-positive and fraction 1-negative Yersinia pestis in African green monkeys (Cercopithecus aethiops). Arch Pathol Lab Med 120: 156–163.

58. Dilks K, Rose RW, Hartmann E, Pohlschroder M (2003) Prokaryotic utilization of the twin-arginine translocation pathway: a genomic survey. J Bacteriol 185: 1478–1483.

59. Ferrandez Y, Condemine G (2008) Novel mechanism of outer membrane targeting of proteins in Gram-negative bacteria. Mol Microbiol 69: 1349–1357.

60. Stanley NR, Palmer T, Berks BC (2000) The twin arginine consensus motif of Tat signal peptides is involved in Sec-independent protein targeting in Escherichia coli. J Biol Chem 275: 11591–11596.

61. Hinsley AP, Stanley NR, Palmer T, Berks BC (2001) A naturally occurring bacterial Tat signal peptide lacking one of the 'invariant' arginine residues of the consensus targeting motif. FEBS Lett 497: 45–49.

62. Bendtsen JD, Kiemer L, Fausboll A, Brunak S (2005) Non-classical protein secretion in bacteria. BMC Microbiol 5: 58.

63. Kato J, Nishimura Y, Yamada M, Suzuki H, Hirota Y (1988) Gene organization in the region containing a new gene involved in chromosome partition in Escherichia coli. J Bacteriol 170: 3967–3977.

64. Ding Z, Christie PJ (2003) Agrobacterium tumefaciens twin-arginine-dependent translocation is important for virulence, flagellation, and chemotaxis but not type IV secretion. J Bacteriol 185: 760–771.

65. He H, Wang Q, Sheng L, Liu Q, Zhang Y (2011) Functional characterization of Vibrio alginolyticus twin-arginine translocation system: its roles in biofilm formation, extracellular protease activity, and virulence towards fish. Curr Microbiol 62: 1193–1199.

66. Galyov EE, Karlishev AV, Chernovskaya TV, Dolgikh DA, Smirnov O, et al. (1991) Expression of the envelope antigen F1 of Yersinia pestis is mediated by the product of caf1M gene having homology with the chaperone protein PapD of Escherichia coli. FEBS Lett 286: 79–82.

67. Runco LM, Myrczek S, Bliska JB, Thanassi DG (2008) Biogenesis of the fraction 1 capsule and analysis of the ultrastructure of Yersinia pestis. J Bacteriol 190: 3381–3385.

68. Felek S, Jeong JJ, Runco LM, Murray S, Thanassi DG, et al. (2011) Contributions of chaperone/usher systems to cell binding, biofilm formation and Yersinia pestis virulence. Microbiology 157: 805–818.

69. Welkos S, Pitt ML, Martinez M, Friedlander A, Vogel P, et al. (2002) Determination of the virulence of the pigmentation-deficient and pigmentation−/plasminogen activator-deficient strains of Yersinia pestis in non-human primate and mouse models of pneumonic plague. Vaccine 20: 2206–2214.

70. Hallett AF, Isaacson M, Meyer KF (1973) Pathogenicity and immunogenic efficacy of a live attenuated plague vaccine in vervet monkeys. Infect Immun 8: 876–881.

71. Cathelyn JS, Crosby SD, Lathem WW, Goldman WE, Miller VL (2006) RovA, a global regulator of Yersinia pestis, specifically required for bubonic plague. Proc Natl Acad Sci U S A 103: 13514–13519.

72. Friedlander AM, Welkos SL, Worsham PL, Andrews GP, Heath DG, et al. (1995) Relationship between virulence and immunity as revealed in recent studies of the F1 capsule of Yersinia pestis. Clin Infect Dis 21 Suppl 2: S178–181.

73. Welkos SL, Friedlander AM, Davis KJ (1997) Studies on the role of plasminogen activator in systemic infection by virulent Yersinia pestis strain C092. Microb Pathog 23: 211–223.

74. Lathem WW, Price PA, Miller VL, Goldman WE (2007) A plasminogen-activating protease specifically controls the development of primary pneumonic plague. Science 315: 509–513.

75. Lathem WW, Crosby SD, Miller VL, Goldman WE (2005) Progression of primary pneumonic plague: a mouse model of infection, pathology, and bacterial transcriptional activity. Proc Natl Acad Sci U S A 102: 17786–17791.

76. Fisher ML, Castillo C, Mecsas J (2007) Intranasal inoculation of mice with Yersinia pseudotuberculosis causes a lethal lung infection that is dependent on Yersinia outer proteins and PhoP. Infect Immun 75: 429–442.

77. Weening EH, Cathelyn JS, Kaufman G, Lawrenz MB, Price P, et al. (2011) The dependence of the Yersinia pestis capsule on pathogenesis is influenced by the mouse background. Infect Immun 79: 644–652.

78. Anderson DM, Ciletti NA, Lee-Lewis H, Elli D, Segal J, et al. (2009) Pneumonic plague pathogenesis and immunity in Brown Norway rats. Am J Pathol 174: 910–921.

79. Price SB, Cowan C, Perry RD, Straley SC (1991) The Yersinia pestis V antigen is a regulatory protein necessary for Ca2(+)-dependent growth and maximal expression of low-Ca2+ response virulence genes. J Bacteriol 173: 2649–2657.

80. Warawa JM (2010) Evaluation of surrogate animal models of melioidosis. Front Microbiol 1: 141.

81. Glomski IJ, Dumetz F, Jouvion G, Huerre MR, Mock M, et al. (2008) Inhaled non-capsulated Bacillus anthracis in A/J mice: nasopharynx and alveolar space as dual portals of entry, delayed dissemination, and specific organ targeting. Microbes Infect 10: 1398–1404.

82. Swedin L, Ellis R, Kemi C, Ryrfeldt A, Inman M, et al. (2010) Comparison of aerosol and intranasal challenge in a mouse model of allergic airway inflammation and hyperresponsiveness. Int Arch Allergy Immunol 153: 249–258.

83. Anderson GW Jr, Leary SE, Williamson ED, Titball RW, Welkos SL, et al. (1996) Recombinant V antigen protects mice against pneumonic and bubonic plague caused by F1-capsule-positive and -negative strains of *Yersinia pestis*. Infect Immun 64: 4580–4585.

84. Worsham PL, Stein MP, Welkos SL (1995) Construction of defined F1 negative mutants of virulent *Yersinia pestis*. Contrib Microbiol Immunol 13: 325–328.

85. Quenee LE, Cornelius CA, Ciletti NA, Elli D, Schneewind O (2008) *Yersinia pestis caf1* variants and the limits of plague vaccine protection. Infect Immun 76: 2025–2036.

86. Cornelius CA, Quenee LE, Elli D, Ciletti NA, Schneewind O (2009) *Yersinia pestis* IS*1541* transposition provides for escape from plague immunity. Infect Immun 77: 1807–1816.

87. Drozdov IG, Anisimov AP, Samoilova SV, Yezhov IN, Yeremin SA, et al. (1995) Virulent non-capsulate *Yersinia pestis* variants constructed by insertion mutagenesis. J Med Microbiol 42: 264–268.

88. Sebbane F, Jarrett C, Gardner D, Long D, Hinnebusch BJ (2009) The *Yersinia pestis caf1M1A1* fimbrial capsule operon promotes transmission by flea bite in a mouse model of bubonic plague. Infect Immun 77: 1222–1229.

89. Berks BC, Sargent F, Palmer T (2000) The Tat protein export pathway. Mol Microbiol 35: 260–274.

90. Kolkman MA, van der Ploeg R, Bertels M, van Dijk M, van der Laan J, et al. (2008) The twin-arginine signal peptide of *Bacillus subtilis* YwbN can direct either Tat- or Sec-dependent secretion of different cargo proteins: secretion of active subtilisin via the *B. subtilis* Tat pathway. Appl Environ Microbiol 74: 7507–7513.

91. Kostecki JS, Li H, Turner RJ, DeLisa MP (2010) Visualizing interactions along the *Escherichia coli* twin-arginine translocation pathway using protein fragment complementation. PLoS One 5: e9225.

92. Deghmane AE, Giorgini D, Larribe M, Alonso JM, Taha MK (2002) Down-regulation of pili and capsule of *Neisseria meningitidis* upon contact with epithelial cells is mediated by CrgA regulatory protein. Mol Microbiol 43: 1555–1564.

93. Koskiniemi S, Sellin M, Norgren M (1998) Identification of two genes, *cpsX* and *cpsY*, with putative regulatory function on capsule expression in group B streptococci. FEMS Immunol Med Microbiol 21: 159–168.

94. Hennequin C, Forestier C (2009) *oxyR*, a LysR-type regulator involved in *Klebsiella pneumoniae* mucosal and abiotic colonization. Infect Immun 77: 5449–5457.

25

Reduction of the Inflammatory Responses against Alginate-Poly-L-Lysine Microcapsules by Anti-Biofouling Surfaces of PEG-b-PLL Diblock Copolymers

Milica Spasojevic[1,2], Genaro A. Paredes-Juarez[2], Joop Vorenkamp[1], Bart J. de Haan[2], Arend Jan Schouten[1], Paul de Vos[2]*

1 Department of Polymer Chemistry, Zernike Institute for Advanced Materials, University of Groningen, Groningen, The Netherlands, **2** Departments of Pathology and Laboratory Medicine, section of Medical Biology, division of immunoendocrinology, University of Groningen, Groningen, The Netherlands

Abstract

Large-scale application of alginate-poly-L-lysine (alginate-PLL) capsules used for microencapsulation of living cells is hampered by varying degrees of success, caused by tissue responses against the capsules in the host. A major cause is proinflammatory PLL which is applied at the surface to provide semipermeable properties and immunoprotection. In this study, we investigated whether application of poly(ethylene glycol)-block-poly(L-lysine hydrochloride) diblock copolymers (PEG-b-PLL) can reduce the responses against PLL on alginate-matrices. The application of PEG-b-PLL was studied in two manners: (i) as a substitute for PLL or (ii) as an anti-biofouling layer on top of a proinflammatory, but immunoprotective, semipermeable alginate-PLL_{100} membrane. Transmission FTIR was applied to monitor the binding of PEG-b-PLL. When applied as a substitute for PLL, strong host responses in mice were observed. These responses were caused by insufficient binding of the PLL block of the diblock copolymers confirmed by FTIR. When PEG-b-PLL was applied as an anti-biofouling layer on top of PLL_{100} the responses in mice were severely reduced. Building an effective anti-biofouling layer required 50 hours as confirmed by FTIR, immunocytochemistry and XPS. Our study provides new insight in the binding requirements of polyamino acids necessary to provide an immunoprotective membrane. Furthermore, we present a relatively simple method to mask proinflammatory components on the surface of microcapsules to reduce host responses. Finally, but most importantly, our study illustrates the importance of combining physicochemical and biological methods to understand the complex interactions at the capsules' surface that determine the success or failure of microcapsules applicable for cell-encapsulation.

Editor: Xiaoming He, The Ohio State University, United States of America

Funding: This work was supported by a project from The Kollf institute and the Juvenile Diabetes research foundation. The funders had no role in study design, data collection and analysis, decision to publish, or preparation of the manuscript.

Competing Interests: The authors have declared that no competing interests exist.

* Email: P.de.Vos@umcg.nl

Introduction

Microencapsulation of therapeutics cells is a promising approach for treatment of endocrine disorders such as anemia [1], dwarfism [2], hemophilia B [3], kidney [4] and liver [5] failure, pituitary [6] other central nervous system insufficiencies [7], and diabetes [8]. The semipermeable membrane allows for diffusion of nutrients and therapeutics, whereas the cells are protected from the immune system. This approach eliminates the necessity for immunosuppression and allows for xenografting. Xenografting may contribute to solving donor shortage.

Alginate-poly-L-lysine capsules have frequently been applied for microencapsulation of pancreatic islets [8]. Alginates are natural, unbranched polysaccharides composed of two monomer units, β-D-mannuronic acid (M) and its C-5 epimer, α-L-guluronic acid (G), connected by 1→4 linkages. They gel under physiological conditions without involvement of any toxic compounds such as harmful solvents. Many groups apply poly-L-lysine (PLL) to

reduce the pore size and to provide immunoprotection [9,10]. Normally unbound PLL is immunogenic [11]; however, to circumvent host responses against PLL, the microcapsules are ionically cross-linked with alginate to induce complexes of superhelical cores of alginate and PLL at the capsule's surface [12,13]. But this process is not straightforward [14,15]. Minor changes in the procedure can result in inadequate binding of proinflammatory PLL with strong immune reactions in the host as a consequence [13,14,16–18]. This was shown recently by our group in a comparison study of the *in vivo* behavior of a series of alginate-PLL capsules that differed only 10% in G-content. The alginate with higher G-content underwent changes *in vivo*, which resulted in the release of proinflammatory PLL followed by a strong tissue response [17].

Many different polycations have been proposed to substitute PLL, designed to provide immunoprotection on alginate matrixes for cell encapsulation [19–22]. Among them are chitosan [20], poly-L-ornithine [21,23], poly-D-lysine [22] and diblock copolymers

[24]. Often, however, new issues are introduced with these alternatives to PLL, leading again to severe inflammatory responses *in vivo* [19]. Partly, this is due to lack of knowledge about how the polyamino acids interact with alginate [14,23,25–27], but it is also due to the enormous lab-to-lab variations in successful formation of immunoprotective membranes [28,29]. These issues led to our current proposal to design means for making capsule's surfaces more biocompatible, while still using PLL for providing immuno-protection because of its well known binding ability to alginate. Introducing diblock copolymers is, theoretically, such an approach, but has been difficult to achieve on the surface of cell-containing hydrophilic capsules. Many procedures to build membranes require harsh chemicals, eliminating them as options as only cell-friendly approaches may be applied to avoid loss of cells. The use of cell-friendly approaches is especially important when cell-sources from rare cadaveric donors are applied such as pancreatic islets for the treatment of diabetes [30]. Any loss of tissue is unacceptable in these types of applications. Here we studied the ability of PEG-b-PLL copolymers to reduce inflammatory responses. The copolymer can be applied as a complete substitute for PLL or as an additional layer on top of a preexisting proinflammatory PLL layer. The PEG-b-PLL copolymers can be bound to the surface of alginate without the application of chemicals that interfere with tissue viability. The PLL-block interacts ionically with the negatively charged alginate-core. The other block, polyethylene glycol (PEG), provides a biocompatible protecting layer on the surface of the capsules.

This study was designed to investigate the application of diblock copolymers in two manners. The first application was as a complete substitute for PLL, forming an immunoprotective membrane as previously suggested [24]. The other application was as an anti-biofouling layer on top of an immunoprotective PLL layer. We choose to use PLL_{100} to study the masking effects of the PEG-b-PLL copolymer. PLL_{100} provokes strong inflammatory responses due to incomplete binding to alginate as will be demonstrated in this study. The adsorption kinetics of the diblock copolymers on the alginate surface was studied by FTIR. The binding of diblock copolymers and surface properties in the absence and presence of the diblock copolymers were character-ized by FTIR and XPS, respectively. Host responses were studied after implanted in the peritoneal cavity of balb/c mice.

Materials and Methods

Materials

Intermediate-G sodium alginate was obtained from ISP Alginates (UK). Poly-L-lysine hydrochloride (PLL_{100}) ($M_n = 16$ kg/mol) and methoxy-poly(ethylene glycol)-block-poly(L-lysine hydrochloride) (PEG_x-b-PLL_y) (x = 454, $M_n = 20$ kg/mol; y = 50 or 100, $M_n = 8$ or 16 kg/mol; PDI = 1.2) were purchased from Alamanda Polymers (USA). Streptavidin fluorescein isothiocyanate (FITC) and Rabbit anti-PEG biotin were purchased from DakoCytomation (Denmark) and Bio-Connect B.V. (The Netherlands), respectively.

Deposition of alginate films on silicon wafers

Prior to applying alginate coatings, double-side polished silicon wafers (Topsil Semiconductor Materials A/S, Frederikssund, Denmark 1000±15 µm thick) were cleaned by subsequent ultrasonication in dichloromethane, methanol, and acetone for 10 minutes. Residual organic contaminants were removed by UV-ozone treatment using an UV-ozone photoreactor PR-100 (Uvikon) for 60 minutes. Due to this treatment, the hydrophilicity of the exposed surface increases. Immediately after cleaning an alginate layer was applied on the surface.

Purified sodium alginate was dissolved in Krebs-Ringer-Hepes buffer (KRH, 220 mOsm) to give a 3.4 w/v % solution. The final alginate layer was obtained by dipping the recently cleaned and vertically aligned silicon wafers (1.5×1.0 cm) into the 3.4 w/v % alginate solution at a constant rate of 1 cm/min. The withdrawal rate was 10 cm/min. Silicon wafers coated with sodium alginate were placed into 100 mM CaCl_2 buffer after which alginate was allowed to cross-link with calcium overnight. Before the alginate gels were exposed to PLL_{100} and copolymer solution, transmission FTIR spectra of the dry alginate layers were recorded.

The binding of copolymers to calcium alginate-PLL_{100} layers was studied as follows. After washing in KRH (containing 2.5 mM CaCl_2) for 1 minute, one portion of alginate gel layers was incubated in PLL_{100} solution (in KRH containing 2.5 mM CaCl_2, PLL concentration $6.25×10^{-8}$ mol/ml) for 10 minutes. Subse-quently the layers were washed four times with KRH, dried under a filtered air stream and measured by FTIR. Alginate-PLL_{100} and the rest of alginate gel layers were incubated in copolymer solutions (in KRH containing 2.5 mM CaCl_2, copolymer concen-tration $3.55×10^{-8}$ mol/ml). After certain time intervals, the wafers were removed from the copolymer solution, washed four times with KRH, dried under a filtered air stream and measured by FTIR. Subsequently the wafers were returned to the copolymer solution in order to continue the adsorption process and to determine the saturation point.

Transmission Fourier transform infrared spectroscopy

The calcium alginate layers, as well as the layers after the pre-treatment with PLL_{100} and/or the adsorption of PEG-b-PLL copolymers, were studied by transmission FTIR. Measurements were performed under vacuum on a Bruker IFS 66 v/S spectrometer equipped with a DTGS detector and OPUS software package. A sample shuttle accessory was used for an interleaved sample and background scanning. A clean silicon wafer was used as a reference. All spectra are averages of 6×120 scans measured at a resolution of 4 cm^{-1}.

The adsorption of PLL_{100} and the copolymer was followed by analyzing the increase in the surface area associated with asymmetric and symmetric C-H stretching vibrations (3000 to 2800 cm^{-1}). In order to quantify the PLL- and copolymer-content on the calcium alginate, the surface area of the symmetric and asymmetric C-H stretching vibrations was determined. This value was reduced for the surface area corresponding to the C-H stretching vibrations of calcium alginate. Thus, the content of polymer attached to calcium alginate for each time point was obtained. These values were plotted as a function of time and the saturation point was determined as the starting point of the plateau.

Microcapsules formation

Only intermediate-G alginates were used and were purified according to literature procedures [31]. Subsequently, capsules were produced based on a previously described procedure with some modifications [32,33]. In some experiments cells were included. To this end, human insulin producing CM cells were cultured in RPMI (Gibco, Breda, The Netherlands) containing 60 kg/mL gentamicin and 10% heat-inactivated fetal calf serum (FCS) [34]. CM cells were always used between passage numbers 5 and 20. The cells were mixed at a concentration of $1×10^6$/ml with 3.4 w/v % sodium alginate solution. The cell containing or empty capsules were formed by converting the 3.4 w/v % sodium alginate solution into droplets using an air-driven generator [35]. The diameter of the droplets was controlled by a regulated airflow around the tip of needle. Alginate droplets were transformed to rigid alginate beads by gelling in a 100 mM CaCl$_2$ solution for at least 10 minutes. The beads were washed with KRH (containing 2.5 mM CaCl$_2$) for 1 minute. One portion of the beads was coated with the PEG-b-PLL copolymer for one hour and subsequently washed four times with KRH. Another portion of the beads was coated with PLL$_{100}$ for 10 minutes (PLL$_{100}$ solution in 310 mOsm KRH containing 2.5 mM CaCl$_2$, PLL concentration 6.25×10^{-8} mol/mL), subsequently washed four times with KRH and in the last step the capsules were coated with the PEG-b-PLL copolymer for as long as required to obtain a saturated surface as monitored by FTIR. Finally, the capsules were washed 3 times with 310 mOsm KRH containing 2.5 mM CaCl$_2$ and stored in this buffer. The diameters of capsules and beads were measured with a dissection microscope (Bausch and Lomb BVB-125, and 31–33–66) equipped with an ocular micrometer with an accuracy of 25 pm. The final diameter of the capsules was 600 μm.

FITC labelling of microcapsules

Fluorescent labeling of microcapsules is a multi-step procedure. Primary antibody was added to a 10% solution of normal rabbit serum in phosphate buffered saline (PBS). The optimal primary antibody concentration was investigated and found to be when the antibody was diluted 500 times. To stain end-groups of PEG, 100 μl of this PBS solution was added to an eppendorf cup with approximately 20 capsules and left to shake for 1 hour at room temperature. The capsules were washed several times with PBS and subsequently incubated in PBS solution of streptavidin FITC (streptavidin FITC/PBS = 1/100) for 30 minutes in the dark. Finally, the capsules were washed several times with PBS, transferred onto a glass slide and studied at room temperature with a Leica TCS SP2 AOBS confocal microscope (50 w Hg lamp, HC PL APO CS 10×/0,30 dry, working distance 11 mm, 5(6)-FITC; FITC excitation wavelength 494 nm, FITC emission wavelength 518 nm). Confocal analyses were performed using the Imaris ×64 version 7.6.4 software.

Testing cell viability

Viability of encapsulated cells was test using a LIVE/DEAD Cell Viability/Cytotoxicity assay Kit from InvitroGen, Life Technologies (New York, USA). Encapsulated cells were incubated for 30 min with Calcein AM (1 mM) and Ethidium Bromide (EB) (2 mM) at room temperature avoiding light. After incubation, the encapsulated cells were washed five times with KRH. Fluorescent confocal microscopy was measured at an emission wavelength of 517 nm (Calcein AM) and 617 nm (EB) using a Leica TCS SP2 AOBS confocal microscope (Wetzlar, Germany)

equipped with an objective HC PL APO CS 10×/0,30, dry immersion, and working distance of 11 mm. Data was analyzed using Imaris ×64 version 7.6.4 software. The number of dead and live cells was quantified by counting at least 500 cells per batch. The fraction of dead cells was expressed as the percentage of the total number of counted cells.

Diffusion characteristics

Permeability of capsules was studied using dextran-f samples of 10, 20, 40, 70, 110, or 150 kg/mol (TdB Consultancy AB, Sweden) as previously described [36–38]. For each dextran, approximately 50 capsules were placed on a microscope slide exposed to 200 μL of 0.1% dextran-f in Krebs Ringer Hepes, promptly covered with a glass coverslip and examined by fluorescence microscopy (Leica TCS SP2 AOBS confocal microscope). These permeability measurements were carried out in triplicate for each dextran-f MW.

X-ray photoelectron spectroscopy (XPS)

In order to quantitatively study the atomic composition, samples of fresh capsules were washed three times with ultrapure water and gradually lyophilized. Samples of lyophilized capsules were fixed on a sample holder. The sample holder was inserted into the chamber of an X-ray photoelectron spectrometer (Surface Science Instruments, S-probe, Mountain View, CA). An aluminum anode was used for generation of X-rays (10 kV, 22 mA) at a spot size of 250×1000 μm. During the measurements, the pressure in the spectrometer was approximately 10^{-7} Pa. First, scans were collected over the binding energy range of 1–1100 eV at low resolution (150 eV pass energy). Next, we recorded at high resolution (50 eV pass energy) C$_{1s}$, N$_{1s}$, and O$_{1s}$ peaks over a 20 eV binding energy range. The polymer content of the capsule's surface was expressed as a percentage of the total C, N, and O content of the membrane.

Animal studies

Wild-type male Balb/c mice were purchased from Harlan (Harlan, Horst, The Netherlands). The animals were fed standard chow and water ad libitum. All animal experiments were performed after receiving approval of the institutional Animal Care Committee of the Groningen University. All animals received animal care in compliance with the Dutch law on Experimental Animal Care. The mice were sacrificed by cervical dislocation.

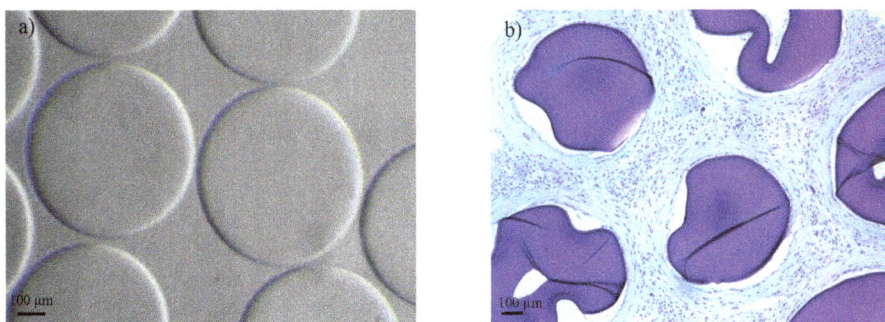

Figure 1. Alginate-PEG$_{454}$-b-PLL$_{100}$ capsules a) before implantation and b) at one month after implantation. GMA-embedded histological sections, Romanovsky-Giemsa staining, original magnification ×10.

a)

b)

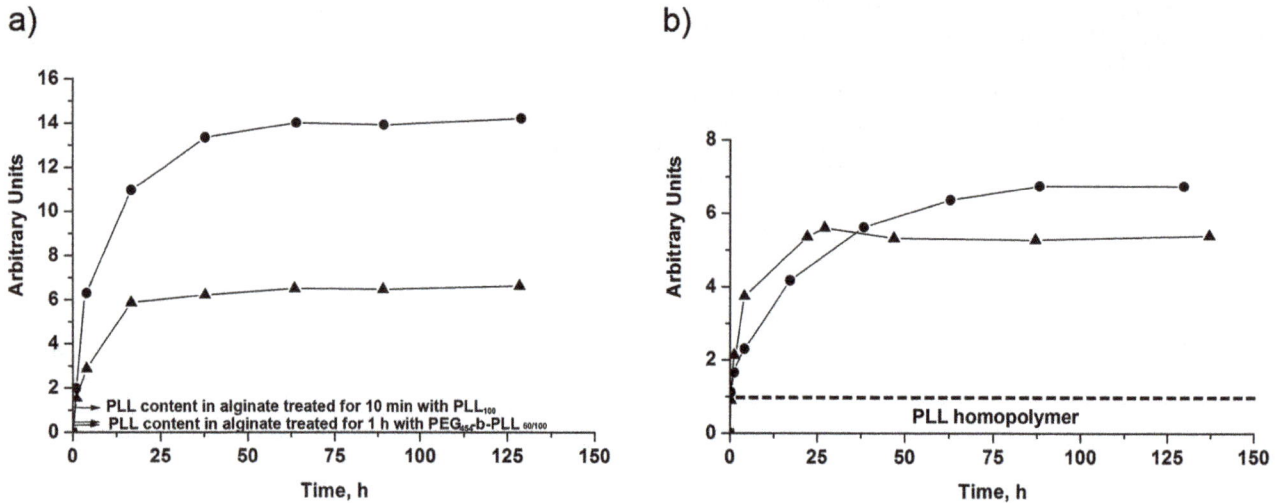

Figure 2. Kinetics of adsorption of the PEG$_{454}$-b-PLL$_{50}$ (•) and PEG$_{454}$-b-PLL$_{100}$ (▲) diblock copolymer on a) the alginate gel and b) the alginate gel pretreated for 10 minutes with PLL$_{100}$.

Implantation and explanation of empty capsules

Capsules were injected into the peritoneal cavity with a 16 G cannula via a small incision (3 mm) in the linea alba. The abdomen was closed with a two-layer suture. The implanted volume was always 0.5 mL as assessed in a syringe with appropriate measure. The transplants contained at least 1000 capsules. The microcapsules were retrieved 1 month after implantation by peritoneal lavage. Peritoneal lavage was performed by infusing 2 mL KRH through a 3 mm midline incision into the peritoneal cavity and subsequent aspiration of the KRH containing the capsules. All surgical procedures were performed under isoflurane anesthesia.

Histology

To assess the integrity of capsules before implantation, the samples of capsules were meticulously inspected for the presence of irregularities or defects in the capsule's membranes by using a dissection microscope.

To detect physical imperfections and to assess the composition and degree of overgrowth after implantation, samples of adherent

capsules recovered by excision and samples of non-adherent capsules were fixed in pre-cooled 2% paraformaldehyde, buffered with 0.05 M phosphate in saline (pH 7.4), and processed for (hydroxyethyl)methacrylate (HEMA) embedding [39]. Sections were prepared at 2 μm, stained with Romanovsky-Giemsa stain and applied for detecting imperfections in the capsule's membrane, for quantifying the composition of the overgrowth and determining the number of capsules with and without overgrowth. Different cell-types in the overgrowth were assessed by identifying cells in the capsular overgrowth with the morphological characteristics of monocytes/macrophages, lymphocytes, granulocytes, fibroblasts, basophiles, erythrocytes, and multinucleated giant cells. To confirm the adequacy of this approach, portions of adherent and non-adherent capsules were frozen in precooled isopropane as described in a previous study [17], sectioned at 5 μm, and processed for immunohistochemical staining and quantification of the different cell types as previously described [40]. The used monoclonal antibodies were: ED1 and ED2 against monocytes and macrophages [41], HIS-40 against IgM bearing B-lymphocytes [42], and R73 against CD3$^+$ bearing T-lymphocytes [43], In control sections we used PBS instead of the first stage monoclonal antibody. Quantification of these cells types after immunocytochemistry was compared with the assessments on the basis of morphological markers and always gave similar results.

The degree of capsular overgrowth was quantified by expressing the number of recovered capsules with overgrowth as the percentage of the total number of recovered capsules for each individual animal.

a)

b)

Figure 3. Illustration of a) alginate-PEG-b-PLL capsules (without PLL$_{100}$ pretreatment) and b) alginate-PLL-PEG-b-PLL capsules (with PLL$_{100}$ pretreatment).

Statistical analysis

Values are expressed as mean ± standard error of the mean (SEM). Normal distribution of the data was confirmed using the Kolmogorov-Smirnov test. As no normal distribution could be demonstrated, we applied the nonparametric Mann Whitney-U test. P-values<0.05 were considered to be statistically significant. The n-values for the animal experiments were based on a mandatory power analysis. The values were 4 mice per experimental group, based on a type I error of 5% and a type II error of 10%.

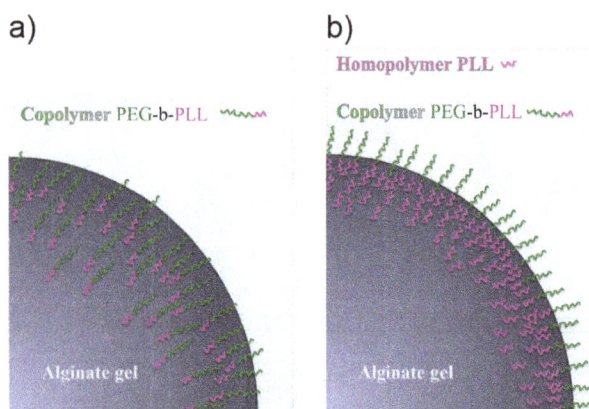

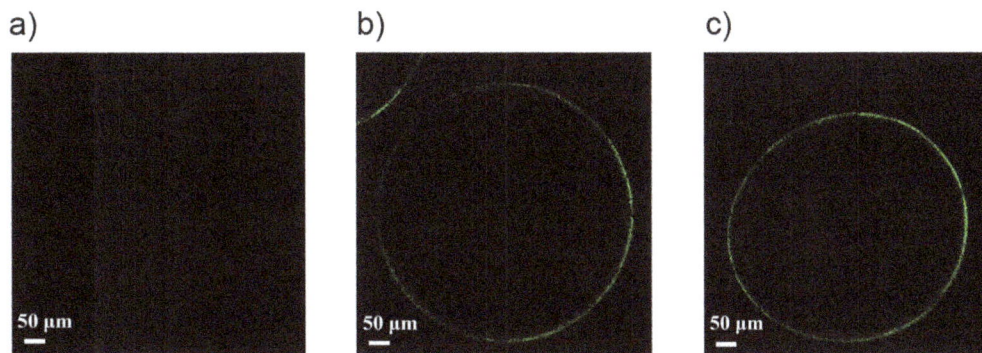

Figure 4. Confocal microscopy images after staining of the PEG blocks. a) Alginate-PLL$_{100}$ capsules, b) alginate-PLL$_{100}$-PEG$_{454}$-b-PLL$_{50}$ capsules and c) alginate-PLL$_{100}$-PEG$_{454}$-b-PLL$_{100}$ microcapsules. Original magnification 10×.

Results

The host responses against alginate-capsules where the PLL layer was completely substituted by PEG$_{454}$-b-PLL$_{100}$ to provide immunoprotection

Based on previous findings [24], we chose the long PEG$_{454}$ for the *in vivo* application because these long chains cannot easily penetrate into the alginate matrix and will stay at the surface. The positively charged PLL blocks are relatively small and will readily penetrate the alginate matrix where the ammonium groups of PLL will ionically interact with the carboxyl groups of alginate. To this end, the two PEG-b-PLL diblock copolymers were allowed to cross-link for one hour. This time period has found to be sufficient to create capsules with a permeability that does not allow entry of molecules larger than 120 kg/mol, which is considered to be an immunoprotective threshold [24,31,44]. Before implantation all capsules were meticulously microscopically inspected. Only perfect capsules with no tails or other imperfections associated with host responses were selected for implantation [45–47] (Figure 1a).

The capsules were implanted in the peritoneal cavity of balb/c mice and retrieved after one month. Macroscopically, the capsules with either an immunoprotective PEG$_{454}$-b-PLL$_{50}$ or PEG$_{454}$-b-PLL$_{100}$ were found in one large clump around the place of implantation. Examination by histology revealed that the capsules were caught in thick layers of fibroblast and were adherent to each other. This may be a sign of an unstable membrane in which positively charged molecules instantly attract inflammatory cells

leading to heavy fibroblast overgrowth (Figure 1b). A series of infrared studies revealed that the relatively short period of incubation (*i.e.* 1 hour), which provides a permeability of 100–120 kg/mol [24] with PEG$_{454}$-b-PLL$_y$ (y = 50 or 100), was too short to allow the formation of a stable membrane (see Figure 2a).

The fact that both PEG$_{454}$-b-PLL$_y$ (y = 50 or 100) cannot adequately substitute PLL in providing an immunoprotective membrane does not imply that they cannot be used for other purposes. The copolymers can be used for the formation of a masking anti-biofouling layer on top of PLL. PEG-b-PLL copolymers have been characterized as polymer with a low immunogenic capacity as they do elicit minor immune activation of nuclear factor NF-κB in THP-1 monocytes [24]. A prerequisite as outlined above, is that the diblock copolymer chains should be adequately bound to the matrix. For these reasons, the next step in our study was to apply PEG-b-PLL copolymers on top of a preexisting immunoprotective layer of proinflammatory PLL. Prior to the copolymer treatment, PLL$_{100}$ was applied to reduce the permeability of the alginate beads. This was done according to the principle illustrated in Figure 3. PLL$_{100}$ efficiently reduces permeability, but PLL$_{100}$ does provoke strong host responses as shown below. In order to determine the time period required to build an effective copolymer layer on top of the alginate-PLL$_{100}$ membrane, we applied FTIR. To this end, one to 1.5 µm thick alginate layers deposited on silicon wafers were incubated in a PLL$_{100}$ solution for 10 minutes, measured by FTIR and subsequently exposed to the copolymer solution and measured again. The kinetics of the adsorption was followed through the increase of

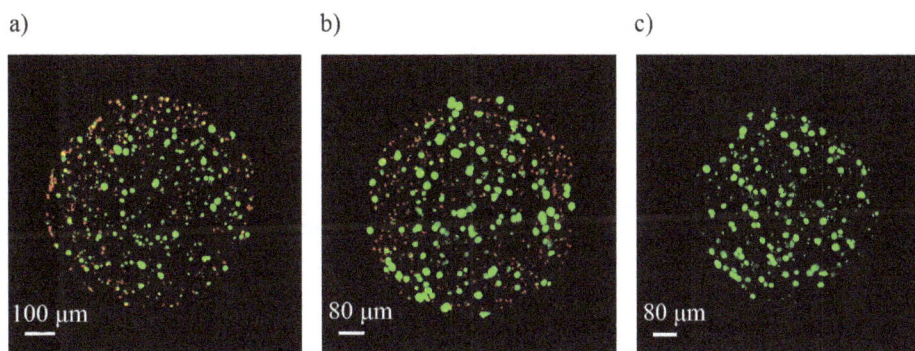

Figure 5. Viability of the insulin producing CM-cells encapsulated in a) alginate-PLL$_{100}$ capsules, b) alginate-PLL$_{100}$-PEG$_{454}$-b-PLL$_{50}$ capsules and c) alginate-PLL$_{100}$-PEG$_{454}$-b-PLL$_{100}$ microcapsules after 5 days of culturing. The remnants and dead cells were still visible in the periphery of the capsules.

Table 1. Percentage of dead CM-cells encapsulated in a) alginate-PLL$_{100}$ capsules (10 minutes incubation), b) alginate-PLL$_{100}$-PEG$_{454}$-b-PLL$_{50}$ capsules (50 hours incubation) and c) alginate-PLL$_{100}$-PEG$_{454}$-b-PLL$_{100}$ microcapsules (50 hours incubation) immediately after encapsulation and after 5 days of culturing (n = 4).

Samples of capsules	Dead CM-cells	
	Direct after encapsulation	Five days after encapsulation
Alginate-PLL100	15.75±1.80	14±3.39
Alginate-PLL$_{100}$-PEG$_{454}$-b-PLL$_{50}$	17.25±3.47	8.5±2.40
Alginate-PLL$_{100}$-PEG$_{454}$-b-PLL$_{100}$	17.75±3.79	12±2.12

the bands that correspond to symmetric and asymmetric C-H stretching vibrations in the FTIR spectrum. Since methyl, methylene, and methine groups do not participate in hydrogen bonding, the position of the bands corresponding to these groups is virtually not influenced by the chemical environment of the measured substance [48]. Therefore, this region was considered as the most reliable to study the quantity of the adsorbed PLL and/or copolymers. The surface area of the C-H bands was determined, reduced for the value which corresponds to C-H vibrations of the alginate gel and plotted as a function of time (see Figure 2).

After the pretreatment of the calcium-alginate layers with PLL$_{100}$, FTIR analysis showed that diblock copolymer chains could still interact and bind to the alginate gels as illustrated in Figure 3b. Binding of copolymers to the alginate-PLL$_{100}$ layer started immediately, continued asymptotically and reached a maximum value after approximately 25 hours for PEG$_{454}$-b-PLL$_{100}$ and 50 hours for PEG$_{454}$-b-PLL$_{50}$ (Figure 2b). Consequently, these time periods were taken as the minimum to achieve a high concentration of copolymers on the capsules' surface and to form an anti-biofouling layer on top of the alginate-PLL$_{100}$ layer.

In the present study we compared the capsules coated with the diblock copolymers for one hour with capsules coated with PLL$_{100}$ (10 minutes) and with PEG$_{454}$-b-PLL$_{50}$ for 50 hours. The reason is that we took the saturation time periods and therefore made this comparison. The alginate-PLL$_{100}$-PEG$_{454}$-b-PLL$_y$ (y = 50 or 100) capsules were prepared by incubating alginate beads in the PLL$_{100}$ solution for 10 min and subsequently in the copolymer solution for approximately 50 hours. To confirm binding of copolymers to PLL$_{100}$-precoated alginate capsules, the staining of the PEG blocks at the surface with antibodies directed against the end group of these blocks (methoxy group) was performed. PLL$_{100}$ capsules were used as negative control. The presence of green fluorescence

on the alginate-PLL$_{100}$-PEG$_{454}$-b-PLL$_y$ (y = 50 or 100) microcapsules demonstrated successful adsorption of diblock copolymers on the surface (Figure 4).

In order to determine whether long incubation times of 50 hours can influence the viability of cells, the insulin producing CM-cells were encapsulated according to this new procedure. CM-cells encapsulated in conventional control alginate-PLL$_{100}$ capsules, that were exposed for only ten minutes to PLL, served as control. The cell-containing capsules were subjected to live-dead staining for studying by confocal microscopy after the encapsulation procedure as well as after culturing for 5 days.. Figure 5 shows the results. The number of dead cells in the capsules was always below 20% and was not different between the freshly encapsulated cells and cells in capsules incubated for 5 days (Table 1). As shown in the enclosed Movie S1 after 5 days of culturing only the remnants of dead cells were still visible. The remnants and dead cells were always in the periphery of the capsules and were observed in all capsule types suggesting that direct interaction with PLL rather than the incubation times is responsible for death of these cells. The same results (data not shown) were obtained for T84 cells which usually are very sensitive for long times of serum deprivation.

The coating procedure had no influence on the permeability of the capsules. The alginate-PLL$_{100}$ capsules, as well as the 25 hours PEG$_{454}$-b-PLL$_{100}$ and the 50 hours for PEG$_{454}$-b-PLL$_{50}$ capsules were tested for permeability with fluorescent dextran with molecular weights of 10, 20, 40, 70, 110, and 150 kg/mol. All three capsule's types were still allowing entry of dextran with a molecular weight of 110 kg/mol but were impermeable for dextran with a Mw of 150 kg/mol (Table 2 and Figure 6). Uncoated, calcium alginate beads were permeable for all samples

Table 2. Permeability of the alginate-PLL$_{100}$, alginate-PLL$_{100}$-PEG$_{454}$-b-PLL$_{50}$ and alginate-PLL$_{100}$-PEG$_{454}$-b-PLL$_{100}$ capsules determined using dextran-f samples.

Dextran Samples, Molecular weight of dextran, kg/mol	Type of the alginate capsules (A)		
	A-PLL$_{100}$	A-PLL$_{100}$-PEG$_{454}$-b-PLL$_{50}$	A-PLL$_{100}$-PEG$_{454}$-b-PLL$_{100}$
10	+	+	+
20	+	+	+
40	+	+	+
70	+	+	+
110	+	+	+
150	−	−	−

a)   b)

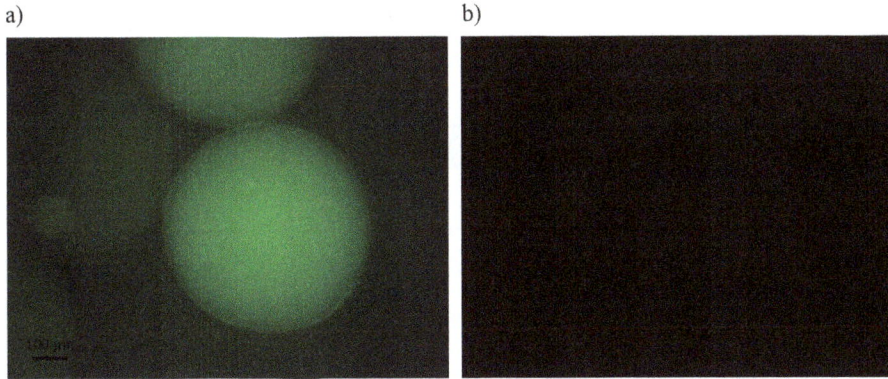

Figure 6. Confocal microscopy images of alginate-PLL-PEG-b-PLL microcapsules after the addition of a) dextran of 110 kg/mol and b) dextran of 150 kg/mol.

of dextran. This illustrated that the initial PLL_{100} incubation is the diffusion-limiting step.

X-ray photoelectron spectroscopy confirms presence of diblock copolymers at the surface

X-ray photoelectron spectroscopy (XPS) is a surface-sensitive quantitative technique for studying elemental composition, chemical, and electronic state of the elements in the material. This technique provides information for the top 2 to 10 nm of any analyzed material. XPS has been extensively used to study the composition of the capsule's surface [15,17,26,49]. To investigate the elemental composition, capsules were analyzed by XPS [17].

The surface elemental composition of the alginate-PLL_{100} and alginate-PLL_{100}-PEG_{454}-b-PLL_y (y = 50 or 100) capsules is presented in Table 3. The ratio of carbon to nitrogen (C/N) for the surface of the PLL-microcapsules was 8.14, whereas the theoretical C/N ratio for PLL is 3. This indicates that 2–10 nm surface layer is composed of both alginate and PLL as shown in our previous studies [17,49]. The C/N ratio for the surface of the alginate-PLL_{100}-PEG_{454}-b-PLL_y (y = 50 or 100) capsules is similar to the theoretical C/N ratio of the corresponding copolymers. Therefore, the XPS analysis confirmed that the surface of these capsules is mainly composed of the diblock copolymers.

Host response against alginate-PLL_{100} and alginate-PLL_{100}-PEG_{454}-b-PLL_{50} capsules

The last step in our study was to investigate whether the copolymer layer, formed after up to 50 hours of cross-linking with alginate-PLL_{100} was functional *in vivo*. We only applied the PEG_{454}-b-PLL_{50} in the *in vivo* study. Alginate-PLL_{100} capsules (*i.e.* controls) and the alginate-PLL_{100}-PEG_{454}-b-PLL_{50} capsules were implanted in the peritoneal cavity of balb/c mice. Before implantation, the grafts (n = 4) were meticulously inspected to ensure that they had a similar mechanical stability and had no broken or imperfect capsules.

The alginate-PLL_{100} capsules without an anti-biofouling layer provoked a very strong inflammatory response as expected. All capsules were found to adhere to the surface of the abdominal organs, which caused a low retrieval rate of the capsules (Figure 7a). In two animals the capsules were found as clumps on top of the liver and were completely caught in thick layers of fibroconnective tissue. Histologically high numbers of macrophages and fibroblasts were found. We also found multinucleated giant cells but no T-cells or B-cells. The few alginate-PLL_{100} capsules that escaped from the host response where mostly caught in the fibrotic clumps.

This was different when the anti-biofouling layer of PEG_{454}-b-PLL_{50} was applied (Table 4). Upon retrieval, 80–100% of the capsule grafts were recovered from the peritoneal cavity, whereas only $2.5 \pm 5\%$ of the alginate-PLL_{100} capsules were recovered (P< 0.01). The alginate-PLL_{100}-PEG_{454}-b-PLL_{50} capsules were mostly

Table 3. Elemental surface compositions of alginate-PLL_{100} and alginate-PLL_{100}-PEG_{454}-b-PLL_y (y = 50 or 100) microcapsules and theoretical atom % of PLL_{100} homopolymer and PEG_{454}-b-PLL_y (y = 50 or 100) diblock copolymers.

Capsules, alginate-	C, %	O, %	N, %	Ca, %	Others (Including Na and Cl), %	C/N ratio
PLL_{100}	58.42	26.97	7.18	1.38	6.05	8.14
PLL-PEG_{454}-b-PLL_{50}	66.38	27.37	6.25	0	0	10.62
PLL-PEG_{454}-b-PLL_{100}	65.70	25.26	9.04	0	0	7.27
Theoretical atom % of						
PLL	66.67	11.11	22.22	0	0	3.00
PEG	66.67	33.33	0	0	0	-
PEG_{454}-b-PLL_{50}	66.67	27.81	5.52	0	0	12.08
PEG_{454}-b-PLL_{100}	66.67	24.49	8.84	0	0	7.54

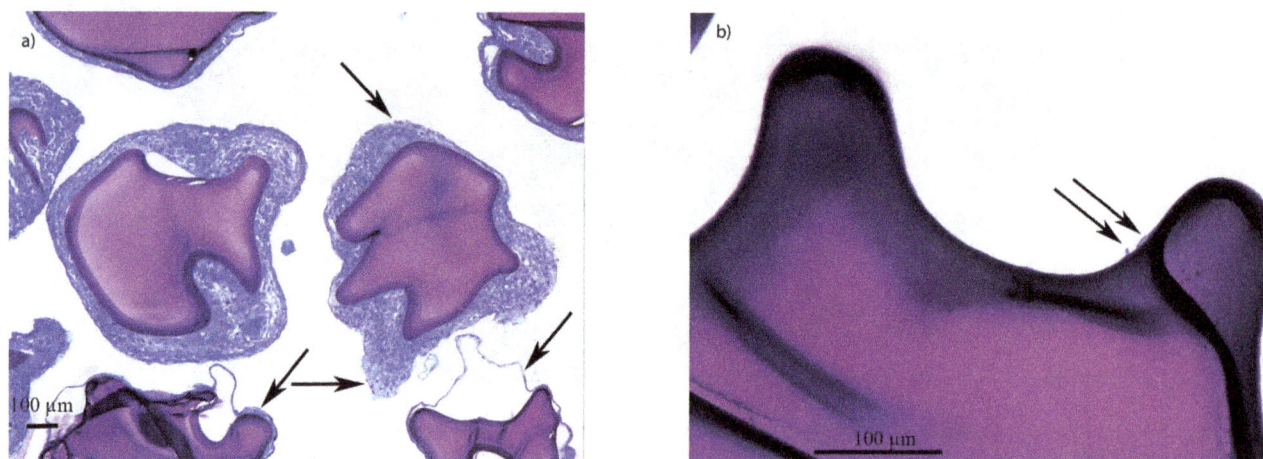

Figure 7. Explanted a) alginate-PLL$_{100}$, (original magnification 10×). Note the macrophages and fibroblasts. b) Alginate-PLL$_{100}$-PEG$_{454}$-b-PLL$_{50}$ microcapsules (original magnification 40×). Only a portion of capsules had inflammatory cells at the surface. Note that the affected capsules in most cases had adherence of a few or sometimes clumps of cells instead of complete coverage as in a). This suggests that local imperfections at the capsule's surface may be responsible for cell adhesion. All capsules were retrieved one month after implantation in the peritoneal cavity of balb/c mice GMA-embedded histological sections, Romanovsky-Giemsa staining.

free-floating and did not adhere to the abdominal organs. The capsules were found in between the intestines and clumping was rarely observed [50]. The percentage of capsules with cellular overgrowth with alginate-PLL$_{100}$-PEG$_{454}$-b-PLL$_{50}$ capsules was 36.25±27.87% whereas with alginate-PLL$_{100}$ capsules it was 97.25±5.5% (P<0.01) at one month after implantation. The capsules' surface was only rarely covered completely with the cellular overgrowth. Mostly, just a few cells were adhered which is usually interpreted as a local imperfection on the capsules' surface. The overgrowth was mainly composed of macrophages and a few fibroblasts (Figure 7b). We found no T-cells or other cells of the adaptive immune system on the capsules or on surrounding tissues that were taken for biopsy.

Discussion

A combined physicochemical and biological approach is still rarely implied in the encapsulation field [28]. The observation that by using diblock copolymers as substitutes for PLL strong inflammatory responses were induced while the diblock copolymers applied on the top of the alginate-PLL$_{100}$ surface reduced inflammatory responses, illustrates the necessity of a multidisciplinary approach in understanding the chemical background of host responses against microcapsules. Our work demonstrates that some polymers such as PEG$_{454}$-b-PLL$_{50}$ or PEG$_{454}$-b-PLL$_{100}$ are not applicable for creating immunoprotective membranes. The relatively short incubation times required to create a membrane impermeable for molecules above 100–120 kg/mol are not

sufficient to provide stable membranes. The same may hold true for many other polymers suggested to substitute PLL [20–23].

In this study, only intermediate-G alginates were applied, as only this type of alginate contains sufficient G-M blocks to bind PLL [17,32]. The diblock copolymer had no effect on the cells in the matrix as demonstrated with insulin producing CM-cells. Moreover, the PEG-b-PLL copolymer has been characterized as a unique polymer with a low immunogenic capacity [24], and PEG is known to provide an anti-biofouling layer in cell microencapsulation [51–56]. Therefore, we did not immediately abandon its application. Instead we studied whether the copolymer can form an anti-biofouling layer on top of the capsules' surface, which should reduce host responses against capsule's components. However, before studying the application of the copolymers as anti-biofouling layer on top of PLL$_{100}$, we first did a chemical analysis of the capsules' surface and determined the requirements for the optimal binding. Transmission FTIR study was applied to determine the time-period required for optimal binding and saturation. Elemental analysis of the capsules' surface in combination with immunocytochemistry demonstrated the efficiency of the bound copolymers to mask proinflammatory PLL. We found that 50 hours of incubation were required to form an efficacious layer on top of the PLL$_{100}$. Such long incubation time-periods may not be applicable for all cell types, but up to now all cells we applied did survive and functioned when cultured for prolonged periods in Krebs-Ringer-Hepes (KRH). KRH is a balanced salt solution that was especially developed for encapsulation of cells [33]. It is serum free but allows for survival of cells for prolonged periods of time.

Table 4. Recovery rates and percentage of alginate-PLL$_{100}$ and alginate-PLL$_{100}$–PEG$_{454}$-b-PLL$_{50}$ capsules with overgrowth, 1 month after implantation in the peritoneal cavity of balb/c mice.

Type of capsules	n	Recovery, %	Overgrowth, %
Alginate-PLL$_{100}$	4	2.5±5	97.25±5.5
Alginate-PLL$_{100}$-PEG$_{454}$-b-PLL$_{50}$	4	95±10	36.25±27.87

The PEG_{454}-b-PLL_{50} binding severely reduced the responses in mice against the alginate-PLL_{100} surfaces. The vast majority of the alginate-PLL_{100}-PEG_{454}-b-PLL_{50} capsules were free of any cell adhesion and free-floating in the peritoneal cavity, whereas nearly all alginate-PLL_{100} capsules without the copolymer were completely overgrown with macrophages and fibroblasts. Notably, however, some attachment of inflammatory cells was still observed on a portion of the alginate-PLL_{100}-PEG_{454}-b-PLL_{50} capsules. This adhesion of cells was different from what we have previously observed [15,57–60]. Complete coverage of capsule with inflammatory cells and fibroblasts, which is indicative for a foreign body response to the capsules, was rarely observed. In most cases, adhesion of groups of macrophages to specific parts of the capsule's surface was seen, suggesting that local imperfections were responsible for immune activation [45,61]. We believe that spatial differences in coating efficacy can be the cause of this type of cell adhesion implying that the system may still be improved in spite of the step-wise chemical approach. For sake of clarity, we counted all the capsules with overgrowth irrespective of the degree of overgrowth. Sometimes just one or two cells were found on the capsules with the PEG_{454}-b-PLL_{50} copolymer (Figure 7b). We believe that these cells will not have an influence on the functional survival of the cells in the capsules [45,61]. The data should therefore be carefully interpreted. The overgrowth is not necessarily having more consequences for cell survival than what was observed in previous studies were around 10% of the capsules were affected but infiltrated with large numbers of inflammatory cells instead of the few cells we found on the affected capsules in this study [44,45,62].

Creating an immunoprotective membrane with PLL without causing an inflammatory response has been shown to be a pitfall in many laboratories [27,63]. Variations in creating an efficacious PLL-membrane that provides immunoprotection without host-responses are one of the major factors responsible for the reported lab-to-lab variations with microcapsules [11,28,44,49,60,64]. The role of PLL in host responses has also been demonstrated in studies that show that calcium alginate normally does not provoke a response, but as soon as a polyamino acid is applied, strong inflammatory responses arise [63]. Adequate binding of PLL on the alginate matrix, which should result in formation of superhelical cores of alginate around PLL, depends on several crucial factors [14,29,65]. It is well recognized that alginate should contain sufficient G-M residues to bind all proinflammatory PLL [17,66]. A seemingly minor difference in G-M content can lead to leakage of PLL *in vivo* with foreign body responses as a consequence [17]. Another factor that is not often taken into consideration is the porosity of the alginate-gel in relation to the size of PLL chain. In our lab the 3.4% intermediate-G alginate gels are commonly used to create an immunoprotective membrane in combination with PLL of 22 to 24 kg/mol [15,17,49]. This relatively large molecule will only bind to sodium-alginate residues at the top 2–4 µm surface of the capsules [15,19,28]. Lower alginate concentrations or smaller PLL molecules can cause incomplete binding of PLL to the alginate core followed by leakage or exposure of unbound PLL at the capsule's surface *in vivo* with eventually host-responses as a consequence [11,13,67]. As shown here, anti-biofouling layers of the PEG_{454}-b-PLL_{50} copolymer may contribute to making PLL binding a less delicate process. Building an efficacious antifouling layer requires however a long incubation period of 50 hours, but it is rather simple as it involves only an incubation step. The binding efficacy can easily be followed through the increase of the bands that correspond to symmetric and asymmetric C-H stretching vibrations in the FTIR spectrum. The simple incubation step requires much less skills and technologies than adequate binding of PLL which depends not only on incubation with PLL but also on exchange of series of ions [14]. The application of this anti-biofouling layer may reduce in the enormous lab-to-lab variations that are considered to be a major threat for progress in the field [17,29,68].

Our study should not be interpreted as a suggestion that PLL binding is the only factor in host-responses against alginate-based microcapsules. Other important issues are the degree of purity of the alginates [16,26,28,65] and the type of alginates [18,32,49,62,64]. Crude alginates contain not only polyphenols but also pathogen associated molecular patterns that are potent stimulators of the immune system [69,70]. Nowadays, only ultrapure alginates are applied and intermediate-G alginates are preferred over high-G alginates despite a better mechanical stability of the high-G alginate gels [32,71–74]. In this study, only pure alginates with no immunostimulatory capacity were applied [24]. Our data showed that in spite of the extreme purity of alginates, inflammatory responses against capsules still occur due to presence of positively charged polyamino acids at the surface of capsules that are not in the required confirmation [12,13].

Conclusions

PEG-b-PLL diblock copolymers may contribute to reduction of host responses against alginate-PLL_{100} capsules by masking proinflammatory PLL_{100} residues. As such, PEG-b-PLL diblock copolymers are effective anti-biofouling molecules. Also, it was demonstrated that PEG-b-PLL diblock copolymers are not suitable as complete substitute for PLL because they provide membranes with the corresponding permeability but are unstable *in vivo*. Our study further illustrates the necessity of combining physicochemical and biological means to understand the complex interactions at the surface of microcapsules and the associated biological responses.

Supporting Information

Movie S1 Viability of the insulin producing CM-cells encapsulated in alginate-PLL_{100} capsules after 5 days of culturing. After 5 days of culturing only the remnants of dead cells were still visible. The remnants and dead cells were always in the periphery of the capsules suggesting that direct interaction with PLL rather than the incubation times is responsible for death of these cells.

Acknowledgments

The authors are grateful to Joop de Vries from Faculty of Medical Sciences, Department of Biomedical Engineering, University of Groningen for performing XPS measurements. This work was supported by a project from The Kolff institute and the Juvenile Diabetes research foundation.

Author Contributions

Conceived and designed the experiments: MS AJS PdV. Performed the experiments: MS GAP-J JV BJdH. Analyzed the data: MS GAP-J JV BJdH AJS PdV. Wrote the paper: MS AJS PdV.

References

1. Koo J, Chang TM (1993) Secretion of erythropoietin from microencapsulated rat kidney cells: preliminary results. Int J Artif Organs 16: 557–560.

2. Chang PL, Shen N, Westcott AJ (1993) Delivery of recombinant gene products with microencapsulated cells in vivo. Hum Gene Ther 4: 433–440.

3. Liu HW, Ofosu FA, Chang PL (1993) Expression of Human Factor IX by Microencapsulated Recombinant Fibroblasts. Hum Gene Ther 4: 291–301.

4. Cieslinski DA, David Humes H (1994) Tissue engineering of a bioartificial kidney. Biotechnol Bioeng 43: 678–681.

5. Uludag H, Sefton MV (1993) Metabolic activity and proliferation of CHO cells in hydroxyethyl methacrylate-methyl methacrylate (HEMA-MMA) microcapsules. Cell Transplant 2: 175–182.

6. Colton CK (1995) Implantable biohybrid artificial organs. Cell Transplant 4: 415–436.

7. Aebischer P, Goddard M, Signore AP, Timpson RL (1994) Functional recovery in hemiparkinsonian primates transplanted with polymer-encapsulated PC12 cells. Exp Neurol 126: 151–158.

8. Lim F, Sun AM (1980) Microencapsulated islets as bioartificial endocrine pancreas. Science 210: 908–910.

9. Leblond FA, Tessier J, Hallé J-P (1996) Quantitative method for the evaluation of biomicrocapsule resistance to mechanical stress. Biomaterials 17: 2097–2102.

10. Robitaille R, Leblond FA, Bourgeois Y, Henley N, Loignon M, et al. (2000) Studies on small (<350 μm) alginate-poly-L-lysine microcapsules. V. Determination of carbohydrate and protein permeation through microcapsules by reverse-size exclusion chromatography. J Biomed Mater Res 50: 420–427.

11. Strand BL, Ryan TL, In't Veld P, Kulseng B, Rokstad AM, et al. (2001) Poly-L-Lysine induces fibrosis on alginate microcapsules via the induction of cytokines. Cell Transplant 10: 263–275.

12. Uludag H, De Vos P, Tresco PA (2000) Technology of mammalian cell encapsulation. Adv Drug Delivery Rev 42: 29–64.

13. Vandenbossche GMR, Bracke ME, Cuvelier CA, Bortier HE, Mareel MM, et al. (1993) Host Reaction against Empty Alginate-polylysine Microcapsules. Influence of Preparation Procedure. J Pharm Pharmacol 45: 115–120.

14. van Hoogmoed CG, Busscher HJ, de Vos P (2003) Fourier transform infrared spectroscopy studies of alginate-PLL capsules with varying compositions. J Biomed Mater Res A 67: 172–178.

15. de Vos P, van Hoogmoed CG, van Zanten J, Netter S, Strubbe JH, et al. (2003) Long-term biocompatibility, chemistry, and function of microencapsulated pancreatic islets. Biomaterials 24: 305–312.

16. de Haan BJ, Rossi A, Faas MM, Smelt MJ, Sonvico F, et al. (2011) Structural surface changes and inflammatory responses against alginate-based microcapsules after exposure to human peritoneal fluid. J Biomed Mater Res A 98A: 394–403.

17. de Vos P, Spasojevic M, de Haan BJ, Faas MM (2012) The association between in vivo physicochemical changes and inflammatory responses against alginate based microcapsules. Biomaterials 33: 5552–5559.

18. de Vos P, de Haan BJ, Kamps JA, Faas MM, Kitano T (2007) Zeta-potentials of alginate-PLL capsules: a predictive measure for biocompatibility? J Biomed Mater Res A 80: 813–819.

19. Ponce S, Orive G, Hernández R, Gascón AR, Pedraz JL, et al. (2006) Chemistry and the biological response against immunoisolating alginate–polycation capsules of different composition. Biomaterials 27: 4831–4839.

20. Orive G, Bartkowiak A, Lisiecki S, De Castro M, Hernández RM, et al. (2005) Biocompatible oligochitosans as cationic modifiers of alginate/Ca microcapsules. J Biomed Mater Res B Appl Biomater 74: 429–439.

21. Basta G, Sarchielli P, Luca G, Racanicchi L, Nastruzzi C, et al. (2004) Optimized parameters for microencapsulation of pancreatic islet cells: an in vitro study clueing on islet graft immunoprotection in type 1 diabetes mellitus. Transpl Immunol 13: 289–296.

22. Bystrický S, Malovíková A, Sticzay T (1991) Interaction of acidic polysaccharides with polylysine enantiomers. Conformation probe in solution. Carbohydr Polym 15: 299–308.

23. Tam SK, Bilodeau S, Dusseault J, Langlois G, Hallé JP, et al. (2011) Biocompatibility and physicochemical characteristics of alginate–polycation microcapsules. Acta Biomater 7: 1683–1692.

24. Spasojevic M, Bhujbal S, Paredes G, de Haan BJ, Schouten AJ, et al. (2013) Considerations in binding diblock copolymers on hydrophilic alginate beads for providing an immunoprotective membrane. J Biomed Mater Res A 102: 1887–1896.

25. Rokstad AMA, Lacík I, de Vos P, Strand BL (2013) Advances in biocompatibility and physico-chemical characterization of microspheres for cell encapsulation. Adv Drug Deliv Rev 67–68: 111–130.

26. Tam SK, Dusseault J, Bilodeau S, Langlois G, Hallé J-P, et al. (2011) Factors influencing alginate gel biocompatibility. J Biomed Mater Res A 98A: 40–52.

27. Rokstad AM, Brekke O-L, Steinkjer B, Ryan L, Kolláriková G, et al. (2013) The induction of cytokines by polycation containing microspheres by a complement dependent mechanism. Biomaterials 34: 621–630.

28. de Vos P, Buèko M, Gemeiner P, Navrátil M, Švitel J, et al. (2009) Multiscale requirements for bioencapsulation in medicine and biotechnology. Biomaterials 30: 2559–2570.

29. Orive G, Emerich D, de Vos P (2014) Encapsulate this: the do's and don'ts. Nat Med 20.

30. Bruns H, Schultze D, Schemmer P (2013) Alternatives to islet transplantation: future cell sources of beta-like cells. Clin Transplant 27: 30–33.

31. De Vos P, De Haan BJ, Wolters GH, Strubbe JH, Van Schilfgaarde R (1997) Improved biocompatibility but limited graft survival after purification of alginate for microencapsulation of pancreatic islets. Diabetologia 40: 262–270.

32. De Vos P, De Haan B, Van Schilfgaarde R (1997) Effect of the alginate composition on the biocompatibility of alginate-polylysine microcapsules. Biomaterials 18: 273–278.

33. de Haan BJ, Faas MM, de Vos P (2003) Factors influencing insulin secretion from encapsulated islets. Cell Transplant 12: 617–625.

34. Smelt MJ, Faas MM, de Haan BJ, Draijer C, Hugenholtz GC, et al. (2012) Susceptibility of human pancreatic beta cells for cytomegalovirus infection and the effects on cellular immunogenicity. Pancreas 41: 39–49.

35. De Vos P, De Haan BJ, Van Schilfgaarde R (1997) Upscaling the production of microencapsulated pancreatic islets. Biomaterials 18: 1085–1090.

36. Vandenbossche GM, Van Oostveldt P, Remon JP (1991) A fluorescence method for the determination of the molecular weight cut-off of alginate-polylysine microcapsules. J Pharm Pharmacol 43: 275–277.

37. Vandenbossche GM, Van Oostveldt P, Demeester J, Remon JP (1993) The molecular weight cut-off of microcapsules is determined by the reaction between alginate and polylysine. Biotechnol Bioeng 42: 381–386.

38. Coromili V, Chang TM (1993) Polydisperse dextran as a diffusing test solute to study the membrane permeability of alginate polylysine microcapsules. Biomater Artif Cells Immobilization Biotechnol 21: 427–444.

39. De Haan BJ, van Goor H, De Vos P (2002) Processing of immunoisolated pancreatic islets: implications for histological analyses of hydrated tissue. Biotechniques 32: 612–614.

40. de Vos P, Smedema I, van Goor H, Moes H, van Zanten J, et al. (2003) Association between macrophage activation and function of micro-encapsulated rat islets. Diabetologia 46: 666–673.

41. Dijkstra CD, Dopp EA, Joling P, Kraal G (1985) The heterogeneity of mononuclear phagocytes in lymphoid organs: distinct macrophage subpopulations in the rat recognized by monoclonal antibodies ED1, ED2 and ED3. Immunology 54: 589–599.

42. Deenen GJ, Hunt SV, Opstelten D (1987) A stathmokinetic study of B lymphocytopoiesis in rat bone marrow: proliferation of cells containing cytoplasmic mu-chains, terminal deoxynucleotidyl transferase and carrying HIS24 antigen. JImmunol 139: 702–710.

43. Huning T, Wallny HJ, Hartly J, Lawetsky A, Tiefenthaler G (1989) A monoclonal antibody to a constant region of the rat TCR that induces T-cell activation. JExpMed 169: 73–78.

44. de Vos P, Faas MM, Strand B, Calafiore R (2006) Alginate-based microcapsules for immunoisolation of pancreatic islets. Biomaterials 27: 5603–5617.

45. De Vos P, De Haan B, Wolters GH, Van Schilfgaarde R (1996) Factors influencing the adequacy of microencapsulation of rat pancreatic islets. Transplantation 62: 888–893.

46. De Vos P, Wolters GH, Van Schilfgaarde R (1994) Possible relationship between fibrotic overgrowth of alginate-polylysine-alginate microencapsulated pancreatic islets and the microcapsule integrity. Transplant Proc 26: 782–783.

47. de Vos P, Van Straaten JF, Nieuwenhuizen AG, de Groot M, Ploeg RJ, et al. (1999) Why do microencapsulated islet grafts fail in the absence of fibrotic overgrowth? Diabetes 48: 1381–1388.

48. Schierbaum (1997) Hesse, M.: Meier, H.; Zech, B.: Spectroscopic Methods in Organic Chemistry (Translated by A. Linden, M. Murray). VIII and 365 pp., 221 fig., 100 tab., Hard cover: DM 168,–/SFr 149,–/ÖS 1226; ISBN 3 13 106 0611; Georg-Thieme Verlag Stuttgart – New York 1997; (New York ISBN 0 86577 6687). Starch - Stärke 49: 257–258.

49. de Vos P, Hoogmoed CG, Busscher HJ (2002) Chemistry and biocompatibility of alginate-PLL capsules for immunoprotection of mammalian cells. J Biomed Mater Res 60: 252–259.

50. Weir GC (2013) Islet encapsulation: advances and obstacles. Diabetologia 56: 1458–1461.

51. Ratner BD, Bryant SJ (2004) Biomaterials: where we have been and where we are going. Annu Rev Biomed Eng 6: 41–75.

52. Sawhney AS, Hubbell JA (1992) Poly(ethylene oxide)-graft-poly(L-lysine) copolymers to enhance the biocompatibility of poly(L-lysine)-alginate microcapsule membranes. Biomaterials 13: 863–870.

53. Sawhney AS, Pathak CP, Hubbell JA (1993) Interfacial photopolymerization of poly(ethylene glycol)-based hydrogels upon alginate-poly(l-lysine) microcapsules for enhanced biocompatibility. Biomaterials 14: 1008–1016.

54. Xu Y, Takai M, Ishihara K (2008) Suppression of Protein Adsorption on a Charged Phospholipid Polymer Interface. Biomacromolecules 10: 267–274.

55. Goto Y, Matsuno R, Konno T, Takai M, Ishihara K (2008) Polymer Nanoparticles Covered with Phosphorylcholine Groups and Immobilized with Antibody for High-Affinity Separation of Proteins. Biomacromolecules 9: 828–833.

56. Holland NB, Qiu Y, Ruegsegger M, Marchant RE (1998) Biomimetic engineering of non-adhesive glycocalyx-like surfaces using oligosaccharide surfactant polymers. Nature 392: 799–801.

57. Bünger CM, Tiefenbach B, Jahnke A, Gerlach C, Freier T, et al. (2005) Deletion of the tissue response against alginate-pll capsules by temporary release of co-encapsulated steroids. Biomaterials 26: 2353–2360.

58. Tatarkiewicz K, Garcia M, Omer A, Van Schilfgaarde R, Weir GC, et al. (2001) C-peptide responses after meal challenge in mice transplanted with microencapsulated rat islets. Diabetologia 44: 646–653.

59. Omer A, Keegan M, Czismadia E, de Vos P, Van Rooijen N, et al. (2003) Macrophage depletion improves survival of porcine neonatal pancreatic cell clusters contained in alginate macrocapsules transplanted into rats. Xenotransplantation 10: 240–251.

60. de Vos P, van Hoogmoed CG, de Haan BJ, Busscher HJ (2002) Tissue responses against immunoisolating alginate-PLL capsules in the immediate posttransplant period. J Biomed Mater Res 62: 430–437.

61. De Vos P, De Haan B, Pater J, Van Schilfgaarde R (1996) Association between capsule diameter, adequacy of encapsulation, and survival of microencapsulated rat islet allografts. Transplantation 62: 893–899.

62. van Schilfgaarde R, de Vos P (1999) Factors influencing the properties and performance of microcapsules for immunoprotection of pancreatic islets. J Mol Med 77: 199–205.

63. Rokstad AM, Brekke O-L, Steinkjer B, Ryan L, Kolláriková G, et al. (2011) Alginate microbeads are complement compatible, in contrast to polycation containing microcapsules, as revealed in a human whole blood model. Acta Biomater 7: 2566–2578.

64. Orive G, Tam SK, Pedraz JL, Hallé J-P (2006) Biocompatibility of alginate–poly-l-lysine microcapsules for cell therapy. Biomaterials 27: 3691–3700.

65. Tam SK, Bilodeau S, Dusseault J, Langlois G, Halle JP, et al. (2011) Biocompatibility and physicochemical characteristics of alginate-polycation microcapsules. Acta Biomater 7: 1683–1692.

66. King GA, Daugulis AJ, Faulkner P, Goosen MFA (1987) Alginate-Polylysine Microcapsules of Controlled Membrane Molecular Weight Cutoff for Mammalian Cell Culture Engineering. Biotechnology Progress 3: 231–240.

67. Vandenbossche GMR, Bracke ME, Cuvelier CA, Bortier HE, Mareel MM, et al. (1993) Host Reaction against Alginate-polylysine Microcapsules Containing Living Cells. J Pharm Pharmacol 45: 121–125.

68. Sobol M, Bartkowiak A, de Haan B, de Vos P (2013) Cytotoxicity study of novel water-soluble chitosan derivatives applied as membrane material of alginate microcapsules. J Biomed Mater Res A 101: 1907–1914.

69. Skjåk-Bræk G, Murano E, Paoletti S (1989) Alginate as immobilization material. II: Determination of polyphenol contaminants by fluorescence spectroscopy, and evaluation of methods for their removal. Biotechnol Bioeng 33: 90–94.

70. Paredes-Juarez GA, de Haan BJ, Faas MM, de Vos P (2013) The role of pathogen-associated molecular patterns in inflammatory responses against alginate based microcapsules. J Control Release 172: 983–992.

71. Thu B, Bruheim P, Espevik T, Smidsrod O, Soon-Shiong P, et al. (1996) Alginate polycation microcapsules. I. Interaction between alginate and polycation. Biomaterials 17: 1031–1040.

72. Stokke BT, Smidsroed O, Bruheim P, Skjaak-Braek G (1991) Distribution of uronate residues in alginate chains in relation to alginate gelling properties. Macromolecules 24: 4637–4645.

73. Thu B, Bruheim P, Espevik T, Smidsrød O, Soon-Shiong P, et al. (1996) Alginate polycation microcapsules: II. Some functional properties. Biomaterials 17: 1069–1079.

74. Thu B, Skjåk-Bræk G, Micali F, Vittur F, Rizzo R (1997) The spatial distribution of calcium in alginate gel beads analysed by synchrotron-radiation induced X-ray emission (SRIXE). Carbohydr Res 297: 101–105.

Permissions

All chapters in this book were first published in PLOS ONE, by The Public Library of Science; hereby published with permission under the Creative Commons Attribution License or equivalent. Every chapter published in this book has been scrutinized by our experts. Their significance has been extensively debated. The topics covered herein carry significant findings which will fuel the growth of the discipline. They may even be implemented as practical applications or may be referred to as a beginning point for another development.

The contributors of this book come from diverse backgrounds, making this book a truly international effort. This book will bring forth new frontiers with its revolutionizing research information and detailed analysis of the nascent developments around the world.

We would like to thank all the contributing authors for lending their expertise to make the book truly unique. They have played a crucial role in the development of this book. Without their invaluable contributions this book wouldn't have been possible. They have made vital efforts to compile up to date information on the varied aspects of this subject to make this book a valuable addition to the collection of many professionals and students.

This book was conceptualized with the vision of imparting up-to-date information and advanced data in this field. To ensure the same, a matchless editorial board was set up. Every individual on the board went through rigorous rounds of assessment to prove their worth. After which they invested a large part of their time researching and compiling the most relevant data for our readers.

The editorial board has been involved in producing this book since its inception. They have spent rigorous hours researching and exploring the diverse topics which have resulted in the successful publishing of this book. They have passed on their knowledge of decades through this book. To expedite this challenging task, the publisher supported the team at every step. A small team of assistant editors was also appointed to further simplify the editing procedure and attain best results for the readers.

Apart from the editorial board, the designing team has also invested a significant amount of their time in understanding the subject and creating the most relevant covers. They scrutinized every image to scout for the most suitable representation of the subject and create an appropriate cover for the book.

The publishing team has been an ardent support to the editorial, designing and production team. Their endless efforts to recruit the best for this project, has resulted in the accomplishment of this book. They are a veteran in the field of academics and their pool of knowledge is as vast as their experience in printing. Their expertise and guidance has proved useful at every step. Their uncompromising quality standards have made this book an exceptional effort. Their encouragement from time to time has been an inspiration for everyone.

The publisher and the editorial board hope that this book will prove to be a valuable piece of knowledge for researchers, students, practitioners and scholars across the globe.

List of Contributors

Carlos C. Goller and Mehreen Arshad
Department. of Pediatrics, Duke University School of Medicine, Durham, North Carolina, United States of America

James W. Noah, Subramaniam Ananthan, Carrie W. Evans, N. Miranda Nebane, Lynn Rasmussen, Melinda Sosa, Nichole A. Tower and E. Lucile White
Southern Research Specialized Biocontainment Screening Center, Southern Research Institute, Birmingham, Alabama, United States of America

Benjamin Neuenswander, Patrick Porubsky, Brooks E. Maki, Steven A. Rogers and Frank Schoenen
Specialized Chemistry Center, University of Kansas, Lawrence, Kansas,
United States of America

Patrick C. Seed
Department. of Pediatrics, Duke University School of Medicine, Durham, North Carolina, United States of America
Department of Molecular Genetics and Microbiology, Duke University School of Medicine, Durham, North Carolina, United States of America
Center for Microbial Pathogenesis, Duke University School of Medicine, Durham, North Carolina, United States of America

Lili Li, Hongli Li, Mingwei Yuan and Minglong Yuan
Engineering Research Center of Biopolymer Functional Materials of Yunnan, Yunnan University of Nationalities, Kunming, Yunnan, China

Qifeng Wang
Department of Radiation Oncology, Sichuan Cancer Hospital, Chengdu, Sichuan, China

Jessica S. Elman, Ryan M. Murray, Fangjing Wang, Keyue Shen and Shan Gao
Department of Surgery, Center for Engineering in Medicine and Surgical Services, Massachusetts General Hospital, Harvard Medical School and the Shriners Hospital for Children, Boston, Massachusetts, United States of America

Martin L. Yarmush
Department of Surgery, Center for Engineering in Medicine and Surgical Services, Massachusetts General Hospital, Harvard Medical School and the Shriners Hospital for Children, Boston, Massachusetts, United States of America
Department of Biomedical Engineering, Rutgers University, Piscataway, New Jersey, United States of America,

Ralph Weissleder
Center for Systems Biology, Massachusetts General Hospital, Harvard Medical School, Boston, Massachusetts, United States of America

Biju Parekkadan
Department of Surgery, Center for Engineering in Medicine and Surgical Services, Massachusetts General Hospital, Harvard Medical School and the Shriners Hospital for Children, Boston, Massachusetts, United States of America
Harvard Stem Cell Institute, Boston, Massachusetts, United States of America

Kevin E. Conway and Bakhos A. Tannous
Department of Neurology, Experimental Therapeutics and Molecular Imaging Laboratory, Massachusetts General Hospital, Charlestown, Massachusetts, United States of America

Gaurav Kwatra, Peter V. Adrian, Tinevimbo Shiri and Clare L. Cutland
Department of Science and Technology/National Research Foundation: Vaccine Preventable Diseases, University of the Witwatersrand, Johannesburg, South Africa,
MRC, Respiratory and Meningeal Pathogens Research Unit, University of the Witwatersrand, Johannesburg, South Africa

Shabir A. Madhi
Department of Science and Technology/National Research Foundation: Vaccine Preventable Diseases, University of the Witwatersrand, Johannesburg, South Africa,
MRC, Respiratory and Meningeal Pathogens Research Unit, University of the Witwatersrand, Johannesburg, South Africa

National Institute for Communicable Diseases: a division of National Health Laboratory Service, Johannesburg, South Africa

Eckhart J. Buchmann
Department of Obstetrics and Gynaecology, University of the Witwatersrand, Johannesburg, South Africa

Charles L. Cantrell
Natural Products Utilization Research Unit, Agricultural Research Service, United States Department of Agriculture, University, Mississippi, United States of America

Valtcho D. Zheljazkov and Ekaterina A. Jeliazkova
Sheridan Research and Extension Center, University of Wyoming, Sheridan, Wyoming, United States of America

Camila R. Carvalho
Natural Products Utilization Research Unit, Agricultural Research Service, United States Department of Agriculture, University, Mississippi, United States of America
Laboratory of Systematic and Biomolecules of Fungi, Microbiology Department, Institute of Biological, Sciences Federal University of Minas Gerais, Belo Horizonte, Minas Gerais, Brazil

Luiz H. Rosa
Laboratory of Systematic and Biomolecules of Fungi, Microbiology Department, Institute of Biological, Sciences Federal University of Minas Gerais, Belo Horizonte, Minas Gerais, Brazil

Tess Astatkie
Faculty of Agriculture, Dalhousie University, Truro, Nova Scotia, Canada

Elien Gevaert and Ria Cornelissen
1 Tissue Engineering Group, Ghent University, Ghent, Belgium

Laurent Dollé and Leo van Grunsven
Liver cell biology laboratory, Vrije Universiteit Brussels (VUB), Brussels, Belgium,

Thomas Billiet and Peter Dubruel
Polymer Chemistry and Biomaterials Research Group, Ghent University, Ghent, Belgium,

Aart van Apeldoorn
Department of Developmental Bioengineering, University of Twente, Enschede, the Netherlands

Ondřej Sglunda, Hana Hulejová, Marké ta Kuklová, Lenka Pleštilová and
Mária Filková Institute of Rheumatology, Prague, Czech Republic

Heřman Mann, Karel Pavelka, Jiří Vencovský and Ladislav Šenolt
Institute of Rheumatology, Prague, Czech Republic Department of Rheumatology, First Faculty of Medicine, Charles University in Prague, Prague, Czech Republic

Ondřej Pecha
Technology Centre ASCR, Prague, Czech Republic

Wang Li and Xiao-Yan Cai
State Key Laboratory of Oncogenes and Related Genes, Renji-Med X Clinical Stem Cell Research Center, Ren Ji Hospital, School of Medicine, Shanghai Jiao Tong University, Shanghai, China

Bo Ye
Department of Thoracic Surgery, Shanghai Chest Hospital, Shanghai Jiao Tong University, Shanghai, China

Jian-Hua Lin
School of Medicine, Shanghai Jiao Tong University, Shanghai, China

Wei-Qiang Gao
State Key Laboratory of Oncogenes and Related Genes, Renji-Med X Clinical Stem Cell Research Center, Ren Ji Hospital, School of Medicine, Shanghai Jiao Tong
University, Shanghai, China School of Biomedical Engineering & Med-X Research Institute, Shanghai Jiao Tong University, Shanghai, China

Subrata Gangooly and Eric Jauniaux
Institute for Women's Health, University College London, London, United Kingdom

Shanthi Muttukrishna
Institute for Women's Health, University College London, London, United Kingdom, Anu Research Centre, Department of Obstetrics and Gynaecology, University College Cork, Cork University Maternity Hospital, Cork, Republic of Ireland

Jiqing Guo and Henry J. Duff
Libin Cardiovascular Institute of Alberta, University of Calgary, Calgary, Alberta, Canada

Laura L. Perissinotti and Sergei Y. Noskov
Centre for Molecular Simulation, Biochemistry Research Cluster, Department of Biological Sciences, University of Calgary, Calgary, Alberta, Canada

Serdar Durdagi
Centre for Molecular Simulation, Biochemistry Research Cluster, Department of Biological Sciences, University of Calgary, Calgary, Alberta, Canada
Department of Biophysics, School of Medicine, Bahcesehir University, Istanbul, Turkey

Mohamed Changalov, Jason M. Hargreaves and Thomas G. Back
Department of Chemistry, University of Calgary, Calgary, Alberta, Canada

Mustafa Mir and Gabriel Popescu
Quantitative Light Imaging Laboratory, Department of Electrical and Computer Engineering, Beckman Institute for Advanced Science and Technology, University of Illinois at Urbana-Champaign, Urbana, Illinois, United States of America

Anna Bergamaschi and Benita S. Katzenellenbogen
Department of Molecular and Integrative Physiology, University of Illinois at Urbana-Champaign, Urbana, Illinois, United States of America

Naoki Ogusu, Junji Saruwatari, Hiroo Nakashima, Madoka Noai, Miki Nishimura, Mariko Deguchi and Kentaro Oniki
Division of Pharmacology and Therapeutics, Graduate School of Pharmaceutical Sciences, Kumamoto University, Kumamoto, Japan

Norio Yasui-Furukori and Sunao Kaneko
Department of Neuropsychiatry, Hirosaki University School of Medicine, Hirosaki, Japan

Takateru Ishitsu
Kumamoto Saishunso National Hospital, Kumamoto, Japan
Kumamoto Ezuko Ryoiku Iryo Center, Kumamoto, Japan

Kazuko Nakagaswa
Division of Pharmacology and Therapeutics, Graduate School of Pharmaceutical Sciences, Kumamoto University, Kumamoto, Japan
Center for Clinical Pharmaceutical Sciences, Kumamoto University, Kumamoto, Japan

Nicola Magrini, Giulio Formoso, Emilio Maestri, Francesco Nonino, Barbara Paltrinieri, Claudio Voci, Lucia Magnano and Anna Maria Marata
Drug Evaluation Area, Emilia-Romagna Regional Agency for Health and Social Care, Bologna, Italy

Lisa Daya and Oreste Capelli
Local Health Authority, Modena, Italy

Cinzia Del Giovane
Department of Clinical and Diagnostic Medicine and Public Health, University of Modena and Reggio Emilia, Modena, Italy

Man Li, Zhen Liang, Xun Sun, Tao Gong and Zhirong Zhang
Key Laboratory of Drug Targeting and Drug Delivery Systems, Ministry of Education, West China School of Pharmacy, Sichuan University, Chengdu, Sichuan, PR China

Nhu-Mai Tran, Murielle Dufresne, Patrick Paullier and Cécile Legallais
UMR CNRS 7338 Biomechanics and Bioingineering, University of Technology, Compiégne, France

Franc¸ois Helle, Thomas Walter Hoffmann, Catherine François, Etienne Brochot, Gilles Duverlie and Sandrine Castelain
EA4294 Department of Fundamental and Clinical Virology, University of Picardie Jules Verne, Amiens, France

Suo-Di Zhai
Department of Pharmacy, Peking University Third Hospital, Beijing, China

Zhi-Kang Ye and Can Li
Department of Pharmacy, Peking University Third Hospital, Beijing, China
Department of Pharmacy Administration and Clinical Pharmacy, School of Pharmaceutical Sciences, Peking University Health Science Center, Beijing, China

Alexander Hoare, Matthew G. Law, David A. Cooper and David P. Wilson
National Centre in HIV Epidemiology and Clinical Research, The University of New South Wales, Sydney, Australia

Stephen J. Kerr
National Centre in HIV Epidemiology and Clinical Research, The University of New South Wales, Sydney, Australia,

The HIV Netherlands Australia Thailand Research Collaboration, The Thai Red Cross AIDS Research Centre, Bangkok, Thailand

Jintanat Ananworanich
National Centre in HIV Epidemiology and Clinical Research, The University of New South Wales, Sydney, Australia
The HIV Netherlands Australia Thailand Research Collaboration, The Thai Red Cross AIDS Research Centre, Bangkok, Thailand
Faculty of Medicine, Chulalongkorn University, Bangkok, Thailand

Kiat Ruxrungtham and Praphan Phanuphak
The HIV Netherlands Australia Thailand Research Collaboration, The Thai Red Cross AIDS Research Centre, Bangkok, Thailand
Faculty of Medicine, Chulalongkorn University, Bangkok, Thailand

Kuan-Yeh Lee
Department of Internal Medicine, National Taiwan University Hospital Hsin-Chu Branch, Hsin-Chu, Taiwan

Sue-Yo Tang
Graduate Institute of Clinical Pharmacy, National Taiwan
University, Taipei, Taiwan,

Shu-Wen Lin
Graduate Institute of Clinical Pharmacy, National Taiwan University, Taipei, Taiwan
Department of Pharmacy, National Taiwan University Hospital and National Taiwan University College of Medicine, Taipei, Taiwan

Hsin-Yun Sun and Wen-Chun Liu
Department of Internal Medicine, National Taiwan University Hospital and National Taiwan University College of Medicine, Taipei, Taiwan

Ching-Hua Kuo
Department of Pharmacy, National Taiwan University Hospital and National Taiwan University College of Medicine, Taipei, Taiwan
School of Pharmacy, National Taiwan University, Taipei, Taiwan

Mao-Song Tsai
Department of Internal Medicine, Far Eastern Memorial Hospital, New Taipei City, Taiwan

Bing-Ru Wu
Department of Clinical Laboratory Sciences and Medical Biotechnology, National Taiwan University College of Medicine, Taipei, Taiwan

Sui-Yuan Chang
Department of Clinical Laboratory Sciences and Medical Biotechnology, National Taiwan University College of Medicine, Taipei, Taiwan
Department of Laboratory Medicine, National Taiwan University Hospital and National Taiwan University College of Medicine, Taipei, Taiwan

Chien-Ching Hung
Department of Internal Medicine, National Taiwan University Hospital and National Taiwan University College of Medicine, Taipei, Taiwan
Department of Medical Research, China Medical University Hospital, Taichung, Taiwan
China Medical University, Taichung, Taiwan

Stian André Engen, Håkon Valen Rukke, Fernanda Cristina Petersen and
Karl Schenck
Department of Oral Biology, University of Oslo, Oslo, Norway

Simone Becattin, David Jarrossay and Federica Sallusto
Institute for Research in Biomedicine, Universitá della Svizzera Italiana, Bellinzona, Switzerland

Inger Johanne Blix
Department of Oral Biology, University of Oslo, Oslo, Norway
Department of Periodontology, University of Oslo, Oslo, Norway

Viktor von Wyl
University College London, Research Department of Infection and Population Health, London, United Kingdom
CSS Institute for Empirical Health Economics, Lucerne, Switzerland

Valentina Cambiano and Andrew N. Phillips
University College London, Research Department of Infection and Population Health, London, United Kingdom

Michael R. Jordan
World Health Organization, Geneva, Switzerland
Tufts University, School of Medicine, Boston, Masschussetts, United States of America

Silvia Bertagnolio
World Health Organization, Geneva, Switzerland

Alec Miners
London School of Hygiene and Tropical Medicine, London, United Kingdom

Deenan Pillay
University College London, Division of Infection and Immunity, London, United Kingdom

Jens Lundgren
Copenhagen University Hospital-Rigshospitalet, University of Copenhagen, Copenhagen, Denmark

Lihan Chen, Øystein Evensen and Stephen Mutoloki
Department of Basic Sciences and Aquatic Medicine, Norwegian University of Life Sciences, Oslo, Norway

Goran Klaric
EWOS Innovation AS, Sandnes, Norway
Department of Mechanical Engineering, University College London, London, United Kingdom

Simon Wadsworth
EWOS Innovation AS, Sandnes, Norway

Suwan Jayasinghe
Department of Mechanical Engineering, University College London, London, United Kingdom

Tsun-Yung Kuo
Department of Animal Science/Institute of Biotechnology, National Ilan University, Taipei, Taiwan

Sing Teang Kong, Wee Beng Lee, Pasikanthi Kishore Kumar and Paul C. Ho
Department of Pharmacy, National University of Singapore, Singapore, Singapore

Hwee Yi Stella Wang, Yan Lam Shannon Ng and Pei Shieen Wong
Department of Neurology, Singapore General Hospital, Singapore, Singapore

Shih-Hui Lim
Department of Neurology, Singapore General Hospital, Singapore, Singapore
Department of Neurology, National Neuroscience Institute, Singapore, Singapore

Department of Neurology, Duke – National University of Singapore – Graduate Medical School, Singapore, Singapore

Hsin-Yi Lo and Tin-Yun Ho
Graduate Institute of Chinese Medicine, China Medical University, Taichung, Taiwan

Chien-Yun Hsiang
Department of Microbiology, China Medical University, Taichung, Taiwan,

Tsai-Chung L
Graduate Institute of Biostatistics, China Medical University, Taichung, Taiwan

Chia-Cheng Li
Graduate Institute of Cancer Biology, China Medical University, Taichung, Taiwan

Hui-Chi Huang
Department of Chinese Pharmaceutical Sciences and Chinese Medicine Resources, China Medical University, Taichung, Taiwan

Jaw-Chyun Chen
Department of Medicinal Botany and Healthcare, Da-Yeh University, Changhua, Taiwan

Joel Bozue, Christopher K. Cote, Todd K. Kijek, Patricia Worsham, Amy Jenkins, Sherry Mou, Krishna Moody and David Fritz
Bac teriology Division, The United States Army of Medical Research Institute of Infectious Diseases, Fort Detrick, Maryland, United States of America

Taylor Chance Camenzind G. Robinson and Todd Bell
Pathology Division, The United States Army of Medical Research Institute of Infectious Diseases, Fort Detrick, Maryland, United States of America

Jeffrey Kugelman
Center for Genome Sciences, The United States Army of Medical Research Institute of Infectious Diseases, Fort Detrick, Maryland, United States of America

Steven J. Kern
Office of Research Support, The United States Army of Medical Research Institute of Infectious Diseases, Fort Detrick, Maryland, United States of America

Milica Spasojevic
Department of Polymer Chemistry, Zernike Institute for Advanced Materials, University of Groningen, Groningen, The Netherlands
Departments of Pathology and Laboratory Medicine, section of Medical Biology, division of immunoendocrinology, University of Groningen, Groningen, The Netherlands

Genaro A. Paredes-Juarez, Bart J. de Haanb and Paul de Vos
Departments of Pathology and Laboratory Medicine, section of Medical Biology, division of immunoendocrinology, University of Groningen, Groningen, The Netherlands

Joop Vorenkamp and Arend Jan Schouten
Department of Polymer Chemistry, Zernike Institute for Advanced Materials, University of Groningen, Groningen, The Netherlands

Index

www.ingramcontent.com/pod-product-compliance
Lightning Source LLC
Chambersburg PA
CBHW061259190326
41458CB00011B/3716